The Physical Basis of
Medical Imaging

The Physical Basis of Medical Imaging

Edited by

Craig M. Coulam, M.D., Ph.D.

Jon J. Erickson, Ph.D.

F. David Rollo, M.D., Ph.D.

A. Everette James, Jr., Sc.M., J.D., M.D.

Department of Radiology and Radiological Sciences
Vanderbilt University School of Medicine
Nashville, Tennessee

APPLETON-CENTURY-CROFTS/New York

81 82 83 84 85 / 10 9 8 7 6 5 4 3 2 1

Prentice-Hall International, Inc., London
Prentice-Hall of Australia, Pty. Ltd., Sydney
Prentice-Hall of India Private Limited, New Delhi
Prentice-Hall of Japan, Inc., Tokyo
Prentice-Hall of Southeast Asia (Pte.) Ltd., Singapore
Whitehall Books Ltd., Wellington, New Zealand

Library of Congress Cataloging in Publication Data
Main entry under title:

The Physical basis of medical imaging.

    Bibliography: p.
    Includes index.
    1. Imaging systems in medicine.   2. Diagnosis,
Radioscopic.   3. Medical physics.   I. Coulam,
Craig M., 1940-   [DNLM: 1. Radionuclide
imaging.   WN 445 P578]
RC78.P45   616.07'572   80-27887
ISBN 0-8385-7844-6

Production Editor: Kevin McLaughlin
Text design: Alan Gold
Cover design: Jean Sabato

PRINTED IN THE UNITED STATES OF AMERICA

Contributors

Donald Baker, Ph.D.
Division of Ultrasound
University of Washington
Seattle, Washington

Gary T. Barnes, Ph.D.
Associate Professor of Radiology
Department of Radiology
University of Alabama Medical Center
Birmingham, Alabama

Michael C. Beachley, M.D.
Professor and Chairman
Department of Radiology
Medical College of Virginia
Richmond, Virginia

Herman A. Bosch, M.D.
Associate Professor of Radiology
Department of Radiology
Medical College of Virginia
Richmond, Virginia

Craig M. Coulam, M.D., Ph.D.
Adjunct Associate Professor of Radiology
Department of Radiology
  and Radiological Sciences
Vanderbilt University School of Medicine
Nashville, Tennessee

Andrew B. Crummy, M.D.
Department of Radiology
The University of Wisconsin
Madison, Wisconsin

Jon J. Erickson, Ph.D.
Assistant Professor of Radiology
Department of Radiology
  and Radiological Sciences
Vanderbilt University School of Medicine
Nashville, Tennessee

Panos P. Fatouros, Ph.D.
Assistant Professor of Radiology
Medical College of Virginia
Radiation Physics Division
Richmond, Virginia

Arthur C. Fleischer, M.D.
Assistant Professor of Radiology
Department of Radiology
  and Radiological Sciences
Vanderbilt University School of Medicine
Nashville, Tennessee

Amil J. Gerlock, Jr., M.D.
Associate Professor of Radiology
Department of Radiology
  and Radiological Sciences
Vanderbilt University School of Medicine
Nashville, Tennessee

S. Julian Gibbs, D.D.S., Ph.D.
Associate Professor of Radiology
Department of Radiology
  and Radiological Sciences
Vanderbilt University School of Medicine
Nashville, Tennessee

John Goddard, Ph.D.
University of Miami Medical School
Mt. Sinai Hospital
Miami, Florida

A. Everette James, Jr., Sc.M., J.D., M.D.
Professor and Chairman
Department of Radiology
  and Radiological Sciences
Vanderbilt University School of Medicine
Nashville, Tennessee

Thomas Jones, M.D.
Department of Radiology
  and Radiological Sciences
Vanderbilt University School of Medicine
Nashville, Tennessee

Philip T. Kan, Ph.D.
Assistant Professor of Radiology
Department of Radiology
Medical College of Virginia
Richmond, Virginia

Charles A. Mistretta, Ph.D.
Department of Radiology
The University of Wisconsin
Madison, Wisconsin

John W. Pagel
Director of Radiation Safety
Vanderbilt University
Nashville, Tennessee

C. Leon Partain, Ph.D., M.D.
Associate Professor of Radiology
Director of the Division
  of Radiological Sciences
Department of Radiology
  and Radiological Sciences
Vanderbilt University School of Medicine
Nashville, Tennessee

James A. Patton, Ph.D.
Associate Professor of Radiology
Department of Radiology
    and Radiological Sciences
Vanderbilt University School of Medicine
Nashville, Tennessee

Henry P. Pendergrass, M.P.H., M.D.
Professor and Vice Chairman
Department of Radiology and Radiological Sciences
Vanderbilt University School of Medicine
Nashville, Tennessee

Ray Powis, Ph.D.
ATL Corporation
Richland, Washington

Ronald R. Price, Ph.D.
Associate Professor of Radiology
Department of Radiology and Radiological Sciences
Vanderbilt University School of Medicine
Nashville, Tennessee

Gopala U. V. Rao, Sc.D.
Professor of Radiology
Radiation Physics Division
Medical College of Virginia
Richmond, Virginia

Charles Robinette, M.D.
Department of Radiology and Radiological Sciences
Vanderbilt University School of Medicine
Nashville, Tennessee

F. David Rollo, M.D., Ph.D.
Professor of Radiology
Director of Division of Nuclear Medicine
Department of Radiology and Radiological Sciences
Vanderbilt University School of Medicine
Nashville, Tennessee

Max I. Shaff, M.D.
Visiting Associate Professor of Radiology
Department of Radiology
    and Radiological Sciences
Vanderbilt University School of Medicine
Nashville, Tennessee

Melvin P. Siedband
Associate Professor
Director, Advisory Center for
    Medical Technology and Systems
University of Wisconsin–Madison
Madison, Wisconsin

Malcolm Sloan, R.T.
Chief Technologist
Department of Radiology
    and Radiological Sciences
Vanderbilt University School of Medicine
Nashville, Tennessee

Kenneth J. W. Taylor, M.D., Ph.D.
Professor
Department of Diagnostic Radiology
Yale University School of Medicine
New Haven, Connecticut

Jack M. Tishler, M.D.
Assistant Professor of Radiology
Department of Radiology
University of Alabama Medical Center
Birmingham, Alabama

William Witt, M.D.
Assistant Professor of Radiology
Department of Radiology
    and Radiological Sciences
Vanderbilt University School of Medicine
Nashville, Tennessee

Contents

Preface

Radiographic, ultrasonic, and nuclear medicine equipment has become more complex. This complexity results directly from increasing demands on medical imaging specialists to detect and evaluate ever smaller lesions and pathologic processes that differ only minimally from surrounding normal tissues. Furthermore, detection and evaluation must be done more reliably than before and with smaller amounts of harmful radiation. Equipment is required that produces images less influenced by the technician, the patient's size or surroundings, or the idiosyncrasies of the equipment itself.

With respect to trends in equipment design, digital circuitry is being used increasingly because of its greater inherent stability and because operational logic can be programmed into it. Thus imaging equipment comes with microcomputer processors, macroprocessors, and minicomputers, transforming the equipment into a "semi-intelligent" device. The mini-, micro-, and macrocomputer systems, in turn, bring their own "language" and servicing problems that are different from the problems of older analog imaging equipment. Thus, to some degree, the imaging specialist must become a computer specialist.

The marriage of digital computers with imaging equipment has introduced new imaging techniques and extended old ones. Computed tomography, digital and real-time ultrasound, as well as multi-gated nuclear medicine cardiac acquisition systems rely heavily on computer manipulation to cosmetically alter the image produced. Nuclear magnetic resonance systems and computerized fluoroscopes are new equipment lines also requiring computer interaction and control. Thus, using digital computers in imaging not only increases the reliability of equipment operation, but expands imaging horizons.

All of this new equipment requires a new or better-informed imaging specialist. The specialist's knowledge of physics must be deeper and broader than before. The same is true for radiology, ultrasound, and nuclear medicine technicians. Furthermore, government regulations and the third-party payer doctrine demand that imaging studies be performed less expensively, less frequently, and with less potential patient danger than before. Therefore, old and new imaging equipment must be correctly and properly applied with respect to patient selection and disease process evaluation. Finally, servicing of equipment is more critical simply because fewer malcalibration errors are allowed.

Because of changes made in imaging equipment lines by commercial vendors, this book is written to help practicing imaging specialists and their trainees become better informed about today's radiographic, ultrasonic, and nuclear medicine imaging methods, and to lay the groundwork for understanding future equipment lines. Furthermore, it attempts to show what trade-offs exist between equipment lines designed for the same job by different manufacturers, so that imagers can move appropriately when selecting equipment.

Since no one is an expert in all the different equipment lines, we sought help from many corners. The chapter authors generously donated their time and efforts. Many equipment manufacturers donated illustrations and offered advice on the layout of the book and toward a better understanding of equipment idiosyncrasies and manufacturer differences. The secretaries and photographers who put the chapters into final form in the end constituted the "basic core." To all these people, we are deeply appreciative. Not to be forgotten are our wives and children, who left us alone long enough to get the book written and who encouraged us when the end was not in sight. To these people the book is dedicated.

The Physical Basis of Medical Imaging

CHAPTER 1

Introduction and Overview

CRAIG M. COULAM
JON J. ERICKSON
A. EVERETTE JAMES, JR.

INTRODUCTION

The field of medical imaging provides an opportunity for advances in physics, engineering, and other basic sciences to be applied directly to diagnosis and treatment of human disease. It is incumbent upon the practitioners of medical imaging to understand the basic principles employed in instruments that image human anatomy and to be aware of any iatrogenic conditions that may be created through their use. In this manner, the instrumentation can be appropriately utilized, and the practitioners can be active participants in its improvement. The purpose of this text is to provide a physical foundation for that understanding.

During the course of initiating and practicing clinical radiology, many different types of imaging equipment must be purchased, maintained, and/or replaced on a periodic basis. Radiographic equipment is always considered to be in a dynamic state by commercial vendors and frequent changes in design may be expected. New and improved features will be offered regularly on "conventional equipment lines" and new products will appear on a regular basis. Because of this constant change, it is necessary for the radiologist to be not only a physician but also a biomedical engineer, accountant, economist, and physicist in order to replace radiographic equipment appropriately, determine if new products represent improvements in methodology, and to make certain the present equipment is maintained in optimal operating condition. This text will review the basic aspects of radiology and radiographic equipment, generally describe present day equipment lines that are commercially available, provide suggestions as to how to maintain equipment in good working order, and present our expectations regarding technology changes that should occur in the next few years. The book is written for practicing diagnostic radiologists who are expanding or updating their equipment, for trainees in the discipline, and for other physicians and scientists who might have an interest in the applications of these techniques. Since the book is primarily intended for nonphysicists and/or nonmathematicians, efforts have been made to minimize theory, to provide practical ideas, to de-emphasize mathematical equations and alternatively to provide charts and graphs, and finally to introduce the fundamental background and concepts necessary so that the reader can understand, utilize, and find helpful the manufacturers' technical specification information.

OVERVIEW

Radiology has a number of commercial features with significant financial implications. Because of this, the practitioner must have a "game plan" as to how much equipment to purchase, given individually varying cash flow problems; when to purchase, given clinical demands and changing diagnostic protocols; and where to purchase, given the introduction of new or modified equipment lines by new or established manufacturers. Other important considerations in this strategic planning relate to the increasing influence of health system agency (HSA) regulations at the federal, state, and local government levels and the third-party payers, who are assuming a greater and greater role in the level of compensation allowable for the delivery of the service. Finally, independent of the major equipment lines that need to be purchased, a number of new and existing accessory and consumable radiological instruments and materials are appearing. These also need to be considered for purchase and involve items of significant allocation, such as digital computers, multiformat cameras, and emergency equipment. These items, in order to be amortized, must be shown to be directly involved in the service aspect of radiology. How one integrates all of these variables into a workable and viable radiology practice is complex and usually requires a unified understanding by the radiologist, the administrative and technical staff, and the local health care planning agencies.

Because of the escalating cost of medical technology, especially sophisticated medical imaging devices, health care planners are using monitoring techniques to discover duplication of expensive equipment between radiology departments and appropriate utilization of existing equipment within a given department. These activities have led to an emphasis on efficacy studies and cost-effectiveness. Considerations of this type generally require a complete line of the most up-to-date equipment in one or more departments in order to make the results of the studies appropriate for the equipment lines that are being purchased by today's radiologists for tomorrow's examinations. Ironically, the third-party payers who wish and need this information in general will not allow total reimbursement for the duplicate examinations necessary to acquire the data. Furthermore, government extramural funding is increasingly difficult to obtain. The radiologist, therefore, in establishing and implementing individual equipment purchases and replacement plans, tends to utilize as a basis the manner in which patients can be most efficaciously evaluated and how different pathological processes can be most accurately and efficiently diagnosed. The equipment line is then modified to include the protocols and desires of referring physicians. This system, although not absolutely precise, does provide for an acceptable level of service both to patients and referring physicians. Generally, this method provides a realistic although personalized approach to minimization of equipment related dollars.

Since specific equipment selection and purchase is generally governed by different types of constraints and demands, the equipment needs of academic and private radiology departments are expected to differ and do, considerably. Academic radiology tends to be less predictable and more dynamic in its equipment needs because changing evaluation protocols from outside the imaging department (eg, surgery, medicine, pediatrics) require that the latest technology equipment be readily available and that innovative use be made of existing equipment. Academic departments require additional staff in order to make professional time available for research and teaching activities. These radiology departments also exist in the university hospital environment where money is generally at a premium, overhead costs are high, and assessments to radiology departments to meet hospital expenditures are large. Consequently, resources for academic equipment purchase are limited and the academic success of the department often becomes closely related to equipment donated for "clinical evaluation" projects by commercial vendors or other parties.

Private hospitals and their radiology departments have needs different from the academic departments. The imaging and disease evaluation protocols tend to be less dynamic and reflect those disease evaluation methodologies that are well established and considered more or less proven. Private radiologists do not generally evaluate prototype equipment because of financial and marketing considerations. The overhead costs for private radiological practice are generally lower. This is because fewer staff are needed since research and teaching activities are not required and because assessments by the institution and medical school for nonrevenue-producing activities are not present. Thus, radiologists in private practice are generally in a better position to finance their own equipment needs than those in an academic department. This difference in private and academic radiology practice sometimes leads to a paradox in that the equipment used during training may not be that later employed in the trainee's private practice.

A factor not generally considered in most efficacy studies is that a difference in information content in an image is sought depending upon whether a disease is being initially diagnosed, is being "staged," or the patient is undergoing serial evaluation. Because of this, the imaging equipment needs of the referring physician and patient change as the patient passes through the detection, evaluation, and treatment phases of the disease process. This time-varying equipment demand usually requires a broad capability and very complete equipment line. This requirement is often met at the expense of nonminimization of equipment related resources.

Beyond the theoretical constraints placed upon the availability of the equipment resources, a circumstance is usually reached in which the necessary monies are available and imaging instrumentation can now be purchased for a specified diagnostic activity or service. All types of equipment are manufactured by many companies, and every company has "optimized" its product line for a slightly different aspect of the intended equipment utilization. In this circumstance, the radiologist must know or be able to determine which is best for a particular environment. One simple solution to this problem is to buy the most complex and sophisticated product, which contains all the "bells and whistles." More often than not, this is an expensive practice requiring years of equipment write-off and amortization. Thus, an alternative method by which equipment is more selectively purchased is usually followed. This activity requires a very thorough knowledge and understanding of each manufacturer's specification sheets. Considerable effort is required by the radiologist to learn and understand the physics and engineering involved in the different equipment designs and manufactures. The radiologist must appreciate the subtleties of the different equipment lines and determine ways to evaluate this equipment individually. Some radiologists, however, feel this activity compromises their professional skills. These persons tend to relegate this activity to other individuals in the department, such as the physicist. This individual, however, may then choose or recommend the equipment on objective engineering criteria without the proper attention to clinical utility. The end result is that the individual who uses the equipment may not necessarily be the one who decides what is optimal for the particular clinical function. Again, while this approach may be functional, the minimization of the equipment-designated dollar and/or optimization for a particular clinical environment may not occur.

Optimal image quality must be arrived at from objective (ie, phantom) data, subjectively from personal perspectives, and be realistically based upon clinical demands. Ideally, those image characteristics will be present if one buys from a manufacturer who has the best equipment and always produces the optimal image quality. Practically, however, the best equipment and the optimal image quality are not always produced by the same manufacturer because quality is dependent upon more than engineering design variables. It is dependent upon individual patient anatomy, differing disease processes, and the ambient departmental working environment. Thus, equipment selection and use needs to be an amalgamation of the radiologists' desires, the objective physical data gathered by the physicist or engineer, the physical constraints of the imaging department, the idiosyncrasies of the technical staff, and the expectations of the referring physician. The image with the greatest aesthetic appeal may not always be optimal because it might be obtained only with equipment that may be difficult to use and service. The equipment may also be more expensive than can be afforded or justified by the institution.

Image quality is inherently difficult to describe since much of this concept depends upon a subjective impression. Attempts to describe and compare images are often made on physical grounds using objective measurements from phantoms and are generally expressed in appropriate engineering or physical terms. Images can be described in terms of spatial, density (contrast), and temporal resolution. Each of these qualities can be defined or quantitated numerically. For example, spatial resolution can be measured by imaging a small, high-density object and then measuring this "point-source" response image in terms of full width half maximum (FWHM), just detectable diameter, or modulation transfer function (MTF) parameters. All of these measurements provide comparable information and can be mathematically converted from one form to another. These conversions do not necessarily result in a straightforward or simple analysis. Similarly, density resolution can be determined by imaging two objects, where one is contained or buried within the other and where the radiographic density difference between the two is minimal. Since the detection of the radiographic density difference is dependent upon image mottle (noise) and the inherent contrast difference, terms such as signal-to-noise (S/N) ratios, and just detectable object-to-background difference (in percent) are generally quoted. Temporal resolution, likewise, is the rapidity with which a system can respond and is generally quoted as images (or scans, frames, etc) per unit time (second) and is a measure of the system "dead time" between rapid exposures. It is important to realize, however, that these three resolution quantities are not independent. In general, images of small objects require large contrast differences and fast system response times (to minimize patient motion). Images of objects having small density differences require larger objects and slower system response times (ie, increased dose or longer data integration time). The optimal image is a compromise of image parameters for a given diagnostic situation or problem.

After the optimal image and best equipment have been selected for individual radiologists in their particular environment, the instrumentation must be kept at this level. All equipment has a tendency either to wear out, drift, or cease functioning during its lifetime. Quality control and preventive maintenance programs need to be established and faithfully adhered to. Objective measurements of image quality need to be made using phantoms and conditions that closely simulate the clinical environment. Anthropomorphic phantoms have been developed to aid in performing this function either by, with, or for the radiologist. It is imperative that the radiologist review this data collection process periodically and totally understand the significance and meaning of any change in the data measurements or equipment function. Ultimately, the radiologist will be responsible for the use of the instrumentation to produce patient images. Excessive patient irradiation, faulty mechanical performance, and improper equipment calibration are not tolerable medically or legally. This requires responsibility on someone's part to see that proper monitoring does not allow these untoward events to occur.

New imaging devices and measurements of anatomy and physiology are often based on entirely new or different methodologies and are continually being made available commercially. Examples of current technology would include infrared images, ultrasound machines (B-mode, bistable, gray scale, M-mode, real time, etc), and computed tomographic scanners, while "new" technology would include nuclear magnetic resonance scanners, digital radiography, positron scanners (eg, Ortec's ECAT scanner), and digital fluoroscopy. In many of these techniques, not only are the physics and operation of the equipment new but also the image information content. The practicing radiologist thus becomes dependent upon physicists and other radiologists to research ways to utilize this technology appropriately. As of late, however, much of the appropriate utilization doctrine is being regulated according to economic considerations by public agencies and not on scientific grounds or according to medical needs by academic institutions. Clearly, some compromise of these differing approaches needs to be reached in the future before technological advancement becomes compromised.

Based upon the philosophy presented above, the integration of bioengineering principles and equipment selection processes is seen to be complex. This means considerable effort is required by the radiologist and all collaborators to arrive at optimal equipment and the best image for any particular circumstance or imaging demand. We have attempted to design the chapters of this text so that the practicing radiologist, administrator, and physicist can understand image production by different instruments. The practical result is a data base that will assist in appropriate selection, acquisition, use, and maintenance of this technology. We have attempted to discuss basic radiological physics, present equipment design, and future equipment needs as part of a continuum of the practice of diagnostic radiology.

CHAPTER 2

Planning, Regulation, Cost, and Efficacy Considerations in the Purchase of Radiological Equipment

HENRY P. PENDERGRASS

The concept of making informed decisions regarding acquisition and purchase of radiology equipment is an essential premise in the design of this volume. With respect to hospital radiology departments, the current posture of public representation in the planning process has introduced some modifications into the traditional interactions between the radiologist, physicist, and departmental planner or architect with the hospital administration and trustee. Representatives of the public and government now participate in the decision-making process for planning and funding health facilities and programs at both local and state or regional levels. These changes are mandated in part by the concept of protection of the public interest. Another major impetus for this additional input by government health planners and the community into the decision-making process is the laudatory desire to control rapidly increasing costs of medical care. Unfortunately, although new technology and duplication of facilities contribute to the increasing costs, a major factor in the current explosion of medical costs is the continuing inflation of our overall economy. Hospitals and physicians must deal in the everyday world for personnel, energy, supplies, and equipment. Key words of the current environment are efficacy, cost containment, cost effectiveness, reasonable cost, alternative approaches, availability of services, and quality health care. This chapter will discuss the status of some of the above phrases and will review the regulatory process and current planning guidelines in historical perspective.

HISTORY OF GOVERNMENT HEALTH ACTIVITIES

EARLY YEARS

Government, at both the national and local levels, has been involved in medical care to some extent since soon after the establishment of constitutional government in the United States.[1] For a century and a half, the major objective of the public health agencies and their physician staffs was in the control and prevention of disease. Major emphasis was placed on improvement of sanitation facilities.* More recently, the public health physician has acquired an expanded role particularly in the area of policy making and planning for health care facilities.

HILL–BURTON PROGRAM

During World War II, construction of hospitals as well as other needed health facilities lagged because of the war effort. After the end of the war, with the obvious need for new hospital construction, Congress was ready and willing to provide federal monies for the universally popular theme of providing modern hospital facilities nationwide. In 1946 Congress passed the Hospital Survey and Construction Act (popularly known as the Hill–Burton program). The program became Title VI of the Public Health Service Act and was administered by the Surgeon General. The role of the federal government under the Hill–Burton program was conceived as that of encouragement in the purchase of new equipment and the modernization of health care facilities with the goal of providing more accessible quality medical services.

Although planning on a nationwide scale was included as a by-product of the Hill–Burton legislation, very little control was initially built into the program. There were requirements for documentation of existing facilities and development of plans for expansion of

---

*As early as 1789, the Congress authorized the US Public Health Service to provide hospital care for merchant seamen. The causative organisms and modes of transmission in epidemic diseases such as yellow fever and venereal disease were identified and controlled—and the diseases treated under the auspices of the US Public Health Service.

facilities based on current deficiencies and future projections. Planning was usually carried out on a statewide rather than on a regional basis. Not infrequently there was ineffective cooperation between government planners and the private hospital and physician sector. In 1961, Somers and Somers noted that

> The American hospital "system" is largely a figure of speech. Our hospitals represent random growth of uncoordinated institutions. Their construction may represent the special motivation of a particular religious denomination or philanthropy, the local pride of a small community, the desire of physicians to have more convenient facilities, or any number of other objectives.[1]

REGIONAL MEDICAL PROGRAM (1965) AND COMPREHENSIVE HEALTH PLANNING AND PUBLIC SERVICE ACT (1966)

Both PL 89-239 (Regional Medical Program) and Pl 89-749 (Comprehensive Health Planing and Public Service Act) provided federal funds for planning purposes but their authority and objectives were sometimes overlapping and contradictory. Somers and Somers observe:

> The planlessness of the planning movement itself is both obvious and disturbing. Conflicts inherited in our fragmented hospital structures are duplicated in the planning laws and agencies. The new regional medical programs, for example, will probably be in frequent conflict with the state-oriented Hill–Burton programs. The new comprehensive state planning bodies, envisaged under PL 89-749, coincide with the Hill–Burton geographical boundaries but encompass far more than facilities in their planning responsibilities.[2]

These authors continued by noting that there was "lots of activity, lots of new planning bodies, a plethora of new and proposed laws, but confused to the point of chaos, with deep-rooted internal contradictions, an image of restrictive negativism, and very limited effectiveness."[2]

MEDICARE

Although the Medicare legislation (PL 89-97, Title XVIII) was designed primarily to provide a reimbursement mechanism for hospital and physician charges to the elderly, the legislation was so all encompassing that, both directly and indirectly, government became increasingly involved in the planning of medical care in the United States. Implicit with planning came control and regulation for both hospitals and physicians. Even though the Medicare patients might involve only 30

percent of the patients treated in the hospital or in physicians' offices, it soon became obvious that it was impossible to provide two separate levels of medical care, one for the elderly and another for the rest of the public. Very rapidly after passage of the Medicare legislation, Medicare guidelines became the standards for medical practice for patients of all ages in the United States.

CERTIFICATE OF NEED LEGISLATION

Over the past several decades, high on the list of priorities for the health planner has been legislation that would require that any institution or individual wishing to purchase or build a health-related facility obtain permission to carry out these purchases or construction. Very specifically, those wishing to construct hospitals or clinics or renovate their health facilities or purchase expensive equipment should be required to obtain the approval of local, state, or regional planning bodies. This approval is usually identified as a certificate of need (CON). Chayet and Sonnenreich observe that "the principal purpose of certificate of need laws is to help control upward spiraling charges for health care by preventing the construction of facilities or the initiation of programs which are unneeded."[3]

In 1964, New York State passed the first of the modern day CON laws (Metcalf–McCloskey Act).[2] Although the Comprehensive Health Planning Act of 1966 (PL 89-749, noted above) was supposed to encourage the development of certificate of need legislation, by the end of 1971 only 15 states had passed such legislation.

THE SOCIAL SECURITY AND PUBLIC HEALTH SERVICE ACTS

Beginning in 1972, the Congress began to pass major legislation designed to control the rapid expansion of medical care costs. The mechanism again was to be certificate of need legislation at the state level. Section 1122 of the Social Security Act required that Medicaid, Medicare, and other federal programs (and of course supporting monies) under the Social Security laws would not be available to certain medical facilities unless they had CON approval. Subsequently, Title XV of the National Health Planning and Resources Development Act of 1974 (PL 93-641) was directed at "new" institutional health services and contained guidelines for the establishment of Health Systems Agencies (HSAs) for health planning and review functions at the state level (Section i). Among other things, this act mandated that each state have a certificate of need legislation operational by October 1980. States that did not have certificate of need legislation operational by that date would not be eligible to receive funds from the Department of Health and Human Services (HHS).* Since every state receives a great deal of federal aid from HHS for health-related matters, there is little doubt that every state will be forced to comply and set up a state-based certificate of need program.

By February 1978, "every state except Missouri had either a CON law, or a Section 1122 agreement or both." Chayet observes that there is overlap and a definite potential for disagreement among the various programs. Section 1122 contains a capital expenditure limitation of $100,000 as opposed to the higher level of limitation ($150,000) in the regulations of Title XV of the Public Health Service Act. The agreements of the various states with the Secretary of HEW may vary in those states that had adopted a certificate of need program prior to Public Law 93-641. An example of the potential problems with different terminology is exemplified by the phrases "capital expenditure" and "new institutional health service." An expenditure can be for a capital expenditure (under Section 1122) without involving a new institutional health service (under Title XV) or conversely a new institutional health service (Title XV) might not involve a capital expenditure within the meaning of Section 1122.[3]

CERTIFICATE OF NEED APPLICATIONS: GENERAL REQUIREMENTS

The certificate of need format usually requires the clinic, hospital, or physician who desires to purchase equipment or to construct a medical facility to document certain basic information along the following lines:

Project description (new, modification, etc)
Location
Costs (in some detail)
Time schedule
Simple line drawing
Impact on health care and/or medical practice
Justification (in some detail)

As noted by Chayet et al, certificate of need is "an expanding regulatory concept." Hospitals and physicians involved in major capital expenditures for equipment must check with their state planning agency for current guidelines because state laws are evolving and changing. One must also be prepared for possible new federal legislation dealing with certificate of need on the national level. In the meantime, some HSAs may be using the current CON guidelines as inflexible laws rather than as general standards or guides. The cost of construction and equipment today has made most single

*Formerly Health, Education and Welfare.

room radiological equipment purchases expensive enough to require CON approval.

The major recommendation to the individual or group planning a purchase or construction that may be subject to CON is that the planning process should be initiated as early as possible. If major radiological equipment purchases are planned, the x-ray companies have knowledgeable specialists who can be most helpful in the CON planning process.

CERTIFICATE OF NEED—CRITICISMS

Participation in the certificate of need planning mechanism can be supported as long as the information required in the public interest is kept within a logical framework and as long as the reviewing agency does not use the certificate of need application process as a mechanism for bureaucratic obstruction of appropriate requests. An editorial in Applied Radiology[4] documents some of the frustration of dealing with certificate of need applications in the state of California. Radiographic fluoroscopic equipment that was 12 years old had a down time of more than 40 percent; $50,000 had been spent in useless "upgrading." A formal request to the state planning agency documented the above and noted the heavy demand on this equipment primarily in the area of GI radiology. A large part of the population served by this equipment was indigent or low-income and supported by some type of government insurance. Because the quality of the service was to be improved (the replacement equipment was to include a modern high milliampere (mA), three-phase generator to replace the obsolete low mA, single-phase equipment) the planning agency required a detailed certificate of need application. After 12 months and an expenditure of $25,000 a certificate of need was obtained. In the meantime, "the costs had risen 16 percent and the total purchase price was $6,000 higher than at the date of the initial application."

Somewhat similar frustrations in dealing with certificate of need applications occurred in the state of Massachusetts. A major teaching hospital in Boston planned an ambulatory care building to provide space for staff physicians who were scattered throughout the community. This project was to replace facilities that were over a century old, and to reduce medical costs by maximizing outpatient and/or preadmission patient activities. The project, initially estimated to cost 22 million dollars, actually cost 33 million dollars, largely due to almost a four-year delay associated with the certificate of need application process. In addition, the hospital's out-of-pocket expenses due to surveys, lawyer's fees, reports, public meetings, general correspondence, etc, approached $800,000.[5] This obviously is an extreme case, but it demonstrates the significant escalation of costs that can occur when a planning agency does not utilize the system as it was intended.

In addition to out-of-pocket costs, current CON guidelines often require that both physicians and hospital administrators spend a great deal of time attending public meetings defending their goal of making quality medical care accessible to the public. It is sometimes difficult to document "unmet needs." Often an extensive demographic survey of the population served is necessary. One may be required to present evidence that there would be no "adverse impact" on any other facility in the same service area. It is appropriate to question how effectively this type of bureaucratic exercise is accomplishing its goal of reducing the cost of medical care. Who should pay for the escalating and excessive costs of preparing the proposals to the local health planning group? At the present time, although society actually pays this cost by indirect means, could the current application costs in some states prohibit individuals and groups from applying?

NATIONAL HEALTH PLANNING AND RESOURCE DEVELOPMENT ACT (1974)

A major thrust of this legislation (PL 93-641, 88 US stat 2225) was to refine further the planning process by "establishing a national network of local and state planning agencies which could establish specific criteria according to broad guidelines developed at the federal level. The local agencies were to collaborate through regional planning councils and to coordinate their activities through state level agencies established as part of the state government structure. By mid-1978 all of the 203 local area planning agencies (Health Service Agencies or HSAs) were established and functioning with some degree of federal support."[6]

Almost two years after passage of PL 93-641, the Health Resources Administration (HRA) circulated a draft of special guidelines for hospital beds; obstetrical, pediatric, and neonatal services; open heart surgery; cardiac catheterization; radiation therapy; and CT scanners. "More than 70,000 responses, many strongly critical,"[11] prompted the HRA to circulate additional revised preliminary drafts; the modified version of the 11 national guidelines was finally published in the Federal Register (vol 3, no 60), March 28, 1978.

Three of the eleven areas involved primarily radiologic services. Linton and Dennis, in discussing this planning emphasis on radiologic facilities note that "neither diagnostic nor therapeutic radiology is regarded as a primary care area, at a time when strong factions outside of medicine have chosen to support a return to primary care emphasis, vis-a-vis further development of consultant's specialties.... [R]egulation was thought to be appropriate because it involved large resource commitments and was difficult to control in a free enterprise format. Control could be effected with

minimal public protest because of a lack of awareness or concern for the discipline involved. The radiologic facilities chosen for regulation, megavoltage radiotherapy equipment, computed tomographic (CT) scanners, and cardiac catheterization facilities, all necessitate substantial capital investments to acquire and comparable financial commitments to operate."[7]

Evens, in his "special article" dealing with *National Guidelines and Standards for Health Planning*, notes that "the guidelines (published in the Federal Register noted above) are the first serious attempt to regulate the productivity of individual medical facilities. Whether the guidelines will be used for guidance or serve as a rigid set of rules that force local medical services and radiologic facilities to fit a national standard is a critical issue.... [A]lthough the concept of the guidelines was to serve as a framework within which HSAs and states could develop plans unique to their population and medical needs, rigid federal control is certainly a possibility."[8]

In his objective critique, Evens lists the major guidelines for cardiac catheterization, megavoltage radiation therapy, and computed tomography scanners as published in the Federal Register. The rationale for the restrictive guidelines recommended for radiation therapy and CT scanners is their high cost. One may assume that if CT and radiation therapy facilities were less costly, guidelines would not be needed. The guidelines for the even more expensive cardiac catheterization facilities, on the other hand, are "designed to encourage the development of diagnostic and treatment facilities in the same institution."

Also noted by Evens are the *rigidity of the guidelines* and the key issue of local versus national responsibility for health planning. The definition of medical terminology at a federal level, specifically with respect to CT and radiation therapy, "may very well influence medical practice without sound medical justification."[12] Institutions and physicians may be influenced by economic considerations to carry out an examination or treatment on two successive days rather than on a single day because of the efforts of the Health Resources Administration to control costs by establishing arbitrary definitions of what constitutes a medical treatment or a diagnostic procedure.

Evens also details other areas where the federal guidelines are inconsistent and may, in fact, tend to limit medical resources, especially in sparsely populated areas. "While cost reduction and high quality can be compatible, often they are not. [While] standards for cardiac catheterization are at a level to encourage quality services, standards for radiation therapy and CT are primarily related to cost containment and define what a health facility can do rather than what it should do. Efficiency is important but an 'assembly line' approach...can result in 'assembly line' medical care.... As currently read, the guidelines clearly reduce accessibility to radiologic services and may reduce their quality."[8]

REPLACEMENT POLICY

Most modern hospital radiology departments are actually minihospitals. They have the same problems with repair and purchase of equipment as do the larger sheltering hospitals. The successful radiology departments usually utilize a combination of modern business and accounting techniques to plan for and fund equipment purchases for both new technology and replacement of obsolete or nonserviceable equipment. Since, as a general rule, radiology departments generate surplus funds, agreement with hospital management for employment of radiology surpluses to maintain and update radiology equipment is fundamental to the long-term growth and survival of radiology in the hospital or medical center.

DEPRECIATION

Webster's New World Dictionary defines *depreciation* as "a decrease in value of property through wear, deterioration or obsolescence, [or] in accounting or bookkeeping, depreciation is the allowance made for this decrease in value." There is general agreement in modern day accounting that durable assets "deteriorate with time and use, and are subject to obsolescence with the development of new technology." The useful life of each particular asset is dependent upon a variable combination of wear and obsolescence factors, but at some point the productive service life of all capital equipment ends. As noted by Terbough, "capital consumption is an inescapable cost of operation. No net gain or profit results until this cost has first been recouped.... It is one thing to agree that depreciation should be charged as a cost of doing business; it is another to say how it should be measured."[9] Meij observes that "there are but few fields in managerial economics where the gap between theory and practice is so wide as that of depreciation of capital assets."[10]

Traditionally depreciation was based on the original or historical cost of the durable asset. In recent years, with the rapid escalation of costs and inflation, there has been a move to base depreciation on current replacement costs rather than on the original cost of the equipment or building. If the replacement cost includes technological advances, the cost of replacement escalates. Since hospital reimbursement rates are based in part on depreciation guidelines, it is important that hospitals and physicians planning expensive equipment purchases remain abreast of current approved methodology.

LEASE VERSUS PURCHASE

As noted by Owen,[11]

the question of whether to lease or purchase medical equipment has no simple answer and each situation needs to be considered on its own merits after a thorough analysis of each alternative....[Listed below] are some of the advantages and disadvantages of leasing:

ADVANTAGES:
Leasing may be the answer where there is a need for modernization but insufficient funds to do so.
Leasing may increase and accelerate third-party reimbursement and the amount could substantially exceed that received from depreciation.
Leasing may be the answer for equipment with rapid obsolescence rates.
Leasing may be a hedge against inflation.

DISADVANTAGES:
Leasing usually costs more than ownership. The residual cost at the expiration of the lease, if written as "fair market value," may be exorbitant.
If third-party reimbursement is not available, it may not be desirable to lease.
Leasing for too long a term may commit the user to obsolescence.

Hospital radiology departments usually generate surpluses or profits. Utilization of departmental depreciation credits and radiology surplus funds should obviate the need for leasing except where decisions are made to utilize radiology funds elsewhere. Perhaps new programs such as expensive CT or cardiac catheterization laboratories will, on occasion, require a leasing arrangement. Since the total cost of leasing will exceed the cost of direct purchase, most radiologic equipment should be purchased, except under circumstances such as discussed above.

INTERNAL CROSS-SUBSIDIZATION

Radiology, pathology, and the pharmacy generate profits or surpluses in most hospitals. For several decades, hospital management has utilized surpluses generated in some hospital units to subsidize losses elsewhere. This widespread practice has been called internal cross-subsidization.[12]

PL 93-641 (National Health Planning and Resources Development Act of 1974) required that HEW develop a uniform institutional rate system designed to reflect the true cost of providing each type of service. Revenues obtained from a profit-making service should not be utilized to subsidize losses incurred from other hospital activities. Profits derived from services to a patient in radiology should not be used to support deficits attributed to patient services in another department.[16] In other words, hospital charges should reflect true costs unit by unit. It would appear that implementation of any policy limiting internal cross-subsidization in hospitals would benefit funding of radiology capital expenditures by requiring that radiology surpluses or profits be utilized by radiology. Implementation of a system requiring identification of true costs of providing services might also result in reduction of current radiology charges; there would be less incentive to raise radiology charges to subsidize income-losing activities elsewhere in the medical center.

EFFICACY

Efficacy is another of the terms utilized by today's health planner. Webster's New World Dictionary defines *efficacy* as "power to produce effects or intended results; effectiveness." In the early 1970s the American College of Radiology, with support from the United States Public Health Service, began to examine the contributions of specific radiologic studies to patient care, given a certain group of symptoms or medical findings. The ACR efficacy study attempted to determine if x-rays were obtained as a defense mechanism because of medico-legal or malpractice fears on the part of the physician—or because of fears of disease on the part of patient or family. Did the information obtained by the x-ray examination change the physician's course of action or merely serve to confirm or substantiate a proposed treatment plan? Are "negative" examinations important? Was the x-ray study really necessary?

Soon after the ACR embarked on its efficacy study, a major new and expensive radiologic technology came into clinical use—the CT scanner. In five short years over 1,000 such costly and sophisticated instruments have been installed and become operational in the United States. The new CT technology, more than anything else, has brought about this classic confrontation between the various elements of society involved with medical care. The hospital, physician, and patient demand that this new technology be made available to all who require it. Cost is important but is probably not the overwhelming consideration for either the patient, with clinical symptoms suggestive of a cerebral vascular accident or a brain tumor, or the physician who orders the necessary diagnostic study (a CT brain scan). The health planner, on the other hand, is concerned with the cost of the study. Perhaps the health planner would be less concerned if the cost of the equipment and the study was significantly less.

Even though the early reports on the clinical ef-

fectiveness of this new CT technology were favorable, there were initially very little data available to test the contributions of this new technology to an "improved health outcome" for society. As noted by Fineberg, "One of the difficulties in evaluating a diagnostic test is its remoteness from health outcome....[S]ensible health planners acknowledged the clinical promise of CT, but greatly feared excessive proliferation and sought some rational basis on which to distribute scanners. Hospital administrators did not want their institutions left behind, but they were concerned about such a large investment in a device whose technological obsolescence may antedate its depreciable life....CT came to symbolize the dilemma posed by expensive new health technology."[13]

Warner, in discussing the effects of hospital cost containment on the development and use of medical technology, concludes that "any serious and effective cost containment policy will have substantial impact on the quantity and use of resources devoted to hospital-based care....Hospital cost containment represents an attempt, albeit imperfect, to reduce or compensate for the discrepancy between the private decision-making costs and the social costs of medical care."[14]

As our societal structure becomes more regulated, we all must be prepared to look critically at the effectiveness of day-to-day contributions to medical care. In addition to the efficacy of radiologic examinations as defined and determined by the ACR, we must carefully examine other factors involved in the delivery of radiologic services. For example, both radiologist and society will have to continue to examine the radiation exposure burden imposed by the x-ray or nuclear medicine examination. Can ultrasound be effectively substituted on occasion for the traditional radiographic study? What are the best film–screen combinations to reduce radiation exposure but still achieve an adequate diagnostic study? Are mammographic screening examinations in asymptomatic women justified? Is there a definable cost–benefit ratio for this procedure? How important is age in determining the appropriateness of the mammographic screening procedure?

What about performance criteria for the very expensive radiologic equipment of this current era? How does one determine if the equipment meets design specifications? Is it reliable? How often does it break down? What are the average repair costs? Should a service contract be purchased?

Will national health insurance significantly increase the utilization of radiologic services so that both available equipment and manpower will not be able to deliver the needed radiologic services? Are we training enough physician radiologists and radiologic technologists to serve the anticipated needs and resources of our society?

It is becoming apparent that the medical care system in the United States may be too complex for a traditional cost – benefit analysis. Schwartz and DesHarnals recommend that efforts be made "to assure that disease is treated with the most effective means available [that will] minimize the cost of such treatment. The method involves such factors as the impact of CT [for example] on the health care system, health outcome of patients, and reduction of hospital occupancy."[15]

Fineberg lists the eight dimensions by which new medical technology can be evaluated:[13]

Technical performance
Clinical efficacy
Resource costs, charges, and efficiency
Safety
Acceptability to patients, physicians, and other users
Research benefits for the future
Larger effects on the organization of health services
Larger effects on society (as pertain, for example, to genetic manipulation technologies)

While methodologies and disciplines to evaluate some of the above criteria are still evolving, it is hoped that this volume will help the formulation of a response to some of these criteria and provide insight on how to approach other questions.

REFERENCES

1. Somers HM, Somers AR: Doctors, Patients & Health Insurance. Washington, DC, The Brookings Institution, 1961, p 83

2. Somers HM, Somers AR: Medicare and the Hospitals: Issues and Prospects. Washington, DC, The Brookings Institution, 1967, p 204

3. Chayet, Sonnereich PC: Certificate of Need: An Expanding Regulatory Concept. Washington, DC, Medicine in the Public Interest, Inc, 1978, p 1

4. Milne EC: On certificate of need (editorial). Appl Radiol, Jan – Feb 1979, p 21

5. Grossman J: Personal communications, April 1979

6. Health Planning Letter, September 11, 1978

7. Linton O, Dennis JM: The government national health care policy. Regulations particularly affecting medical imaging. In James AE, Jr (ed): Legal Aspects of Diagnostic Imaging. Baltimore, Urban and Schwarzenberg, April 1980

8. Evens RG: National guidelines and standards for health planning: their relation to radiology. Am J Roentgenol 131: 1101–1104, 1978

9. Terbough G: Realistic Depreciation Policy. Chicago, Machinery and Allied Products Institute, 1954, pp 1–10

10. Meij JL (ed): Depreciation and Replacement Policy. Chicago, Quadrangle Books, 1961, pp 1–5, 15–23, 26–31, 106–112, 178–185

11. Owen RD: General Electric Co, Personal communication, March 16, 1979

12. Havighurst CC, Blumstein JF, Bovbjerg R: Strategies in underwriting the cost of catastrophic disease. Law and Contemporary Problems 40 (4): 122–195, 1976

13. Fineberg HV: Evaluation of compiled tomography: achievement and challenge. Am J Roentgenol 131: 1–3, 1978

14. Warner KE: Effects of hospital cost containment on the development and use of medical technology. Milbank Memorial Fund Quarterly/Health and Society 56 (2): 208, 1978

15. Schwartz R and DesHarnals S: Computed tomography: the cost-benefit dilemma. Radiology 125: 253–254, 1977

CHAPTER 3

Atomic and Nuclear Physics

F. DAVID ROLLO
RONALD R. PRICE
JAMES A. PATTON

ATOMIC PHYSICS

DEFINITIONS

Matter is defined to be anything that occupies space. The smallest subdivision of matter that retains the original physical and chemical properties is referred to as a molecule. Molecules of an element (eg, hydrogen or potassium) contain but a single type of atom, while molecules of compounds (eg, potassium chloride) are composed of different types of atoms.

In this text the Bohr atomic structure is used. The Bohr atom consists of a central nucleus, which contains protons and neutrons. Both particles have masses approximately 2,000 times that of the electron; thus the nucleus is considered to contain almost all of the mass of the atom. The neutron has a neutral charge, while the proton has a positive charge.

Electrons having a negative charge revolve about the nucleus in discrete energy levels, or orbits. In the neutral atom, the number of electrons exactly equals the number of protons in the nucleus. The electron orbits are grouped in shells, which contain no more than some maximum number of electrons defined by the relation $2n^2$, where n is the principal quantum number assigned to a given shell. The quantum numbers are integers, beginning with 1 for the innermost shell and increasing by unity for each succeeding shell outward. Thus, there can be no more than two electrons in the first shell, eight in the second, eighteen in the third, and so on. The shells are also identified by letters of the alphabet, with the innermost being K, the next L, and so forth. The basic atomic configuration is shown in Figure 3.1.

The number of protons within the nucleus is the atomic number Z. This number is different for each element and distinguishes one atom type from another. Different elements are typically identified by using a chemical symbol as well as a subscript. The subscript is simply the Z number. For example, carbon is written as $_6$C and helium as $_2$He. The neutron number N is used to indicate the number of neutrons within the nucleus of a given atom. For a given element having a specific atomic number, it is possible to have several different neutron numbers. Nuclides that have the same Z but a different N are referred to as isotopes. Isotopes therefore have the same chemical properties, since the total number of protons and thus the arrangement of electrons are the same. They simply differ in the total number of particles contained in the nucleus. The total number of particles within the nucleus is the mass number A. Thus,

$$A = N + Z. \tag{1}$$

To distinguish one isotope from another, a superscript designating the A number is added to the nomenclature presented above. A generalized expression for identifying an isotope having the chemical symbol X, atomic number Z, and neutrons number N

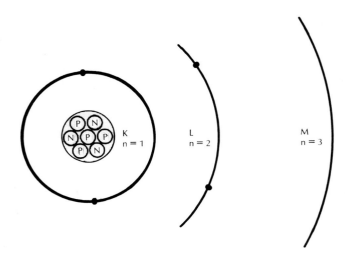

Figure 3.1. Schematic of Bohr atom. Nucleus contains protons and neutrons, while electrons revolve in discrete energy levels about nucleus. By convention, electron energy levels are assigned either letters (K, L, M...) or an integer ($n = 1, 2, 3...$).

would be $^A_Z X$. Therefore, $^{12}_6 C$ and $^{14}_6 C$ identify isotopes of carbon, which by definition have the same Z number but a different N number.

Several nuclides have the same neutron number. Such nuclides are isotones. For example, $^{14}_6 C$ and $^{15}_7 N$ are typical isotones that have the same N number but different A and Z numbers.

Also, several nuclides have the same mass number. Such nuclides are called isobars. For example, $^{15}_8 O$ and $^{15}_7 N$ are isobars that have the same A number but different Z and N numbers.

The proton, the neutron, and the electron are considered the primary building blocks of the atom. Experiments have established that the electron has a charge of 1.602×10^{-19} coulomb (C) and a mass (m_e) of 9.109×10^{-31} kg. The electron mass m_e is used as a reference in atomic and nuclear theory. For example, the mass of the proton (m_p) is expressed as $1836\ m_e$ and the mass of the neutron (m_n) as $1839\ m_e$. Similarly, the charge of the electron is used as a reference charge. Thus, by selecting the electron charge to be -1, the charge of the proton becomes $+1$. The neutron, as the name suggests, is neutral and hence has a charge of 0.

PERIODIC TABLE

All of the elements can be arranged in an orderly series, called the periodic table, in accordance with their increasing atomic number. There are nine vertical groups and seven horizontal periods. The groups are families of elements with similar chemical properties (ie, they react chemically in a similar fashion). The periods consist of elements that have the same number of electron shells about the nucleus but different chemical properties. Elements in a given group have similar chemical properties because they have the same number of electrons in their outer shells. For example, lithium, sodium, and potassium each have a different number of shells, but each has only one electron in its outermost shell. Thus, since electron configuration determines the chemical properties of an atom, all three should and, in fact, do have similar chemical behavior.

The valence of a given element is determined by the number of electrons in the outermost shell, the so-called valence shell. Typically, valence is determined by the ease with which a given atom can fill its outermost shell or subshell. An outer shell is in an especially stable condition when it contains multiples of eight electrons. Thus, elements such as lithium, sodium, and potassium are said to have a valence of $+1$ because they can most easily end up with a filled outer shell by giving up the single electron in their outermost shell. This loss of an electron causes the atom to have an excess of positive charges, thus the positive sign for the valence.

Likewise, elements such as fluorine, chlorine, and bromine have seven electrons in their outermost shell and can most easily saturate the outer shell by accepting an electron. This results in a valence of -1, since the resulting atom will have one more electron than proton. Similar statements can be made for the remainder of the elements in the periodic table.

It should be noted in the periodic table that there is a group of elements whose outer electron shells are filled. This group is referred to as the inert elements, since they do not readily participate in chemical reactions because of their filled outer shells.

From this discussion it should be concluded that the chemical properties of an element depend on its valence, which in turn depends on the number of electrons in the outermost shell or subshell.

EXCITATION AND IONIZATION

In the normal state the Bohr atom contains the same number of protons and electrons and thus has a neutral charge. Normally, each electron within the atom will remain in its lowest energy state, the so-called ground state. If energy is supplied to the electron from an outside source, it may be raised to a higher energy level. If the electron is raised to a higher level within the atom, the atom retains its neutral charge but is said to be excited. This process is referred to as excitation. Excitation is illustrated as Process A in Figure 3.2.

If the electron receives energy in excess of its potential energy, it will leave the atom. The process, called ionization (Process B in Figure 3.2), leaves the atom with a net positive charge. The free electron and the positively charged atom are collectively called an ion pair.

In both the excitation and the ionization processes, the atom will eventually return to the ground state. This involves electrons falling from higher energy levels to fill the vacancy left by the elevated electrons. When this occurs, a photon will be emitted in accordance with Bohr's postulate: radiation is emitted as a photon from an atom only when an electron changes from one stationary state to another of lower energy. The energy of the emitted photon will be equal to the difference in energy between the initial and final energy states of the electron.

This energy difference is constant for a given element (ie, the magnitude will be a characteristic of the element involved). Therefore, x-rays produced by the transition of an electron from one energy level to another are called characteristic x-rays. Characteristic x-rays are identified according to the name of the subshell in which the original vacancy existed. The K series, for example, arise when electrons fall to fill vacancies in the K shell. When this is accomplished by electrons falling from the L or M shells, the corresponding x-rays are called K_α and K_β respectively. Similarly, L-shell vacancies filled from the M shell are referred to as L_α x-rays. With regard to characteristic x-rays, shells above M are considered so close together in energies that they are treated collectively as a single shell at infinity. Therefore, the filling of the K, L, and M shells by electrons from infinity are referred to as K_γ L_β, and M_α x-rays respectively.

It is important to note that x-rays are extranuclear in origin. It will be pointed out later that gamma rays and x-rays have the same physical properties. They differ only in their source, with gamma rays being intranuclear in origin.

NUCLEAR PHYSICS

NUCLEAR FORCES

The basic question of nuclear composition was resolved in 1932 when Chadwick identified the neutron. In the same year Werner Heisenberg used this discovery when he hypothesized that the proton and neutron are the basic building blocks of the nucleus.

The nature of the forces that hold neutrons and protons together in the nucleus is still not well understood. It is clear, however, that the force is not electric in origin, since the neutron carries no charge. It also appears that the required nuclear binding energy is not supplied by gravitational forces, since such forces are considered too weak by several orders of magnitude.

In 1935 Yukawa proposed that the nuclear binding force is an exchange force similar to that involved in molecular binding. For example, in the case of molecular hydrogen H_2, the hydrogen atoms are bound by the exchange, or sharing, of electrons between the two nuclei. This sharing leads to a lower energy state and hence to a binding energy, which does not exist if each electron remains permanently attached to one proton only.

Yukawa suggested that a similar process occurred within the nucleus, with the proton and neutron sharing a then undetected nuclear particle. This particle was later named the pi (π) meson or pion.

The Yukawa theory proposes that the proton and the neutron continuously change identity by the exchange of pions from one nucleon to another. The energy change from such a transfer is:

$$\Delta E = m_\pi c^2 = 135 \text{ meV} \tag{2}$$

where m_π is the mass of the pion.

This exchange phenomenon is thought to create a resonant condition which provides the stability observed in the nucleus.

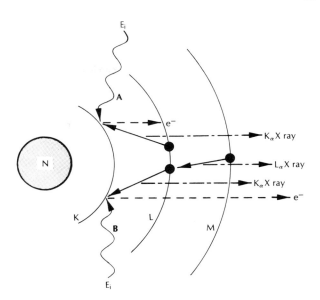

Figure 3.2. (Process A) Photon having incident energy E_i is shown to interact with K shell electron. Process is referred to as excitation because electron only receives sufficient energy to be elevated to L shell. Vacancy in K shell is filled by electron from L shell. In the process, energy lost by transition is emitted as K x-ray. (Process B) Photon having incident energy E_i is shown to interact with K shell electron. Process is referred to as ionization because electron receives sufficient energy to be ejected from atom, thus forming ion pair. Vacancy in K shell is filled by electron from L shell, with subsequent emission of K x-ray. Vacancy created in L shell is then filled by electron from M shell, which results in emission of L x-ray. Finally, electron from outside atom will fill M shell vacancy with emission of M x-ray (not shown). This last event is required to return excited atom to its ground state (ie, balance in number of electrons and protons).

NUCLEAR STABILITY

Neutron–Proton Ratio. Certain combinations of protons and neutrons within the nucleus produce stable nuclei; others do not. Those that are not stable transform or decay spontaneously to achieve a more stable combination of neutrons and protons. This process of decay, referred to as radioactivity, can involve the emission of alpha particles, beta particles, and in certain cases gamma rays, depending on the type of nuclear instability involved.

One factor that appears to be important in nuclear stability is the neutron–proton ratio. The importance of this ratio is illustrated in Figure 3.3, which is a plot of the neutron number N versus the atomic number Z for the relatively stable nuclei. The stable nuclei fall along a relatively narrow band called the line of stability. Initially the slope of this line is approximately unity because of the tendency for light nuclei to contain equal numbers of protons and neutrons. It can be seen

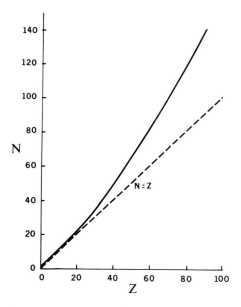

Figure 3.3. Plot of neutron number N versus atomic number Z for relatively stable nuclei is shown as solid line. For comparison, plot of $N=Z$ is shown as dotted line.

Z	N	Number of Stable Nuclei
Even	Even	164
Even	Odd	55
Odd	Even	50
Odd	Odd	4

TABLE 3.1. **Even-Odd Rules**

that as Z increases, the N/Z ratio increases to about $1:5$. This addition of extra neutrons can be explained intuitively as a need to increase the average distance between protons within the nucleus, thereby reducing the repulsive coulombic force acting between these particles, in accordance with the inverse-square law. If a nuclide is too rich in either protons or neutrons, it is said to have an unfavorable N/Z ratio. Such nuclides are unstable. Stability may be achieved by spontaneous emission of particles from the nucleus, which in turn changes the identity of the nuclide, to obtain a more favorable ratio. For example, a nuclide too rich in neutrons will undergo the conversion

$$N \rightarrow p + \beta^- + \bar{\nu} \tag{3}$$

which converts a neutron to a proton with the emission of a beta particle, β^-, with the extra energy of the reaction represented by $\bar{\nu}$, the antineutrino.

On the other hand, a nucleus too rich in protons will undergo the conversion

$$p \rightarrow n + \beta^+ + \nu \tag{4}$$

where a proton is converted to a neutron with the emission of a positron, β^+, and extra energy represented by ν, the neutrino.

In both cases, the N/Z ratio is changed in a favorable direction (ie, toward the stability diagonal).

Shell Model. Examination of the Z and N numbers of all the stable nuclei shows a tendency of nucleons to pair, as illustrated in Table 3.1. The grea-

test number of stable nuclei have both Z and N numbers that are even, whereas only four of the stable nuclei have both Z and N values that are odd. The predominance of even Z and even N in stable nuclei also suggests that the nucleus may contain shells or energy levels similar to those in the extranuclear portion of the atom. In this so-called shell model of the atom, stability appears to occur when a shell in a given level is filled.

Further support for the shell model of the nucleus is obtained from the observation that nuclei containing certain numbers of protons or neutrons appear to be extremely stable. The numbers, referred to as magic numbers, are 2, 8, 20, 28, 50, 82, and 126. Multiple examples support this observation. Helium 4 contains two protons and two neutrons (ie, both particles are represented by the magic number 2). This element is inert and constitutes about 100 percent of natural helium. Oxygen 16 and calcium 40 are two other extremely stable nuclides, which have magic numbers of 8 and 20 respectively for both Z and N.

Binding Energy. All nuclei contain protons and neutrons. It has been established that if the sum of the Einstein mass–energy equivalents of these individual nucleons within a given nucleus is greater than the mass–energy equivalent of the composite nucleus, the element will be stable. This implies that a portion of the nuclear mass is converted to energy, which serves to bind the nucleus together.

If the mass converted to energy is m, the energy equivalent of this mass loss, E, is given by Einstein's mass–energy equation:

$$\Delta E = \Delta mc^2 \tag{5}$$

For convenience, all units of mass in nuclear physics are expressed in terms of the atomic mass unit, amu, which is defined to be $1/12$ the mass of the ^{12}C atom. Thus, 1 amu $= 1.661 \times 10^{-24}$ g. Substituting this mass in equation 5, with the appropriate conversion factors, gives 1 amu $= 931.48$ meV. Thus, if Δm in amu is known, the energy equivalent in meV can be obtained by simple multiplication.

There are several methods of expressing the loss of mass in the formation of a nucleus. One measure is the mass deficit, which is the difference between the mass of the entire atom M and the sum of the free masses of its constituents W. This can be expressed

$$\delta = W - M \tag{6}$$

where $W = Zm_p + Nm_n + Zm_e$.

In these equations Z and N are the atomic and neutron numbers respectively and m_p, m_n, and m_e the mass of the proton, neutron, and electron respectively. Note that M, the measured mass of the atom, includes the mass of the electrons. Thus, W must also include the mass of the electrons if the true mass deficit is to be calculated.

For ^4_2He, where $Z = N = 2$, the mass deficit is calculated as:

$$W = 2(1.007276) + 2(1.008665) + 2(0.0005487)$$

$$W = 4.032979 \text{ amu}$$

The measured atomic mass is $M = 4.002603$ amu. Hence

$$\delta = 4.032979 - 4.002603$$

$$\delta = 0.030376 \text{ amu}$$

The energy equivalent $= (0.030376 \text{ amu}) (931.48 \text{ meV}/\text{amu})$

$$E_B = 28.28 \text{ meV}$$

E_B is referred to as the binding energy of the nucleus and represents the energy equivalent of the mass deficit. E_B is the energy that would be radiated from the atom during the formation of the nucleus from the constituent nucleons. In general, nuclei having large values of E_B are most stable against the loss of a neutron or a proton from the nucleus. However, this does not necessarily imply stability against all forms of nuclear decay. For example, several alpha emitters have higher binding energies than do some stable nuclei.

It has been found very useful to consider E_B to be uniformly distributed over all of the constituent nucleons. This results in an important quantity referred to as the binding energy per nucleon, E_b, which is

$$E_b = 931.48(W - M)/A \tag{7}$$

E_b represents the energy required to extract a single nucleon from the nucleus of an element having a mass number of A.

A plot of E_b versus A is shown in Figure 3.4. Elements having intermediate mass numbers are the most stable. It is interesting to note that in a plot more refined than that shown in Figure 3.4, discontinuities are found to occur at Z or N values of 2, 8, 20, 28, 50, 82, and 126, the magic numbers. The corresponding elements happen to be extremely stable, suggesting that a closure of nuclear energy shells occurs at these values

in a manner analogous to the closure of orbital shells in the extranuclear portion of the atom $Z = 2$, 10, 18, and so forth.

NUCLEAR REACTIONS

Spontaneous Reactions. Unstable nuclei undergo either radioactive decay or spontaneous fission in an attempt to become stable. In general, such spontaneous reactions are exoergic; that is, they involve the release of energy.

The process of radioactive decay can involve the release of particles or gamma rays from the nucleus. For example, those nuclei that have an N/Z ratio that is too large attempt to attain a more stable state by the emission of a beta particle. Nuclei having a ratio that is too small either emit a positron or capture an orbital electron in an effort to improve the neutron-proton balance. In general, unstable elements that have Z greater than 82 use alpha decay as their mechanism for achieving a more stable state. In any of these reactions, gamma ray emission can be an accompanying process.

Fission is a process that involves the splitting of a nucleus into two nuclei of roughly the same size. The process may occur spontaneously in very heavy nuclei, where the mutual force of repulsion of the protons approaches the magnitude of the cohesive forces that hold the nucleus together. The addition of energy, such as that provided by neutron bombardment, may also cause more stable nuclei to undergo fission. There are four basic methods of artificially inducing bombardment: with thermal neutrons, fast neutrons, charged particles, or high-energy photons.

Thermal neutrons are neutrons that have lost sufficient energy through collisions to cause them to come

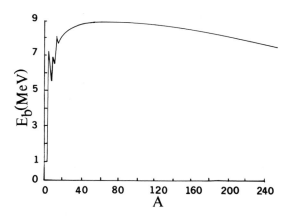

Figure 3.4. Plot of binding energy per nucleon E versus mass number A for all elements. Nuclei having intermediate mass numbers are more stable than those having either very low or high A values. Process of fusion involves light nuclei (low A), whereas fission is predominant in heavy nuclei (high A).

into thermal equilibrium with their surroundings at room temperature. The fission of uranium 235 and plutonium 239 by thermal neutrons are the most important reactions leading to the release of nuclear energy. It is important to note that while thermal neutron fission occurs readily in ^{235}U, this is not the case in ^{238}U, primarily because the N/Z ratios present in the nuclei of these two nuclides create two different energy states. In ^{235}U the energy provided by thermal neutrons is sufficient to cause fission. However, the energy of these same neutrons is not sufficient to disrupt the nucleus of ^{238}U. Neutrons having higher energy content are required. Such neutrons are called fast neutrons.

Elements having atomic numbers above 90 have been successfully fissioned by bombardment with protons, deuterons, and alpha particles. This process is called charged-particle fission.

When fission is induced by high-energy photons, the process is called photofission.

A number of nuclides, such as natural uranium, undergo spontaneous fission. In almost all cases this process is in competition with alpha emission, which is the predominant mode of decay.

The fission of a uranium nucleus or one of its neighbors typically results in a total energy release of about 200 meV. Most of this energy is released as the kinetic energy of the fission products, while some is released as gamma rays at the instant of fission. The remaining energy is released over an extended period by the radioactive decay process of the unstable daughter nuclei.

Fusion. Fusion is a process in which light nuclei combine to form a heavier nucleus. For the most part, fusion reactions, like fission reactions, are exoergic, ie, energy is released. This is evident from the binding energy curve in Figure 3.4, which shows that the release of energy per nucleon by fusion (low A) may be several times that available from fission (high A).

The fusion reaction is the process by which the sun produces energy. The reactions involve the fusion of hydrogen at temperatures sufficient to sustain the reaction, typically several million degrees. Some fusion reactions and the corresponding energies released are

$$^2H + {}^2H = {}^3He + {}^1n + 3.25 \text{ meV} \tag{8}$$
$$^2H + {}^3H = {}^4He + {}^1n + 17.6 \text{ meV} \tag{9}$$
$$^2H + {}^3He = {}^4He + {}^1p + 18.3 \text{ meV} \tag{10}$$

If reactions of this type could be harnessed, the energy problems of the world could be resolved. To date, several laboratories have been able to achieve instantaneous fusion reactions, but none have been able to create a sustained reaction. The technical problems associated with creating and maintaining the high temperatures required for a sustained fusion reaction appear to be so complex that no one forsees this process as being a major source of energy in the very near future.

Nuclear Equations. Most commercially available radioisotopes are produced by means of nuclear reactions. This involves bombarding the nucleus of a selected element with a particle to cause formation of a new element that is radioactive. Such reactions can be expressed by nuclear equations, such as

$$^{A_1}_{Z_1}X + P_i \rightarrow {}^{A_2}_{Z_2}Y + P_0 \tag{11}$$

where X is the element bombarded, P_i is the bombarding particle or photon, Y is the element formed, and P_0 is any particle or photon emitted in the process. It is important that the A and Z numbers be balanced on either side of the equation. This involves combining the A and Z values of the elements and the particles on either side of the equation and making sure they are equal. Some typical nuclear reactions include:

$$^{40}_{20}Ca + {}^1_0n \rightarrow {}^{37}_{18}Ar + {}^4_2\alpha \tag{12}$$
$$^{32}_{16}S + {}^1_0n \rightarrow {}^{32}_{15}P + {}^1_1P \tag{13}$$
$$^{197}_{79}Au + {}^1_0n \rightarrow {}^{198}_{79}Au + {}^0_0\gamma \tag{14}$$

For convenience, the above can be expressed in shorthand as

$$^{40}Ca(n, \alpha)^{37}Ar \tag{15}$$
$$^{32}S(n, p)^{32}P \tag{16}$$
$$^{197}Au(n, \gamma)^{198}Au \tag{17}$$

The target nucleus precedes the parenthesis, the formed nucleus follows the parenthesis, and the bombarding particle and the particle or photon produced appear within the parenthesis.

Chart of the Nuclides. The isotopes of all of the elements are combined on a single chart, the chart of the nuclides. The chart is arranged with the atomic number plotted vertically and the neutron number horizontally. This arrangement demonstrates the continuity in the composition of the nuclides, which progresses from the lightest to the heaviest element. For a given Z, the chart indicates all of the possible isotopes for that element.

Each specific nuclide is represented on the chart of the nuclides by a block. The shading and labeling of each block is used to specify certain information concerning the properties of the nuclide. For example, a gray block denotes a stable nuclide, whereas a white block indicates an artificially produced radioactive nuclide. White blocks with a black corner are used to designate an artificially produced radionuclide resulting from fission, and gray blocks with a black band denote a naturally occurring radionuclide. Each of these block types is illustrated in Figure 3.5.

Each block contains important information regarding the nuclide. For example, the blocks of all nuclides include the chemical symbol, the mass number, percent abundance, activation cross section, and atomic weight. For radioactive nuclides, information regarding the half-life, mode of decay, radiation type, and energy is also provided.

A line drawn through the stable nuclides extends from the lower left to the upper right corner of the chart of the nuclides. Nuclides below this line are characterized by an excess of neutrons and in general are beta emitters. Nuclides above the line are characterized by an excess of protons and decay by either positron emission or K capture.

The chart of the nuclides provides a compact summary of the important information needed by those involved in the application of radioisotopes.

RADIOACTIVE DECAY

Radioactivity is the spontaneous emission of particles or radiation from the nucleus of an atom. The process is said to be spontaneous because it is not induced by external means. Certain nuclides are radioactive; others are not. The most important factors for stability are: (1) favorable N/Z ratio; (2) pairing of nucleons; and (3) high binding energy per nucleon.

The greater the variance from these three factors, the greater the tendency of a nuclide to be unstable. If unstable, the nuclide undergoes any one of a number of decay processes to attain a stable N/Z ratio. In this section the various modes of decay are presented.

DECAY SCHEMES

All modes of decay can be conveniently represented on decay schemes, which provide a detailed description of how a parent radionuclide decays to the ground state of the daughter. Decay by positive-particle emission is indicated by an arrow drawn down and to

SYMBOLS

RADIATIONS AND DECAY

α   alpha particle
β⁻   negative electron
β⁺   positron
γ   gamma ray
n   neutron
p   proton
ε   electron capture
σ   neutron cross section
IT   isomeric transition
D   radiation delayed
SF   spontaneous fission
E   disintegration energy

TIME

μs   microseconds (10^{-6} s)
s   seconds
m   minutes
h   hours
d   days
y   years

Figure 3.5. Example block types and symbols used to define characteristics and properties of each nuclide shown in chart of the nuclides. (Reproduced with permission from the Chart of the Nuclides, distributed by Educational Relations, General Electric Co., Schenectady, N.Y.)

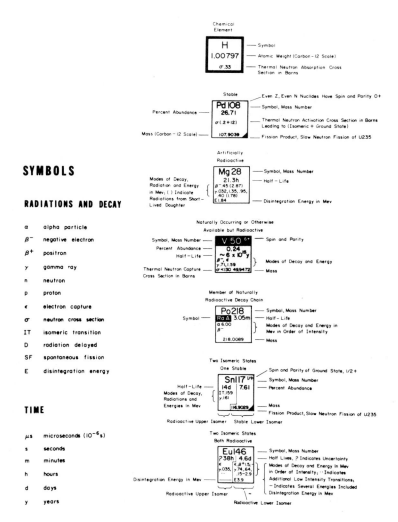

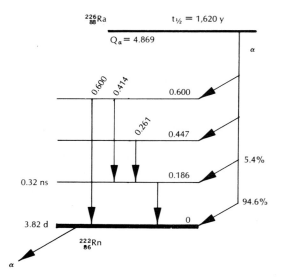

Figure 3.6. Alpha decay scheme illustrated by decay of ^{226}Ra. Process involves emission of alpha particle having any one of four different possible energy values. Better than 94 percent of the time, alpha emission places daughter directly in ground state. In all other cases, alpha emission requires one or more subsequent gamma emissions to achieve ground state.

the left, as shown in Figure 3.6. Negative-particle emission is represented by an arrow drawn down and to the right, as shown in Figure 3.7. Gamma emission is indicated by arrows drawn straight down, as shown in both figures. Energy levels in the daughter nucleus are represented by horizontal lines. Each level is labeled with its energy in meV, relative to the ground state of the daughter. The relative percentage of the time each emission type occurs, the half-lives of each radionuclide, and Q, the total energy released in the nuclear transaction are the other important features shown on the decay scheme. Occasionally, particle emission lines are shown without a percentage designation (Fig. 3.6).

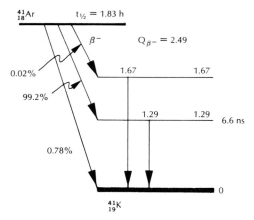

Figure 3.7. Beta decay scheme illustrated by decay of ^{41}Ar. Major decay process involves emission of beta particle followed by emission of 1.29 meV gamma ray.

This implies that the decay process can occur, but very infrequently. Usually, gamma ray energies are indicated on the diagram; when they are not given, the value can be obtained by determining the difference between the two energy states involved.

Decay schemes are a very convenient method of presenting the details of a given decay process. While this information is useful in understanding decay schemes, the data is considered essential in absorbed-dose calculations.

DECAY PROCESS

Alpha Particles. The emission of alpha particles from the nucleus of an atom is represented by the general nuclear equation

$$_Z^A X \rightarrow {}_{Z-2}^{A-4}Y + {}_2^4\alpha + \gamma + Q \qquad (18)$$

In this relationship, X represents the parent radionuclide and Y the daughter product.

It should be noted that the atomic number of the daughter is two less than that of the parent. Thus, when an alpha particle is emitted, the atom must promptly lose two electrons in order for the orbital structure to agree with the new nuclear configuration. In many cases, the emission of an alpha particle leaves the nucleus in an excited state. In such cases, one or more gamma rays will be emitted to drop the daughter to the ground state. When alpha emission places the daughter directly in the ground state, no gamma ray release is required.

In the equation, Q represents the total energy released in the transition from parent to daughter. This includes the kinetic energy of the alpha particle as well as the energy of recoil imparted to the newly formed daughter nucleus.

Virtually all nuclei that decay by alpha emission have an atomic number greater than 82.

Beta Particles. The emission of a beta particle from the nucleus of an atom is represented by

$$_Z^A X \rightarrow {}_{Z+1}^A Y + {}_{-1}^0\beta^- + \bar{\nu} + \gamma + Q \qquad (19)$$

It should be noted that the daughter nucleus has a gain of one in atomic number. This is explained on the basis of the nuclear conversion

$$_0^1 n \rightarrow {}_1^1 p + e^- + \bar{\nu} + Q \qquad (20)$$

where the electron shown becomes the emitted beta particle. Thus, beta emission is found in those unstable nuclides that have an unfavorably high N/Z ratio (ie, too few protons or an excess of neutrons). Such nuclides achieve greater stability by converting a neutron into a proton by the process of emitting a beta particle.

The Q in this equation represents all of the energy available from the nuclear arrangement required to complete the transition from the parent to the daughter state.

Initially it was thought that the kinetic energy of the ejected beta particle plus the energy of any associated gamma rays should equal Q, the energy of transition. However, in practice this does not occur. Observed beta particles are found to have a continuous spectrum of energies ranging from 0 to a maximum of E_{max}, where $E_{max} = Q$ when there are no gamma rays involved.

In 1931, Pauli suggested an explanation for this observation. He postulated that the constant amount of energy available for each beta transition, E_{max}, is shared between an antineutrino and a beta particle. This point is illustrated in Figure 3.8, which shows a typical beta spectrum and the division of energy between the beta particle and the antineutrino.

In those cases where the beta emission does not place the daughter nucleus directly in the ground state, the particle emission will be followed by subsequent gamma emissions; otherwise, no gamma emission occurs.

Positron Particles. Unstable nuclides having an N/Z ratio that is too low are either neutron deficient or have too many protons. Such nuclei attempt to gain a more stable configuration by means of the nuclear reaction:

$$_Z^A X \rightarrow _{Z-1}^A Y + _1^0\beta^+ + \nu + Q \tag{21}$$

The basis for this transformation is the nuclear conversion

$$_1^1 p \rightarrow _0^1 n + e^+ + \nu + Q \tag{22}$$

A proton is converted to a neutron with the release of a positron, the antiparticle of the electron.

The spontaneous decay of a proton indicated in this reaction is energetically impossible, since the sum of the neutron and positron masses exceeds the proton mass. However, since the reaction does occur, it must be concluded that the required energy is supplied by the other nucleons of the nucleus. The equation also shows that a neutrino is emitted in the conversion process.

As with beta emission, positron particles have an associated continuous spectrum, with the difference between the particles' maximum expected energy, E_{max}, and the observed energy being attributed to the neutrino.

Also as with beta particle emission, certain transitions may require gamma ray release in order to bring the daughter to the ground state.

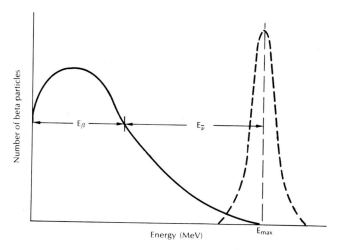

Figure 3.8. Example beta spectrum. Beta particle energies are shown to have continuous spectrum from 0 to maximum beta energy E_{max}, rather than appearing as single peak about mean energy E_{max} (dotted curve). For each beta particle having an observed energy E, corresponding antineutrino has energy $\bar{E}$; thus, $E + \bar{E} = E_{max}$.

Unlike beta particle emission, in order for positron emission to occur a daughter mass requirement must be met. Since the positron is antimatter, additional energy must be supplied by the nucleus to allow the creation of the antimatter particle. This energy corresponds to the mass of the particle plus its pair in matter, the electron. The rest mass of each is m_e, so the energy required is $2m_e c^2$. Therefore, unless the daughter atomic mass is at least two electron masses lighter than its parent, positron emission cannot occur. Where daughter mass is greater than this required minimum, the nuclide decays by electron capture, which is an alternative method of correcting a neutron deficiency.

Electron Capture. A number of radionuclides have an unfavorably low N/Z ratio and daughter products whose mass is greater than the maximum acceptable for positron emission. Such nuclides decay by the process of electron capture.

Electron capture is a nuclear transition in which a nucleus captures one of its own orbital electrons and emits a neutrino. Approximately 90 percent of the captures involve K-shell electrons, and the process is therefore commonly referred to as K capture. The general equation for electron capture is

$$_Z^A X + e^- \rightarrow _{Z-1}^A Y + \nu + \gamma + Q \tag{23}$$

The daughter produced by electron capture is the same as that resulting from positron decay.

The neutrino emissions, however, are different in the two modes of nuclear transition. In positron emission, the energy of nuclear transition is divided between the positron and the neutrino. In electron capture, when the nucleus acquires an electron it immediately combines with a proton to form a neutron, thus reducing the atomic number by one. At the same time, a neutrino having an energy less than or equal to Q is emitted, the neutrino depending on whether a gamma ray emission is involved.

Thus, in contrast to the positron reaction, neutrinos emitted in the process of electron capture do not always share the energy of nuclear transition with a particle but may carry the energy by themselves.

For completion, the equation allows for gamma ray release as a possible accompanying process to neutrino emission. As before, gamma ray emission is not always required.

Deexcitation Process. The electron capture process leaves a vacancy in one of the orbital electron shells, which must be filled by electrons from outer orbits. This filling process results in the emission of x-rays characteristic of the daughter nuclide. This type of x-ray emission is referred to as fluorescence, and the x-rays themselves as fluorescent photons. The detection of fluorescent photons is the principal method of proving that the electron capture process has occurred.

In certain cases the emitted fluorescent photons interact with one of the orbital electrons. If the energy exchange is sufficient to eject the electron from the atom, the process is referred to as an internal photoelectric effect, and the electron is called an Auger (pronounced "oh-zhay") electron.

Fluorescence and the Auger effect compete for the deexcitation of atoms.

Isomeric Transition. All decay processes can place the daughter nuclide directly in the ground state. When an excited state persists for a measureable length of time, the decay process is considered to have two energy states. The intermediate energy state is referred to as a metastable state. The occurrence of this state is indicated by adding an m to the mass number designation of the nuclide (eg, technetium 99m or cobalt 60m).

The deexcitation of a nucleus to the ground state involves a release of energy but no change in the atomic or mass numbers of the nuclide. Such nuclides are called nuclear isomers, ie, same Z or N but different quantum states. The process of nuclear deexcitation is called isomeric transition and may be accomplished by means of either internal conversion or gamma ray emission.

Internal Conversion. The deexcitation of a nucleus from an excited state may result in the emission of a gamma ray. In certain cases, the nuclear deexcitation energy can eject an orbital electron from the atom. This process is referred to as internal conversion. It should

be noted that internal conversion electrons differ from Auger electrons in that the former receive their energy directly from the nucleus, whereas the latter receive their energy from an extranuclear source, namely fluorescent photons.

Gamma Ray Emission. In all decay processes the daughter can go directly to the ground state with the emission of a particle. When excitation of the daughter nucleus persists following the emission of the particle, gamma emission is available as a mode of nuclear deexcitation. This process is the most important method by which nuclear deexcitation occurs. In general, the photon emission will follow the particle within 10^{-6} seconds. Occasionally, however, the emission may be delayed for hours or even days. In such cases, the excited nuclide is said to be in a metastable state.

In all nuclear deexcitation, the nuclear transition followed by gamma ray emission is analogous to the orbital electron rearrangement followed by x-ray release, which occurs when an excited atom returns to the ground state.

ACTIVITY EQUATIONS

The earliest studies of radioactive materials showed that each radionuclide type is characterized by its own fractional decay rate. It was also shown that the rate at which a number of atoms are decaying, (dN/dt) is proportional to the number of atoms available for decay (N) in accordance with the relationship:

$$A = \frac{dN}{dt} = -\lambda N \tag{24}$$

In this equation, A is the activity in disintegration per unit time, λ is a proportionality factor called the decay constant, and the minus sign is used to indicate that the total number of atoms is decreasing with time.

Integration of this equation yields $N = N_O e^{-\lambda t}$ where N_O is the number of atoms present at $t = 0$, and e is the base of the natural logarithm. It should be noted that the decay constant must have units of reciprocal time to cancel the units used for t in the equation.

Activity is defined to be the number of atoms disintegrating per second. It therefore follows that the absolute activity A at any time t is proportional to N, the number of radioactive atoms present at that time. This same relationship should also hold for any observed counting rate R, provided the source/detector geometry is maintained constant for each measurement. Therefore,

$$\frac{N}{N_O} = \frac{A}{A_O} = \frac{R}{R_O} = e^{-\lambda t} \tag{25}$$

and

$$A = A_o e^{-\lambda t}$$

or

$$R = R_o e^{-\lambda t}$$

In general, A is expressed in disintegrations per unit time or fractional curies, while R has units of counts per unit time.

A plot of activity versus time results in a characteristic exponential decay curve such as that shown in Figure 3.9.

Half-life. The half-life of a radionuclide is the time required for the activity to decrease to one half its initial value. This time can be found by substituting $A = A_0/2$ into the activity equation and solving for time. The resulting half-life $t_{1/2}$ is given by

$$t_{1/2} = \frac{0.693}{\lambda} \qquad (26)$$

Mean Life. Mean life has been found useful in describing radioactive decay. It is assumed that the number of radioactive atoms remain constant at N_o until time τ, when all atoms decay simultaneously. In this sense, τ represents the mean life of the decaying atoms.

Effective Half-life. In most dose-estimate calculations, the physical half-life as well as the biologic half-life must be taken into account. While physical half-life relates to the time required for the nuclide to decay to one half its initial value, biologic half-life refers to the time required for the body to biologically

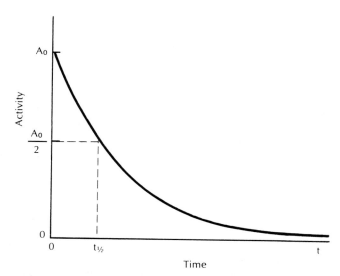

Figure 3.9. Plot of activity versus time using linear scales results in characteristic exponential decay curve. Half-life $T_{1/2}$ is time at which activity has decreased to one half its initial value.

eliminate one half of the amount of the agent that was initially administered. It is usually assumed that biologic elimination occurs in an exponential fashion. The combination of these two half-lives can be represented by a single time referred to as the effective half-life T_{eff}, which is expressed

$$\frac{1}{T_{eff1/2}} = \frac{1}{t_{p1/2}} + \frac{1}{t_{B1/2}} \qquad (27)$$

or

$$T_{eff1/2} = \frac{(t_{p1/2})(t_{B1/2})}{t_{p1/2} + t_{B1/2}} \qquad (28)$$

where $t_{p1/2}$ is the physical half-life and $t_{b1/2}$ the biologic half-life. In dose-estimate calculations, the mean effective life $\bar{T}_{eff}$ is most commonly used, where:

$$\bar{T}_{eff} = 1.44 T_{eff1/2} \qquad (29)$$

The mean effective life has found particular application in equations used to make does estimates for the total decay of the nuclide.

Radioactive Equilibria. In many cases, the daughter formed by a decay process is also radioactive. When this occurs, the following general equation applies:

$$A \xrightarrow{\lambda_1} B \xrightarrow{\lambda_2} C \qquad (30)$$

where A represents the parent radionuclide, B the radioactive daughter, and C the resultant stable nuclide. The decay constants for the transition from A to B and B to C are λ_1 and λ_2 respectively.

If it is assumed that the number of radioactive atoms of A and B are $N_1 = N_{10}$ and $N_2 = 0$ respectively at $t = 0$ and N_1 and N_2 at a later time t, then, the equation

$$N_2 = \frac{\lambda_1}{\lambda_2 - \lambda_1} N_{10}(e^{-\lambda_1 t} - e^{-\lambda_2 t}) \qquad (31)$$

applies to three special types of radioactive equilibria: secular equilibrium, transient equilibrium, and no equilibrium.

Secular equilibrium is characterized by a parent that has an extremely long half-life in comparison with its daughter. As a general rule, the half-life of the parent must be at least 10^4 times as long as that of the daughter. For this case:

$$N_2 \lambda_2 = \lambda_1 N_1 \qquad (32)$$

Then, since the terms on either side of the equation are the respective activities of the daughter and parent, it follows that

$$A_2 = A_1 \qquad (33)$$

This equation indicates that in secular equilibrium the relative number of atoms of parent and daughter are inversely proportional to the ratio of their decay constants. If the log of the activities of the parent and daughter is plotted against time for this condition of secular equilibrium, the curves look as shown in Figure 3.10. The curves show that in secular equilibrium the daughter has an apparent half-life equal to that of the parent. The most important application of this latter point is in radium 226 therapy sources, where the short-lived buildup product radon 222 assumes essentially the same half-life as the long-lived parent. This ensures the source of a constant specific activity over a very long life.

Transient equilibrium differs from secular equilibrium in that the half-life of the parent is greater than that of the daughter by a factor of 10. In this case, λ_1 is only slightly smaller than λ_2. Thus

$$N_2 = \frac{\lambda_1}{\lambda_2 - \lambda_1} N_{10} e^{-\lambda_1 t} \tag{34}$$

and

$$N_2(\lambda_2 - \lambda_1) = N_1 \lambda_1 \tag{35}$$

or

$$A_2 - N_2 \lambda_1 = A_1 \tag{36}$$

A plot of the log of activity versus time for transient equilibrium is presented in Figure 3.11. It can be appreciated from this figure that transient equilibrium is similar to secular equilibrium in that when equilibrium is established, the activities of both parent and daughter decrease at equal rates, with the actual rate being a function of the parent half-life. The two types of equilibrium differ in that the transient equilibrium shows a constant decrease in activity with time, primarily because of the smaller difference between the half-lives of the parent and daughter in this equilibrium type. In addition, in transient equilibrium

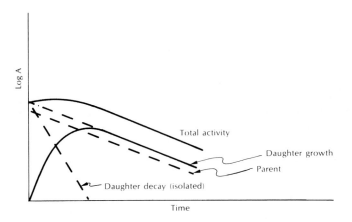

Figure 3.11. Plot of log activity versus time for parent and daughter satisfying conditions for transient equilibrium. Activities of both parent and daughter decrease at equal rates, with actual rate being a function of parent half-life. Daughter activity is actually higher than that of parent at equilibrium.

the activity of the daughter is actually higher than that of the parent during the equilibrium phase.

The condition of transient equilibrium has found an extremely valuable application in nuclear medicine generators such as the molybdenum 99–technetium 99m system. In this case, ^{99m}Tc has a half-life of 6 hours, while ^{99}Mo has a half-life of 66 hours. The plot of log of activity versus time for this parent–daughter combination is shown in Figure 3.12. In this case the

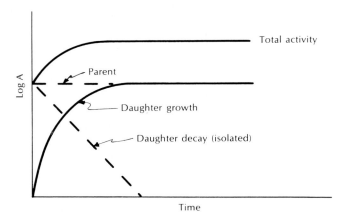

Figure 3.10. Plot of log activity versus time for parent and daughter satisfying conditions for secular equilibrium. At secular equilibrium, relative activities of parent and daughter are same.

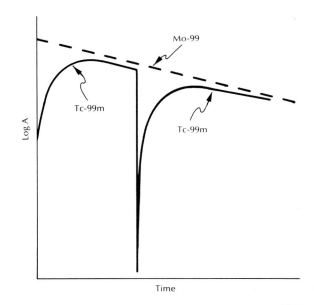

Figure 3.12. Plot of log activity versus time for ^{99m}Mo–^{99m}Tc generator system. Although parent–daughter relationship satisfies definition of transient equilibrium, daughter activity is always less than that of parent because 14 percent of the time ^{99}Mo decays directly to ^{99}Tc without going through isomeric state. Sharp decrease in ^{99m}Tc activity illustrates effect of elution on daughter activity.

^{99m}Tc activity remains below that for ^{99}Mo. This varies from the expected because approximately 14 percent of the ^{99}Mo nuclei decay promptly to ^{99}Tc without passing through the isomeric state of ^{99m}Tc. In Figure 3.13, the elution of ^{99m}Tc from the generator is indicated by a sharp decrease in the ^{99m}Tc activity level, followed by a prompt return to the equilibrium state.

In no equilibrium, the parent half-life is shorter than that of the daughter; thus, $\lambda_1 > \lambda_2$. The daughter activity rises to a maximum and then decreases, eventually assuming its own half-life. For relatively short times, N_2 must be calculated from the general equation. For long times, the condition $\lambda_2 > \lambda_1$ can be applied to the general equation to obtain the following result for determining N_2:

$$N_2 = N_{10} \frac{\lambda_1}{\lambda_1 - \lambda_2} e^{-\lambda_2 t} \qquad (37)$$

SUMMARY

This chapter discusses the theory associated with atomic and nuclear models. In addition, the basic concepts associated with nuclear reactions, and the structure of the chart of its nuclides is explained. Finally, radioactivity and its associated decay schemes and decay equations are presented. This chapter is intended to provide a review of the basic atomic and nuclear physics theory required for an understanding of the physics of diagnostic radiology in general.

REFERENCES

1. Chase GD, Rabinowitz JL: Principles of Radioisotope Methodology. Minneapolis, Burgess Publishing Co, 1970
2. Friedlander G, Kennedy JW: Nuclear and Radiochemistry. New York, John Wiley & Sons, Inc, 1964
3. Lapp RE, Andrews JL: Nuclear Radiation Physics. Englewood Cliffs, NJ, Prentice-Hall, Inc, 1972
4. Rollo FD: Atomic and nuclear physics. Chapter 1 in Rollo FD (ed): Nuclear Medicine: Physics, Instrumentation and Agents. St Louis, CV Mosby, 1977
5. Rollo FD: Radioactivity and properties of nuclear radiation. Chapter 2 in Rollo FD (ed): Nuclear Medicine: Physics, Instrumentation and Agents. St Louis, CV Mosby, 1977

CHAPTER 4

Interactions of Radiation with Matter

RONALD R. PRICE
F. DAVID ROLLO

The term *radiation* is used to describe either a stream of particles or electromagnetic radiation (Table 4.1) propagating through space. The particles may be either charged or uncharged and possess kinetic energy ranging from a few electron volts (eV) to billions of electron volts (BeV). Similarly, electromagnetic radiation may possess very little energy per photon (low energy x-rays, light photons, radio waves) or relatively large amounts of energy per photon (gamma rays).

If the space through which the radiation passes is occupied by matter, interactions will occur that result from collisions of the radiation with the atoms composing the matter. More specifically, the interactions will either take place with the nuclei or orbital electrons. The mode by which the radiation may interact as well as the probability of the interaction depend upon the type of radiation, the kinetic energy of the radiation, and the properties of the matter being irradiated. The result of these interactions may be the absorption of the incident radiation, a scattering of the incident radiation from its initial direction, the ionization or excitation of the atoms composing the matter, or the conversion of the incident radiation into another type of radiation. Collisions that result in no change in either the internal energy of either participant or the total kinetic energy of the colliding pair are said to be elastic. Inelastic collisions, on the other hand, result in a change in the energy of at least one of the colliding particles or quanta as well as a change in the total kinetic energy of the system. The probability of occurrence for a collision of a given type may be represented by the apparent cross sectional area that the target presents to the bombarding particle. The unit of cross section is the barn (1 barn = 10^{-24} cm^2).

INTERACTIONS OF PARTICULATE RADIATION

HEAVY, CHARGED PARTICLES

Within the category of heavy, charged particles are included alpha particles, protons, deuterons, tritons, and ionized atoms. The interactions of these particles with matter is a random process. For charged particles, the energy transfer is usually the result of the interaction of the electric fields surrounding the interacting particles rather than a direct physical contact. Energy is lost primarily through inelastic collisions with the electrons of the medium through which the particle is passing. Because of the great mass of these particles, relative to the electron mass, their paths are almost straight lines. Collisions in which the electron receives only enough energy to be raised to a higher level within the atom (ie, less tightly bound) are said to degrade the energy of the incident particle by excitation. A collision that results in an electron being stripped from its atomic orbit is referred to as ionization. An ionization process will result in the formation of a positive and negative ion (ion pair). Sometimes electrons that have been freed (ie, received energy in excess of their binding energy) in an ionization process will receive enough surplus energy to in turn initiate an ionization process. These energetic electrons are referred to as delta rays and may be observed in photographic emulsions or cloud chambers that have been exposed to radiation. The energy required to strip an electron from its atomic orbit in a gas is between 25 and 40 eV (average of 34 eV/ip). The average energy expended per ion pair produced in a medium is referred to as the W-quantity. For alphas irradiating air, the W is on the average 32.5 eV. In general, it will not take 32.5 eV to strip a given electron from either oxygen or nitrogen. The additional energy included in the W-quantity goes into excitation of other atoms and molecules and into the kinetic energy of the ejected electron.

Specific ionization is defined as the number of ion pairs produced per unit length of path of the incident particle. A related quantity, the linear energy transfer (LET), is defined as the energy deposited in the absorbing material per unit path length. The concept of LET is especially important in radiation biology because of the dependence of tissue damage upon the LET of the incident particle.

The rate of energy loss of a charged particle depends upon its charge and velocity. As a particle loses energy and slows down, the electrons of the material

TABLE 4.1. **Types of Radiation in Common Use**

Radiation	Charge	Approximate Energy Range	Primary Source
Particles			
Alpha	$+2$	3–9 meV	Radioactive decay of heavy nuclei
Beta	-1	0–3 meV	Radioactive decay
High-energy electrons	-1	0–20 meV	Accelerators
Positron	$+1$	0–15 meV	Radioactive decay
Neutrons	0	0–10 meV	Nuclear bombardment (decay of some heavy nuclei)
Protons	$+1$	0–30 beV	Nuclear bombardment
Mesons	$+1, 0, -1$	0–5 beV	Nuclear bombardment
Numerous other common subatomic particles	—	—	Nuclear bombardment
Electromagnetic Radiation			
X-rays	0	few eV–100 keV	Orbital electron transitions
Gamma rays	0	10 keV–10 meV	Radioactive decay (Nuclear transition)
UV, IR, micro- and radio waves	0	10^{-10} eV–1 eV	Atoms, molecules, oscillators

are subjected to the electric field of the particle for a longer time. As a result, the number of ion pairs formed per unit distance increases. The increase in the specific ionization at the end of the path is referred to as the Bragg peak (Fig. 4.1). The incident particle will no longer create ion pairs when it ultimately comes to rest and is neutralized by the addition of electrons from the medium.

The range of an alpha particle in air is roughly proportional to its energy. Energetic alpha particles may travel a few centimeters in air. In tissue, however, their range is only a few microns and is easily stopped by a sheet of paper.

NEUTRONS

Neutrons are produced by three general processes: (1) nuclear bombardment, (2) fission in a reactor, and (3) decay via spontaneous fission of heavy nuclei (eg, Californium 252).

Neutrons are classified according to their kinetic energy (ie, velocity), since $KE = 1/2\ mv^2$. Although the classifications are somewhat arbitrary, very low energy (slow) neutrons with average energies equal to the average kinetic energy of gas molecules at room temperature are referred to as thermal neutrons (0.025 eV at 22°C). Neutrons with energies between 0.5 eV and 10 keV are referred to as intermediate, neutrons within the energy range of 10 keV to 20 meV are called fast, and neutrons above 20 meV are called relativistic.

Since the neutron is uncharged, the electrostatic field surrounding the atomic nucleus will not prevent neutrons from colliding with the nucleus. Neutrons may be captured by a nucleus or may collide either elastically or inelastically. Elastic scattering is the primary mechanism for slowing down fast neutrons. This process is referred to as moderation. Nuclei that are nearly the same mass as the neutron make the most

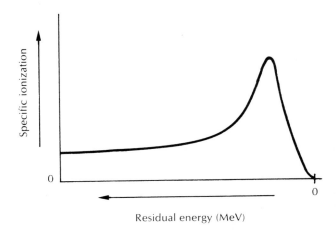

Figure 4.1. A plot of the specific ionization versus the residual kinetic energy of an alpha particle traveling through matter. The residual kinetic energy is inversely related to the distance traveled. The region of increased specific ionization just before the particle loses all of its kinetic energy is referred to as the Bragg peak.

effective moderators. Materials rich in hydrogen and carbon are most frequently used.

When a nucleus captures a neutron, the internal energy of the nucleus will generally increase by about 8 meV (the average binding energy per nucleon for most nuclides) plus the kinetic energy of the neutron. In the capture of a slow neutron, the excess energy is usually not sufficient to eject a particle, and therefore, the excited nucleus will generally release its excess energy in the form of electromagnetic radiation. This type of reaction is called (n, γ) and is a common reaction used to produce radionuclides, that is, activation. This form of activation results in the production of an isotope of the same chemical element as that being bombarded by the neutrons. Capture processes involving intermediate, fast, and relativistic neutrons may result in the ejection of one or more nuclear particles depending upon the excess kinetic energy. When these ejected particles are protons, deuterons, or alphas, the remaining nucleus will be a different element from that which was bombarded.

Some elements such as lithium, boron, and cadmium exhibit very high capture cross sections for slow neutrons. Some heavy nuclei such as ^{235}U and ^{239}Pu will undergo spontaneous fission after the capture of a neutron.

ELECTRONS

In general, beta particles and positrons undergo the same types of interactions with matter as do heavy, charged particles. However, because of the smaller mass of these particles, there are some important differences. The electron (positron) has less mass than a proton or an alpha particle by a factor of 1,800 and 7,000 respectively. Because of this smaller mass, the electron travels at much greater velocity than the larger particles in order to possess a kinetic energy equivalent to that of the more massive particles. Classically, the kinetic energy of a particle is given by the expression:

$$E = 1/2\, mV^2 \qquad (1)$$

where E is the kinetic energy, m is the mass of the particle, and v is the velocity. This equation is valid for velocities that are small with respect to the speed of light. At high velocities, the effective mass depends upon the velocity and a relativistic correction to the mass, as proposed by Einstein.

Electron collisions are primarily the result of electrostatic (coulombic) interactions. As with heavier particles, the rate of energy loss for any electron is inversely proportional to its velocity. However, unlike those involving heavy particles, electron collisions, because of the small mass relative to the target, frequently result in a larger percentage of the energy of the

incoming particle being transferred to the target particle. Thus, the path of an electron as it traverses a medium is very tortuous, reflecting the large angular deflections that result from the interactions.

The repulsive coulombic force between an electron traversing a substance and the orbital electrons in the substance may be sufficient for either excitation or ionization of the target atom. If the interaction is with a more tightly bound electron such as in the K, L, or M shells, characteristic x-rays are produced as outer orbit electrons fall back to re-establish the ground state. In the reconfiguration process, occasionally the excess energy, which is usually released in the form of an x-ray, may be transferred directly to an orbital electron. The result is the appearance of a monoenergetic electron from the atom. Electrons produced in this manner are called Auger electrons.

Elastic collisions of an electron with the electric field of a nucleus are referred to as Rutherford scattering. When an electron undergoes an inelastic collision with the coulombic field of a nucleus, the electron will be slowed down and deflected and electromagnetic radiation will be produced. This radiation is called *bremsstrahlung* (braking radiation). Bremsstrahlung radiation is characterized by a continuous band of energies ranging from zero to the maximum energy of the incident electrons. The intensity of bremsstrahlung is proportional to the square of the atomic number of the material (Z) and to the square of the particle charge (e) and inversely proportional to the square of the particle mass (m). That is:

$$\text{Intensity} \propto \frac{Z^2 e^2}{m^2} \qquad (2)$$

The small mass of the electron makes this particle much more effective in producing bremsstrahlung radiation than heavy charged particles. From equation 2, it should be recognized that bremsstrahlung production is enhanced by target materials with high Z. This process accounts for the production of x-rays in an x-ray tube. Bremsstrahlung production is a very inefficient process in that only about one percent of the total energy of an electron beam will be converted to bremsstrahlung radiation. From the above discussion, it should be obvious why it is customary to use materials of low atomic number to shield against electrons. Plastics and glass provide adequate absorption while keeping the bremsstrahlung production at a minimum.

In any medium, an electron may travel at a velocity that is greater than the speed of light in that medium. In this circumstance, Cerenkov radiation will be produced. Cerenkov radiation is the bluish light seen around the core of swimming pool reactors.

As indicated above, positrons may undergo the same types of interactions as electrons. However, unlike electrons or beta particles, a positron will also undergo annihilation after coming to rest. That is, a positron after losing all kinetic energy will combine with a free electron to annihilate and form two 0.511 meV photons. The photons are given off at 180-degree angles from each other with a combined energy that equals the rest mass of the electron–positron pair.

INTERACTIONS OF PHOTONS (ATTENUATION)

Photons (x-rays or gamma rays) may interact with matter by means of one of five basic processes. These are:

1. Coherent scattering
2. Photoelectric effect
3. Compton scattering
4. Pair production
5. Photodisintegration

Each of the above mentioned processes will have a probability of occurrence or cross section associated with it. The probability that a photon will traverse a given thickness of material is equal to the product of the probabilities that the photon does not interact by any of the five processes.

The probability $[P(x)]$ that a particle will not interact in a thickness (x) is given by the expression

$$P(x) = e^{-\mu x} \tag{3}$$

where e is the base of the natural logarithm (e = 2.71), x is the thickness of the material, and μ is the total linear attenuation coefficient. The quantity μ is dependent upon the energy of the photon and the material being traversed. The total linear attenuation coefficient in units of inverse distance is equal to the sum of the linear attenuation coefficients of each of the five processes

$$\mu = \Omega + \tau + \sigma + k + \pi, \tag{4}$$

where Ω, τ, σ, k, and π represent the attenuation of coherent scattering, photoelectric effect, Compton scattering, pair production, and photodisintegration respectively. It follows that

$$e^{-\mu} = (e^{-\Omega x})(e^{-\tau x})(e^{-\sigma x})(e^{-kx})(e^{-\pi x})$$

$$= e^{-(\Omega + \tau + \sigma + k + \pi)x} \tag{5}$$

The attenuation of a beam consisting of N photons encountering an absorber of thickness x can now be described mathematically. The number of unattenuated photons N left in the beam after traversing the material is given by the following expression:

$$N = N_o e^{-\mu x} \tag{6}$$

It is important to note that the linear attenuation coefficient (μ) is for monoenergetic radiation and that its value is dependent on both the energy of the photon and the type of absorbing material and its physical state (gas, liquid, or solid).

The thickness of material that will reduce the number of transmitted photons to exactly one half of the incident number is called the half-value thickness or half-value layer (HVL).

$$\frac{N}{N_o} = 1/2 = e^{-\mu \text{HVL}} \tag{7}$$

$$\text{HVL} = \frac{ln2}{\mu} = \frac{0.693}{\mu} \tag{8}$$

The concept of mass attenuation coefficient μ_m has been instituted to describe the attenuation of materials independent of their physical state. That is, a material has the same mass attenuation coefficient regardless of whether it is a solid, liquid, or gas, whereas the linear attenuation coefficient would be greatly different for a solid and a gas. The mass attenuation is found simply by dividing the linear attenuation coefficient by the density of the material ($\mu_m = \mu/\rho$, ρ = density).

As was implied earlier, the x-ray beams produced in x-ray tubes are, for the most part, a continuum of energies (polychromatic) as a result of the bremsstrahlung interaction. There will be some monoenergetic characteristic x-rays included in the beam resulting from collisions with orbital electrons. It has been found empirically that the average energy of a polychromatic beam of x-rays produced in an x-ray tube will be somewhere between one-third and one-half the maximum energy of the bombarding electrons.

If one measures the number of transmitted photons as a function of increasing absorber thickness for both a monoenergetic beam and a polychromatic beam, curves similar to those shown in Figure 4.2 will be found.

For monoenergetic beams, the HVL remains constant at all absorber thicknesses. For polychromatic beams, the HVL (penetrating ability) increases continuously with absorber thickness since the lower energy x-rays are being selectively removed from the beam. The phenomenon of selective removal of the lower-energy photons is referred to as beam hardening.

Attenuation implies that photons within a beam have undergone some form of interaction that has caused a change in the properties of the incident photons. This change could be complete absorption of a photon, the scattering of a photon to a new direction with no loss in energy, or scattering with a loss in energy.

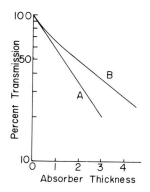

Figure 4.2. **A**. Semilogarithmic plot of the percent transmission of a beam of monoenergetic photons as a function of the thickness of an absorber. **B**. Semilogarithmic plot of the percent transmission of a beam of polychromatic photons as a function of the thickness of absorber. The deviation from a straight line indicates the presence of low energy photons that are selectively removed at small absorber thicknesses (beam hardening).

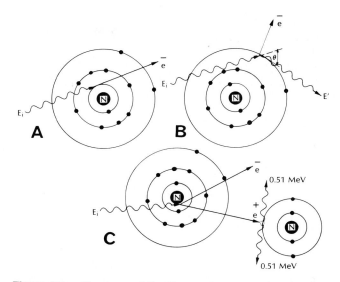

Figure 4.3. Diagrams of the three principal modes of interaction of photons with matter. **A**. Photoelectric effect. **B**. Compton scattering. **C**. Pair production followed by the annihilation of the positron.

COHERENT SCATTERING

Coherent scattering is the name given to that class of interactions in which the incident radiation undergoes a change in direction with no loss in energy. Since the energy of a photon is directly proportional to its wavelength, this implies no change in wavelength after the interaction. Coherent scattering is sometimes referred to as classical scattering since it can be explained completely by classical physics. Thus, the quantum nature of the photon need not be invoked. Since no energy is transferred to the target electron, coherent interactions will not produce ionization and the only effect is a change in the direction of the incident radiation.

There are two types of coherent scattering: (1) those in which a single orbital electron is involved (Thomson scattering) and (2) those in which orbital electrons behave as a single unit (Rayleigh scattering). Coherent scattering is most important at low energies. However, it accounts for only a small percentage of the total interactions. In general, coherent scattering rarely results in the photon being scattered through more than a few degrees.

PHOTOELECTRIC EFFECT

In a photoelectric interaction, shown diagrammatically in Figure 4.3.A, the total energy of an incident photon is transferred to an inner shell electron. The electron (called the photoelectron) is then ejected with kinetic energy E_e, which is equal to the difference between the incident photon energy $h\nu$ and the binding energy of the electron E_B.

$$E_e = h\nu - E_B \qquad (9)$$

The photoelectric interaction occurs most commonly with the inner most lightly bound electrons, the K, L, M, and N orbits. However, the process cannot take place unless the incident photon energy is greater than the binding energy of the particular shell involved. With the ejection of the photoelectron, the atom is left as a positively charged ion with a vacant inner shell that must be filled. An electron from a nearby less tightly bound shell will immediately drop into the void. When this outer electron becomes more tightly bound to the nucleus, it gives up energy in the form of a characteristic x-ray or releases an Auger electron. The energy of the x-ray photon is equal to the energy difference in the two shells of the atom. This energy difference is characteristic for each element.

In Figure 4.4 the mass attenuation coefficient for lead is plotted as a function of the incident photon energy. The discontinuities seen in the curve at approximately 85, 20, and 10 keV where the attenuation coefficient suddenly increases are termed absorption edges. These edges occur when the photon energies just equal the binding energy of the inner electron shells. Photons with energy equal to or slightly greater than the K-shell binding energy interact predominantly with K-shell electrons. Similarly, photons with energies near the L-shell binding energy but less than the K-shell binding energy interact predominantly with the L-shell electrons since they cannot interact with the K-shell electrons.

It was stated earlier that the photoelectric effect is most probable with tightly bound electrons. Elements

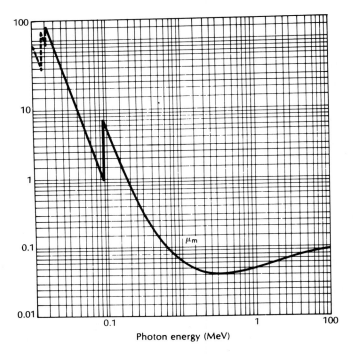

Figure 4.4. Total mass attenuation coefficient for lead versus the energy of the incident photon beam. K and L absorption edges are depicted.

COMPTON SCATTERING

In Thomson scattering, the photon interacting with the electron results in the electron being set into oscillation. In those interactions in which the electron receives a net energy transfer from the incident photon, the electron will recoil from the point of interaction. In 1923 Compton was the first to predict this type of interaction. The kinetic energy acquired by the electron (E_e) has been transferred from the photon; therefore, the photon must leave the site of the collision with less energy (E'). From conservation of energy requirements

$$E = E' + E_e. \tag{10}$$

Since Compton interactions take place with free or loosely bound electrons, the electron binding energy is ignored in the energy conservation equation. "Loosely bound" means that the binding energy is small with respect to the energy of the incident photon energy. Within the diagnostic energy range (20 to 150 keV), even the inner shell electrons of the low-Z elements found in soft tissue would be considered free.

As shown diagrammically in Figure 4.3.B, the electron recoils at some angle θ with respect to the incident direction, and the photon will similarly be scattered at an angle ϕ. The electron angle is constrained to be in the range 0° to 90°; however, the photon angle may be as great as 180° (backscatter). Both θ and ϕ tend to decrease with increased energy of the incident photon. That is, both the recoil electron and the scattered photon will tend to be scattered in the forward direction in interactions involving high-energy photons.

Because momentum must also be conserved in the interaction, equations can be written that relate the energy of the scattered photon ($E_{\gamma'}$) to its angle of scatter (ϕ).

$$E_{\gamma'} = \frac{E_\gamma}{1 + \frac{E_\gamma}{m_0 c^2}(1 - \cos\phi)} \tag{11}$$

where $m_0 c^2$ is the rest mass of the electron (0.511 meV). Equation 11 can be used to show that no matter how large the energy of the incident photon, the maximum energy of a photon scattered at 180° will be 255 keV. Similarly, it can be shown that the maximum energy of a photon scattered at 90° will be 511 keV. Using the formula keV $= 12.4/\lambda$, where λ is expressed in angstroms, one can rewrite the above equation in terms of the difference in wavelength ($\Delta\lambda$) between the incident and scattered photon:

$$\Delta\lambda = \lambda' - \lambda = 0.024(1 - \cos\phi) \tag{12}$$

This is commonly called the Compton wavelength.

Almost all the scattered radiation produced in di-

with high atomic numbers (Z) bind their electrons more tightly, thus it is reasonable to expect that the probability of the photoelectric effect increases as the Z of the absorber increases.

It has been found that the photoelectric effect is approximately proportional to the third power of Z: photoelectric effect $\propto Z^3$. The probability of occurrence of the photoelectric effect is roughly proportional to the inverse of the third power of the photon energy (E): photoelectric effect $\propto 1/E^3$.

As shown in Figure 4.5, the photoelectric effect is most likely to occur with low energy photons irradiating high Z materials, provided, of course, that the energy of the photon is greater than the electron binding energy.

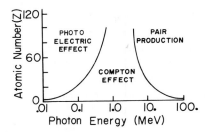

Figure 4.5. Relative importance of the three principle modes of interactions of photons in matter as a function of photon energy and the atomic number (Z) of the absorbing material. Note that the photon energy scale is logarthmic.

agnostic radiology or nuclear medicine procedures is the result of Compton interactions. Since the Compton interaction involves an electron as its scattering center, the probability of a Compton interaction depends directly upon the total number of electrons in the absorber.

PAIR PRODUCTION

Pair production is possible only with photons having energies greater than 1.02 meV. In the vicinity of a strong electromagnetic field (such as that surrounding the atomic nucleus), the energy of the photon may be converted directly into an electron–positron pair. Photon energy in excess of 1.02 meV will appear in the form of kinetic energy of the electron and positron. When the positron comes to rest, it undergoes annihilation with the release of two photons at 180° with respect to each other, and each with an energy of 0.511 meV (Fig. 4.3.C).

PHOTODISINTEGRATION

Photodisintegration reactions are important only for photons of very high energy. Since the threshold energies required for these reactions are well above the diagnostic energy range, photodisintegration reactions will not be discussed.

RADIATION DOSE

UNITS

Before discussing radiation dose and how it is measured, it is necessary to define three basic units of radiation measurement: the roentgen, the rad, and the rem.

The roentgen is the unit of radiation exposure. Radiation exposure is defined only when the medium that is being irradiated and absorbing energy from the radiation field is air. As discussed previously, the transfer of energy from the radiation field to the air will manifest itself by ionization of the atoms in the air. The amount of energy absorbed by the air can be related to the number of ion pairs created. In a small volume of air mass M, the radiation exposure χ is

$$\chi = \frac{Q}{M} \tag{13}$$

where Q is the total charge of either sign of the ion pairs created. The roentgen (R), the unit of radiation exposure, is defined to be equal to a liberated charge of 2.58×10^{-4} coulombs per kilogram of air. A new international system of radiation units (SI) has been proposed for adoption. In the SI system the unit of exposure is 1 coulomb/kilogram of air rather than the

roentgen. We will continue to use the traditional units in this chapter. The roentgen is applicable only to x and γ radiation below 3 meV. The roentgen specifically is not applicable to charged particle beams or photons above 3 meV. To put the roentgen into perspective, the exposure at the surface of the body for an AP film of the abdomen is approximately 1 R.

The rad (radiation absorbed dose) is the unit of absorbed dose for any ionizing radiation. The rad is defined as the deposition of 100 ergs of energy in 1 gram of any material being irradiated by any type of ionizing radiation. Thus, the rad can be defined independent of the type of radiation, the energy of the beam, and the type of material being irradiated. The newly proposed SI unit of absorbed dose is the gray (Gy). The gray is defined a 1 joule/kg. Thus 1 gray is equivalent to 100 rads. In relating the number of rads deposited per R of exposure, one must take into account both the material being irradiated and the energy of the radiation beam. In general, the absorbed dose is proportional to the attenuation of the beam in the medium. That is, one would expect a higher dose in bone than in soft tissue at diagnostic energies due to greater attenuation. The dose deposited in soft tissue at diagnostic energies is about 0.95 rad per roentgen and decreases as the energy of the beam increases. Similarly the energy deposited per roentgen would be much higher for lower energies and for more dense materials such as bone.

The rem is the unit of dose equivalent (DE). The dose equivalent (DE) is defined as the absorbed dose (D) in rads multiplied by a quality factor (QF).

$$DE(\text{rem}) = D(\text{rad}) \times \text{QF} \tag{14}$$

In the SI system of units, the unit of DE is the sievert (Sv). The DE expressed in sieverts is equal to the product of the absorbed dose in grays and the QF (1 Sv = 100 rem).

The rem has been defined because it has been found that for equal absorbed dose, the various types of ionizing radiation—ie, those with different linear energy transfer (LET)—often differ in the efficiency with which they produce a particular biologic or chemical response. A list of QF as a function of LET is found in Table 4.2. It should be noted that for all photon energies used in diagnostic procedures, the QF is equal to one. Thus the number of rems associated with a particular procedure is numerically equal to the number of rads.

The QF actually represents an approximation to the more specific quantity, the RBE (relative biologic effectiveness). The RBE is defined by the following:

$$\text{RBE} = \frac{\text{Dose of reference radiation to produce specific response}}{\text{Dose of radiation under study to produce the same response}} \tag{15}$$

TABLE 4.2. **Quality Factors (QF) for Different LET Radiations**

Radiation	QF
X-rays, gamma rays, & beta particles with $E_{max} > 0.03$ meV	1.0
Beta particles with $E_{max} \leqslant 0.03$ meV	1.7
Neutrons and protons $\leqslant 10$ meV	10 (30 for the eye)
Alpha particles from natural radionuclides	10

From Kereiakes JG: *Radiation Biology*, Continuing Education Lectures 1. Southeastern chapter SNM publication, pp 9-1 to 9-40.

The RBE dose is also expressed in rem.

$$\text{RBE dose (rem)} = \text{Absorbed dose (rad)} \cdot \text{RBE} \qquad (16)$$

INTERNAL DOSIMETRY

The techniques used to estimate doses from internal sources of radiation (radionuclides) have been generally accepted as those recommended by the Medical Radiation Dose (MIRD) Committee of the Society of Nuclear Medicine.

If one imagines a large volume of soft tissue in which a radioactive material is uniformly distributed, then the dose rate (D) to the tissue would vary directly as the amount of activity per unit mass (A/M) and the amount of energy released by each decay of the radioactive nuclei (E).

$$D = CE\left(\frac{A}{M}\right) = \Delta\left(\frac{A}{M}\right) \qquad (17)$$

where C is a constant.

For a particular radionuclide, E is also a constant and when combined with C defines another constant Δ. The Δ symbol was chosen by MIRD and is called the equilibrium dose constant; it has units of gram·rads per microcurie·hour.

MEASUREMENT OF DOSE

The instrument used to determine the absorbed dose to a material is referred to as a dosimeter. The dosimeter is designed to respond to the amount of energy absorbed within the medium. Specifically, the dosimeter must be designed to absorb an amount of energy equal to that which is absorbed by the medium displaced by the dosimeter. This is referred to as tissue equivalence. Numerous types of dosimeters have been designed and used to make radiation dose measurements. These include the use of photographic emulsions, radiation sensitive chemical reactions,

thermoluminescent materials such as lithium fluoride (LiF), photoluminescent materials, and direct calorimetric techniques.

The ionization chamber is probably the most commonly used instrument for estimation of radiation exposure. The use of an ionization chamber to make exposure estimates depends upon the Bragg-Gray principle.

Bragg-Gray Principle. The Bragg-Gray principle assumes the dosimeter to be a very small gas-filled cavity within the medium and as such does not affect the number or energy of the electrons that are liberated from the medium at the location of the cavity. The Bragg-Gray principle states that if the gas-filled cavity were replaced by an equal volume of the medium, the energy that would be absorbed in the medium D_m is related to the energy absorbed in the gas cavity D_g by the ratio of the mass stopping powers of the medium and the gas for the liberated electrons.

$$D_m = \frac{\mu_m}{\mu_g} D_g \qquad (18)$$

where μ_m is the mass stopping power (rate of energy loss along its path) and μ_g is the mass stopping power for the gas.

Referring back to the discussion of the roentgen, it was indicated that it would be necessary to collect all electrons liberated at a location. Since some electrons may be energetic enough to travel some distance from the site of production, it must be assumed that an equal number of electrons created at other sites terminate at the measurement site in order to have an accurate estimate of dose. This criterion is referred to as electron equilibrium. Ionization chambers are designed with special air equivalent walls at specific energies to assure that electron equilibrium is established. Thus the ionization chamber can be calibrated to read in units of roentgens, assuming the beam energy is known.

If a radionuclide decay results in a number of different radiations, then a Δ would exist for each radiation. Then the dose rate to the tissue from all types of radiation would be given as:

$$\dot{D} = \frac{A}{M}\Delta = \frac{A}{M}(\Delta_1 + \Delta_2 + \cdots + \Delta_n) \qquad (19)$$

or

$$\dot{D} = \frac{A}{M}\sum_{i=1}^{n}\Delta_i \qquad (20)$$

In the case of finite sized human beings, some photons originating within an organ in the body will not be absorbed. Thus, we must know the fraction of the time that a photon emitted from a particular organ will actually get absorbed in that organ or another

TABLE 4.3 Some Reactor-Produced Radionuclides

Radionuclide	$T_{1/2}$	Reaction
^{24}Na	15 hours	^{23}Na$(\eta, \gamma)^{24}$Na
^{42}K	12.4 hours	^{41}K$(\eta, \gamma)^{42}$K
^{47}Ca	4.5 days	^{46}Ca$(\eta, \gamma)^{47}$Ca
^{51}Cr	27.8 days	^{50}Cr$(\eta, \gamma)^{51}$Cr
^{59}Fe	45 days	^{53}Fe$(\eta, \gamma)^{54}$Fe
^{75}Se	120 days	^{74}Se$(\eta, \gamma)^{75}$Se
^{99}Mo	67 hours	^{98}Mo$(\eta, \gamma)^{99}$Mo
^{198}Au	64.8 hours	^{197}Au$(\eta, \gamma)^{198}$Au
^{203}Hg	46.6 days	^{202}Hg$(\eta, \gamma)^{203}$Hg

TABLE 4.4. Some Accelerator-Produced Radionuclides

Radionuclide	$T_{1/2}$	Possible reactions
^{11}C	20.3 min	^{11}B$(p, n)^{11}$C ^{11}B$(d, 2n)^{11}$C ^{10}B$(d, n)^{11}$C ^{12}C$(p, pn)^{11}$C
^{13}N	10.0 min	^{12}C$(d, n)^{13}$N ^{16}O$(p, \alpha)^{13}$N
^{15}O	2.0 min	^{14}N$(d, n)^{15}$O
^{18}F	110 min	^{16}O$(\alpha, pn)^{18}$F ^{19}F$(p, pn)^{18}$F
^{67}Ga	78 hr	^{66}Zn$(d, n)^{67}$Ga ^{65}Cu$(\alpha, 2n)^{67}$Ga
^{85m}Kr	4.4 hr	^{84}Kr$(d, n)^{85m}$Kr
^{81}Rb	4.7 hr	^{79}Br$(d, 2n)^{81}$Rb
^{123}I	13 hr	^{122}Te$(d, n)^{123}$I ^{123}Te$(p, n)^{123}$I ^{121}Sb$(\alpha, 2n)^{123}$I
^{201}Tl	74 hr	^{200}Hg$(d, n)^{201}$Tl ^{201}Hg$(d, 2n)^{201}$Tl

organ. MIRD has called this quantity the absorbed fraction and has represented it by the symbol ϕ. The absorbed fraction will depend upon the energy of the radiation, the size of the organ, and its location in relationship to another organ if the other organ is the source of radiation and the attenuating characteristics of the target organ.

Radiation may be classified as either nonpenetrating or penetrating. Nonpenetrating radiation deposits its energy in the immediate vicinity of its origin while penetrating radiation may travel long distances before depositing all of its energy. Electrons, positrons, internal conversion electrons, Auger electrons, and very low energy photons (< 11 keV) are classified as nonpenetrating radiation. All photons above 11 keV are classified as penetrating radiation.

The general dose-rate equation for a specific target–source organ pair is given as:

$$\dot{D}(T \leftarrow S) = \frac{A_s}{m_T} \sum \Delta_i \phi_i (T \leftarrow S) \qquad (21)$$

where $(T \leftarrow S)$ signifies that the source of radiation is in organ S and the dose-rate is being calculated to target organ T, the activity is the source organ A_S while m_T is the mass of the target organ. The absorbed fraction $\phi(T \leftarrow S)$ describes the specific geometry between source and target. In many cases the target and source are the same organ. In this case $\phi = 1$ for the nonpenetrating radiations. In those cases when the target and source organs are different than $\phi = 0$ for the nonpenetrating radiation.

The total dose ($\bar{D}$) is derived from $\dot{D}$ by integrating the dose over the entire time the radioactivity is present. The activity may diminish by either physical decay of the radionuclide or through the biological elimination of the material from the body.

$$\bar{D}(T \leftarrow S) = \frac{\tilde{A}_s}{m_T} \sum \Delta_i \phi_i (T \leftarrow S), \qquad (22)$$

where $\tilde{A}_s$ is the cumulative activity, that is, the activity summed over time.

RADIONUCLIDE PRODUCTION

A very important application of the concepts of the interactions of radiation with matter is radionuclide production. Radionuclide production is accomplished by bombarding materials with either neutrons produced in nuclear reactors or with charged particles (photons, deuterons, or alphas) from a particle accelerator. Some radioisotopes are also obtained from the separation of fission products produced in the fission of ^{235}U or ^{239}Pu.

The amount of radioactivity produced in a target material being bombarded by neutrons is given by the following equation:

$$A = \frac{N \phi \sigma}{3.7 \times 10^{10}} \left(1 - e^{\frac{-0.693t}{T_{1/2}}} \right) \qquad (23)$$

where N is the number of atoms of the target material, ϕ is the neutron flux in terms of n/cm/sec^2, σ is the cross section for the reaction in barns, $T_{1/2}$ is half-life of the radionuclide produced, and t is the length of time of the irradiation.

The principal reaction used in large scale production of radionuclides is the neutron capture reaction— (n, γ). In the (n, γ) reaction, the target nucleus captures a neutron and then decays via the emission of a photon. In this case, the new nuclei are isotopes of the original target nuclei. Other decay modes are also possible after the neutron capture. However, generally speaking neutron bombardment will create an unstable nucleus with an excess of neutrons. A nucleus in this state most often decays via beta decay or electron capture in an attempt to gain more protons. A list of typical reactor-produced radionuclides is shown in Table 4.3.

The cyclotron is the primary particle accelerator used for medical radionuclide production. The cyclotron is usually simpler and less expensive than a linear accelerator. In a cyclotron, particles are accelerated in a helical trajectory between four D-shaped electromagnets. Ions are injected at the center of the evacuated Ds and accelerated toward the outside by means of alternating fields in the electromagnet. Once the particles reach the outer edges of the electromagnets, they have gained enough energy to overcome the electrostatic repulsion of the positively charged nuclei of the target and thus can undergo a nuclear collision with the target nuclei.

The decay characteristics of the radionuclides produced are generally those of proton-rich materials. Proton-produced radionuclides often decay via positron emission or electron capture and are generally very short lived, eg, ^{11}C, ^{15}O, and ^{13}N. A list of common accelerator-produced radionuclides is found in Table 4.4.

REFERENCES

1. Chase GD, Rabinowitz JL (eds): Principles of Radioisotope Methodology. Minneapolis, Burgess, 1964, pp 111–158
2. Hendee WR (ed): Medical Radiation Physics. Chicago, Year Book Medical Publishers, 1979, pp. 40–50, 96–183
3. Rollo FD: Radioactivity and properties of nuclear radiation. In Rollo FD (ed): Nuclear Medicine: Physics, Instrumentation and Agents. St. Louis, Mosby, 1977
4. Christensen EE, Curry TS, Dowdy JE (eds): An Introduction to the Physics of Diagnostic Radiology. Philadelphia, Lea and Febiger, 1979, pp 49–58
5. Barberio HC: Production of radionuclides. In Rocha AFG, Harbet JC (eds): Philadelphia, Lea and Febiger, 1978

CHAPTER 5

Production of X-Rays

JON J. ERICKSON
CRAIG M. COULAM

The production of x-rays is basic to all radiographic procedures. An understanding of the techniques used to facilitate their production and control their characteristics is important for the successful application of present-day equipment to clinical procedures. This chapter will introduce the theoretical basis for x-ray production from high-energy electrons and discuss the practical aspects of various equipment components.

BASIC PHYSICS

When high-energy electrons impinge on a target material, two physical processes take place that produce x-rays. Figure 5.1 illustrates the end results of these processes and shows a typical distribution of x-ray photons as a function of energy. The electron is a charged particle and as such interacts with the electric fields of atoms in the target. As the electron passes through the target it has a finite probability of passing very near the nuclei of target atoms. When this happens the strong positive charge of the nucleus causes the negatively charged electron to deviate from a straight line. In doing so it loses kinetic energy in the form of electromagnetic radiation. This radiation is called bremsstrahlung or braking radiation. The straight-line distribution in Figure 5.1 represents the bremsstrahlung radiation produced at the tube anode. If the electron–nucleus interaction is sufficiently strong, the electron can become trapped and give up its total kinetic energy in bremsstrahlung. In this case, the wavelength of the emitted radiation can be found by the simple relationship:

$$\lambda = \frac{12.4}{E} \tag{1}$$

where λ is the wavelength in Angstrom units and E is the electron energy in keV. Note that the wavelength of the emitted bremsstrahlung radiation decreases as the energy of the incoming electron increases. The bremsstrahlung emitting interaction can only occur with elec-

trons whose energies are high enough to allow them to penetrate the orbital electrons (or electron cloud) surrounding the target nucleus.

The second mode of interaction takes place between the incoming electrons and the orbital electrons surrounding the target atom. In this case, the incoming electron transfers its energy through a collision process to one of the orbital electrons. The orbital electron may be completely ejected from the atom or simply raised to a higher energy orbit. The ejected electron will continue on through the target material and undergo subsequent interactions as though it were an original

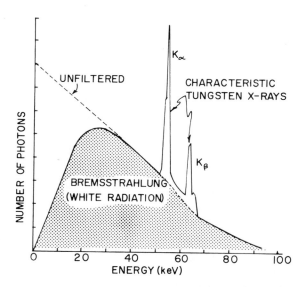

Figure 5.1. A plot of x-ray photon energy versus the number of photons produced at a specific energy secondary to bremsstrahlung radiation in an x-ray tube. The dotted line is the relationship generated at the x-ray tube anode. The solid line is the relationship outside the x-ray tube housing following low-energy photon filtration by the tube housing itself. The sharp peaks in the solid line are the photopeaks of energy, called characteristic radiation, which are secondary to electron shell changes in the anode and are characteristic of the material of the target, such as tungsten.

incoming electron. The excited atoms will lose their energy to the surrounding media in the form of heat. At an electron energy of 100 keV, less that 1 percent of the energy of the incoming electron beam is converted to bremsstrahlung. The remaining 99 percent is converted to heat in the target material and must be dissipated by cooling of some form. As the energy of the incoming electron increases, an ever larger percentage of the energy is dissipated as bremsstrahlung. The ratio of collisional (heat) energy loss to radiation energy loss also decreases as the density of the target material increases. This is simply a result of the fact that more dense materials have fewer electrons per gram of material and are more tightly bound to the nucleus. Thus the nuclear interactions that produce bremsstrahlung become more prominent. The collisional losses for lead and tungsten are about one half that of water.

CHARACTERISTIC RADIATION

If a collisional interaction occurs between an incoming high-energy electron and an orbital electron such that the latter is ejected from the atom, a vacancy is left in the orbital structure. This vacancy is normally filled by an electron from a higher shell dropping into the lower energy shell. When this happens, an amount of energy equal to the difference in the binding energies of the two shells is emitted in the form of electromagnetic radiation. This radiation is named for the shell from which the original electron is ejected; ejection of a K electron results in radiation of K x-rays and ejection of an L electron results in radiation of L x-rays. In order for characteristic radiation to be produced, the incoming electrons must have sufficient energy to eject the orbital electron in the first place. Thus to produce K x-rays from a target of tungsten, the incoming electrons must have an energy of at least 69.51 keV. Characteristic radiation lines at 58 and 68 keV are shown in Figure 5.1.

When the incoming electrons have sufficient energy to eject an orbital electron from a given level, all of the characteristic radiations resulting from refilling the vacancy are present. The relative intensities of the four K lines remain constant independent of the energy of the incoming electrons.

Of particular interest to radiology are the bremsstrahlung and characteristic radiations of tungsten as this is the primary material used as a target material. The dashed line in Figure 5.1 shows that the quantity of bremsstrahlung radiation increases linearly as its energy decreases. However, the existence of the tube housing and its filtration effects reduce the low-energy radiations so that the bremsstrahlung or "white" radiation has the shape shown in this figure. The characteristic radiations of tungsten result primarily from ejection of the K and L shell electrons. It should be noted however that M and N shell electrons are also ejected from the tungsten atom, but these result in characteristic radiations of 10 keV or less and contribute little to the tube output because they are either absorbed in the target material or are filtered in the tube housing. The K radiation lines shown at approximately 58 and 68 keV are known as K_α and K_β respectively. Each of these peaks is actually two radiation lines. The $K_{\alpha 1}$ (59.3 keV) and $K_{\alpha 2}$ (57.9 keV) result from L_{III} and L_{II} electrons filling vacant K shells. The $K_{\beta 1}$ (67.2 keV) and $K_{\beta 2}$ (69.1 keV) result from M_{III} and M_{II} to K transitions. In the diagnostic energy range, the ratio of characteristic radiation to bremsstrahlung may be as high as 30 percent.

X-RAY TUBES

Figure 5.2 is an illustration of a basic x-ray tube construction showing all of the components essential to the production of medical x-rays. The purpose of the tube is to provide a means of producing and controlling a stream of high-energy electrons, which impinge on a target to produce the x-rays. The source of electrons in all x-ray tubes (with the exception discussed below) is a heated filament. When the filament is heated to approximately 2,000°C, electrons are boiled off in the process of thermionic emission. The filament is usually made of tungsten wire to enable it to withstand this high temperature. The high voltage potential between the filament cathode and the anode target draws the electrons from the filament as they are emitted. This flow of electrons is seen in the external circuit as an electrical current. The actual current flow in this circuit is relatively small, seldom greater than 200 milliamperes. The current flow can be limited by the temperature of the filament, which controls the number of electrons available to be accelerated to the anode.

A second effect which also limits the flow is the space charge effect. When electrons are emitted from the filament and the positive attraction to the anode is not sufficient to remove them immediately from the vicinity of the filament, they form a cloud of negative charge. This charged cloud around the filament prevents the emission of more electrons unless they have acquired sufficient thermal energy to overcome the repulsion of the electrons already emitted. This space charge effect is a self-limiting process and prevents the tube current from increasing unless the acceleration potential is increased. Figure 5.3 illustrates a typical tube current versus tube potential curve. At an anode potential of less than 30 to 40 kilovolts (peak) (kVp), the space charge limits the current flow, while at the higher anode potential the flow is essentially limited to

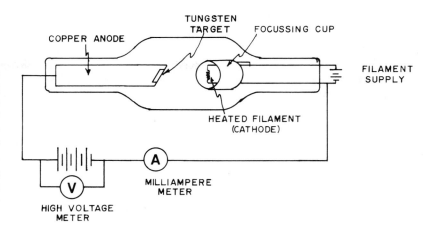

Figure 5.2. Typical anode–cathode x-ray tube relationship. The anode is composed of a high melting point, high-Z material such as tungsten and connected to a copper anode for heat dissipation. The cathode filament is linear in construction and mounted in a cup in order to minimize and focus the space charge electrons boiled off the hot filament by thermionic emission. Electrons accelerate across the space between the cathode and anode under a high voltage potential.

the number of electrons made available by the temperature of the filament. Unless the filament temperature is increased, the current flow is relatively independent of the tube potential once the saturation region is reached.

The inside of the x-ray tube must be maintained at a high vacuum, since the presence of gas of any kind in the tube affects the tube operation in two different ways. First, the gas can provide a conductive path for an electric arc within the tube when the high voltage is applied. This is a serious problem and can destroy both the tube and the generator control system. Second, the gas molecules can act as targets for the accelerating electrons, causing the production of spurious low-energy x-rays and the scattering of electrons from their path to the anode; thus the tube output is reduced. Tubes that must be operated at high potential, where arcing can be a problem, are "warmed up" before use by operation for an extended length of time at less than the normal operating potential. As the warm-up proceeds the

potential is slowly increased to the operating level. This procedure allows any gas present in the tube to be ionized at the lower potential and the resultant ions to be swept out of the space leaving a clean high vacuum.

The electrons are released from the filament in all directions. After release, they are attracted to the anode and move away from the filament. If the filament was in free space the electron cloud would be fairly large and difficult to control. Because of this, the filament is enclosed in a metal cup, which in turn is electrically connected to the filament. By this connection the focusing cup becomes negatively charged and repels the electrons that have been emitted from the filament. As a result, the electron cloud is more concentrated and smaller before being accelerated to the anode. The net result is a much smaller electron beam impinging on the target. As will be discussed below, this is an absolute requirement for high-quality radiographic studies.

TARGET

When the stream of electrons, having been accelerated by the potential between the cathode and anode, strike the anode and undergo deceleration and absorption, they produce x-rays. The x-rays generated are emitted isotopically, but only those emitted in the direction of the surface of the target escape from the target material. In order to produce x-rays in a useful beam configuration, the target is oriented at an angle relative to the direction of the incoming beam as shown in Figure 5.4. The use of the slanted anode surface actually serves another important purpose in the production of medical images. In order to provide sufficient electron current to generate a usable x-ray beam, it is necessary to use an electron beam whose geometric dimensions are less than optimum. The slanted target allows the x-ray beam produced to appear as though it were generated from a much smaller electron beam. This focusing effect can be understood from Figure 5.4.

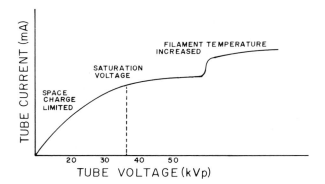

Figure 5.3. Plot of a typical tube current versus tube anode voltage relationship. The number of electrons available to be accelerated to the anode is limited by the number of electrons boiled off the filament by thermionic emission and by the effect of an ambient space charge that surrounds the filament. Electrons with energies greater than the ambient space charge are available for acceleration to the anode.

The electron beam of width x impinges on the target oriented at angle θ with respect to it and emits the x-rays at 90°. By simple geometric considerations it can be seen that the x-ray beam will have a width of $x \cdot \sin\theta$. As θ decreases so does the apparent width of the x-ray beam.

The angle cannot, however, be made equal to zero because only a very small number of x-rays emitted by the target would appear in the beam exiting the tube. With the exception of the so-called micro focus x-ray tubes, modern tubes have angles in the range of 16° to 18°. Notice that the focusing mechanism—often referred to as line focus technique—affects only the apparent height of the electron beam and not the width of the beam. In order for the thinnest beam from the filament to be obtained, tubes are manufactured such that the filament coil is aligned with the vertical dimension of the electron beam. This allows the use of a filament large enough to produce both the required electron current and a relatively small effective beam size.

The trade-offs between available x-ray fluence and apparent focal spot size, as produced by line focusing, make it necessary to manufacture x-ray tubes that contain two filaments. One filament is shorter and hence produces a smaller apparent focal spot. Because of its smaller size, it cannot produce the electron flux necessary for high x-ray loads. For the higher tube output in instances where a less well focussed image is acceptable, the larger filament is used.

TARGET CONSTRUCTION

Design considerations of modern x-ray tubes deal for the most part with dissipating the tremendous amount of heat generated by absorption of the high-

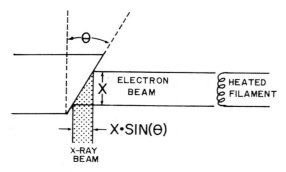

Figure 5.4. The apparent height of the x-ray beam is controlled by the angle θ of the anode inclination. The apparent width of the beam is controlled by the linear height of the filament. Smaller x-ray beams are made by changing the height of the filament winding and not by changing the anode construction; the trade-off is a smaller x-ray flux for a smaller or narrower x-ray beam.

energy electrons in the target. In order that the maximum efficiency in x-ray production be obtained, a target of the highest possible atomic number (Z) is used. However, the heating considerations require a material with a high melting point. This trade-off between physical characteristics results in the almost exclusive use of tungsten ($Z=74$, melting point = 3,370°C) as target material. Targets are not constructed as solid tungsten because it is less than satisfactory as a heat conductor. This causes the region on which the electron beam impinges to become extremely hot; thereafter it cools slowly. To overcome this difficulty, several anode designs have come into common use. The simplest construction consists of a large copper anode in which the target area is replaced by a small block of tungsten. For infrequent, short exposures the copper can remove the heat from the tungsten target and cool it adequately by radiation of the heat into the surrounding space. For longer, more frequent exposures, cooling by conduction and radiation is not adequate. In this case a cooling fluid, usually a nonconducting mineral oil, is pumped around the tube and over the end of the anode to remove the generated heat more quickly.

For longer exposures such as those used in fluoroscopic and angiographic studies, even the heat exchanging cooling system is not adequate. When the electron beam is focussed on a small target area to produce the small focal spot required for high resolution radiography, it can very quickly overheat the target and produce severe surface irregularities. The rotating anode tube was designed to overcome this rapid surface destruction due to overheating. In this design, as shown in Figure 5.5, the anode is constructed on the end of a rotating disc mounted on bearings in the tube. The coils mounted on the outside of the tube housing are energized to cause the rotor to spin at high speed. Once the rotor is spinning at the desired speed, the exposure can be started. The rotation of the anode allows the generation of a small focal spot x-ray beam while at the same time increasing the area on which the electron beam impinges. The rotor is normally operated at rotational speeds as high as 10,000 rpm. The effectiveness of this technique for reducing spot heating can be seen in an example comparing static to rotating anodes. A typical static anode tube will irradiate a target area 7 mm by 2 mm or 14 mm². If the exposure pulse lasts 1/60 of a second and the rotating anode spins at 3,600 rpm, the exposure lasts for one entire revolution of the anode. A typical anode diameter ranges between 75 and 100 mm. At a 100-mm diameter the 7-mm-high focal spot is spread over a 314-mm length or a total area of approximately 2,200 mm². This obviously reduces requirements for high heat transfer rate from a single point on the anode.

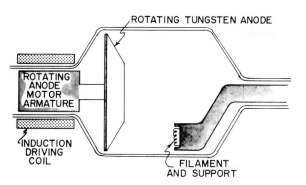

Figure 5.5. Typical rotating anode x-ray tube housing construction. The tube anode is fixed to the armature of an electric motor, which is rotated at high speeds using an induction coil mounted external to the tube housing. High-energy electrons are generated at the filament at the opposite end of the tube. The tube housing is sealed and air removed so the electrons generated at the filament can travel to the anode in a nearly complete vacuum. Tube cooling is maintained by the passing of nonconducting oil over the external surface of the tube housing.

Because the anode is rotating at extremely high speed, special mechanical problems are created in the tube design. The tube must maintain the vacuum to operate properly and so, dry, nonvaporizing lubricants must be used in the bearings. Most modern rotating anode tubes use stainless steel bearings lubricated with metallic silver. The clinical environment in which this type of tube is used causes a great deal of heat to be generated in the anode. In order to protect the bearings from this heat and the resultant changes in mechanical tolerances, material with low thermal conductivity, usually molybdenum, is used for the construction of the main shaft of the anode. The large mechanical stresses induced by the high rotational speed coupled with the thermal expansions produced by the generation of x-rays require very careful monitoring of the tube's operation. X-ray generators designed for use with this type of tube incorporate an interlock system, which prevents any electron flow to the anode unless the anode is rotating at the proper speed. Failure of this interlock can result in destruction of the anode surface at the point where the electron beam strikes, thus making an otherwise adequate x-ray tube completely unacceptable for clinical use. With a little experience one can tell by the sound of the tube when the anode is rotating. If there is any variation from the normal operating sound, the tube should be shut down and examined by qualified personnel. It is not unknown for the rotating anode to disintegrate and send parts through the glass tube wall and the heavy metal tube enclosure.

A variation of the rotating anode has been developed by Machlett (Dynamax 100) that is designed to overcome some of the mechanical problems of the classical rotating anode. It consists of a cup-shaped, lightweight graphite anode into which are mounted small tungsten elements. This design structure serves two purposes. The mounting of the tungsten target elements inside the rotating cup causes them to be forced against their mounts during rotation. In the standard design, the surface must be one integral piece because the rotation would tend to throw off the small individual elements due to centripetal force. The second purpose served by the individual elements is that the spaces between the elements function as expansion joints allowing the anode to absorb more heat and not be subjected to the mechanical stresses inherent in the single unit tube. Besides these mechanical considerations, the graphite construction allows the tube to absorb more heat than the conventional molybdenum construction. Depending on design details of the conventional anode, the Dynamax 100 rotating anode has a heat capacity 1.5 to 2 times greater. The design of this anode also allows a more compact tube construction.

SPECIAL PURPOSE TUBES—FIELD EMISSION—MICRO FOCUS

In most tubes the electron stream is generated by thermionic emission from a heated filament. The thermal inertia of the hot filament makes the generation of short, well controlled bursts of x-rays difficult without design compromises. The field emission tube shown in Figure 5.6 does not employ a heated filament. Very high field strengths around the points of the cathode needles draw electrons from the needle points to the cylindrical anode. The focal spot is, in this case, roughly doughnut shaped and circularly symmetric. Except for high kVp chest radiographs, field emission tubes have not found many applications in conventional radiographic procedures.

The use of x-rays in magnification radiology to produce highly detailed images of small structures has led to the development of microfocus x-ray tubes. In this design the electron beam is focused by use of multiple focusing grids in a manner analogous to that used in cathode ray tube displays. The focusing process produces a very small, highly intense electron beam at the surface of the anode. While this produces the very small apparent focal spot required for magnification radiography, it does place very severe stresses on the anode structure. Because the heating is so concentrated, the anode is usually cooled by an active cooling system in which cooling oil is pumped through channels in the anode itself. Even with this cooling, the tube is normally limited to low-power studies (ie, below 90 kVp and 3 mA), effectively eliminating its use in clinical angiographic work where its imaging properties would be very desirable.

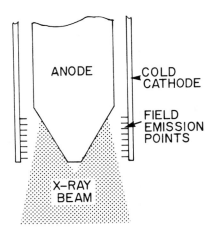

Figure 5.6. Field emission tubes differ from cathode-filament tubes in that electrons are drawn off multiple small "cathode needles" by the high voltage of the anode. No heat is applied to the cathodes. The trade-off necessitated is that higher kVp operating voltages must be used (and thus higher kVp x-ray photons are produced). Also, the x-ray focal spot is doughnut shaped rather than more or less rectangular. Field emission tubes are used primarily for high kilovoltage radiology work, such as for 350 kVp chest x-ray units.

HEATING UNITS AND TUBE RATINGS

As must be obvious by now, one of the primary concerns of tube and system design is the dissipation of heat. The conventional unit used in radiography is the heat unit (HU), which is defined as the product $mA \cdot kVp \cdot$ exposure time in seconds. The amount of heat in heat units that is produced by x-ray generation can be controlled by any combination of these three variables. The ability of the anode to dissipate heat determines the limitations under which these parameters may be varied. As will be seen, a tube able to withstand an exposure of 120 kVp $\cdot$ 150 mA $\cdot$ 1/20 sec = 900 HU may not be able to handle one of 100 kVp $\cdot$ 200 mA $\cdot$ 1/20 sec = 1000 HU. The reason for this is that the anode simply cannot dissipate the heat fast enough to keep the area exposed to the electron beam below the 3,000° C melting point of tungsten. Because this problem is universal, rating charts are usually provided by x-ray tube manufacturers from which it is possible to determine allowable exposure parameters.

Three types of charts are available from which it is possible to determine tube limitations for almost any clinical situation. The simplest chart is that used for single exposure. Figure 5.7 is a typical example. This is a plot of a family of curves each member of which represents an mA value for tube operation. The axes on this graph depict the other two parameters involved in the exposure, time and kVp. This chart is used to determine allowable combinations of kVp and time for

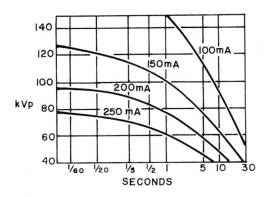

Figure 5.7. A typical exposure chart for x-ray tubes. The actual heating rate must be balanced against the tube cooling rate in order to avoid tube damage. The tube operation must therefore be limited by appropriate use of the kVp and mAs operating stations. These can be chosen from this chart by first picking an operating kVp and exposure time and then using a filament mA less than or equal to the curvilinear mA line lying on the intersection point of the chosen kVp and exposure time values.

a chosen mA. Any combination of kVp and time is allowed as long as lines drawn horizontally and vertically from the respective axes intersect on or below the chosen mA line. A variation of this chart is sometimes used in which mA is substituted for kVp as the vertical axis. In this case, the family of curves represents allowable limits for kVp.

In many instances x-ray systems must operate under very heavy thermal loading resulting from a combination of spot films and fluoroscopic viewing. In such use, the ability of the tungsten target to withstand the instantaneous heating of the single exposure is not usually the limiting factor. Rather, the entire tube assembly and its ability to dissipate heat begins to limit operation. If the tube assembly is allowed to get hot, several undesirable things can take place. Unequal thermal expansion of the glass envelope and the metal components that pass through the glass can cause the joints to crack and the tube to lose its vacuum. In rotating anode tubes, the rotating member and its bearings can become warped and permanently damaged. The total thermal load of the anode assembly can be determined from a chart known as an anode heat storage chart. Figure 5.8 is typical of this type of chart. This chart contains two curves: a cooling curve representing the anode's ability to dissipate heat, and a family of heating curves used to determine the total heat increase due to a given heat deposition rate. In this example the tube assembly has a maximum capacity of 150,000 heat units as shown by the point at which the cooling curve crosses the zero-time vertical axis. The use of this chart is best illustrated by an example. Consider a radiological examination that requires 5 minutes of fluoroscopic viewing and five spot films to

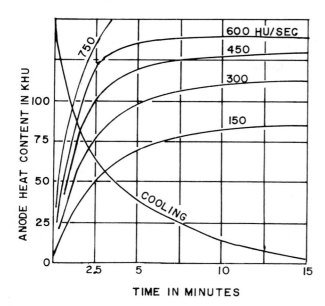

Figure 5.8. Typical anode heat storage chart. The total anode heat generation following a single exposure or multiple repetitive exposures cannot exceed the anode cooling rate without tube damage. Charts of this type must be used with fluoroscopy or angiography equipment because of their continuous and/or repetitive operating procedures.

complete the study. If the fluoroscopic procedure were done at 100 kVp and 4.5 mA the heat load for this input is 100 kVp·4.5 mA = 450 HU/sec. The total heat input for this is found by following the 450 HU/sec curve to 5 minutes and then tracing horizontally back to the vertical axis to find a total of 120,000 heat units. If the spot films are taken with a technique that produces 5,000 heat units per film, they result in an increase in heat load of 25,000 units. The total heat load on the tube at the end of this study is thus 145,000 heat units, well within the tube capabilities. However, should the study require a 6 mA fluoroscopic procedure because of patient size, the tube would be overloaded at the end of the five spot films.

X-RAY GENERATORS

The production of x-rays requires the acceleration of electrons through potentials of several hundreds of kilovolts. This potential is created from the incoming 110 or 220 volt line voltage through the use of transformers. It is not necessary to understand fully the laws of induction and all their ramifications to understand the operation of a transformer. When a wire conductor moves through an electromagnetic field, an electrical current is caused to flow in the conductor. Actually, it makes no difference whether the wire moves and the field is stationary or the wire is stationary and the field moves. A current is induced in the wire in any

case. The amount of current is directly proportional to the rate at which the electromagnetic field lines are passed by the moving wire. Conversely, if a current is passed through a wire, an electromagnetic field is created in the space about a wire. Combining these two aspects of electromagnetism allows one to produce a transformer that will either step up or step down from one voltage level to another. The transformer shown schematically in Figure 5.9 consists of an iron core on which are wound two coils of wire. The primary coil or winding is the input while the secondary winding is the output. The purpose of the iron core is to increase the efficiency of energy transfer between the primary and secondary windings. The ratio of the voltage between the primary and the secondary windings is directly proportional to the ratio of the number of turns in the primary and secondary windings, that is,

$$\frac{V_1}{V_2} = \frac{N_1}{N_2} \qquad (2)$$

where V_1 and V_2 are the primary and secondary voltages respectively and N_1 and N_2 are the number of turns in the respective windings. If V_2 is greater than V_1, it is termed a step-up transformer. The transformer does not generate electrical power, and ignoring small losses, the power output of the transformer is equal to the power input where power in watts is defined as the product of voltage times current. This means that the equation $V_1 I_1 = V_2 I_2$ is accurate. Practically, it means that if the voltage on one side of the transformer is increased, the current on the same side of the transformer must necessarily be reduced.

Figure 5.10 shows the arrangement of transformers commonly used in diagnostic x-ray systems. The autotransformer shown in this illustration is simply a spe-

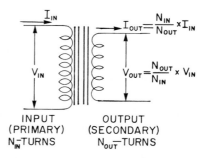

Figure 5.9. A simple (but workable) transformer. Current is generated at the output side of the transformer coils by the electromagnetic field created by the current in the input coils. The voltage on the output transformer side is related to the voltage on the input side through the ratio of the number of windings on the output and input sides respectively. The output current is related to the input current through the ratio of the input to output voltages respectively.

cial case of the dual winding transformer in which a limited range of output voltages is provided with only a small loss in power due to inefficiencies in the transformer. The various taps on the autotransformer represent the various kVp ranges available on most modern systems. In some systems the variable adjustment of the kVp in each range is provided by the voltage divider rheostat shown here. Other systems may smoothly move the tap on the autotransformer between settings. The actual construction will depend on the individual manufacturer. The autotransformer output is fed to the primary of the high-voltage transformer, which actually produces the accelerating potential for the x-ray tube. This two-part design allows the construction of a control panel containing only relatively low voltage (220 to 440 volts); the high voltage transformer can be separated and placed in an oil-filled tank. The oil reduces the chances of arcing in the transformer. The meters monitor the voltage and current supplied to the x-ray tube. The kVp meter can be placed in the primary of the high-voltage transformer because the output voltage can be calibrated so that the meter reads accurately. The mA meter, on the other hand, must be in the secondary of the transformer because losses in the transformer make this parameter difficult to calibrate without actual measurement. The high-voltage transformer shown in Figure 5.10 is a center tap configuration. In this type of configuration, only half of the total accelerating potential appears across any portion of the circuitry. If a noncenter tap configuration is used, one side of the transformer is tied to the circuit ground while the other swings between plus and minus 150,000 volts. In the center tap configuration, one end of the transformer is at minus 75,000 volts while the other is at plus 75,000 volts. This provides the 150 kVp for tube operation but requires only half the insulating capability.

RECTIFICATION

Figure 5.11 (top line) shows the type of waveform produced by the output of the high voltage transformer. It is seen that during one half of the cycle the potential is negative with respect to the circuit ground. If this voltage is applied directly to the x-ray tube, the electrons liberated from the heated filament will flow from cathode to anode during the positive half of the cycle, ie, while the anode is positive with respect to the cathode. However, during the negative phase, no current will flow in the x-ray tube because there is no source of electrons in the anode. This circuit produces what is known as self-rectification in that the x-ray tube itself rectifies the alternating current (AC) voltage from the transformer and converts it to direct current (DC). This configuration has two serious drawbacks. The x-ray flux produced by the tube is a function of both the voltage and the current. The actual flux has a

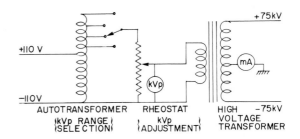

Figure 5.10. A transformer configuration commonly used in diagnostic equipment. This transformer configuration differs from that of Fig. 5.9 in that a variable adjustment of the input voltage is made possible through use of a rheostat, thereby providing some control over the output voltage. Alternatively, changes in the tap on the autotransformer settings allow incremental or step changes in the output voltage levels. Generally, the tap changes are used for large voltage level changes and the rheostat for small and/or continuous voltage level changes.

time variance shape shown in Figure 5.11 (second line). This rapid fluctuation as a function of time makes it very difficult to produce uniform exposures as well as sequential images of short duration. The second difficulty with this circuit is the fact that the target may actually become hot enough to emit electrons by ther-

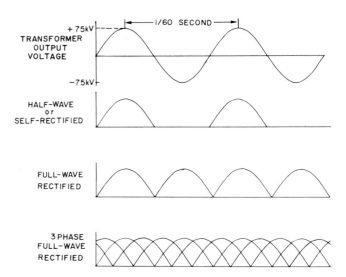

Figure 5.11. Voltage rectification diagrams. The output voltage of the transformer is of the alternating type and must be converted into the direct or constant potential type. This is done through use of full-wave rectifying circuits operating on single or three-phase transformer outputs. Three-phase, full-wave output voltage can be further classified as 6 pulses per cycle or 12 pulses per cycle depending upon the number of voltage peaks per cycle. Twelve pulses per cycle operation requires special circuitry but less dead time before the first pulse (peak) voltage is available for x-ray generation.

mionic emission. In this case, the tube will conduct during the negative phase of the voltage cycle. If this current is large enough, the flow of electrons striking the filament will be strong enough to destroy it and make the tube unusable. For these reasons, self-rectification is not used even though it is very simple.

By inserting electronic devices specially designed to rectify voltage in the anode and cathode portions of circuit, the reverse bias (ie, the negative voltage phase) does not appear across the x-ray tube, thus preventing the anode to cathode current flow. Until recently these devices were vacuum tube rectifiers capable of handling the high power required of diagnostic x-ray systems. These tubes are called thyrotrons. Modern solid-state electronics has produced solid-state rectifiers that are replacing thyrotrons in diagnostic x-ray systems. Even though only one rectifier is required to prevent the reverse bias from reaching the tube, two are normally used. This is simply for the sake of safety and increased reliability; should one of the rectifiers fail, the second will still protect the tube. In addition, the presence of a rectifier in each leg of the circuit prevents the entire tube assembly from having a potential placed on it during the nonconducting phase.

The rectifying circuit removes the possibility of reverse conduction in the x-ray tube but does not change the wave form of the potential applied to produce x-rays. Several modifications to this circuit can be made that will smooth out the potential applied to the tube. The use of full wave rectification is shown in Figure 5.11 (third line). This voltage wave form is called single cycle full wave rectified. In order to further flatten this voltage, it is common practice to combine the output of several rectifiers such that each is slightly shifted in time with respect to the others. Most hospital electrical systems can supply three-phase power, ie, three 60-cycle power lines each 120° out of phase with the other two. Three-phase x-ray generators produce the wave form shown in Figure 5.11 (fourth line).

Combining the three wave forms following full wave rectification will produce a voltage with six pulses or peaks in 1/60 of a second. By appropriately connecting the three phases with large capacitors, it is possible to produce 12 pulses per 1/60 of a second. These multiphase generators make possible the production of short pulses of x-rays with reliable and uniform intensity. They also decrease the "wait time" required for maximum kVp to be available at the tube.

The voltage output of these x-ray power supplies depends on the incoming voltage from the hospital. If the x-ray system requires very stable power supplies for extended lengths of time, it is common practice to use a motor–generator system. The line voltage is used to drive a synchronous motor whose rotational speed is determined by the line frequency. The motor in turn drives a generator, whose output voltage depends on its rotational speed. Because the line frequency is controlled much more accurately than is its amplitude, this system results in a very stable x-ray tube voltage, which is also immune to electrical noise on the power line.

X-RAY CONTROL PANEL

In recent years, regulation and control of the kVp, mA, and time of exposure have been relegated to microprocessor computer circuits. These small logic circuits use modern computer processing methods and memory to take much of the guesswork out of x-ray tube control. These circuits can compute instantaneously the heat units that the tube will be subjected to, given any chosen operating conditions. If the tube ratings have been exceeded, not only will the logic circuits inform the technician of this fact, but they can also suggest alternative, viable operating conditions similar to the original parameters. Through the expanded use of computer memory circuits, many pre-programmed techniques can be set up on the control panel as push-button options to minimize operator set-up time. Further development of these "intelligent" control panels can be expected in future radiographic equipment in order to make x-ray exposures safer and more easily controllable.

SUMMARY

In conclusion, the anode voltage must be of a very large and constant potential (or nearly constant) for proper x-ray tube operation. This requires use of a transformer to create the large potentials and a rectifier system to make it essentially constant in value. With this arrangement, x-rays can be produced at the anode through bombardment of the target material by electrons generated at the cathode (filament) via thermionic emission and accelerated toward the anode by the large anode kilovoltage. Heat generated at the tube must be removed by circulating oils external to the tube housing or inside the anode itself. Failure to cool the tube properly results in shortened tube life and the tube's eventual destruction.

CHAPTER 6

Radiographic Films and Screen-Film Systems

GOPALA U.V. RAO
WILLIAM WITT
MICHAEL C. BEACHLEY
HERMAN A. BOSCH
PANOS P. FATOUROS
PHILIP T. KAN

A typical radiographic examination consists of irradiating the patient with a uniform beam of x-rays and recording the emerging information—carrying intensity distribution—on a double emulsion film sandwiched between a pair of intensifying screens. The screens, composed of phosphor of a high atomic number (Z), convert the absorbed x-rays into a light photon distribution, which in turn exposes the photographic emulsion of the x-ray film. It is possible to expose the film directly to the emergent x-ray beam but the sensitivity will be lower by a factor of 20 to 30, and thus requiring proportionally larger radiation exposures to obtain a satisfactory image. Also, the characteristics of radiographs made with a nonscreen film are strikingly different from those made with a pair of intensifying screens sandwiching the film. In general, nonscreen film radiographs yield better resolution than those made with a screen–film combination. However, the latter usually have a higher contrast. For these reasons, the use of nonscreen film is often limited to peripheral bone radiology, where high resolution is important for detecting subperiosteal resorption or erosion, as is found in hyperparathyroidism or inflammatory arthritic disease. Until recently nonscreen films were also used extensively in mammography, where the visualization of microcalcifications is crucial to early cancer detection. However, with the advent of xeroradiography and single coated films used in conjunction with single intensifying screens, nonscreen films have become nearly obsolete even in these applications.

COMPOSITION OF X-RAY FILM

A double coated x-ray film consists of a transparent plastic support, called the base, both sides of which are coated with photographic emulsion. The base is typically about 150 microns thick. The emulsion is about 10 microns thick for films used with intensifying screens and considerably thicker for nonscreen films. The emulsion consists of silver halide crystals and a gelatin, which serves as a binder. The crystals, or grains as they are sometimes referred to, are about 0.1 to 1 micron in diameter. The absorption of a few photons by one of the grains produces a few metallic silver atoms, which in turn lead to the release of about 10^9 atoms of silver when the grain is developed. The silver halide crystals can be produced in many different shapes and sizes, depending on how they are grown. In general, large grains with large cross-sectional areas produce emulsions with higher speed than do small grains. While the inherent photographic speed is dependent on grain size, photographic contrast is dependent on the grain-size distribution. High-contrast emulsions have a narrower size distribution than low-contrast emulsions. The use of large grains produces considerable density variations in the exposed film, leading to what is commonly referred to as graininess. However, the density variations due to the statistical fluctuations in the incident x-ray beam (quantum mottle) are more pronounced than those due to film graininess.

X-ray films intended for use with intensifying sources are sometimes coated with a thin layer of light-absorbing dye between the emulsion and the base. This helps to reduce crossover effects.[1] Crossover exposure arises because some of the light emitted by the front screen and not absorbed by the front side of the film emulsion may cross over the film base and be absorbed by the emulsion on the other side. Likewise, some of the light from the back screen may be absorbed by the front emulsion of the film. The elimination of crossover obviously increases screen–film resolution. An x-ray film that incorporates a crossover-reducing dye is the XUD film made by 3M.

SENSITIVITY OF X-RAY FILM

X-ray films are more sensitive to light than ordinary photographic films by several orders of magnitude. This is due to the fact that the emulsion layer is considerably thicker and the fact that the base is often coated on both sides with emulsion. The mechanisms by which light photons and x-ray photons affect the film are also different. In the case of x-rays, the incoming x-ray photons interact with the silver and halogen atoms within the emulsion by photoelectric and Compton effects. The electrons produced in this manner ultimately result in energy absorption within the grains of the emulsion and produce the latent image.

Since the K shell binding energy of silver and bromine are 25.5 keV and 13.5 keV respectively, x-ray films exhibit a much higher sensitivity at these energies than at others. Figure 6.1 illustrates the relative sensitivity of x-ray films as a function of x-ray photon energy. The sensitivity of x-ray films may also be increased substantially by increasing the development time and/or developer temperature. These two factors also bring about increases in the background fog and film contrast. Background fog usually sets an upper limit to the sensitivity increases that can be obtained through increased developer temperature and development time.

X-RAY INTENSIFYING SCREENS

As already stated, the x-ray film is quite frequently sandwiched between a pair of intensifying screens made of luminescent phosphors. A typical phosphor layer consists of the phosphor particles dispersed in a low-Z matrix. The thickness ranges from 100 to 300 microns depending on the desired combination of sensitivity and resolution. Other parameters that may be varied include the distribution of phosphor grain size and the introduction of dyes. For screens of equal thickness, the light output increases with increasing grain size; this results in increased screen speed. The addition of dyes to the screen leads to preferential absorption of light that would otherwise travel laterally and thereby decrease sharpness. Since the dyes absorb part of the emitted light, they are more effective in phosphors with high x-ray to light conversion efficiency. As will be discussed in detail later, both the sensitivity and resolution of x-ray intensifying screens depend critically on the thickness of the phosphor layer and the dyes present. In general, the use of a thicker screen results in increased x-ray absorption, thus enhanced sensitivity. However, the lateral diffusion of light is greater for a thicker screen. Sensitivity and resolution are inversely related, and the desired compromise is usually dictated by clinical requirements. Between the plastic support of the screen and the phosphor coating is a thin coating (about 1 ml) of light-reflecting material such as titanium dioxide. The purpose of this layer is to reflect the light emitted in the backward direction by the phosphor material and thereby enhance the sensitivity. The entire screen surface is also coated with a protective layer of clear plastic to reduce static and to protect the phosphor material from wear and tear while cleaning the screens.

X-RAY ABSORPTION

An essential property of a good screen is high x-ray absorption. This requires the use of high atomic number phosphors. Until recently, calcium tungstate ($CaWO_4$) phosphors were used almost exclusively in diagnostic radiology. The K-absorption edge of tungsten is at 69.5 keV, which is relatively high compared to the energy of most of the photons in a typical diagnostic x-ray spectrum. This means that these x-rays will not interact with tungstate K shell electrons, and hence absorption is low. On the other hand, the new rare-earth phosphors exhibit increased x-ray absorption due to the K-absorption edges of lanthanum and gadolinium. The K edges of these elements are 39 and 50 keV respectively. Calculated x-ray absorption factors for 10 mil screens as a function of photon energy are shown in Figure 6.2.

Since the K edges of the phosphor elements are widely different, the variation of their x-ray absorption

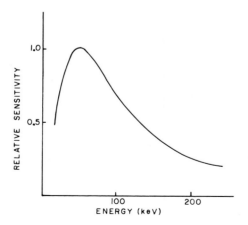

Figure 6.1. Relative sensitivity of x-ray film as a function of photon energy.

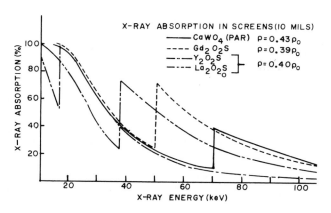

Figure 6.2. Calculated absorption factors for 10 mil screens as a function of photon energy (from Sklensky[2]).

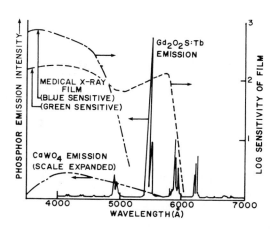

Figure 6.3. Light sensitivity of typical x-ray films and spectral emission of $CaWO_4$ and Gd_2O_2S:Tb screens (from Buchanan[3]).

coefficients with photon energy varies considerably from material to material. In a typical diagnostic x-ray examination, the transmitted x-ray beam consists of a large percentage of x-rays with energies less than 50 keV. Since rare-earth phosphors have a higher absorption coefficient than calcium tungstate at energies less than 60 keV (Fig. 6.2), the sensitivity of rare-earth screens is considerably higher than that of calcium tungstate screens. With the same phosphor material, screen sensitivity obviously is a function of screen thickness. However, the greater the thickness, the lower the resolution.

Phosphor conversion efficiency is defined as the fraction of absorbed x-ray energy that is emitted as light energy. The conversion efficiency of calcium tungsten is typically 3 to 5 percent as compared to 13 and 18 percent for La_2O_2S:Tb and Gd_2O_2S:Tb respectively.

Another characteristic that affects the speed of an x-ray screen–film combination is the degree of matching between the light output of the screen and the spectral sensitivity of the film. Conventional x-ray films (such as DuPont Cronex 4 or Kodak XRP) are sensitive primarily to ultraviolet and blue light (Fig. 6.3). These films are designed to be used with calcium tungstate screens, which emit primarily blue light (Fig. 6.3). Rare-earth screens, on the other hand, emit primarily green light; the film used with these screens should therefore be green sensitive.

RECIPROCITY LAW

The reciprocity law for x-ray films states that the optical density of the film depends only on the product of the intensity of the x-ray beam and the time of exposure, and not on their respective values. Reciproc-

ity failure represents a loss in speed at either high or low intensity levels (Fig. 6.4). No reciprocity law failure is observed in the case of nonscreen exposures.

THEORETICAL CONSIDERATIONS OF SCREENS AND FILMS

Radiographic image quality is governed by a complex interplay of five basic characteristics: (1) average film density, (2) contrast, (3) latitude, (4) resolution, and (5) noise. In this section, we will discuss the role of the characteristics of films and film–screen systems discussed in the previous section in the optimization of radiographic image quality with respect to these five characteristics of the image. In the following discussion the term *image receptor* will be used when referring to film–screen combinations.

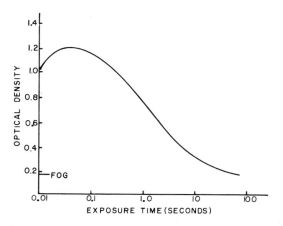

Figure 6.4. Reciprocity law failure in x-ray films.

DENSITY

Film density is by far the most important of the five basic characteristics. The radiographic density D at a given point on a processed film is a measure of the degree of blackening at that point. It is defined by the expression

$$D = \log_{10} \frac{B_I}{B_T} \qquad (1)$$

where B_I is the brightness of the light from the illuminator on which the film is viewed and B_T is the brightness on the observer's side of the film.

A plot of density against the logarithm of the x-ray exposure responsible for the density is called the characteristic curve of the image receptor. Typical characteristic curves are shown in Figure 6.5.

The x-ray exposure reaching the film itself depends on the body part being examined, its thickness, the projection used, and the technical factors involved in making the exposure and developing the film. The technical factors are the kVp, the type of generator (single phase or three phase), mA, focus-to-film distance, field size, filter in the beam, grid (if any), image receptor sensitivity, film development temperature, and processing time.

When the exposure is optimal, the density of the film will follow that portion of the characteristic curve that has the maximum slope and is reasonably straight.

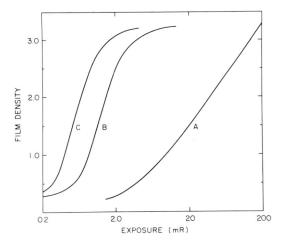

Figure 6.5. Typical characteristic curves for x-ray image receptors. Curve A is for a typical x-ray film used without intensifying screens, curve B for the same film when used with medium-speed screens, and curve C when used with high-speed screens. Notice that curves B and C have the same general shape, indicating that the curve depends mainly on the film used. The slope of the curve, however, decreases considerably if the film is used without intensifying screens (curve A).

Variations in transmission through different parts of the body result in substantial changes in density, and a good radiograph is obtained. If the film is underexposed, the densities correspond to the toe region of the characteristic curve. The net result is that density variations for the same relative variations in x-ray transmission are much smaller and contrast between various structures is reduced. If the film is overexposed, the densities correspond to the shoulder region of the characteristic curve, again resulting in reduced contrast. Figures 6.6 and 6.7 illustrate these principles.

The useful portion of the characteristic curve can be represented by the equation

$$D = \gamma \log_{10} E + C \qquad (2)$$

where D is the density above base plus fog, γ is the slope, often referred to as the film gamma, E the exposure to the image receptor, and C a constant.

The speed S of an image receptor is defined as the reciprocal of the exposure in milliroentgens required to produce a density of 1.0 above base plus fog. With this definition, it follows that

$$1.0 = \gamma \log_{10} \frac{1}{S} + C \qquad (3)$$

Subtracting equation 3 from equation 2 and simplifying, we get

$$D = 1.0 + \gamma \log_{10} SE \qquad (4)$$

Equation 4 relates the density D at any given point of an exposed radiograph to the exposure E that caused it. Using this equation, the entrance exposure E at any point on the radiograph can be calculated. This in turn can be used to determine the skin exposure and the exposure to different tissues in the path of the beam from a knowledge of the patient thickness and the beam HVL for soft tissue (usually between 3.0 to 5.0 cm in the diagnostic range).

In using equation 4, it must be remembered that the speed S of the image receptor depends on the film emulsion and its characteristics, the light conversion efficiency of the screens and their spectral emission characteristics, the dye used in the screens, the spectral sensitivity of the film, the x-ray absorption factor of the screens, sensitivity of the film to direct x-ray exposure, and the effectiveness of the reflective layer in the screens. It also varies considerably with the spectral composition of the x-ray beam incident on the image receptor, the type of developer, development time and temperature, exposure time (due to reciprocity law failure), and the time interval between exposure and processing (due to latent image fading). Screen–film speed may also vary from batch to batch and with age.

Figure 6.6. Radiographs illustrating the influence of optimal exposure and underexposure on image interpretation. When exposure is optimal, the densities on the film will correspond to that portion of the characteristic curve that has the maximum slope. Variations in transmission through different parts of the body result in substantial changes in density, and a good radiograph is obtained. **A.** The optimally exposed PA chest radiograph shows obliteration of a portion of the descending thoracic aorta, indicating an alveolar process in the posterior basal segment of the left lower lobe. **B.** This radiograph was made on the same patient but is underexposed and some of the densities correspond to the toe region of the characteristic curve. The net result is that density variations for the same relative variations in x-ray transmission are much smaller. Hence, contrast between the various structures is reduced. Note that margins of the descending thoracic aorta are barely perceptible and a diagnosis of alveolar infiltrate in the left lobe cannot be made from this film.

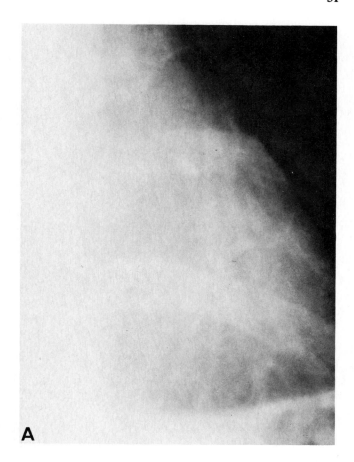

A

Furthermore, the speed of a screen relative to any other screen is essentially independent of the film with which it is used.[5] Similarly, the speed of a film relative to any other film is essentially independent of the screen with which it is used (Tables 6.1 through 6.6).* Figures 6.8 to 6.10 show the variation of speed with kilovoltage (assuming heavy filtration) for a number of commercial screens. These figures are based on published data by Rossi.[6]

*In Tables 6.1 to 6.5, the nonitalic numbers in the body of the table are the relative speeds normalized to a value of 0.8 for par speed screens used with XRP film. These numbers can also be interpreted roughly as the absolute speeds in mR^{-1} at 80 kVp (40 kVp constant potential in Table 6.5), heavy filtration (3.5 cm Al), and narrow beam geometry. The speeds at other kilovoltages (heavy filtration) can be obtained from Figures 6.1 to 6.3.

$$\text{Average Gradient} = \frac{1.75}{\log E_2 - \log E_1}$$

$$\text{Latitude} = \log E_2 - \log E_1$$

where E_1 and E_2 are the relative exposures required to produce film densities of 0.25 to 2.0 respectively above base plus fog; f_{50} and f_{10} are the spatial frequencies in cycles per mm at which the MTF is 0.5 and 0.1 respectively. N_e is the equivalent passband in cycles/mm calculated using the formula

$$N_e = 2 \int_0^\infty |M(f)|^2 \, df$$

where $M(f)$ is the MTF and f the spatial frequency. The italic numbers in the body of the table are a measure of the quantum mottle and represent the product $N_e \sqrt{S/\varepsilon}$ where S is the speed in mR^{-1} and ε the screen absorption factor.

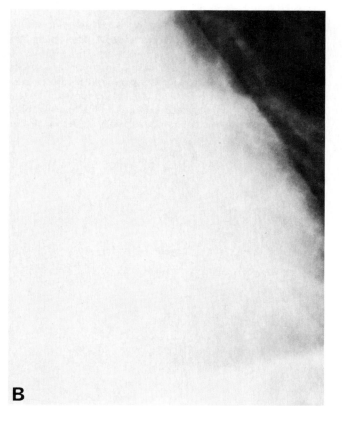

B

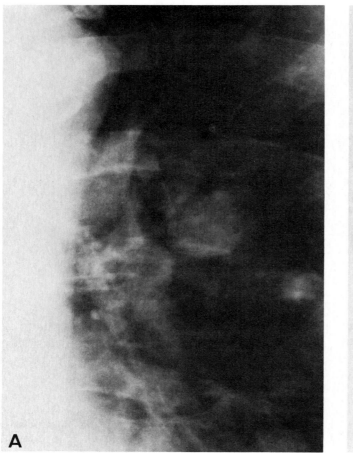

Figure 6.7. Radiograph illustrating the influence of optimal exposure and overexposure on image interpretation. **A.** The optimally exposed film shows multiple metastatic nodules in the left lung field. **B.** The nodules are barely perceptible, since the lung field is overexposed and the film densities correspond to the shoulder region of the characteristic curve, again resulting in reduced contrast. However, visualization of the air in the left main stem bronchus is better since this corresponds more closely to the linear portion of the characteristic curve. It is for this reason that the lung fields may have to be deliberately overexposed occasionally to demonstrate pathology in the mediastinum.

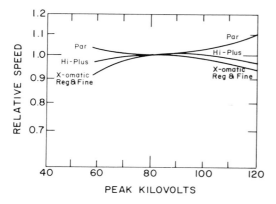

Figure 6.8. Variation of speed with kilovoltage for specified intensifying screens. (Courtesy of Investigative Radiology)

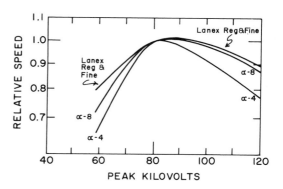

Figure 6.9. Variation of speed with kilovoltage for specified intensifying screens. (Courtesy of Investigative Radiology)

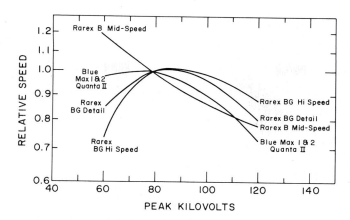

Figure 6.10. Variation of speed with kilovoltage for specified intensifying screens. (Courtesy of Investigative Radiology)

TABLE 6.1. **Physical Characteristics of Selected X-ray Screen–Film Systems**

DuPont Screens	ε	f_{50}	f_{10}	N_e	Cronex 4	Cronex 6	Cronex 6 Plus	Cronex 7
				Average Gradient	3.0	2.2	2.6	3.0
				Base + Fog	0.2	0.2	0.2	0.2
Detail (calcium tungstate)	0.19	2.5	10.5	3.8	0.2, *3.9**	0.2, *3.9*	0.2, *3.9*	0.1, *2.8*
Fast Detail (calcium tungstate)	0.14	1.8	6.5	2.8	0.4, *4.7*	0.4, *4.7*	0.4, *4.7*	0.2, *3.3*
Par-Speed (calcium tungstate)	0.21	1.4	5.0	2.0	0.8, *3.9*	0.8, *3.9*	0.8, *3.9*	0.4, *2.8*
High Speed (barium lead sulfate)	0.30	1.0	3.2	1.6	1.2, *3.2*	1.2, *3.2*	1.2, *3.2*	0.6, *2.3*
Hi-Plus (calcium tungstate)	0.34	1.1	3.3	1.8	1.6, *3.9*	1.6, *3.9*	1.6, *3.9*	0.8, *2.8*
Lightning Plus (calcium tungstate)	0.43	0.9	3.0	1.4	2.4, *3.3*	2.4, *3.3*	2.4, *3.3*	1.2, *2.4*
Quanta II (barium fluorochloride)	0.38	1.1	3.5	1.8	3.2, *5.2*	3.2, *5.2*	3.2, *5.2*	1.6, *3.7*
Quanta III (lanthanum oxybromide)	0.45	0.8	2.5	1.2	6.4, *4.5*	6.4, *4.5*	6.4, *4.5*	3.2, *3.2*

*See footnote on p. 51 for explanation of italic and nonitalic numbers.

CONTRAST

Next to film density, image contrast and image latitude are the most crucial technical parameters influencing image interpretation. Contrast and latitude go hand-in-hand. In general the higher the contrast, the narrower the latitude. These characteristics can be manipulated by changing the beam quality and/or the radiographic film. Image contrast is also influenced by the grid used and airgap, if any. Differences in contrast and latitude cannot be appreciated unless the radiographs in question have identical optical densities at specified reference points. Wide-latitude films permit simultaneous visualization of a range of anatomical details. For example, in high-contrast chest films, either the lung is overexposed or the mediastinum underexposed. However, in wide-latitude chest films both areas may be adequately exposed simultaneously and the

TABLE 6.2. **Physical Characteristics of Selected X-ray Screen–Film Systems**

Kodak Screens	ε	f_{50}	f_{10}	N_e	Kodak Film		
					X-omat RP	X-omat G	Ortho G
X-omatic Fine (BaSrSO$_4$)	0.20	3.1	9.7	4.8	0.3, *5.9**	0.15, *4.2*	0.12, *3.7*
X-omatic Regular (BaSrSO$_4$)	0.37	1.5	4.8	2.2	1.6, *4.6*	0.80, *3.2*	0.60, *2.8*

*See footnote on p. 51 for explanation of italic and nonitalic numbers.

TABLE 6.3. **Physical Characteristics of Selected X-ray Screen–Film Systems**

				Kodak Film		
				X-omat RP	Ortho G	Ortho H
Average Gradient				2.8	—	—
Base + Fog				0.2	—	—

Kodak Screens	ε	f_{50}	f_{10}	N_e	X-omat RP	Ortho G	Ortho H
Lanex Fine	0.34	2.1	7.8	3.2	0.6, *4.3**	0.8, *4.9*	1.6, *6.9*
Lanex Regular	0.62	1.1	3.3	1.8	2.0, *3.3*	3.2, *4.1*	6.4, *5.8*

*See footnote on p. 51 for explanation of italic and nonitalic numbers.

TABLE 6.4. **Physical Characteristics of Selected X-ray Screen–Film Systems**

3M Screens	ε	f_{50}	f_{10}	N_e	3M Film				
					XUL	XUD	XDL	XD	XM
Trimax 2	0.28	—	—	3.4	0.4, *4.1**	0.4, *4.1*	0.8, *5.7*	0.8, *5.7*	1.6, *8.2*
Trimax 4	—	1.4	6.0	2.0	0.8	0.8	1.6	1.6	3.2
Trimax 8	0.48	1.0	4.0	1.8	1.6, *3.3*	1.6, *3.3*	3.2, *4.6*	3.2, *4.6*	6.4, *6.6*
Trimax 12	—	0.9	3.7	1.6	2.4	2.4	4.8	4.8	9.6

*See footnote on p. 51 for explanation of italic and nonitalic numbers.

chance for technologist error is less. Proper interpretation of all the structures within the exposed region can be ensured, but subtle changes within a given region may be more difficult to analyze because of insufficient contrast in that region. High-contrast films make it easier to appreciate subtle density differences in properly exposed regions.

The radiographic image is caused by differential absorption of x-rays by the tissues of the body. The ratio of the exit x-ray exposure difference between any two neighboring regions of the body, ΔE, to the average exit exposure, E, is called exposure contrast.

$$\text{Exposure Contrast} = \Delta E / E \qquad (5)$$

Because the attenuation coefficient for soft tissue increases rapidly as x-ray energy decreases, the exposure contrast increases with decreasing kVp.

The ability of a film or film–screen combination to translate changes in exposure to changes in density depends on the shape of its characteristic curve.

Taking the differential of equation 2, which relates density to exposure, one obtains:

$$\Delta D = \frac{\gamma}{2.3} \left(\frac{\Delta E}{E} \right) \qquad (6)$$

ΔD is usually referred to as the density contrast. It is also sometimes called the image contrast.

TABLE 6.5. **Physical Characteristics of Selected X-ray Screen–Film Systems**

Screens	ε	f_{50}	f_{10}	N_e	Film — Kodak MR (SO-442)	Film — DuPont Cronex Lo-dose
				Average Gradient	2.3	1.8
				Base + Fog	0.17	0.22
DuPont Lo-dose I (CaWO$_4$) yellow dye	0.38	4	13	5.8	—	0.05, *2.1**
DuPont Lo-dose II (CaWO$_4$) no dye	0.40	3	9	4.4	—	0.10, *2.2*
Kodak Min-R (SO-299) (La$_2$O$_2$S : Tb Gd$_2$O$_2$S : Tb) no dye	0.40	3	10	4.6	0.11, *2.4*	—

Courtesy of *Investigative Radiology*.

*See footnote on p. 51 for explanation of italic and nonitalic numbers.

TABLE 6.6. **Intercomparison of Relative Speeds of Selected Intensifying Screens**

Screens	N_e* (c/mm)	$S^{\dagger}$ (mR^{-1})	QMI‡
Kodak X-omatic Fine	4.8	0.3	5.9
DuPont Detail	3.8	0.2	4.0
3M Trimax 2	3.4	0.8 (XD film)	5.7
Kodak Lanex Fine	3.2	0.6	4.3
DuPont Par	2.0	0.8	3.9
DuPont Hi-Plus	1.8	1.6	3.9
Kodak Lanex Regular	1.8	2.0	3.3
3M Trimax 12	1.6	4.8 (XD film)	—
DuPont Quanta III	1.2	6.4	4.5

*$N_e = 2 \int_0^{\infty} |M(f)|^2 df$ (overall resolution measure).

†S = Screen Speed at 80 kVp, heavy filtration when used with Kodak XRP, Dupont Cronex 4, 6, 6+ or 3M Type R film, unless otherwise specified.

‡QMI = Quantum mottle index $+ N_e \sqrt{S/\varepsilon}$ where ε is the screen absorption factor at 80 kVp, heavy filtration. QMI values listed apply when used with Kodak XRP, Dupont Cronex 4, 6, 6+ or 3M Type R film, unless otherwise specified.

The average exposure, E, at any given location on the exit side of the patient is governed by the beam quality (determined by the kVp and filtration), focus-to-film distance, and the mAs used in making the exposure. However, the exposure contrast, $\Delta E/E$, depends on beam quality alone. The exposure at any location determines the density at that location as per equation 2 above. The exposure contrast, $\Delta E/E$, between any two structures determines the density contrast, ΔD, as described by equation 6 above. Density contrast or image contrast can be altered by changing either the beam quality, which changes the exposure contrast, or the film gamma. This is illustrated in Figures 6.11 and 6.12.

As stated before, the gamma is defined as the slope of the straight line portion of the characteristic curve. Sometimes, other measures are used to describe the characteristic curve. The term *contrast factor* is often used to specify the slope of the curve at a density of 1.0 above base plus fog. The term *average gradient* is used to specify the slope of the straight line drawn on the characteristic curve between points on the curve at densities of 0.25 to 2.0 respectively above base plus fog. That is,

$$\text{Average Gradient} = \frac{2.00 - 0.25}{\log_{10} E_2 - \log_{10} E_1} \tag{7}$$

where E_1 and E_2 are the exposures required to produce film densities of 0.25 to 2.0 respectively. Any of the above terms is adequate to describe the ability of the system to translate exposure variations into film density variations. Following recent trends, the average gradient is listed in Tables 6.1 through 6.5.

Scattered radiation can be an important cause of poor image quality. If the exposure contrast is $\Delta E/E$ in the absence of scattered radiation, it will be reduced to $\Delta E/E(1+S/E)$, S being the amount of scattered radiation reaching the film. Scatter thus reduces contrast to a fraction $1/(1+S/E)$ of what it would have been in its absence. S/E ranges anywhere from 2 to 10 depending on beam quality, patient thickness, and field size. With large patients, large field sizes, and high beam qualities, ie, high average energy, scattered radia-

tion is often reduced by the use of a grid. The effectiveness of a grid to eliminate scatter depends on its ratio and its lead content. Figure 6.13 illustrates the effect of scattered radiation on diagnostic image quality. Scattered radiation can also be reduced by the use of air gap or magnification techniques.

LATITUDE

Image latitude (sometimes called the gray scale) can be defined as the range of anatomical details that can be simultaneously visualized on a radiograph.

Since the normal useful range of densities found in radiographs is 0.25 to 2.0, image latitude can be defined quantitatively as the difference in soft tissue thickness that will result in densities of 0.25 and 2.0. If E_1 and E_2 are the exposures resulting in densities, it follows from equation 2 that

$$0.25 = \gamma \log_{10} E_1 + C \tag{8}$$

$$2.00 = \gamma \log_{10} E_2 + C \tag{9}$$

from which it is seen that

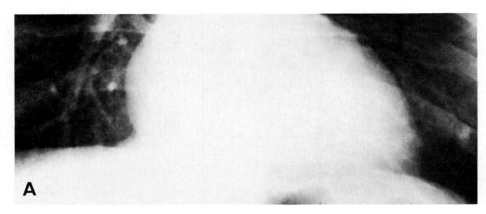

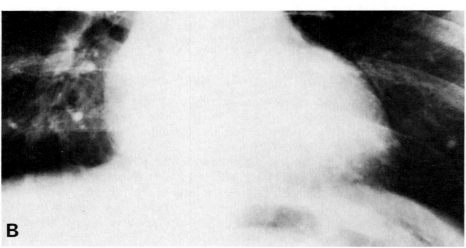

Figure 6.11. Radiographs illustrating the influence of beam quality on image contrast. The film made at 120 kVp (**A**) exhibits less contrast than the one which was made at 80 kVp (**B**) (5 and 25 mA respectively). Notice the clarity of the calcified granulomata in the film in (**B**). In general, however, a low kV technique tends to produce an underexposed mediastinum when the exposure is designed for analysis of the lung, as illustrated by this example. Notice that the azygoesophageal line is barely perceptible in (**B**) while it is seen with excellent clarity in (**A**). Films made at 120 kVp in general provide a larger latitude, showing both soft tissue and pulmonary pathology simultaneously with reasonable clarity.

$$\log_{10} E_2 - \log_{10} E_1 = \frac{1.75}{\gamma} \qquad (10)$$

or

$$\frac{E_2}{E_1} = 10^{1.75/\gamma} \qquad (11)$$

The quantity $\log_{10} E_2 - \log_{10} E_1$ in equation 10 above represents the exposure change in log units to bring about a density change from 0.25 to 2.0. This is often referred to as the film latitude. From equation 10, it is seen that film latitude is inversely proportional to the film gamma or the average gradient. For this reason one of the factors is sufficient to specify both. In Tables 6.1 to 6.5, only the average gradient is listed. Notice that it is listed as a characteristic of the film alone and is independent of the screens with which the film is used. This is because, as shown by Bates,[5] the average gradient and film latitude are governed by film only and are independent of the screens and beam quality, provided that film darkening due to direct x-ray absorption in the film is negligible compared to that due to light emission from the screens.

E_1 and E_2 are related to the incident exposure E_0 through the equations

$$E_1 = E_0 e^{-\mu T_1} \qquad (12)$$

and

$$E_2 = E_0 e^{-\mu T_2} \qquad (13)$$

where T_1 and T_2 are the soft tissue thicknesses in the patient that result in exit exposures E_1 and E_2 and the corresponding film densities 0.25 and 2.0, and μ is the linear attenuation coefficient of the incident x-ray beam in soft tissue.

From equations 12 and 13, on simplification one obtains

$$T_1 - T_2 = \frac{2.303 \cdot 1.75}{\gamma \mu} \qquad (14)$$

Using the relationship between the linear attenuation coefficient and the soft tissue half value layer (ie, $\mu = .693/(HVL)_{ST}$), the soft tissue latitude (STL) is seen to be equal to

$$STL = \frac{1.75}{\gamma} \cdot 3.323 (HVL)_{ST} = \frac{5.82}{\gamma} (HVL)_{ST} \qquad (15)$$

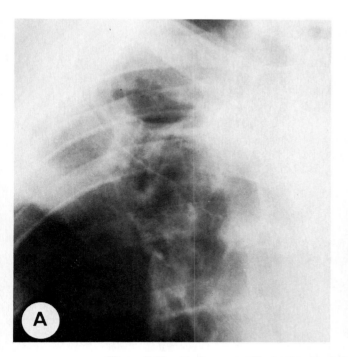
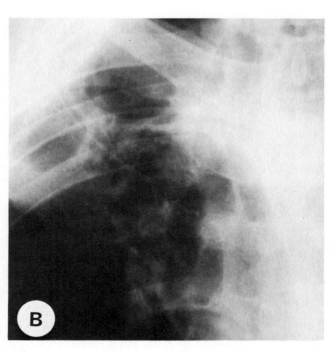

Figure 6.12. Radiographs illustrating the influence of film gamma on image contrast. The two images shown here were made on the same patient using the same factors: 120 kVp and 5 mA. The one on the left (**A**) was made with Kodak XRP film and the one on the right (**B**) with Kodak XL film, which has the same speed as XRP but a lower gamma (wider latitude). DuPont Hi-Plus screens were used in each case. Notice that the XRP film (**A**) is quite good for pulmonary pathology but the mediastinum is relatively underexposed. Small pulmonary densities seen in this film are less apparent in the XL film (**B**). However, since it has a lower gamma, the XL film provides a better visualization of the mediastinal structures at the expense of reduced contrast in the lung fields.

The quantity 3.323 $(HVL)_{ST}$ is referred to as the exposure latitude or the subject latitude as opposed to the factor $1.75/\gamma$, which represents the film latitude. The overall soft tissue latitude is the product of the film latitude and the exposure latitude, just as image contrast was shown in the previous section to be the product of the exposure contrast and the film gamma. For a given beam quality (that is, a given value of $(HVL)_{ST}$), a smaller film gamma implies a greater film latitude. The greater the latitude, the less the local contrast in a given region. While a wide-latitude radiograph permits interpretation of a comparatively wide range of anatomy, it makes it difficult to appreciate subtle changes in isolated areas of tissue with similar absorption characteristics. For example, in a wide-latitude chest radiograph, all the structures within the mediastinum, the lungs, the ribs, and the clavicles are simultaneously displayed. A high-contrast chest radiograph, on the other hand, will be either too dark in the lung fields or too light in the mediastinal region. However, subtle changes can be better appreciated in those regions that are properly exposed.

Figures 6.12 and 6.14 show radiographs illustrating the inverse relationship between latitude and contrast.

Film latitude and average gradient are subject to considerable variations depending on development conditions.[5] Furthermore, in an actual radiographic situation, the range of tissue densities displayed in different regions of the radiograph and the contrast differences between them are determined primarily by

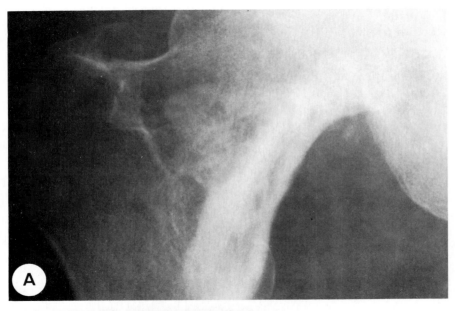

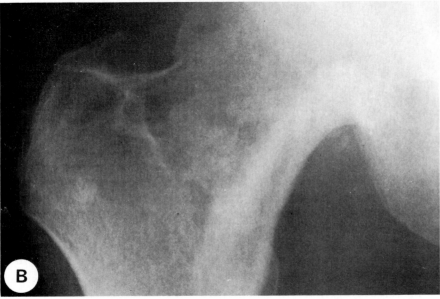

Figure 6.13. Radiographs illustrating the effect of scattered radiation on image quality. These AP films of the hip were made at 75 kVp with appropriate compensation in mA. The presence of scattered radiation in film **B** obliterates much of the fine trabecular detail in the femoral neck and in the endosteal thickening along the medial aspect of the femoral neck. Radiation exposure is three times higher with the grid.

the incident beam characteristics. At low kVp, contrast is higher but the latitude is lower. At higher kVp, the latitude is larger and the contrast lower. In an underexposed or an overexposed radiograph, variations in tissue density are not displayed as proportional variations in film density because of the toe and shoulder regions of the characteristic curve. Small differences in the average gradient and latitude of the film are not clinically significant. The average gradient of most x-ray films when exposed with intensifying screens is between 2.2 and 3.2.

RESOLUTION

A sharp line of demarcation in the tissues of the body such as a bone–soft-tissue interface may appear as a diffuse border in the radiographic image. Also if the objects of interest are small and positioned near each other as in the case of miliary lung densities in chest radiography or the blood vessels in angiography, they may fuse into each other in the image. These are examples of suboptimal resolution and the terms *unsharpness*, *resolving power*, *line pair resolution*, and *modulation transfer function* are used to describe these features of the image. Of these, modulation transfer function, or MTF, is the most recent and the most useful. The MTF, in simple terms, is a graph showing fractional contrast in the image of a test pattern, of sinusoidal transmittance plotted against the number of cycles per millimeter in the pattern, the pattern being imaged under the same circumstances as the region of the radiograph in question.

In the case of radiography of stationary objects,

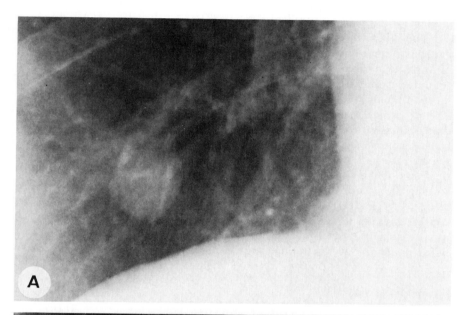

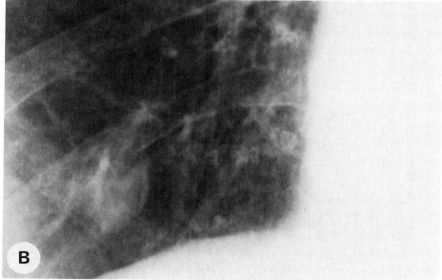

Figure 6.14. Radiographs illustrating the inverse relationship between latitude and contrast. The 120 kVp film (**A**) has a wider latitude but lower contrast than the 80 kVp film (**B**). In **A**, the right lower lobe pulmonary nodule is seen with sufficient clarity and at the same time the mediastinum is sufficiently penetrated in that the dorsal spinal disc interspaces are just perceptible. The high-contrast technique (**B**) reveals more interstitial lung structure, but the mediastinum is less penetrated since the technique has been adjusted for interpretation of the lungs. Wide-latitude films and high-kV techniques also provide a large margin of technologist error.

the focal-spot size, the characteristics of the intensifying screens, and the magnification factor for the structures of interest determine the overall MTF. It can be shown[7,8,9] that the MTF of x-ray focal spots is given by the equation

$$M(f) = \frac{\text{Sin } \pi f_0 a(m-1)}{m} \bigg/ \frac{\pi f_0 a(m-1)}{m} \quad (16)$$

where f_0 is the spatial frequency (cycles per mm) in the plane of interest at right angles to the x-ray beam, a is the effective focal spot size, and m the magnification factor. Figure 6.15 shows the MTFs of 0.25 and 0.50 mm focal spots for different values of the magnification factor, m. The methodology for determining the MTFs of focal spots that are not rectangular is described elsewhere.[10] Figure 6.16 shows the effect of focal-spot size on image resolution in clinical radiographs.

The MTF of an x-ray film–screen combination depends primarily on the screens used and to an insignificant degree on the film used. This is because the resolution capabilities of x-ray films are far superior to those of intensifying screens. The MTF of radiographic screens is determined by the degree of light diffusion that occurs between the screen and the film. This in turn is governed by the chemical composition of the screen material, size of the crystals, screen thickness, tightness of the packing, and the presence of any absorbing dye. Poor film–screen contact is a common cause of MTF degradation; thus excellent film–screen contact is important in all MTF measurements. This is usually achieved by using vacuum cassettes. The detailed methodology for the determination of the MTF

of x-ray intensifying screens is described elsewhere.[11,12] Figure 6.17 shows the MTF curves for typical image receptors. Figures 6.18 and 6.19 show the effect of image receptor on image resolution.

Although the resolution characteristics of x-ray intensifying screens are best specified by the complete MTF curve, in practice it is adequate to quote only one or two points on the curve. Tables 6.1 to 6.5 present those values of the spatial frequency (cycles/mm) at which the MTF becomes 0.5 and 0.1. These are referred to as f_{50} and f_{10} respectively. Another single-number measure of image sharpness is the equivalent passband N_e, defined as the integral of the squared MTF:

$$N_e = 2 \int_0^\infty (M(f))^2 \, df \quad (17)$$

The values listed for f_{50}, f_{10}, and N_e in Tables 6.1 to 6.5 were obtained directly from experimentally measured MTF data. Notice that these three numbers are listed as characteristics of the screens only. This is because standard x-ray films have an MTF close to unity up to about 15 to 20 cycles/mm while the MTF of intensifying screens falls to 50 percent at about 1 to 3 cycles/mm. The MTF curves used in this study were obtained either from the manufacturer or from a recent paper by Arnold et al.[14] N_e values were calculated from the MTF curves by numerical integration.

The equivalent passband N_e of an intensifying screen with a given phosphor material is inversely proportional to the square root of its speed, ie, $N_e \sqrt{S} =$ constant. Straight lines through the origin are obtained when one plots $1/N_e$ against $\sqrt{S}$. The slope of the

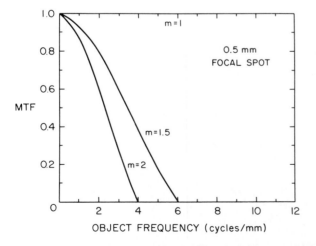
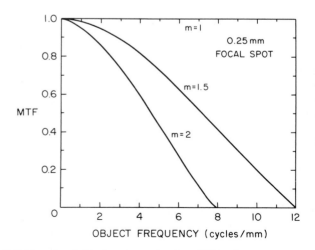

Figure 6.15. MTFs of 0.25 mm (right) and 0.50 mm (left) focal spots for different values of the magnification factor m defined as $(d_1 + d_2)/d_1$, where d_1 is the focus-to-object distance and d_2 is the object-to-film distance. Notice that when $m = 1$, the focal-spot size has no effect on image resolution; in other words, the MTF is unity at all spatial frequencies. As the magnification factor increases, the focal spot MTF decreases. For magnification factors greater than 1, the smaller focal spot, the better the MTF.

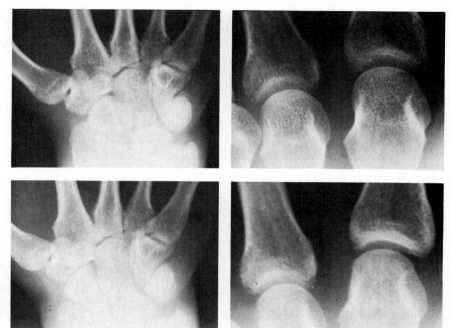

Figure 6.16. Clinical radiographs illustrating the influence of focal-spot size on image resolution. Notice that when $m=1$ (left), there is no perceptible difference in resolution regardless of focal spot size. However, when $m=2$ (right), resolution is much better with the smaller focal spot (upper right).

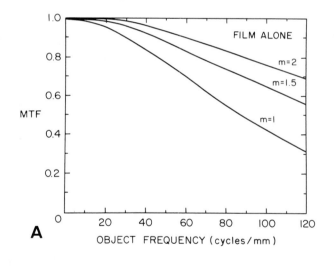

A

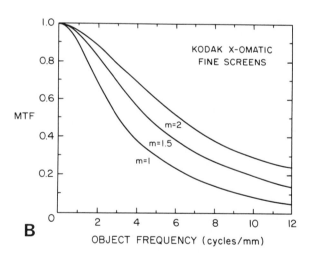

B

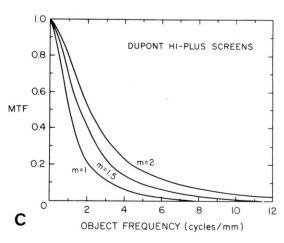

C

Figures 6.17. MTF curves for nonscreen film (**A**) and two types of screens at different magnification factors (**B,C**). In each case, the larger the magnification, the larger the image that is presented to the image receptor, resulting in an apparent increase in resolution.

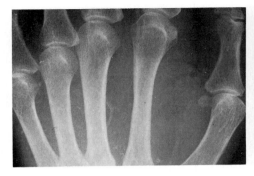

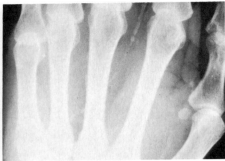

Figure 6.18. Radiographs illustrating the difference in resolution between nonscreen film (left) and screen film (right). Notice the increased resolution of fine trabeculae in the distal metacarpal heads but lower contrast of vascular calcification with the nonscreen technique on the left. Radiation exposure with the nonscreen technique is 20 times higher.

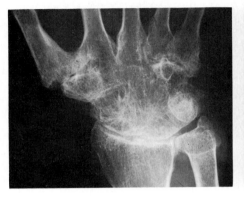

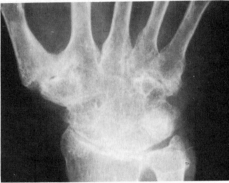

Figure 6.19. Radiographs illustrating the difference between high detail screens (left) and high-speed screens (right). Because the film is the same, no differences in gamma are involved. Notice the increased resolution with X-omatic Fine screens (left). This increase in resolution may be of advantage in evaluating patients with osteopenia. Radiation exposure is 7.5 times higher with the high-resolution screens.

straight line for a given phosphor material depends on the film used and the quality of the x-ray beam incident on the image receptor.[15,16] This relationship is applicable when comparing screens of the same phosphor, ie, thicker versus thinner screens. It is not directly applicable when two different phosphors are compared on the basis of their speed alone, eg $CaWO_4$ versus $La_2O_2S:Tb$.

Composite MTF for Stationary Objects. In the case of stationary objects, the composite MTF is obtained by multiplying together the appropriate values of the MTF of the focal spot and of the screens at each of several points on the spatial frequency scale. Shown in Figure 6.20 are the overall MTFs of Hi-Plus and X-omatic fine screens, used with different focal spots and magnification factors. Hi-Plus screens are about 7.5 times faster than X-omatic screens.

In Figure 6.21 are shown a number of radiographs illustrating the significance of these concepts in practical radiography.

Composite MTF for Moving Objects. Patient motion is a common cause of poor image resolution. When significant motion is involved, the interplay among focal-spot size, magnification, and screen MTF becomes exceedingly complex (as illustrated in Fig. 6.22). The loss of resolution due to patient motion is dependent on the velocity of motion, the type of mo-

tion, and the exposure time. The exposure time in turn depends on the focal-spot size. The larger the focal-spot size, the larger the maximum tube current that can be used, and therefore the shorter the exposure time. On the other hand, the larger the focal-spot size, the greater is the loss of resolution due to geometric factors. The loss of resolution due to geometric factors also depends on the magnification involved in imaging. The larger the magnification factor, the greater is the geometric unsharpness. On the other hand, the larger the magnification factor, the larger the image presented to the image receptor and the better its apparent resolution. The loss of resolution due to the image receptor also depends on the nature of intensifying screens used. In general, for a given phosphor, the faster the screen the poorer the resolution. However, the faster the screen the smaller is the exposure required, thus decreasing the loss of resolution due to patient motion.

Two examples have been chosen to illustrate the value of MTF analysis in specific radiographic studies. The first (Table 6.7) is the case of cerebral angiography in adults at a focus to film distance of 40 in. The patient is assumed to be close to the image receptor and the MTFs are calculated at a magnification factor of 1.2. The examination is to be carried out at 100 kVp, a decision based on contrast and latitude requirements. An 8:1 grid is to be used to reduce the effect of scattered radiation. The calculations are made at a spatial frequency of 2 cycles/mm, using a Machlett

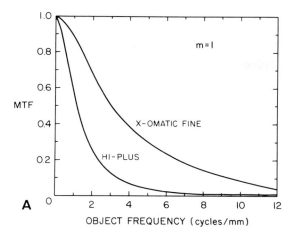

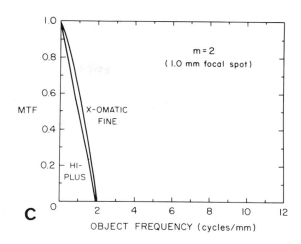

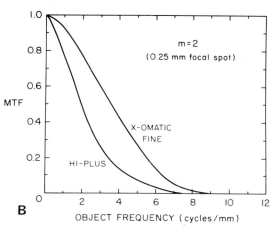

Figure 6.20. Composite MTFs for Hi-Plus and X-omatic Fine screens, used with different focal spots and magnification factors. Hi-Plus screens are about 7.5 times faster than X-omatic screens. **A.** The large separation between these MTF curves indicates much better resolution capabilities for the X-omatic Fine screens at no magnification. **B.** At 2× magnification and small focal spot, the resolution rendered by X-omatic Fine screens is still better than that by Hi-Plus. But the difference is not as large as for *m*=1. This is reflected in a narrower gap between the MTF curves. **C.** At 2× magnification and large focal spot, the MTF curves approach one another, indicating equally poor resolution for both systems.

Dynamax 61 tube with 0.25- and 1.0-mm focal spots. Two types of screens, DuPont Detail and DuPont High Speed, are considered. The calculations include a 0.5 mm focal spot because it is not uncommon to find that the equivalent focal-spot size is substantially larger than the manufacturer's stated value. With a 0.25-mm focal spot, the maximum current at which the tube can be operated is only 100 mA. With a 1.0-mm focal spot, the tube current can be raised to 1,000 mA with a proportional decrease in exposure time. The calculation shows that if the velocity of patient motion is negligible, the best MTF is obtained by using the 0.25-mm focal spot and detail screens. On the other hand, if patient motion is close to a millimeter per second, the best MTF is obtained by using the 1.0-mm focal spot and detail screens.

Table 6.8 shows the results in a similar situation but using a magnification technique (*m*=2). In this case, a 0.25-mm focal spot with detail screens still gave the best MTF as long as the velocity of patient motion was negligible. On the other hand, if the velocity of motion had been close to a millimeter per second, the best MTF would have been obtained by the use of high-speed screens and a 0.25-mm focal spot.

Dependence of Image Sharpness on Contrast and Density. The modulation transfer function (MTF) of an x-ray imaging system is independent of beam quality. It is also essentially independent of the film used since the predominant factors that determine system MTF are screens, motion, focal-spot size, and magnification. However, image sharpness, as visualized on a radiograph, depends on not only the system MTF but also image contrast, which in turn depends on beam quality, the characteristic curve of the film–screen combination, and the ratio of scatter to primary radiation at any point in the image. Image sharpness also depends on the average density at the point of observation. Obviously, if the film is either too light or too dark, visualization of image sharpness is seriously hampered. Figure 6.23 shows radiographs that illustrate these principles.

RADIOGRAPHIC NOISE

Perception of large low contrast details such as tumor masses and tuberculous lesions as well as the visualization of interstitial parenchyma, trabecular pat-

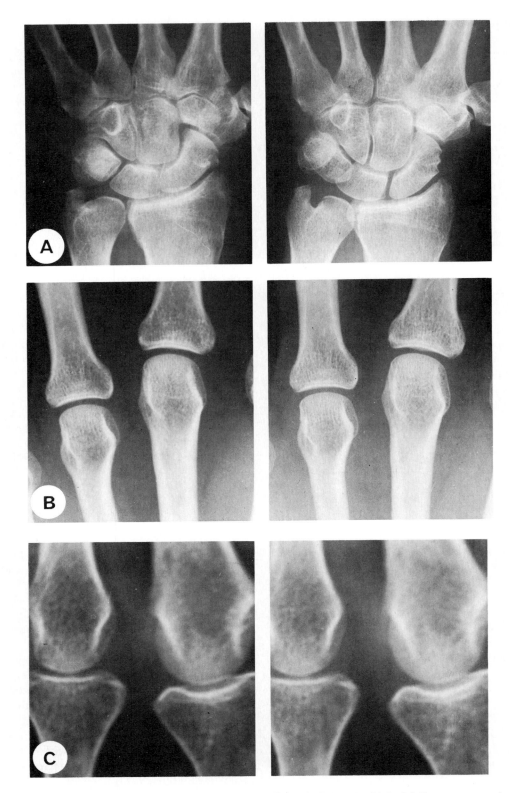

Figure 6.21. Radiographs illustrating the difference between high-detail screens and high-speed screens when used with different focal spots and different magnification factors. **A.** When $m=1$ (unmagnified), X-omatic Fine screens (right) yield much better resolution than Hi-Plus screens (left). This is true regardless of focal-spot size. In this case, a focal-spot size of 0.25 mm was used. **B.** When $m=2$, X-omatic Fine screens (right) still give significantly sharper images than Hi-Plus screens (left), provided the focal spot is small, as illustrated here. Focal spot size = 0.25 mm. **C.** When $m=2$ and the focal spot is large, geometric unsharpness is so dominant that image resolution is about the same with either screen. Focal-spot size = 1.0 mm.

TABLE 6.7. **MTF Calculations for Cerebral Angiography at** $m = 1.2$ *

	Composite MTF at Object Frequency of 2 Cycles/mm	
	0mm/sec	1mm/sec
Detail Screens, 8 : 1 Grid		
0.25mm Focal Spot (100 KVP, 100mA, 0.5sec)	0.70	0
0.50mm Focal Spot (100 KVP, 100mA, 0.5sec)	0.67	0
1.0mm Focal Spot (100 KVP, 1000mA, 0.05sec)	0.58	0.56
High Speed Screens, 8 : 1 Grid		
0.25mm Focal Spot (100 KVP, 100mA, 0.25sec)	0.57	0.36
0.50mm Focal Spot (100 KVP, 100mA, 0.25sec)	0.55	0.35
1.0mm Focal Spot (100 KVP, 1000mA, 0.25sec)	0.47	0.47

*See text for discussion
m = 1.2, FFD = 40″

TABLE 6.8. **MTF Calculations for Cerebral Angiography at** $m = Z$ *

	Composite MTF at Object Frequency of 2 Cycles/mm	
	0mm/sec	1mm/sec
Detail Screens, No Grid		
0.25mm Focal Spot (100 KVP, 100mA, 0.25sec)	0.70	0.45
0.50mm Focal Spot (100 KVP, 100mA, 0.25sec)	0.48	0.31
1.0mm Focal Spot (100 KVP, 1000mA, 0.025sec)	0	0
High Speed Screens, No Grid		
0.25mm Focal Spot (100 KVP, 100mA, 0.125sec)	0.64	0.57
0.50mm Focal Spot (100 KVP, 100mA, 0.125sec)	0.44	0.39
1.0mm Focal Spot (100 KVP, 1000mA, 0.0125sec)	0	0

*See text for discussion
m = 2.0, FFD = 40″

terns, and microvasculature can be influenced by radiographic noise.

The noisy appearance (radiographic mottle) of uniformly exposed x-ray film sandwiched between a pair of intensifying screens is known to be due to three factors[23]: (1) quantum mottle, which arises from the random spatial fluctuations in the x-ray photons absorbed and the light photons emitted; (2) screen mottle, which is due to structural inhomogeneities in the phosphor material of the screens; and (3) film graininess, which is due to the random distribution of exposed grains in the film.

The quality control in the manufacture of screens is generally good so the mottle due to structural inhomogeneities can be neglected. Thus, the spatial variation of the density on a film exposed in contact with a

Object Motion	Velocity of Motion
	Time of Exposure
Geometric	Focal Spot Size
	Magnification Factor
Image Receptor	Magnification Factor
	Nature of the Screens

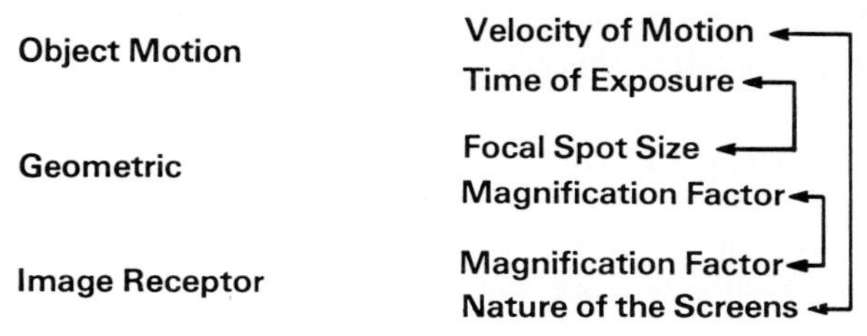

Figure 6.22. Interplay of factors affecting image sharpness. See text for discussion.

pair of intensifying screens consists of a coarse pattern caused by the quantum mottle superimposed on the fine grain pattern of the film. Manifestation of the quantum mottle itself depends not only on the number of x-ray quanta absorbed in the screens per unit area but also on the MTF of the screens. The better the MTF of the screen, the more faithful is the transmission of the quantum mottle to the film. The manifestation of quantum mottle is also influenced by the film's characteristic curve and the film density at the point of observation. Quantum mottle makes bone appear washed out in a pattern suggesting demineralization as in osteomalacia. Similarly, mottle can interfere with interpretation of the interstitial pattern within the lung and the soft tissues. However, interference by mottle usually can be compensated for by the radiologist since the mottle is visible over the entire film. Figure 6.24 shows chest radiographs that illustrate the effect of quantum mottle on image quality.

When a fast screen–film combination is used, the x-ray exposure needed to obtain an adequate density will be small, and this will result in large photon fluctuations across the exit beam. If, in addition, the screen–film combination has a good MTF, these fluctuations will be faithfully reproduced on the film. This will result in poor visualization of low-contrast objects but will not interfere with the visualization of high-contrast objects (Fig. 6.25, right). When a relatively slow screen–film combination is used and at the

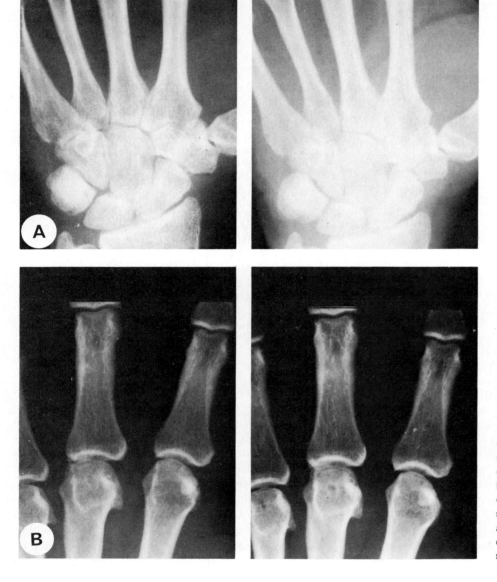

Figure 6.23. Radiographs illustrating the dependence of image sharpness on density and contrast. **A.** These two radiographs were made with the same screens, same kVp, and same geometry. However, the image on the left was made with a higher contrast film (XRP) and appears to be sharper. **B.** These two radiographs were made using the same screens, same film, and same geometry (that is, same MTF). Hence they are expected to yield equally sharp images. However, since the film on the left was made at a lower kVp, it has a higher contrast and appears to be sharper.

same time the MTF is poor (Fig. 6.25, right), the statistical fluctuations displayed on the image will be small. Low-contrast objects will be better seen, but high-contrast objects will not be, because of the poor MTF.

The overall mottle in an exposed film can be measured in terms of the Selwyn noise index.[17] This is defined as the quantity $A(\sigma_D)^2$ where σ_D is the standard deviation of a number of density measurements on the film and A is the area of the aperture used in making the measurements. This is a gross index and does not reveal the spatial frequency content of the noise and its dependence on the MTF of the screens. The random distribution of the x-ray photons absorbed in the screen corresponds to a "white noise" whose manifestation on the film depends on the MTF of the screens and the

gradient of the film's characteristic curve. For this reason, a more sophisticated method, involving the conversion of the density fluctuations on a uniformly exposed film into their Fourier components, is often used to characterize the noise in it. The square of the Fourier transform of the measured density fluctuations is referred to as the Wiener spectrum, which provides a complete description of the spectral composition of noise.

Wagner et al[18,19] and Doi et al[20] have recently measured the Wiener spectra for a number of modern x-ray film–screen combinations. Figure 6.26 shows a typical Wiener spectrum taken from a recent paper by Wagner et al.[18] It can be seen that the noise is high at low spatial frequencies and falls off gradually with increasing spatial frequency due to MTF degradations

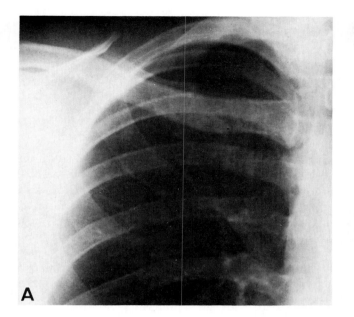

A

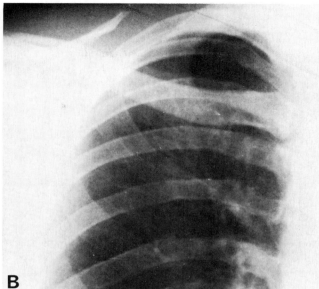

B

Figure 6.24. PA chest radiographs of the same patient using 120 kVp. **A.** Film on the left was made with Hi-Plus screens. **B.** Film on the right with Quanta III screens. A four-fold reduction in exposure was accomplished using Quanta III screens. However, there is now considerable quantum mottle. Notice the pronounced mottle in the film on the right giving the appearance of demineralized bone. An experienced radiologist will not, however, mistake that as such, since the mottle is present throughout the film, including the soft tissue regions.

eventually reaching the film granularity level. Alpha 8 screens, which are twice as fast as Alpha 4 screens, have a slightly higher low frequency noise. However, the high frequency noise is larger in the case of Alpha 4 screens because of their superior MTF.

The integral of the Wiener spectrum above the film granularity level is a measure of the total quantum mottle. Intuitively, one can expect that the quantum mottle will depend on the number of x-ray photons

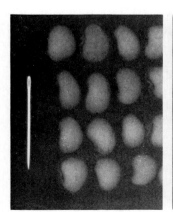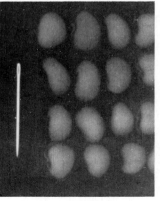

Figure 6.25. Radiographs illustrating the influence of system MTF on radiographic mottle. See text for explanation.

absorbed per unit area in the screens. This number in turn will depend on the system speed and the screen absorption factor. In general, faster systems will be noisier because they will require fewer x-ray quanta to yield a given density. The quantum mottle will also be proportional to the system's resolution since a sharper system will transmit input noise more faithfully to the film. More detailed considerations[17] show that the quantum mottle at a film density of 1.0 above base plus fog is proportional to $\left(\gamma N_e \sqrt{S/\varepsilon}\right)^2$ where ε is the screen absorption factor, N_e the equivalent passband, S the speed of the screen–film combination, and γ the slope of the H and D curve at the point of interest. Even though the quantity $\gamma N_e \sqrt{S/\varepsilon}$ is an accurate measure of the mottle that would be observed on a uniformly exposed film, in reality the quantity of significance is $N_e \sqrt{S/\varepsilon}$. This is because the signals in the radiologic image and the noise are equally influenced by the film gamma, and hence the signal/noise ratio is independent of it. This quantity is called the quantum mottle index (QMI). The small numbers in the body of Tables 6.1–6.5 represent calculated values of the QMI.

When film–screen systems are evaluated for quantum mottle, they are exposed uniformly to a density of 1.0 above base plus fog. However, the mottle at any given point in a clinical radiograph depends on the

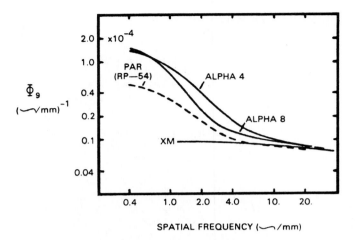

Figure 6.26. Measured Wiener spectra for Alpha 4 and Alpha 8 screens using XM film. (Courtesy of R F. Wagner[18] and Radiology).

exposure at that point. If the density is D, then the exposure, E, that resulted in that density is obtained from equation 4 and is given by

$$E = \frac{1}{S} 10^{\frac{D-1.0}{\gamma}} \qquad (18)$$

Taking this into consideration, it follows that the radiographic mottle at a density D, different from 1.0, at any given point of a patient radiograph is proportional to

$$\gamma N_e \sqrt{S/\varepsilon 10^{\frac{D-1.0}{\gamma}}} \qquad (19)$$

Noise and Magnification. Radiographic noise in itself is unaffected by magnification. However, since the image is larger than the object by a factor of m^2 in area, the size of the noise relative to the magnified object is reduced compared to the size of the same noise relative to the size of the original object under contact exposure. Also, spatial frequency in the object plane and that in the image plane are different by a factor of m. Taking these two considerations into account, Doi and Imhof[21] have shown that the effective Wiener spectrum $\phi_{eff}(f_x, f_y)$ and the true Wiener spectrum $\phi(f_x, f_y)$ are related to each other by the equation

$$\phi_{eff}(f_x, f_y) = (1/m^2)\phi(f_x/m, f_y/m) \qquad (24)$$

Thus the effect of radiographic magnification on the Wiener spectrum is twofold: (1) the Wiener spectral value decreases by a factor equal to the square of the magnification factor; and (2) the spatial frequency increases by a factor equal to the magnification factor.

In conclusion, radiographic image quality is a complex entity that depends on the image latitude and the density, contrast, resolution, and noise at the point of interest. All of these parameters interact with each other in a complex manner as outlined in this chapter.

CLINICAL APPLICATIONS

A radiographic study of good quality performed in the appropriate clinical setting forms the cornerstone of the art and practice of radiology. To obtain such a study requires the complex interaction of many variables discussed in this chapter and throughout the remainder of the text. The film or, more appropriately, the film-screen combination represents the final common path of these interactions and is a register of our understanding and application of the interplay of variables that ultimately produces a radiographic image. If our understanding is sufficient and our choice of applications wise, the result will be good; if not, it will be poor.

It is and should be the goal of all members of the radiologic team—physicist, radiographer, and radiologist—to produce the highest quality diagnostic image possible in any given set of circumstances. However, it is the special burden of the radiologist to see to and insist that a patient be given only the radiation exposure necessary to achieve his diagnostic conclusion. For the radiologist to do otherwise is to shirk his responsibility as a physician. Unfortunately, these objectives may seem to work at cross-purposes, eg, the obtaining of additional views to enhance diagnostic quality of a study. If they are obtained to increase diagnostic certainty or influence the therapeutic approach, the reason is laudable although the patient dose is higher. If they are obtained to make an unusual case more spectacular, such a reason should be deprecated.

It is beyond the purview of this chapter and text to enter into an in-depth discussion of the philosophy of good radiologic practice, but it is within the context of this chapter to bring into agreement the objectives of high-quality images and reduced patient exposure. This has been shown to be clearly achievable with modern film-screen technology—chiefly rare-earth screens and appropriate film combinations. The remainder of this chapter will be devoted to examples of clinical trials assessing the trade-off between diagnostic radiographic quality and reduced exposure.

ANGIOGRAPHY

The need and use of rare-earth phosphors has been most clearly indicated and widely adopted in angiography. This is because patient exposures are large,[25,26] the demand on tube and generator is high, and the time of exposure must be brief. Furthermore, the contrast between opacified vessel and surrounding tissue is high and, hence, a larger amount of mottle can be tolerated. Magnification is occasionally required, and the desired beam quality is in the 60 to 80 kVp range. All these factors favor the use of faster and more efficient rare-earth screens. Ovitt[27] et al have evaluated MTF, absorption efficiency, quantum mottle, and speed of rare-earth systems (Alpha 4 or Alpha 8 with XM film) versus fast $CaWO_4$ systems (Siemens SHS, Radelim STF, DuPont Hi-Plus, Lightning Plus, and Kyokko). MTF and quantum mottle were quite similar in all systems. The Alpha 8 screens were 10 kV faster throughout the 75 to 90 kVp range due to increased absorption efficiency.

Resolution with 1.37 magnification was also greater with the rare-earth system due to decreased mA requirements (from 700 mA to 100 mA), which allow the use of a 0.6-mm focal spot instead of a 1.0-mm focal spot. Our experience has been with Lanex regular (Kodak) screens and OG film (small and medium-sized patients) or OH film (large patients), with excellent results. These systems are two- and four-fold faster, respectively, than $CaWO_4$ screens of similar thickness. Quantum mottle is quite noticeable with OH film but acceptable due to decreased subject motion in large patients (Fig. 6.27.A, B, C).

UROGRAPHY

As with angiography, enhanced subject contrast makes the application of rare-earth intensifying screens to excretory urography both feasible and desirable. Stables et al[28] evaluated several rare-earth systems (Alpha 4/XD, Alpha 8/XD, Alpha 8/XM, Quanta 2/XRP-1) versus $CaWO_4$ (Par/XRP-1, Hi-Plus/XRP-1) for speed, detail, motion, mottle, and overall

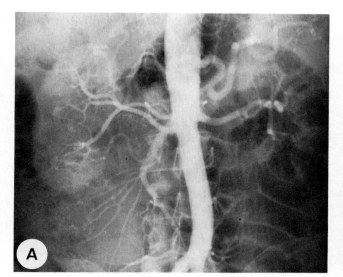

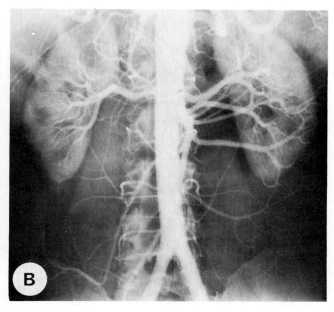

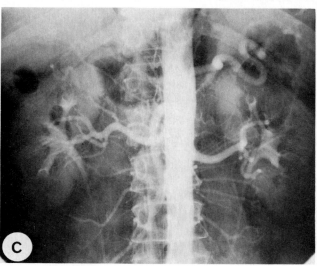

Figure 6.27. Routine aortography with various screen–film systems. **A.** Dupont Hi-Plus/RPO—800 mA 1/10 sec 78 kVp. **B.** Lanex Reg/OG—800 mA 1/20 sec 68 kVp. **C.** Lanex Reg/OH—600 mA 1/40 sec 63 kVp.

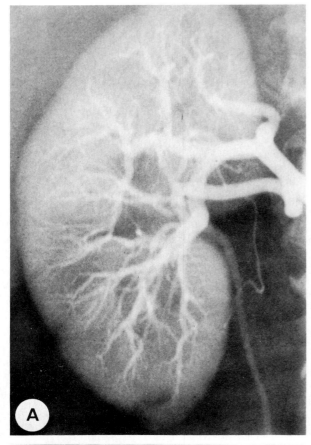

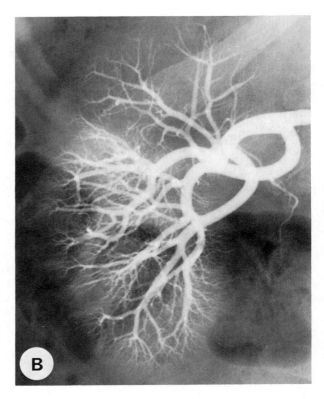

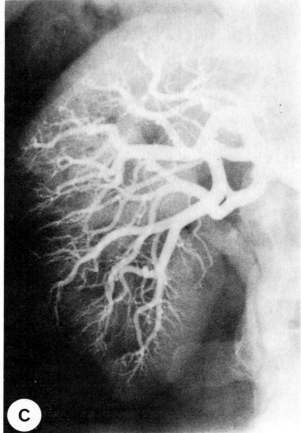

Figure 6.28. Magnification (2×) renal arteriography with various screen–film systems. Grid-biased tube with 0.25 mm focal spot is used. **A.** Dupont Hi-Plus/RPO—100 mA 3/20 sec 82 kVp. **B.** Lanex Reg/OG—100 mA 1/10 sec 75 kVp. **C.** Lanex Reg/OH—50 mA 1/10 sec 68 kVp.

quality. Speed was lowest (two- to twelve-fold) and detail greatest with the Par speed system, but motion unsharpness caused all rare-earth systems, with the exception of Alpha 8/XM, to be 1.67 to 1.83 times "better in overall quality" than the Par/XRP-1 system. The Alpha 8/XM system was not favored due to unacceptable mottle. Patient dose reduction was two- to five-fold. Similar results were obtained by Thornbury et al[29] comparing Lanex/OG with Hi-Plus/RPL with no significant difference in quantum mottle, "diagnostic certainty," or detail. Mean exposure was reduced to 50 percent with the Lanex/OG system. Our experience has been with the Lanex/OG system with 50 percent reduction in patient dose and no sacrifice in image quality (Figure 6.28.A, B, C).

CHOLANGIOGRAPHY

Reported applications of rare-earth systems to cholangiography are limited in the literature but considerations similar to those in urography apply. Large body thicknesses are involved and motion is an important consideration in the use of $CaWO_4$ screens. Since 60 to 80 kVp are generally used in the energy

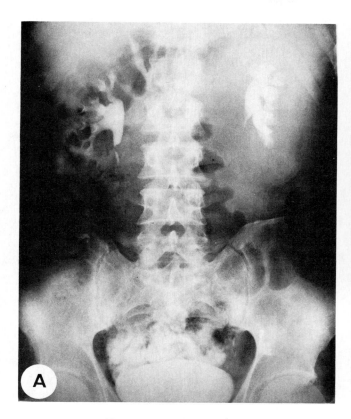
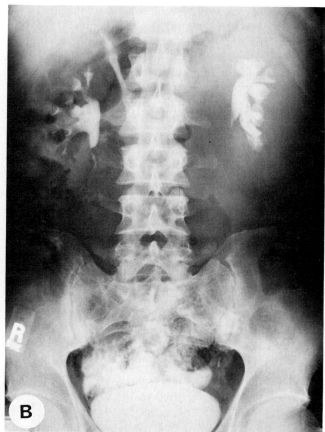

Figure 6.29. Urography with various screen–film systems. Same patient with Page kidney. **A**. Dupont Hi-Plus/Cronex—200 mA 2/10 sec 65 kVp. **B**. Lanex Reg/OG—200 mA 1/10 sec 65 kVp.

range where rare-earth screens have the optimal speed as shown in Figure 6.2, the use of rare-earth screens will significantly reduce motion. Imhof et al[30] compared Par/RP with Alpha 8/XM systems taking advantage of the improved image of rare-earth systems with 2× magnification. The overall MTF of the Alpha 8/XM system was slightly better and diagnostic accuracy was similar but favored the Alpha 8/XM system. Mean dosage was reduced from 390 mR to 190 mR.

SKELETAL RADIOLOGY

The uses of rare-earth phosphors in this area are somewhat circumscribed. In small part examinations, doses are usually small and fine detail is necessary. These factors favor Par or Hi-Plus screens. However, in examining the lumbosacral spine and pelvis, large part thickness leads to marked increase in exposure factors and therefore patient dose. This dosage increase is also applied to more radiosensitive organs—vertebral marrow and gonads. Also, the pathology sought is often less subtle. For these reasons, use has been made of the Lanex/OG system with beneficial results in decreased exposure and no noticeable sacrifice in quality. This is

especially applicable in scoliosis, with which children and adolescents would be subjected to repeat studies. Newlin[31] reports similar experience with lumbosacral spine work in a student health center where mAs and, therefore, patient dose were decreased 50 to 85 percent with improved film quality due to decreased motion unsharpness. Her experience also points out the effect film–screen combinations can have on major equipment purchases, eg, being able to maintain and use a 300 mA single phase generator, which would not be adequate with slower recording systems.

Fine detail work with the fast $CaWO_4$ screen is possible using 4× magnification.[32] Comparable results could probably be obtained with many rare-earth systems but this has not been documented.

PEDIATRICS–OBSTETRICS

Here the requirement for the lowest possible exposure dose is the overriding consideration since the radiation burden will be borne longer by this group than any other segment of the population. In the case of the fetus and neonate, large portions of the body are often included in a single study. From the standpoint of diagnostic quality, the single most important factor is motion unsharpness. These requirements are best met with fast film–screen systems. Wesenberg et al[34,35] have applied the Alpha 4/XD system to greater than 20,000 pediatric examinations from newborn chests and abdomens to outpatient GI examinations. They have accomplished an across the board 25 to 50 percent exposure reduction without sacrifice in quality compared to Par speed systems.

CHEST

Chest films taken "within the department" are in most instances performed in the range of 100 to 350 kVp. The radiation dose to the patient is small and the exposure time is brief; thus a wide variety of film–screen systems could be employed. However, optimum energy absorption is obtained using $CaWO_4$ phosphors rather than rare-earth phosphors (Fig. 6.2).

GASTROINTESTINAL STUDIES AND ABDOMINAL FILMS

Clinical studies reported in the literature are lacking in this area, with the exception of pediatrics,[33,34] in which case Alpha 4/XD performs well with a 50 percent dose reduction when compared to par speed systems. This speed and dose reduction would be comparable to that of a Hi-Plus/$CaWO_4$ system. Due to the high contrast differences between barium and soft tissue, rare-earth systems with speeds two to five times that of Hi-Plus should be applicable in a fashion similar to the urography studies reported above.

Plain abdominal films present a more difficult problem. Here the subject contrast is often low and, therefore, signal-to-noise ratios must be kept low; this in turn excludes very fast rare-earth systems. Favorable results should be obtainable with faster $CaWO_4$ systems (Hi-Plus) or slower rare-earth systems (Alpha 4/XD, Lanex/OG, Quanta II/Cronex 4).

PORTABLES

Due to the limited power of portable generators, exposure factors are limited and patient motion becomes the major cause of image degradation in portable examinations. Under these circumstances, even very fast systems (Lanex/OH, Alpha 4/XM or Alpha 8/XM, Quanta III/Cronex 7) with their inherent increased quantum mottle are probably superior to slower systems with larger exposure times. No records of clinical trials except in the pediatric age group are available in the literature.

MAMMOGRAPHY

Probably no area of radiology has generated more debate or public awareness of the risks of radiation exposure than this one. There have been major advances in dosage reduction in this area[35] with the evaluation of Min-R, Lo Dose II, Alpha 4, Rarex B and the monitoring of a high diagnostic reliability detecting microcalcifications >300 μ or low-density masses (nylon beads) to a size of 2 mm. None of the conventional techniques, however, will provide the soft-tissue details of xeroradiology (chapter 19). Since the major thrust of mammographic screening and evaluation is the detection of occult malignancy, xeroradiography is the method preferred by these authors. Exposure for xeroradiography would be $\sim$1 rad as compared to $\sim$0.2 rad for the film–screen combinations above.[36]

GENERAL CONSIDERATIONS

We have briefly surveyed the use and effectiveness of a variety of film–screen combinations keeping in mind two requirements: (a) high-quality radiography and (b) reduction in patient exposure. In most instances these requirements can be met using some combination of rare-earth intensifying screens and matched films of various speeds. The advantages and disadvantages of beginning with or converting to such systems are:

ADVANTAGES
1. Reduction in patient dose[31,33,34,37]
2. Reduction in personnel exposure by as much as 60 percent[37,38]
3. Increased tube life by approximately 50 percent[37]
4. Use of smaller generators due to reduced exposure factors[31]
5. Reduction in patient motion exposure with portable examinations improving quality and reducing the number of repeat examinations[37]
6. Reduced kVp with increased subject contrast
7. Reduced mA allowing small focal spot use and decreased geometric unsharpness

DISADVANTAGES
1. Increased quantum mottle
2. Increased cost (two to three times for rare-earth phosphors)
3. Conversion of safelight to accommodate green-sensitive film
4. Variation in speed of system with kVp
5. Possibility of mismatched films and screens, eg, departments using both $CaWO_4$ and rare-earth screens in the same darkrooms

REFERENCES

1. Rao GUV, Fatouros PP: Evaluation of a new x-ray film with reduced crossover. Medical Physics 6: 226–228, 1979
2. Sklensky AF, Buchanan RA, Maple TG, Bailey HN: IEEE Trans Nucl Sci NS 21: 685, 1974
3. Buchanan RA: IEEE Trans Nucl Sci NS 19: 81, 1972
4. Rao GUV, Beachley MC, Kan PT: Characteristics of screen–film systems for chest radiography. Proc of DHEW Symposium on Optimization of Chest Radiography, Madison, Wisconsin, 1979
5. Bates LM: Some physical factors affecting radiographic image quality: their theoretical basis and measurement. Public Health Service Publication No 999-RH-38, 1969
6. Rossi RP, Hende WR, Ahrens CR: An evaluation of rare-earth screen–film combinations. Radiology 121: 465, 1976
7. Rao GUV, Clark R, Gayler B: Radiographic magnification—a critical theoretical and practical analysis (Part 1). Appl Radiol 37–40, Jan–Feb 1973
8. Rao GUV, Clark R, Gayler B: Radiographic magnification—a critical theoretical and practical analysis (Part 2). Appl Radiol 25–33, Mar–Apr 1973
9. Rao GUV, The importance of focal-spot characteristics in clinical radiographs. Proc Soc Phot-Opt Instrumentation Engineers 47: 214–217, 1974
10. Rao GUV, Bates LM: The modulation transfer functions of x-ray focal spots. Physics in Med Biol 14: 93–106, 1969
11. Morgan RH, Bates LM, Rao GUV, Marinaro A: Frequency response characteristics of x-ray films and screens. Am J Roentgenol 92: 426, 1964
12. Rossmann K, Lubberts G, Cleare HM: Measurement of the line spread function of radiographic systems containing fluorescent screens. J Opt Soc Am 54: 187, 1965
13. Rao GUV, Jain VK: Gaussian and exponential approximations of the modulation transfer function. J Opt Soc Amer 57: 1159, 1967
14. Arnold BA, Eisenberg H, Biarngard BE: The LSF and MTF of rare-earth oxysulfide intensifying screens. Radiology 121: 473, 1976
15. Rao GUV, Fatouros PP: The relationship between resolution and speed of x-ray intensifying screens. Medical Physics 5: 205–208, 1978
16. Rao GUV, Fatouros PP, James AE: Physical characteristics of modern radiographic screen–film systems. Inv Radiol 13: 460–469, 1978
17. Rao GUV, Fatouros PP: Quantum fluctuations in radiographic screen–film systems. Med Physics 6: 118–122, 1979
18. Wagner RF, Weaver KE: Prospects for x-ray exposure reduction using rare-earth intensifying screens. Radiology 118: 183, 1975
19. Wagner RF: Fast Fourier digital quantum mottle analysis with application to rare-earth intensifying screen systems. Med Physics 4: 157, 1977
20. Doi K, Rossmann K: Measurements of optical and noise properties of film–screen systems in radiography. Proc Soc Phot-Opt Instrumentation Engineers 56: 45, 1975
21. Doi K, Imhof H: Noise reduction by radiographic magnification. Radiology 122: 479–487, 1977
22. Rao GUV: Do high detail screens always yield better resolution than high speed screens? Am J Roentgenol 112: 812–817, 1971
23. Doi K, Rossman K: Measurement of optical and noise properties of screen–film systems in radiographs. SPIE 56: 45, 1975
24. Rossman K: Effect of quantum mottle and modulation transfer on the measurement of radiographic image quality. In Mosley, Rust (eds), Diagnostic Radiologic Instrumentation. Springfield, Ill: Charles C Thomas, 1965, p 356
25. Seidlitz L, Margulis AR: Doses to the vertebral marrow during common x-ray examinations in clinical situations. Investigative Radiology 9: 419, 1974
26. Bengtsson G, Blomgren PG, Bergman K, Aberg L: Patient exposures and radiation risks in Swedish diagnostic radiology. Acta Radiol 17 (Fasc 2): 81, 1978
27. Ovitt TW, Moore R, Amplatz K: The evaluation of high-speed screen–film combinations in angiography. Radiology 114: 449, 1975
28. Stables DP, Rossi RP, Caruthers SB, Anderson N: The application of fast screen–film systems to excretory urography. Am J Roentgenol 128: 617, 1977
29. Thornbury JR, Fryback DG, Patterson FE, Chiavarini RL: Effect of screen–film combinations on diagnostic certainty: Hi-Plus/RPL versus Lanex/Ortho G in excretory urography. Am J Roentgenol 130: 83, 1978
30. Imhof H, Doi K: Application of radiographic magnification technique with an ultra-high-speed rare-earth screen–film system to oral cholecystography. Radiology 129: 173, 1978
31. Newlin N: Reduction in radiation exposure: the rare earth screen. Am J Roentgenol 130: 1195, 1978
32. Genant HK, Doi K, Mall JC: Optical versus radiographic magnification for fine-detail skeletal radiography. Invest Radiol 10: 160, 1975
33. Wesenberg RL, Rossi RP, Hilton SW, Blumhagen JD, Gilbert JM, Chionis ML: Low dose radiography in pediatric radiology. Am J Roentgenol 128 (6): 1066, 1977
34. Wesenberg RL, Rossi RP, Hendee WR: Radiation exposure in radiographic examinations of the newborn. Radiology 122: 499, 1977
35. Arnold BA, Webster EW, Kalisher L: Evaluation of mammographic screen–film systems. Radiology 129: 179, 1978
36. Chang CHJ, Sibala JL, Martin NL, Riley RC: Film mammography: new low radiation technology (work in progress). Radiology 121: 215, 1976
37. Campbell J: X-ray efficiencies achieved by linking changer to fast screen–film combination. Southern Hospitals, 1978
38. Eskridge M: Comparison of departmental radiation doses before and after use of rare-earth screens. Appl Radiol Nov–Dec 1970

CHAPTER 7

Fluoroscopic Imaging

MELVIN P. SIEDBAND

The production of an excellent fluoroscopic image requires that each of the subsystems of the fluoroscopic chain be understood and operated in optimal fashion. It is instructive therefore to evaluate each of these subsystem elements in detail and determine how they affect the overall system response. First the overall fluoroscopic chain will be reviewed and then the individual subsystem elements will be examined as they are found sequentially in the chain. These elements are the image intensifier, the optical coupling subsystem, the television subsystem, and the automatic brightness control. A few comments on fluoroscopic quality assurance programs will conclude the discussion.

As previously discussed in Chapter 5, x-rays are produced by bombarding a heavy-metal target with a beam of electrons. The x-rays are emitted with an essentially uniform intensity in all directions. That portion of the beam to be used is allowed to exit through a hole in the lead shielding surrounding the x-ray source. In practice, the tube is housed in a lead-lined aluminum case and an adjustable collimator or beam definer is used to determine the x-ray field size.

The x-ray beam is not homogenous; that is, it contains a broad distribution of x-ray energies. Since patients absorb the lower energy photons more readily than the higher energy photons, most of these lower energy photons will never exit from the patient and are therefore useless. It is possible to reduce patient exposure to the x-rays by adding aluminum filtration to the collimator and thereby attenuating the low-energy spectrum of the beam.

Three things happen to the x-ray photons that enter a patient. Some are absorbed totally through the photoelectric effect. Some are partially absorbed. In this case a portion of the initial energy of the photon is converted into electrons that are in turn absorbed, and the remaining energy is converted into a new x-ray photon known as scattered radiation (Compton absorption). Finally, some of the x-ray photons pass through the patient unimpeded.

The photons that exit from the patient pass through the table-top material and the grid to arrive at a scintil-lator, which is located in the x-ray image intensifier. In the scintillator, the x-rays may be absorbed by the photoelectric effect, produce scattered radiation by means of the Compton effect, or be transmitted unaltered. When electrons are produced by the photoelectric or by the Compton effect, they displace other electrons in the scintillator material. When these electrons are replaced, the scintillator produces visible light.

A photocathode is in intimate contact with the scintillator and produces free electrons when illuminated. These free electrons are then accelerated by means of the electric field within the image intensifier, and when they impinge upon the output phosphor, they produce a smaller but brighter light image. The small image at the output phosphor of the image intensifier can be lens- or fiberoptically coupled to a variety of devices. A mirror viewer will permit the radiologist to see the image directly. Alternatively, the image can be directed to a television camera for viewing on a television monitor or for recording on a video tape or video disc recorder. Electronic systems permit the manipulation of the televised image for image subtraction, edge enhancement, or other types of video processing (see Chapter 9). The image may also be lens-coupled to film cameras including various types of motion picture cameras. The output image may also be coupled to light-sensing devices, such as photomultiplier tubes, which provide the control signals to automatic brightness stabilization systems for maintaining the image constant during fluoroscopy or to automatic exposure controls needed when photographing the image of the output phosphor.

Other elements of the system are important for the production of a good image. If the x-ray tube focal-spot size is large, spatial resolution will be degraded, and it will be impossible to see fine structures. Degradation of object contrast (density resolution) is adversely affected by scattered radiation. Object contrast can be improved initially by choosing a proper kilovoltage so as to achieve a reasonable contrast for the object to be viewed. The use of a grid or airgap technique to reduce scattered radiation arriving at the scintillator will reduce the probability of scattered radiation reaching the image intensifier tube. Finally, minimizing the dimensions of the field of the x-ray beam by collimation prevents Compton scatter from other elements of the patient from creating spurious light photons from within the scintillator.

As the position of the patient within the beam changes, areas of greater or lesser beam attenuation may be interposed and the brightness of the image will also change. An automatic brightness control can be used to monitor the image brightness, which may be altered by changing the intensity of the x-ray beam by adjustment of beam current or tube voltage.

IMAGE INTENSIFIERS— THE REASON FOR THE TUBE

Early attempts at x-ray image intensification were based on optical coupling of the image on a fluoroscopic screen to a high-sensitivity television camera tube by means of an extremely fast lens. The first systems were modification of photofluoroscopic chest-filming devices. Figures 7.1 and 7.2 illustrate such systems. Later systems used an ingenious reflective-refractive optical system developed by Bouwers for coupling to optical image intensifiers and image orthicon or isocon television camera tubes. The drawback to lens-coupled systems is illustrated in Figure 7.3.

In this system, the lens that couples the scintillator to the camera tube may be thought of as an element on the surface of a sphere having its center on the scintillator. If the light is emitted equally in all directions, the lens will gather light in proportion to the ratio of the solid angle subtended by the lens to the total hemisphere.

It was originally thought that the low level of light passing through the lens could be increased by the use of light or optical image intensifiers. Such intensifiers were developed for night viewing of military targets. Unfortunately this approach is not feasible because the lens will not gather enough of the light produced by

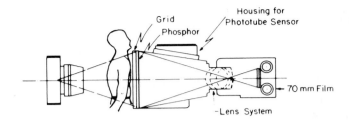

Figure 7.2. Photofluorographic system.

each x-ray scintillation to meet the statistical requirements of image formation. For example, an f/1.0 lens is able to couple 0.1 percent of the 500 or so light photons produced per x-ray scintillation to the film. The mean number of photos, u, collected is $(500)(0.001) = 0.5$. Using Poisson statistics the probability of collecting n photons is:

$$P_n = \frac{e^{-u}u^n}{n!} \tag{1}$$

The probability of collecting *no* photons is:

$$P_0 = e^{-0.5} \tag{2}$$

$$= 0.607 \tag{3}$$

The probability of collecting exactly one photon is:

$$P_1 = e^{-0.5}(0.5) \tag{4}$$

$$= 0.304 \tag{5}$$

And the probability of collecting two or more photons is:

$$P_{2+} = 1 - P_0 - P_1 \tag{6}$$

$$= 0.089 \tag{7}$$

These numbers mean that (1) about 60 percent of the available statistical information is not seen at all by the camera tube, and (2) about one-third of the information seen is of higher amplitude by at least a factor of two and dominates the noise statistics. Thus it is as if the detection efficiency was closer to the value of P_{2+}. For conventional screen-film cassettes, the P_0 is infinitesimal; the film is certain to receive some light photons from each scintillation. In the lens-coupled case of this example, the camera tube exposure would have to be increased by the factor of $1/0.089$ or at least 11 times over the conventional radiographic exposure for equivalent image noise. The reciprocal of P_{2+} is thus a measure of the minimum factor by which the radiation to a camera tube must be increased to match reasonably the scintillation or quantum noise of a conventional radiograph.

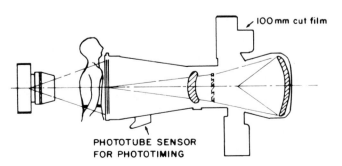

Figure 7.1. Photofluorographic system.

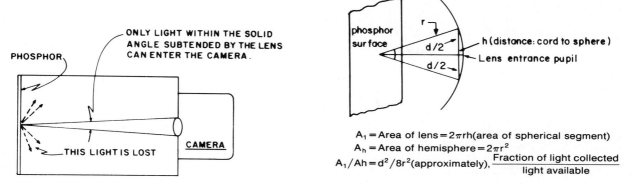

Figure 7.3. Lens-coupled screen.

A_1 = Area of lens = $2\pi rh$(area of spherical segment)
A_h = Area of hemisphere = $2\pi r^2$
$A_1/A_h = d^2/8r^2$(approximately), $\dfrac{\text{Fraction of light collected}}{\text{light available}}$

The first x-ray image intensifiers developed by Coltman avoided the optical coupling losses by placing the scintillator screen and a vacuum tube photocathode on the two surfaces of a thin film of glass. Figure 7.4 illustrates the construction of the earlier image intensifiers. Most of the x-rays penetrated the glass input window of the x-ray tube and were able to reach the phosphor layer. The phosphor, a scintillator of zinc cadmium sulfide, had to be thick enough to stop effectively the x-ray photons and convert them to light, yet thin enough to afford adequate resolution by minimizing the lateral scatter of light. The result was that only about 20 percent of the arriving x-ray photons were effective in producing visible light photons. The light from the scintillator would excite the photocathode to produce free electrons, which were then accelerated across the tube by means of the high voltage of the electron lenses, and a smaller and brighter image was formed at the output phosphor. The output phosphor was aluminized to prevent light feeding back from the output phosphor to the input photocathode. Because the photocathode was in intimate contact with input screen, more than half of the visible light photons were accepted by the photocathode, and about 20 percent of these were effective in producing photoelectrons. Thus,

for the average burst of visible light photons produced per accepted x-ray photon, about 50 photoelectrons are produced. Under such conditions, P_0 is infinitesimal. For all practical purposes, the quantum efficiency of the input screen is the quantum efficiency of the image intensifier tube, quite unlike the situation in the photofluorographic geometry (Fig. 7.4).

The first significant improvement in x-ray image intensifier tube design involved the incorporation of the rare-earth phosphors, oxysulfides of gadolinium and lanthanum, which made it possible to reduce the thickness of the input screen and have higher quantum efficiencies (Fig. 7.5). Such tubes had substantially improved resolving capabilities and effective quantum efficiencies as high as 40 percent. The newest tubes use scintillators of deposited cesium iodide, which has the interesting characteristics of forming needles or optical fibers such that an input phosphor can be quite thick with little lateral light transfer (Fig. 7.6). This means that quantum efficiencies greater than 60 percent can be achieved with high resolution.

The electron lens system of the earlier tubes permitted single mode operation; that is, the input phosphor image could be transferred to a specific area at the output phosphor. Improvements in design make it

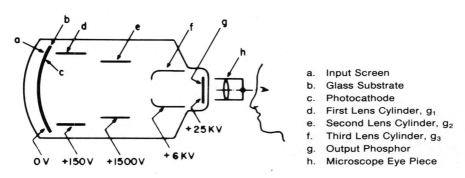

a.	Input Screen
b.	Glass Substrate
c.	Photocathode
d.	First Lens Cylinder, g_1
e.	Second Lens Cylinder, g_2
f.	Third Lens Cylinder, g_3
g.	Output Phosphor
h.	Microscope Eye Piece

Figure 7.4. Basic image intensifiers.

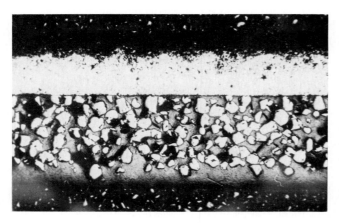

Figure 7.5. Powder screens—ZnCdS crystals; microscopic, cross-sectional view.

possible to change the voltages applied to the electron lens elements so that the output image size can be varied to magnify the image at the output screen. Such variable magnification schemes make it possible for the radiologist to adjust simultaneously the collimator shutters for a smaller field of view and the magnification of the image intensifier so that the image area always fills the fluoroscopic television monitor or a cine film frame. The output phosphors of the image intensifiers have also been modified in recent years: lateral light scatter in the output phosphor degrades image contrast. Lateral light scatter can occur through the phosphor itself or through multiple reflections in the output faceplate or glass window of the image intensifier tube. The use of optical absorbers in the glass and in the phosphor (dark screens) can substantially reduce this lateral light transfer.

It is also possible to manufacture the x-ray image intensifier tube with a fiberoptic input window. The x-ray scintillator is coated on the outside surface of the input window and the fiberoptic faceplate couples

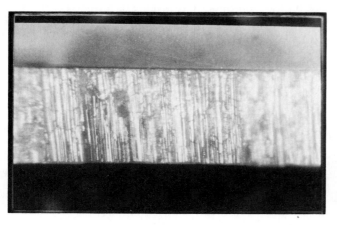

Figure 7.6. Powder screens—CsI crystal; microscopic, cross-sectional view.

the light to the photocathode. Fiberoptic tubes are usually used for small format imaging and hold promise for special procedures, microsurgery, or dental fluoroscopy. The input image diameters of such tubes range between 18 and 100 mm.

When image intensifier tubes are made in very large formats, above 250 mm input diameter, the glass window of the tube becomes prohibitively thick and results in excessive x-ray attenuation. Therefore, tubes in the 250 to 375 mm range are made with input windows of stretched titanium or other metal foils. The use of a very thin foil rather than a glass window results in less x-ray beam attenuation prior to interaction with the input phosphor.

CHARACTERISTICS OF THE X-RAY IMAGE INTENSIFIER

FORMAT

The mechanical characteristics of the tube, the dimensions of the input screen and of the output phosphor, and the optical characteristics are defined as the *format*. A standard 6-inch intensifier tube with a 0.5-inch output window can be defined as a 150/13, which means that the input image is 150 mm in diameter and the output image is 13 mm in diameter. Some tubes have magnification capabilities, that is, they can be operated in two modes, one in which the full input diameter of the image is mapped to the output phosphor, and the other a magnification mode in which only part of the input is mapped to the full output phosphor. Because very fast lenses are sensitive to the optical characteristics of the tube, especially the thickness of the glass window, they must be closely controlled and made part of the design of the optical coupling system. Image intensifier tubes are now being made with the output phosphor coating the inside of a fiberoptic output window. This permits direct coupling (without lenses) to a television camera tube having a fiberoptic input window.

GAIN

The total brightness gain of the image-intensifying tube consists of several components. The quantum gain or quantum detection efficiency, QDE, is the measure of the probability of capturing x-ray photons and converting them to light. The noise characteristics of the tube and the minimum patient exposure requirements are determined by the QDE of the input screen. The conversion efficiency of the input screen is a measure of the number of light photons produced per captured x-ray photon. The photocathode efficiency is a measure of the number of photoelectrons produced per incident light photon. The photoelectrons are accelerated across the electric field of the image intensifier, typically 25 kV, to strike the aluminized output phosphor, which converts the incident electrons to visible light photons. The energy conversion efficiency of the output phosphor is a measure of the number of visible light photons expressed in units of energy to the energy of the arriving electrons. The brightness gain of the tube is a measure of the visible light photons per unit area of output screen to visible light photons per unit area of the input screen. In order to compare one tube with another, the brightness of the output screen is compared to the brightness of a standard input reference (Patterson CB2 screen). The conversion factor is a measure of the output screen luminance to the exposure dose rate and is expressed in cd/m·mR·s, candles per square meter (brightness) per milliroentgen per second (radiation level). The intensification factor or brightness gain is the result of three principal elements: the quantum gain, the electron gain (which contains all of the conversion factors of the input screen, output screen, and electric field), and the minification gain (the ratio of the input screen area to the output screen area).

Once the brightness exceeds a certain value, approximately 2,000, additional brightness gain will not result in a significant improvement in image quality, the quantum gain being the more significant factor. Quantum gain or quantum detection efficiency can be measured by comparison with a single crystal detector of assumed unity gain. Such detectors are made of thick crystals of cesium iodide or sodium iodide closely coupled to a photomultiplier tube. A thick lead sheet with a small pinhole is placed in front of the large single crystal, which is exposed to x-rays. The signal-to-noise ratio at the output of the photomultiplier tube is measured. Next the x-ray image intensifier tube is substituted for the single crystal detector and the same photomultiplier tube used to measure the signal-to-noise ratio of the pinhole image at the output phosphor of the image intensifying tube. The quantum detection efficiency of the image intensifier tube is then:

$$QDE = \left[\frac{(S/N)\ tube}{(S/N)\ cell} \right]^2 \tag{8}$$

MODULATION TRANSFER

The modulation transfer function is a measure of the spatial frequency response of an optical device to a sinusoidal bar pattern. Since such bar patterns are hard to produce, two alternative techniques are used. One method measures the square wave response to a pattern of lead strips that vary in spatial frequency. For example, strips 5 mm wide with 5 mm space between them would have a spatial frequency of 0.1 line pair per mm.

Strips of 0.5 mm with 0.5 mm of space between them would have a square wave spatial frequency of 1 line pair per mm. Test objects are made with lead strips having square wave spatial frequencies ranging from 0.1 line pair per mm to 10 line pairs per mm. The test objects are placed in front of the x-ray image intensifier and the output amplitude versus frequency measured using a device consisting of a microscope lens, a slit, and a photomultiplier tube. The results are fed to a recorder. The recorded square wave function is then analyzed in terms of its sine wave components by means of a Fourier-series expansion. Analysis of Fourier-series expansions of square wave terms will yield an equation defining sine wave amplitudes in terms of the square wave amplitudes. In the following formula, $S(f)$ represents the amplitude of the sine wave at frequency f obtained by substituting measured values $M(f)$ of the square wave amplitudes at f, $3f$, $5f$, etc.

$$S(f) = \frac{4}{\pi} M(f) - \frac{M(3f)}{3} + \frac{M(5f)}{5} - \frac{M(7f)}{7} \dots \tag{9}$$

A second technique for obtaining the modulation transfer function is the line spread function. Here, a fine slit is used to expose the image intensifier to a single line of x-rays. The output image is scanned with a device similar to that described for measurement of the square wave response, and the line spread function is recorded. By integrating over the product of the line spread function and spatial frequency as shown in the following equation, the modulation transfer function may be obtained directly.

$$\text{Amplitude of MTF at } f = \frac{\int_{-\infty}^{\infty} A(x)\cos(2\pi f x)\, dx}{\int_{-\infty}^{\infty} A(x)\, dx} \tag{10}$$

$A(x)$ is the line spread function amplitude at distance x, and f represents the spatial frequency. Several integrations are performed to yield the amplitude term for each spatial frequency.

Each element of the image-intensifying tube contributes to the overall modulation transfer function. The thickness of the input screen, the characteristics of the electron lenses, and the characteristics of the output screen all contribute to the shape of the modulation transfer function. In general, the principal factor in the degradation of the MTF and image contrast lies in the light scatter in the input and output screens, which in turn is a function of screen thickness and lateral light attenuation. The limiting resolution of the tube is taken as that spatial frequency of the modulation transfer function where the amplitude of the signal has fallen to 5 percent. Because the overall performance of any imaging system will be the product of all the elemental MTFs and the contrast of the object being visualized, limiting resolution of the intensifier tube is not useful in describing performance. Noise content per unit bandwidth of any system is related to the square of the signal amplitude. When the frequency response is reasonably smooth, a noise equivalent frequency, N_e, is found by integration of the modulation transfer function $g(f)$.

$$N_e = \int_0^\infty [g(f)]^2 \, df \qquad (11)$$

where $g(f)$ is the amplitude response normalized to 1.0 at $f=0$. The N_e is a better term for defining system performance than limiting resolution, as its reciprocal is directly related to the dimensions of the smallest object visible in a practical system. In a practical system, limiting resolution will usually occur at the spatial frequency corresponding to about the 40 percent amplitude level of the tube. For that reason, an image intensifier tube having a modulation transfer function that maintains a high amplitude and then falls suddenly at the higher frequencies is much preferred over a tube that has a very high value of limiting resolution and a more modest value of low frequency contrast.

OPTICAL SYSTEMS

The simplest image-intensifier system would consist of the intensifying tube and a simple eyepiece for viewing the image at the output phosphor. This type of system, while offering superb optical properties, forces the radiologist to occupy a position that may be inconvenient given different patient positions. An improvement is a mirror viewer. In this system, a fast lens is used to collimate the image of the output phosphor. Collimation means that the object (the output phosphor) is placed in the focal plane of the lens so that the image is focused at infinity. The objective lens of the optical viewer forms the real image so that it appears to be the same size and distance from the observer as the patient's body part would appear. Field lenses serve to direct the light from the collimating lens to the observer's eyes. The mirrors, of course, direct the image, invert and position it for convenience.

Figure 7.7 illustrates a mirror viewing system. The image intensifier with the collimating lens assembly may be coupled to a television camera by means of an objective lens at the camera, as shown in Figure 7.8. The image size at the retina of the television camera tube will be the same as the output image of the image intensifier tube multiplied by the ratio of the focal lengths of the lenses. The objective lens of the television camera, since it is seeing a collimated light source, will be focused at infinity. The spacing between the two lenses is not critical, although if too great, there will be

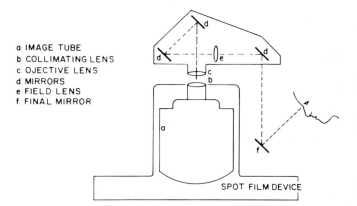

a. IMAGE TUBE
b. COLLIMATING LENS
c. OJECTIVE LENS
d. MIRRORS
e. FIELD LENS
f. FINAL MIRROR

SPOT FILM DEVICE

Figure 7.7. Mirror viewer.

some vignetting or loss of brightness at the outer edges of the image. A small lens with a mirror or prism can be used to focus the image of the output phosphor onto an aperture plate behind which is located a photomultiplier tube. By forming the image over an aperture plate, the hole in the plate can be made about one-half the size of the full image, so that as the radiologist uses the shutters to diminish the illuminated field size, the central portion of the image will be unaffected. In other words, adjustment of the shutters to less than one-half the image area will not affect the signal being received by the photomultiplier tube and thus will not affect the automatic brightness stabilization circuits.

In a collimated light system, it is possible, to interpose a partially silvered beam-splitting mirror so that 90 percent of the light is reflected and 10 percent of the light transmitted. A drive mechanism can position the mirror into the system when required so that most of the output light of the collimator can be fed to a film camera and a portion of the light fed to the television camera for monitoring during the procedure. Switches can change the output of the photomultiplier tube to stabilize the system for automatic timing of the exposures to the film cameras. Various configurations

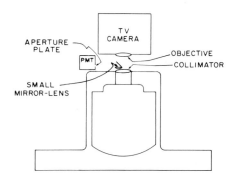

TV CAMERA

APERTURE PLATE

PMT

OBJECTIVE
COLLIMATOR

SMALL MIRROR-LENS

Figure 7.8. Simple TV coupled to intensifier.

incorporating partially silvered mirrors, optical cubes, and other schemes can be used to direct the light to different ports of two- or three-port systems for multiple applications of cineradiography, large format fluoro-spot-filming, and so forth (Fig. 7.9).

The collimating lens is very fast. Many lenses have speeds ranging from $f/0.68$ to $f/1.0$ to maximize the light coupled from the output phosphor to the rest of the system and to permit very large diameter collimating lens, which in turn permits separation between the collimating and objective lenses without vignetting. The spacing between the collimating lens and the faceplate of the intensifier tube is on the order of 1 mm or less, so that the thickness of the faceplate of the tube becomes a critical element in the design of the lens. Because expansion of the glass envelope of the intensifier tube and various mounting elements defocuses the lens, most systems have a mechanical arrangement for holding the collimating lens directly to the intensifier tube. Focusing adjustments of the collimating lens can be made only with special optical tools to prevent collision between the lens and the faceplate of the tube, which could result in destruction of the intensifier tube.

IMAGE NOISE

Fluoroscopic images are limited by both noise and spatial resolution. If we raise the sensitivity of the detector, the image amplifier–television combination, the fluoroscope will show a grainy, busy image; the effect called quantum mottle. The scintillations of the input phosphor responsible for producing this quantum mottle will tend to mask small differences of contrast in the fluoroscopic image. It is interesting to note that the number of photons per picture element required merely for a particular contrast difference to be seen is the same regardless of the size of that element. For objects of small size, contrast differences of less than ap-

proximately 5 percent are imperceptible. The number of photons per picture element, pixel, as a function of contrast can be approximated by the formula

$$N = \frac{50}{(C - 0.05)^2} \qquad (12)$$

where N is the number of photons, and C is the contrast. Objects of 100 percent contrast will require approximately 50 photons per picture element, while objects of 10 percent contrast require almost 20,000 photons per picture element.

At 80 kVp, 1 R of radiation flux will be equivalent to about 2×10^8 photons/mm^2. Thus the exposure required to produce a radiograph in the diagnostic range can be estimated:

$$R/_{\text{image}} = \frac{2 \times 10^{-7}}{(QDE)(RL)d^2(C - 0.05)^2} \qquad (13)$$

where QDE is the quantum detection efficiency, RL is the radiolucency of the patient, d is the diameter of the object of interest in mm, and C is the contrast. Table 7.1 shows some values of incident exposure estimated from this formula.

As long as the image-intensifying tube has adequate light gain, the quantum detection efficiency, element size, and contrast will determine the minimum radiation requirements for visualization. To illustrate a common mistake, examine the following: during cineradiography the lens of the motion picture camera is set to full aperture on the false assumption that this will permit a reduction of patient exposure. When this is done, the radiation level must be reduced to prevent overexposure of the film, but the film will appear very noisy or grainy and the object of interest will disappear into the noisy background. It is best to estimate the radiation requirements by the use of the formula and set the lens iris to achieve the level of film darkening appropriate for that particular film. To emphasize the point, the lens setting is determined by the sensitivity of the film and the radiation level determined by the requirements of the object of interest within the patient, its size, its contrast, and the quantum detection

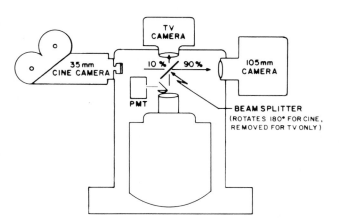

Figure 7.9. Three-port optical system.

TABLE 7.1. Relative Exposure per Image

Application	QDE	RL	d	C	Exposure
	(%)	(%)		(%)	
Chest film	15	3.0	0.7 mm	10	35 mR
Head film	10	1.0	0.5 mm	10	320 mR
Tomography	10	0.5	0.5 mm	3	1.8 R
Airport package	30	25.0	3.0 mm	50	1.5 μR

efficiency of the detector, with due allowance for grids, attenuation of table tops, and so forth.

A similar situation exists in conventional radiography: screens should be chosen as a function of the resolution requirements of the object size and the film chosen to have a sensitivity that will permit use of the appropriate radiation level. If, for example, a film of too high a sensitivity is used, the radiation level will be forced too low and objects of interest will disappear in the noise or graininess of the radiograph. Film of insufficient sensitivity will produce excellent images but at increased exposure levels to the patient. One of the fundamental reasons for the success of the rare-earth screens is that they have a higher QDE than the old-style calcium tungstate screens for the same thickness. It is the higher QDE vs thickness that results in the improvement. A number of years ago, one manufacturer offered rare-earth screens with higher sensitivity films and claimed an order of magnitude reduction of patient exposure. Unfortunately, the noise on the radiographs was excessive and the films were not acceptable to most radiologists. The same manufacturer now offers the improved screens with standard speed or even slightly slower films, and there is still a net gain in image quality with a more than two to one reduction of patient exposure.

There are many film-speed-enhancing chemicals and intensifiers for the salvaging of underexposed films. Obviously, it is a simple matter to reduce patient exposure by such underexposure–overdevelopment photographic techniques. Of course, the use of such methods will result in an increase in the noise and grain of the films, and objects of interest will disappear.

In image-intensification systems, instead of film sensitivity being varied, the iris of the objective lens is adjusted. Some camera tubes have an internal electrical means for controlling sensitivity. The iris of the objective lens to a Vidicon camera can be operated wide open and the electronic circuits will set the gain of the camera tube. On the other hand, fixed sensitivity tubes such as the Plumbicon or other lead oxide camera tubes must have the objective lens iris set to that value yielding a good compromise between tube sensitivity and image noise for best results.

Because the requirements for imaging vary as a function of the body part being examined, the lens adjustments are not fixed functions of the machine design but are determined by the user requirements. As most manufacturers have standardized installation techniques and tests to verify that the apparatus is functioning properly, it is up to the user to verify proper operation for each individual application. This can be achieved by taking test films of test objects (patient phantoms) or by examining patient films and then closing the lens one stop and doubling exposure per frame, and opening the lens one stop and halving

patient exposure per frame, followed by a critical examination of the films to determine which noise level and contrast appearance is best for a given application. When in doubt, it is best to open the lens more and reduce patient exposure to that point at which image noise just becomes objectionable. In this way, a good compromise between equipment loading, heat dissipation, and patient exposure may be achieved.

TELEVISION SCANNING

A television camera must convert the image on a surface to a signal that can be passed through a wire. It does this by moving the point of sensitivity across the input surface or retina of a camera tube until the entire surface of the image is scanned or swept out. In the case of most camera tubes, the scanning uses a beam of electrons to read the charge on the surface of a semiconductor, which varies in conductivity as a function of light. The basic problem pertaining to the spatial resolution of scanning is the need to have a sufficient number of scanning lines to count a given number of objects in the field. An image will have a surface of a given dimension and will have its information capacity defined in terms of spatial resolution expressed in line pairs per mm. Resolution is defined in line pairs per mm because objects and spaces between objects must be counted equally. One object and one space will be defined as one line pair in the direction of scanning. If we were to examine a copper mesh having ten holes per centimeter, or 100 holes per cm^2, the system must resolve one pair per mm and have two picture elements or pixels per mm to display each mesh hole and mesh wire. Separable, countable objects require at least one line pair or two pixels on each axis so that the space between objects as well as each object may be resolved. Figure 7.10 shows the image of a set of round objects to be scanned.

The first problem is to determine the number of scanning lines required. Obviously, one must direct a scanning line through each of the round objects. If the round object is white, the output signal is assumed to be positive. If the object is dark, the output signal is negative. For a succession of horizontal white objects with dark spaces between them, each object will produce a positive half-cycle and each space a negative half-cycle of the signal; thus each line pair or object will represent one whole cycle of the electrical signal pass band. To determine whether or not there is a space between vertical objects, it is necessary to have a scanning line for the spaces. Thus, for a row of N objects arranged vertically, there must be at least $2N$ scanning lines. However, when objects are vertically disposed randomly it is possible for the scanning lines to scan in such a way by grazing the tops and bottoms

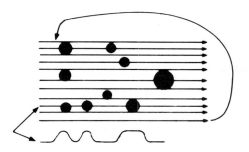

Figure 7.10. Scanning round objects.

of the objects that we still cannot determine whether there is a space between them. For this reason, the number of scanning lines is increased by the factor $\sqrt{2}$ so that for N objects arranged vertically, there will be $2N\sqrt{2}$ or 2.8 scanning lines per object. If there are a total of N^2 objects in the field, the system would have to have approximately $2N\sqrt{2}$ scanning lines to detect both the objects and the spaces between the objects and N cycles of pass band per scanning line, or a total image pass band of $2N^2\sqrt{2}$ cycles per image. The blanking time, the time when the scanning beam is turned off to allow the deflection circuits to reset the beam position back to the start of each line and to the upper lefthand corner of each frame, accounts for a factor of about 15 percent of the available time.

Alternatively, we can take a given television system and evaluate it for its total image passband. A standard 525-line United States television system will have approximately 480 scanning lines visible in the scene (since about 10 percent or 45 lines are used in the deflection circuitry). Dividing that number by $2\sqrt{2}$ means that about 180 countable objects can be resolved in the vertical direction. In order to have equal vertical and horizontal resolution, the $3:4$ aspect ratio (that is, the width is four-thirds the height of the image) would dictate that the horizontal resolution must correspond to about 240 countable objects. In order to reduce flicker and to make the image stationary with respect to 60-cycle power line magnetic field interference, each $1/30$ of a second picture frame consists of two fields, each $1/60$ of a second in time and consisting of $262\ 1/2$ interlaced scanning lines. Some stray magnetic fields due to nearby motors, fluorescent lights, or common power wiring, however, will continue to produce a stationary, slight distortion in the image. This is preferable to a slow, moving distortion through the image, which would occur without the interlaced fields. Because common television can resolve 180 objects vertically and 240 objects horizontally, if the television chain is presented the image of the output of a 15-cm x-ray image intensifier, imaging a piece of copper mesh, the system should be able to resolve 12 mesh holes per cm since this corresponds to the 180 mesh holes across

the field of view of the tube. It may see a slightly higher value of mesh if the mesh is turned so that the diagonal axis of the mesh is the vertical axis of the television system. This is the same as 30 mesh holes per inch at the face of a 6-inch image intensifier tube.

We define a space on the surface of the image of a linear dimension as equal to a half-cycle of bandwidth or as one pixel. We can define the pixel requirements as having the dimension of the smallest object we wish to resolve, in that image. This does not mean that if we have an object smaller than the pixel it will not be detected. It does mean that the contrast of an object smaller than the pixel dimension will be spread over the pixel dimension. For example, if a system has a pixel dimension of 0.5 mm, and we examine single pieces of copper wire of 0.1 mm, instead of appearing as high contrast objects of 0.1 mm, they will appear as lower contrast objects of 0.5 mm in dimension. The television system will be optimized for objects equal to or larger than one cycle of horizontal bandwidth. Smaller objects will lose contrast.

There are several ways of overcoming this difficulty. One approach would be to use a zoom lens between the television camera tube and the image intensifier. Unfortunately, zoom lenses have a great number of optical elements; the extra glass means that additional light scatter within the lens will degrade the image contrast.

Another approach would be to increase the number of scanning lines and the bandwidth of the system to improve resolution. One disadvantage of the use of nonstandard scanning systems is that accessory items such as television monitors, video tape recorders, and various amplifiers will have to be modified and become more expensive. However, the higher line rate systems have additional disadvantages; the greater number of scanning lines means that the information per original pixel size on the retina of the camera tube must be subdivided into a greater number of pieces according to the increased number of scanning lines, thus the signal level is diminished. As the signal level diminishes, the image information approaches the image noise or mottle in intensity. This can be more quantatively examined since the noise in electronic systems is defined by the following formulas for current noise (14) and thermal noise (15):

$$i_n = \sqrt{2ei\Delta f} \tag{14}$$

where i_n is the noise current, e is the charge of an electron (1.6×10^{-19} coulomb), f is the bandwidth, and i is the device operating current or peak signal current, and

$$e_n = \sqrt{4kT\Delta fR} \tag{15}$$

where e_n is the noise voltage, k is the Boltzmann

constant (1.38×10^{-23} JK^{-1}), T is the absolute temperature, and R is the load resistor or output impedance of the device. From these equations, it can be seen that increasing the system bandwidth increases the noise level of the system. Thus, tube operation at higher bandwidths means a diminished signal and increased noise, resulting in a degradation of the signal-to-noise ratio, an important measure of the performance of the camera system. In general, television camera systems are operated such that the sum of electrical noise introduced by the television chains of the two formulas is less than the quantum noise, the fundamental noise of fluoroscopic imaging. If the TV chain is operated at high bandwidths, the noise introduced can result in higher patient exposures. Most television camera tubes are designed for optimum performance slightly above the US standard of 525 lines per image. Only in exceptional situations is operation at the higher numbers of scanning lines—higher bandwidth—a reasonable and correct approach.

Another approach to improving image spatial resolution is the use of a zoom intensifier tube so that when the output image of the intensifier tube is in the large-field mode, the resolution in line pairs per mm measured at the face of the intensifier will be low, and when the image is magnified by operating the intensifier in the small-field mode, the resolution will be much higher. The radiologist surveys a 22-cm field of interest, and when an object of particular interest is sighted, the image can be magnified for more detailed evaluation. The collimator shutters are closed to the area of interest so that less scatter reaches the system. Therefore, contrast is improved, and since a smaller field of view is mapped to the surface of the camera tube, the resolution of objects within the patient is much improved.

TELEVISION SUBSYSTEMS

After the above review of the overall TV scanning systems, it is now instructive to examine each of the TV subsystem components in greater depth. The TV subsystem consists of a camera tube, the camera electronics, a monitor, and a recording or storage medium such as video tape or video discs.

TELEVISION CAMERA TUBES

TV camera tubes used for medical fluoroscopy will have a retina or active element of a very thin, light-sensitive material. In order to have maximum sensitivity, it is necessary that each element of the retina be active and sensitive to light at all times and not only at the instant of interrogation by the scanning electron

beam. The general principle of operation is that the scanning electron beam places a charge on the surface of the retina. Light-induced conductivity of the retina discharges surface electrons in proportion to the light striking that element. As the scanning electron beam sweeps by, it replaces the light-conducted charge, and a resistor in series with the retina reads the charging current. This signal is then fed to a series of amplifiers and eventually controls the beam of electrons used to illuminate the surface of the television display tube.

The principal difference between the common Vidicon camera tube, the Plumbicon and other types of lead oxide surface tubes, the Saticon, the Newvicon, and the silicon Vidicon are in the materials and construction of the retina, not in the basic operation of the tube itself. The construction of such tubes is shown in Figure 7.11. A hot cathode produces the scanning beam of electrons. G1 controls the beam of electrons, G2 accelerates the beam and defines the beam diameter, G3 produces an electric field required for keeping the beam in focus, and G4 controls the beam landing angle at the retina of front of the tube. Magnetic deflection coils positioned around G3 focus and deflect the beam in the scanning of the retina. The semiconductor materials used in the common Vidicon tubes change resistance as a function of illumination. The materials used in the lead oxide tubes, such as the Plumbicon or in certain other camera tubes, change in their ability to conduct a specific number of electrons as a function of illumination. This difference between resistance and conductivity is important since it means that the Vidicon types can be altered in sensitivity by changing the supply voltage to the retina, whereas the lead oxide tubes will have a fixed-gain. The surface of the Vidicon tube is analogous to a film having variable film speed from, say, ASA 10 to ASA 100,000 while the lead oxide and similar tunes have a fixed sensitivity of ASA 1,000. The camera circuits using the Vidicon tubes can contain a circuit for monitoring the picture level to develop an automatic gain control; AGC voltage sets the camera tube target voltage for varying light levels. The fixed-gain camera tubes cannot be used in

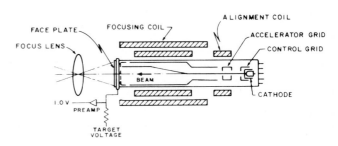

Figure 7.11. Camera tube construction.

this way, and instead such camera AGC circuits can control only the iris of the lens or the gain of the video amplifier for varying conditions of illumination.

The output signal level of a Vidicon camera and the fixed-gain camera tubes are shown in Figure 7.12. The measure of the change of the picture signal versus change of illumination is called gamma and is defined as:

$$\gamma = \log(i_s)/d\log(E) \tag{16}$$

The gamma of the fixed-gain tubes approaches 1.0, while that of the Vidicon tubes is closer to 0.7. This is analogous to the gamma or average gradient of photographic film, and is a measure of contrast. It means that the fixed-gain tubes such as the Plumbicon will produce a higher contrast picture but with a smaller dynamic range than the Vidicon. The Vidicon, however, has the advantage of operating over varying conditions of light intensity. The Vidicon can be used in fluoroscopy systems that do not have automatic brightness stabilization circuits because the dynamic range of the Vidicon camera is so great. On the other hand, the fixed-gain tubes require that the image brightness presented to the camera tube be maintained over a very narrow range. If this is done, the constant-gain tubes will present a picture of greater contrast.

Even though the image of the camera tube is read out at a rate of one complete image in 1/30 of a second (or alternatively, two interlaced fields at 1/60 of a second each), the picture-time constant of the camera tube is somewhat longer than this. For the common Vidicon, this time constant is on the order of 1/5 to 1/10 of a second. This means that if the camera lens were shuttered, the image would persist for about that length of time. When examining moving objects with the Vidicon, there will be two to four times more blur in the image than with the fixed-gain tubes. However, the longer time constant of the Vidicon means that there will be a time averaging of the scintillation noise so that the image will appear quieter. From the point of view of applications this means that Vidicon is better suited for the less complex systems used for viewing higher contrast objects, such as barium studies of the gastrointestinal tract, for example, and in situations where motion stopping is not required. It is also less expensive.

The fixed-gain tubes, such as the Plumbicon and the special target Vidicons, require the use of an automatic brightness stabilizer. The images will appear noisier, requiring the observer to use mental time averaging to see through the noise. These faster time constant tubes permit the use of video tape and disc recorders for frame-by-frame analysis of images. Such

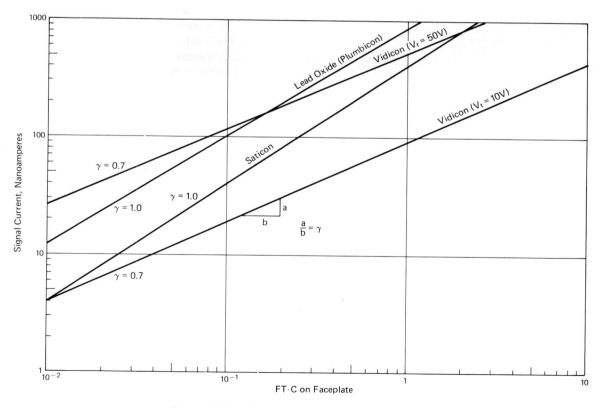

Figure 7.12. Output vs light for camera tubes.

tubes also work well when used as back-up viewers during cineradiology to ascertain whether the movie camera is recording the data. Such cameras and tubes are more expensive than the common Vidicon cameras but offer the advantages of higher contrast imaging and the ability to visualize subtler objects.

TELEVISION CAMERAS

Figure 7.13 shows a block diagram of a camera used for medical television. The small output signal at the viewing resistor is brought up to a standard level (usually about one volt) by the preamplifier. The frequency and phase response of the signal are adjusted to produce an equal emphasis of all spatial frequencies with the absence of streaking effects. Because the scanning beam is stopped at the edges of the picture, there is a tendency for a white line to appear at the edges; therefore, a video blanking circuit cuts off the signal just inside all four edges; The synchronizing generator starts with a master oscillator at twice the horizontal line frequency, divides this signal by two to produce the horizontal line frequency, and also divides the master oscillator by 525 to produce the vertical scanning frequency. This will produce a ratio of horizontal to vertical pulses of 262.5. Thus two interlaced fields will be produced per full frame and the vertical field rate will be the same as the power line frequency, 60 Hz. The vertical frequency is compared to the power line frequency to develop a signal that is fed back to control the master oscillator. In this way, the vertical scanning frequency is forced to be identical to the power line frequency. Therefore, power line interference, such as stray magnetic fields, will not produce an image or line crawl, which can be very distracting to the viewer who must scrutinize small areas of the image. Vertical and horizontal synchronizing signals are used to drive the deflection circuits and to produce synchronizing signals, which are mixed with the output video signal from the camera tube. The vertical and horizontal synchronizing signals are also used to turn off the electron beam during the time the beam is retracing.

The composite video contains a mixture of the amplified camera tube signal, the blanking signals, and the synchronizing signals. The monitor will extract the synchronizing signals, which are used to drive the monitor deflection circuits, and the video signals, which are used to drive the kinescope beam. In many cameras the synchronizing signals and the video signals are fed through a gate circuit, which is energized only during the time of the central portion of the image. In this way, the video signal level is compared to a reference to develop the AGC signal from the center area only. More elegant cameras generate circular blanking and beam control signals that permit a larger area of the retina to be used for imaging purposes.

Television cameras used for fluoroscopic imaging should have special modifications. For example, a conventional TV camera will see objects as they exist in nature, ranging from black to white. Because of the reduced contrast of fluoroscopic images, fluoroscopic cameras must have video-gain circuits of extended range and a means for setting the black level of the picture when the actual input is gray.

Another more serious problem, however, is related to the nature of the image itself. In an everyday scene, the light photons are independent of each other. In the output image of the x-ray tube, the light photons occur in bursts of about 10^5 per scintillation. If the camera circuit has been tuned excessively to compensate for losses of the high spatial frequencies resulting from low voltage operation of the Vidicon camera tubes, then the camera will emphasize the scintillation noise of the image and produce an excess noise or "waterfall" effect. High spatial frequency compensation of TV cameras is accomplished by tuning the amplifiers to improve the image along the direction of scanning. The

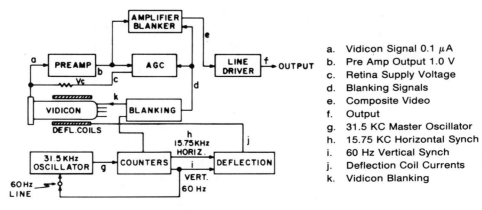

Figure 7.13. TV camera block diagram.

a. Vidicon Signal 0.1 μA
b. Pre Amp Output 1.0 V
c. Retina Supply Voltage
d. Blanking Signals
e. Composite Video
f. Output
g. 31.5 KC Master Oscillator
h. 15.75 KC Horizontal Synch
i. 60 Hz Vertical Synch
j. Deflection Coil Currents
k. Vidicon Blanking

medical TV camera should operate the camera tube at the higher allowed voltages to obtain the high spatial frequency enhancement in both direction with a reduced need for such amplifier tuning. The output phosphor thickness of the image intensifier tubes and the characteristics of the fast lenses can be partially compensated for by adjustment of the spatial frequency response of the medical television camera. The fluoroscopic image is intermittent during the examination, and the AGC circuits of the camera must be designed to accommodate this type of operation. Finally, the electrical environment of an x-ray room means that strong electrical and magnetic interference problems must be accommodated by the TV circuits.

TELEVISION MONITORS

The signal from the television camera is fed to the monitor through a coaxial cable having an impedance of 75 ohms. The camera has a source impedance of 75 ohms, and the cable must be terminated with a resistance of 75 ohms. If this is done, all of the energy transmitted by the camera will go to the end of the cable to be totally dissipated. If the end of the cable is terminated in other than 75 ohms, energy will be reflected toward the television camera and produce ghost images. Several monitors, video tape recorders, and other devices can be placed along the cable as long as the line terminates in a 75-ohm resistor. Branching of the line requires isolation amplifiers. The input to the isolation amplifier is an open circuit, which will not load the line, and the output is a 75-ohm source similar to that of the camera. The output of the isolation amplifier cable must also be terminated by a 75-ohm resistor. It is possible, by following some simple rules, to send camera video information over coaxial cable for distances of about 1,000 meters and, with special amplifiers, for distances of several miles.

The size, centering, and stability controls of the monitor have obvious functions. The two user controls are brightness and contrast. To permit optimum visualization of the image, the brightness of the screen should be set at a level just above that of the normal room light. It is important that the room not be totally darkened but set to a comfortable moderate level. If this is done, the observer's eyes will remain in cone vision rather than rod vision, and subtle details will be more discernible. The observer will not have to accommodate changes in brightness between observation of the patient and observation of the monitor.

The contrast should be set so that the darkest object in the scene is just below the black level on the monitor and the bright objects of interest do not completely saturate or white out such that details in image are lost. It is appropriate, when viewing objects of low contrast within the patient, to adjust the contrast and brightness controls to maximize the object's visibility even at the expense of increased noise.

Under conditions of moderate light, the human eye is capable of resolving one minute of arc. Thus, in order merely to resolve the 480 visible scan lines of a standard television monitor, the monitor should subtend an 8° solid angle. If the monitor subtends a larger angle, the observer will be able to resolve the lines but obtain no additional information. Since there are 2.8 scanning lines on the monitor for each vertical, countable object, there is no need to resolve the scanning lines to discern the objects. For reasonable distance accommodation, the monitor will most often be located between 4 and 5 feet from the observer and a 12- to 14-inch diagonal image monitor will be near optimum. If the monitor is to be closer to the observer, a smaller screen must be used; if farther, a larger screen. Since monitors are inexpensive compared to the rest of the fluoroscopic equipment, it is expedient to have additional monitors arranged for multiple viewing.

VIDEO RECORDERS

Video tape recorders for medical x-ray systems should have several characteristics beyond those of home video recorders. First, they must be capable of remote-control operation between standby and record. When installed, the video tape recorder can record automatically as the operator depresses the fluoroscopic control switch. Following or during an examination, a study can be re-examined without exposing the patient to x-rays. Second, the medical image is very noisy. For this reason, a medical-quality tape should be used. Some video tape recorders will allow slow motion or field-by-field observation of the image. When used with fast time constant cameras, the video tape recorder can monitor an injection sequence also recorded by a cineradiographic camera. The video tape can be reviewed immediately to determine whether the injection was adequate or if a repeat study in another projection is required.

Video disc recorders are used to record either single fields, single frames, or a short sequence (Fig. 7.14). Some video disc recorders have removable discs so that a sequence of images can be recorded and removed. One application of the video disc recorder is called "sticky" fluoroscopy. The machine records the last full frame of information during a fluoroscopic sequence and displays that frame when the fluoroscopic switch is released. During the procedure the radiologist presses the foot switch and real-time information is displayed; when he releases the foot switch, the last image freezes and remains on the screen when the x-rays are off. During an examination the radiologist can momentar-

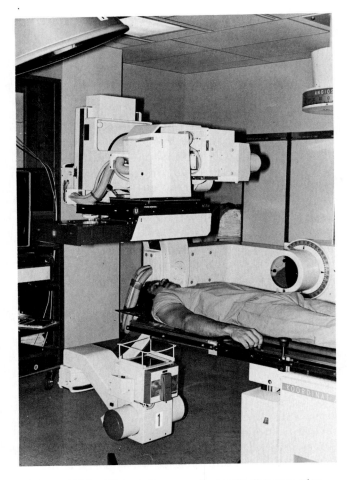

Figure 7.14. Biplane fluoro system with disc recorder.

ily remove his foot from the switch and then depress it to record a single frame of information. During an upper gastrointestinal examination, for example, an object of interest may be seen on the screen. The radiologist momentarily removes his foot, presses it down again, and then, when the x-rays are off, he can manually go back to the disc recorder and display that field or frame for closer scrutiny. At the end of a fluoroscopic sequence, the recorded information can be examined one image at a time, very much like a conventional slide show.

It is also possible to use recorded information on the disc or a specially recorded synchronizing track to lock the image of the television camera to the stored image on the disc. In this way a scout image can be recorded and subtracted from real-time images of the TV camera obtained during an injection. A video tape recorder can then record the difference images, which will have the same appearance as a sequence of subtraction films. When disc recorders are used with C-arm assemblies, one image can be recorded with the image intensifier vertical and the second image recorded and displayed with the assembly horizontal to produce image pairs, or as necessary for stereotaxic views. A biplane system can also be made to time-share one generator by using a disc recorder to store the image of the nonenergized plane.

New developments in electronic memory circuits for computers have led to digital image storage devices. Such devices can record one or two frames of information and take image differences or enhance the edges of displayed objects and, in general, perform many of the functions of the disc recorder. While limited to recording only a few frames, memory circuits have no moving parts and potentially can be produced at low cost.

AUTOMATIC BRIGHTNESS STABILIZATION

The automatic brightness stabilizer (ABS) is that part of the fluoroscopic control system that keeps the light output of the image intensifier constant over variations of patient attenuation and system geometry. Portions of the system may be shared with automatic exposure control systems, which maintain constant film density of cineradiographic or fluoroscopic spot films. A properly designed ABS must accomplish the following objectives:

1. It must hold the image brightness constant for variations of patient thickness and attenuation.
2. It must ignore information at the image margins, such as the bright flash around the patient's neck during an upper GI series.
3. It must operate to preserve image contrast and minimize image noise.
4. It must keep the operation within the ratings of the x-ray tube.
5. It must effect a reasonable compromise between patient exposure and image quality.
6. It must keep the patient exposure to within the Bureau of Radiological Health limits of 5 R/min except when an override mode of operation is selected by the operator.
7. It must respond fast enough to track during an examination but slowly enough to avoid hunting between bright and dark portions of the image.
8. It must compensate for system variables, such as the magnification at the image intensifier and the use of disc recorders.
9. It must be capable of being disabled or "held" at a particular equilibrium value prior to injection of contrast media.
10. It must be capable of being shut off to permit the manual control of factors.
11. It must display the operating factors and modes of operation to the radiologist.

BRIGHTNESS VARIATION WITH X-RAYS FACTORS

To a first approximation, the brightness of the image varies directly as mA and as the fifth power of kVp. Thus, as the kVp would vary from 80 to 88, a ten percent change, there would be a 50 percent change of brightness. Operation of the system at higher kVp will result in increased transmission of the beam by the patient so that less radiation is required. However, contrast degrades as kVp increases. Thus, one should operate at high values of kVp for reduced patient exposure and at low values of kVp for best image contrast. Clearly, a compromise is required. When viewing low contrast objects in fluoroscopy, the system should be operated at the lower kVp. This is particularly true when using iodine-based contrast media as in arteriography or in cholecystography. On the other hand, when examining the lower bowel, particularly when using barium-based contrast media, operation at high kVp is better; the images are of fairly high contrast and patient exposure is reduced.

Constant image brightness can be achieved by adjustment of either kVp or mA. Table 7.2 shows the results of an experiment using a pressed wood phantom of various thicknesses to yield cine exposures of constant density. For each image mAs per frame and system kVp were varied. For the 18 cm thick phantom, a value of brightness was obtained by operation at 120 kVp at 0.1 mA per frame; the same brightness was also obtained at 70 kVp at 0.9 mA per frame. Operation at the higher kVp would result in less than one-third the patient exposure per frame as operation at the lower kVp. The operator must be able to select operation at low, medium, and high kVp appropriate to the particular study.

BRIGHTNESS SENSING

Image brightness can be sensed several ways.

Image Intensifier Photocathode Current. The photocathode of the image intensifier is normally connected to ground and the final anode of the tube connected to a source of 25 to 30 kV. The ground connection can be removed and fed to a current amplifier so that the amplifier output is proportional to the radiation input to the intensifying tube. The disadvantage of this type of system is that photocathode current will be related to the average image brightness over the entire surface of the photocathode. When coning is limited to a small bright area, the average current will be related to the average image brightness over the entire surface of the photocathode. In this case, the average current could be the same as that

TABLE 7.2 Mesh Resolution of Image Systems

| | Field Size (Center/Edge) | | |
	9+ inch (22+ cm)	6–7 inch (15–17 cm)	~ 4 inch (~10 cm)
Image tube	40/35	50/40	60/50
TV monitor	24/20	30/24	40/35
16-mm film	35/30	40/35	50/40
35- to 105- mm film	40/35	50/40	60/50

produced by a dim image over the full field. It is possible to compensate for small-area imaging by the use of additional circuits to measure the settings of the shutters over the x-ray tube. However, bright flashes at the margins of the image would still be detected and cause an undesired response in the ABS circuits.

TV Camera Signal Sensing. Most TV cameras have automatic gain control (AGC) circuits for controlling the camera tube target voltage or the gain of video amplifiers in order to provide a constant output signal over variations of image brightness. The AGC signal can be used to control the generator as well. Electronic circuits in the TV camera can be used to select only the center portion of the image for operation of these sensing circuits so that marginal flashes will be ignored. One disadvantage of this type of system is that the camera tube is in the servo loop, thus variations of the camera tube sensitivity with temperature or variations between tubes at the time a camera tube is replaced will cause light-level sensing variations in the system. Gain control signals from such systems are not suitable for sharing between fluoroscopic ABS systems and exposure control systems for filming, such as fluoro-spot-filming of cineradiographic systems.

Lens-Coupled Photo Tube Sensing. This method uses a lens often combined with a prism or mirror so that the collimated light from the image intensifier is sampled and the image of the output phosphor is formed over an aperture plate in front of a photomultiplier tube. The hole size of the aperture plate in front of a photomultiplier tube is such that about one-half of the image diameter is used for the ABS circuit. This system can then compensate for coning effects, field-size changes, and mode changes of the image intensifier tube and will ignore bright flashes at the margin. The gain of the photomultiplier tube can be controlled by adjustment of its power supply voltage so that it may be shared between the fluoroscopic ABS circuits and the various filming systems.

Other Sensing Systems. Simple systems for measuring the overall light output of the output phosphor, for examining the video output of the television camera, or for sensing the signal received from an input-mounted ion chamber are also used in certain specialized systems.

TYPES OF BRIGHTNESS-STABILIZATION CIRCUITS

Operation of a fluoroscopic system with iodine-based contrast media must be between 60 and 80 kVp for best contrast. Operation of the system for best viewing using double contrast techniques in a lower GI series may force the system to stabilize somewhere near 110 kVp. The operator must have control of the system to force its operation into the required region. Brightness stabilizers can be classified in terms of the variable controlled by the brightness sensor.

Type 1. Variable mA, Preset kVp. In this system, the operator presets the kVp, and the brightness sensor controls the tube current over a range of about 20 to 1. Thus, the operator can set this system to the kVp required for the particular examination, and the brightness sensor will automatically adjust mA to yield an image of contrast brightness. However, a 20 to 1 range of mA may not be sufficient to cover the full range of patient thicknesses or the attenuation difference in panning from chest to belly. If a low kVp is selected, operation in a thick portion of an obese patient may force the mA to exceed the 5 R/min BRH limit, and the image will fade unless the operator adjusts the system for operation above the limit. Some of the earlier mA-only stabilizers operated over a range of 1 to 5 mA, and had an even smaller dynamic range. Another problem is that mA-only systems are limited by the time constant or cooling time of the x-ray tube filament. The time constant for a change of 50 percent brightness is on the order of 0.4 seconds. Some variable mA systems operate by adjustment of the on-time or duty cycle of the tube instead of adjustment of tube emission by variation of the tube filament temperature. For duty-cycle control, the tubes are grid-pulsed and average tube current is adjusted by the setting of the pulse width; for example, a tube having a peak current of 10 mA is pulsed on for 10 percent of the time (1 ms pulses, 9 ms apart) so that the average tube current is 1 mA. Adjustment of the pulse width has the effect of adjusting average mA without the disadvantage of the long time constant of the tube filament. With some x-ray tubes the focal spot has a tendency to grow at very low values of tube current. Pulsing of these tubes means that the focal spot can be preserved at the expense of circuit complexity.

Type 2. Variable mA with kVp Following. This system operates by varying the mA as a function of the brightness sensor, but it has an additional circuit that senses if an upper or lower bound of mA has been exceeded and then controls the adjustment of kVp through a motor-driven variable transformer. Thus, if the mA rises above a certain preset value, the motor will drive the kVp value higher. This will, of course, force the mA value down, and the system will be stabilized at a higher kVp. Similarly, if the mA falls below a certain value, the kVp drive motor will once again be energized and the kVp will be forced downward until the mA reaches a value within its operating range. Such systems have a kVp hysteresis since they perform differently as a function of whether the operating point is approached from above or below. The time constant of such systems is also slow since the filament time constant dictates the minimum response time of the kVp follower. If the kVp follower moves too swiftly, the filament control of the stabilizer will be unable to respond in time and the system will overshoot. They have the advantages, however, of being inexpensive to produce and having large dynamic ranges. Unfortunately, there is no way that such systems could be set optimally for all modes of operation, and they are best suited for simple systems used for single applications, such as GI examination.

Type 3. Variable kVp with Selectable mA. In this system, the brightness sensor controls the kVp of the system. The operator will have previously selected the value of mA required. If a motor-driven variable transformer is used to select kVp, the system has the additional advantage of remembering the last operating point as the operator energizes the system with the foot switch; thus restabilization of the system between scenes is very rapid. The operator can select a low mA, which will force the brightness stabilizer to operate at a higher kVp for GI examinations, or a high mA, which will force the kVp of the system downward for best contrast when viewing iodine-based contrast media.

Type 4. Variable kVp, Variable mA. In this system, the output of the brightness sensor controls both kVp and mA in order to maintain either constant image noise or constant image contrast. Unfortunately, such systems make it difficult for the operator to select the mode of operation best suited for the particular examination. Because the brightness stabilizer must operate by averaging the brightness of the image over the selected area, and because of limitations of motor speed, tube time constant, problems of flashing at the margins of the image, the characteristics of image panning, and so on, this brightness stabilizer is a compromise design. Automatic gain control circuits of the television camera can be used to cover local variations of image brightness and to prevent saturation of the image in the event of marginal flashes or saturation of the central image, as during the instant of injection of contrast media in a catherization procedure.

ABS PERFORMANCE REQUIREMENTS

Vidicon cameras have a broader dynamic range than the fixed-gain camera tubes, such as the Plumbicon or Newvicon; thus Vidicon cameras can tolerate overall scene brightness variation of as much as 10 to 1 without losing the image, whereas the fixed-gain tubes can operate only over a range of approximately four to one in brightness. Film cameras usually have a ± 1 stop latitude, which corresponds to a total brightness range of about four to one. However, a frame-by-frame analysis of low-contrast scenes on film dictates that a one-half stop variation or total excursion of two to one is all that can usually be tolerated. In other words, the brightness stabilizer design requirements for systems with Vidicon tubes are far less stringent than for systems with Plumbicon or similar tubes or with filming systems. An ideal brightness stabilizer would probably be the Type 3 and would have front panel controls visible and accessible to the operator that would permit one to select the value of mA, permit the system to override the BRH limits when required for obese patients, permit manual operation for exceptional situations, and permit hold operation so that the system could be held at a stabilized value just prior to injection of contrast media (Fig. 7.15). It would display actual kVp; the display of mA would be implicit in the selection switches at the front panel control and would be clustered with all of the other fluoroscopy and spot-film camera controls so that the operator could tell at a glance what the system would do when one pressed the foot switch.

TESTING FLUOROSCOPIC SYSTEMS

Once a fluoroscopic system has been purchased and installed, the complexity and number of adjustments make it inevitable that portions of the system will fail or fall out of adjustment. Slow changes of image quality will occur and reduce the probability of a correct diagnosis long before system failure is suspected. For that reason, routine tests of system performance must be conducted. Such tests must be simple, relatively nontechnical, understandable by the user, and noninvasive, that is, none of the panels needs to be removed or sensitive adjustments made by the user. If the tests detect substandard operation, then technically qualified servicemen can make the adjustment. The most common problems of fluoroscopic systems are the obvious mechanical ones, such as a defective mounting device or support. Such mechanical defects can be discovered by operation of the system followed by a physical inspection. Most of the other problems will

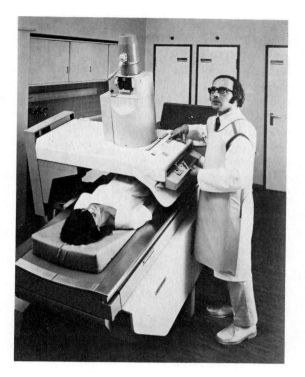

Figure 7.15. System fluoro control panel.

involve the intensifier or camera focus, or the generator will have drifted out of calibration, or the tube will have been abused in a cineradiographic run and no longer will have a small enough focal-spot size. To test the system for focus, a copper mesh tool can be used. This is placed in front of the image intensifier tube with a copper plate used as a beam attenuator placed at the table top or as close to the x-ray tube as possible. The x-ray system should be energized in the fluoroscopic mode and the collimator set to an inscribed square at the tube input field. If possible, the grids should be removed or slid back. Table 7.2 lists the mesh patterns in holes per inch that should be visible when the system is in proper focus. It is a good idea to incorporate small pieces of mesh in the construction of patient identification devices that are used for identifying the leader of cine films by radiographing the device when the room is being made ready to receive the patient.

A penetrameter may be used to evaluate the contrast performance of the system. One type of penetrameter consists of two aluminum plates, each about 17 cm × 17 cm × 2 cm, used with a third plate about 17 cm × 17 cm × 0.8 mm, with holes of 1.6-mm, 3.2-mm, 4.8-mm, and 6.4-mm diameters. The holes in the 0.8-mm plate represent a 2 percent change of thickness of the entire assembly, hence this device is called a 2 percent penetrameter. A simple test consists of placing the entire assembly on the table and operating between 80 and 100 kVp at about 1 mA and observing the image of a 10 cm × 10 cm square of the phantom.

All systems should display the two larger holes, better systems will display the three larger holes, and a superior system will display all of the holes. The image will be noisy so it will take some effort to see the holes. Operation of the brightness stabilizer may be checked by observing the density and apparent contrast of the image of the penetrameter with both heavy aluminum plates and with one aluminum plate without adjustment of the controls. The system should not saturate. Other routine tests by the x-ray technologist, as well as more sophisticated tests by qualified engineers and physicists, should be performed on a scheduled basis.

REFERENCES

1. Rose A: Vision—Human and Electronic. New York, Plenum Press, 1973
2. Coltman JW, Anderson AE: Noise limitations to resolving power in electronic imaging. Proc. of the IRE 48 (5): May 1960
3. Coltman JW: The scintillation limit in fluoroscopy. Scientific Paper No 1815, Westinghouse Research Laboratories, Pittsburgh, 1954
4. Dainty JC, Shaw R: Image Science. New York, Academic Press, 1974
5. Siedband MP: How the user may specify and measure the performance of image intensifier systems. Proceedings of the SPIE, 56: 1975
6. Schade OH Sr: Medical x-ray photo-optical system evaluation. Department of Health, Education and Welfare Publication (FDA) 76-8020, October 1975
7. Stober EV: Lock Your Eyes in Cone Vision. Machlett Laboratories 24 (3), Stamford, Conn., Cathode Press, September 1967
8. Siedband MP: Choosing and setting up TV systems for fluoroscopy. Proc SPIE 35: 1972
9. Gebauer A, Lissner J: Schott, Roentgen Television. New York, Grune and Stratton, 1974
10. Siedband MP: Automatic brightness stabilizers. Proc SPIE, Medicine III 47: 1974
11. Siedband MP: Limitations of exposure reduction during fluoroscopy by image storage. Proc SPIE 43: 1973
12. Siedband MP: Quality assurance measurements in diagnostic radiology. National Bureau of Standards, Special Publication 456, 1976

CHAPTER 8

Fluoroscopic Image Quality and Its Implications Regarding Equipment Selection and Use

GARY T. BARNES
JACK M. TISHLER

The configuration of a modern fluoroscopic imaging system (Fig. 8.1) consists of an undertable x-ray source assembly, an overtable image intensifier, and a viewing system. The image intensifier and viewing system are supported on the spot-film device. The function of the image intensifier is to convert the x-ray image emerging from the patient into a light image and then to amplify it. In a remote-controlled system the location of the source assembly and image intensifier are reversed. The control console in a remote system is usually located at some distance from the x-ray table. The primary advantage of such an arrangement is that the x-ray tube can also be used for conventional radiography after or during the fluoroscopic exam. The disadvantages of remote-controlled fluoroscopes are increased cost and complexity and high radiation levels in the vicinity of the x-ray table when the x-ray tube is energized. A remote-controlled unit requires closed-circuit TV viewing systems while the more common configuration of Figure 8.1 can employ either a TV or mirror system. The essential elements of both viewing systems are depicted in Figure 8.2. The mirror viewing system is simpler since it does not require a video chain and is, therefore, more reliable, and less expensive.

The objectives of this chapter are to review the various factors that affect fluoroscopic and spot-film image quality, analyze equipment parameters that affect these factors, discuss the choices and trade-offs that can be made in the selection and use of a fluoroscopic system, and finally discuss the type of choices that one might make for different clinical applications. These objectives will be accomplished by description of equipment function and performance from a conceptual point of view. The operational details of the various imaging system components and an explanation of how design parameters affect component performance will be discussed in the following chapter.

FACTORS AFFECTING FLUOROSCOPIC IMAGE QUALITY

BRIGHTNESS

The perception of anatomical detail in a fluoroscopic image depends on four basic factors: brightness, contrast, sharpness, and noise. That is, for a sufficiently bright fluoroscopic image, a border between anatomical regions is easier to see if their difference in illumination is great, abrupt, and not degraded by excessive noise. As illustrated in Figure 8.3 the luminance of a fluoroscopic image should be greater than 1 candela per square meter (cd/m^2) to achieve the satisfactory visual performance. The luminance depends on several factors: image intensifier exposure rate and conversion factor, the efficiency and f-number of the display optical coupling, the size of the displayed image, and, if viewed on a TV monitor, the sensitivity of the TV pickup tube and the amount of video amplification. Luminance can be expressed as

$$L = \dot{X} \cdot G_x \cdot \xi \cdot g / M^2 \tag{1}$$

where L, $\dot{X}$, G_x, ξ, and g are, respectively, the image luminance, input phosphor exposure rate, image intensifier conversion factor, optical coupling efficiency, and display light gain. M is the image magnification (or minification) that occurs in the optical coupling and video stages. For a mirror viewing system, g is set equal to one and M reduces to the magnification of the optical coupling stage.

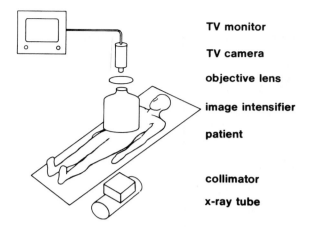

Figure 8.1. Components of a fluoroscopic imaging system.

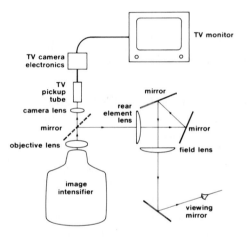

Figure 8.2. Components of mirror and TV viewing systems.

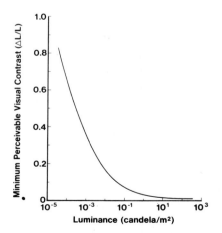

Figure 8.3. Plot of visual contrast threshold versus image background luminance. Based on the data of Blackwell, for an object subtending a $\sim 1/2°$ visual angle.[1] Similar curves have been obtained for visual acuity as a function of image luminance.[2]

The conversion factor is a measure of the light output of an image intensifier for a given radiation input and is usually expressed in units of candela per square meter divided by milliroentgens per second or $(cd/m^2)/(mR/sec)$. Its value depends on the radiolucency of the image intensifier's entrance window, the x-ray absorption efficiency of the input phosphor, the phosphor light conversion efficiency, the voltage between the photocathode and anode, and the minification gain.* The use of cesium iodide as an input phosphor was introduced in the early 1970s and resulted in increased absorption for a given phosphor coating thickness and increased phosphor light conversion efficiency.[3] More recently the perfection of cesium iodide columnar crystal growth technology[4] and increased entrance-window radiolucency along with improvements in photocathode and output phosphor efficiencies have resulted in even greater conversion factors without loss of resolution.[5] Typical values currently range from 100 to 200 $(cd/m^2)/(mR/sec)$ for nominal 6-in and 9-in diameter input phosphor intensifiers with a minification gain of ~ 120.[6] Smaller values result, due to decreased minification gain, when the magnification mode is employed on a dual (or triple) field intensifier.

Tandem (infinity conjugate) lens systems are currently employed to couple the image intensifier and TV pickup tube. Such lens systems allow parallel optical coupling of video and film cameras with independent control of the speed and magnification of each receiver channel. The efficiency of the lens system depends usually on the f-stop employed for the camera or receiver lens. As the f-stop of this lens is decreased (ie, the size of the lens aperture is increased) the amount of light getting through the lens system increases. An approximate expression for the efficiency of a lens optical coupling system (ratio of the number of light photons arriving at the image plane to the number emitted by the output phosphor) is

$$\xi \simeq M_o^2 \cdot T/(8 \cdot f^2) \tag{2}$$

where f refers to the f-number of the optical system, M_o is the optical magnification that occurs in the lens system, and T is the optical transmission of the lens elements. The simplifying assumptions underlying equation 2 are that the objective lens is larger than the image intensifier output phosphor and that there is little light lost due to vignetting. In well designed systems a large objective lens is necessary so that the receiver lens (TV or film camera) sees little or no vignetting.

*Specified conversion factors are generally measured with a 7-mm Al HVL beam quality and a 1 mR/sec input phosphor exposure rate.[7] In clinical use the value will vary due to differences in beam quality.

For a mirror viewing system, the optical and image magnification are the same ($M = M_o$), and equations 1 and 2 can be combined and reduced to

$$L \simeq \dot{X} \cdot G_x \cdot T/(8 \cdot f^2) \qquad (3)$$

where f now refers to the f-number of the field lens, which is usually around 1. Substituting in typical values of $\dot{X} = 0.05$ mR/sec, $G_x = 180$ (cd/m^2)/(mR/sec), and $T = 0.6$, one obtains a resultant image luminance of ~ 1 cd/m^2 for such a system. Referring to Figure 8.3 one can see that such a fluoroscopic image luminance is sufficient to achieve reasonable visual performance. The brightness obtained with a mirror viewing system can be increased either by increasing the exposure rate or by employing an image intensifier with a higher conversion factor.

A monitor luminance of ~ 50 cd/m^2 is typically obtained with a closed-circuit TV system.[8] Manufacturers set up such a system for a certain input phosphor exposure rate. The f-stop of the TV camera lens is then adjusted to match the light input with the sensitivity of the pickup tube and achieve the desired video signal. With this approach f-stops ranging from 4 to 8 are usually obtained, indicating a TV system light gain of $\sim 10^5$ for a typical fluoroscope ($X = 0.05$ mR/sec, $G_x = 180$ (cd/m^2)/(mR/sec), $M_0 = 1$, and $M = 10$). The large light gain and bright fluoroscopic image are two advantages of a TV display over a mirror viewing system.

CONTRAST

The visual contrast of an object imaged fluoroscopically depends on its luminance relative to that of its surroundings or, expressed alternatively, the fractional variation of luminance associated with the object, $\Delta L/L$. Fluoroscopic visual contrast depends on display contrast and subject contrast.[9] That is

$$\Delta L/L = \gamma_{dis} \cdot SC \qquad (4)$$

Display contrast, γ_{dis}, is a property of the display modality employed, and subject contrast, SC, depends on patient attenuation differences and the relative amount of scatter imaged. Subject contrast can be expressed mathematically as

$$SC = \Delta\mu \cdot t \cdot SDF \qquad (5)$$

where $\Delta\mu$, t, and SDF are, respectively, the difference in the effective linear attenuation coefficients of the object and the surrounding area, the thickness of the object, and the scatter degradation factor. $\Delta\mu \times t$ is the primary beam subject contrast, and the SDF is the fraction of the possible or primary beam subject con-

trast that is imaged due to scatter.[9,10] The scatter degradation factor is given by

$$SDF = 1/(1 + S/P) \qquad (6)$$

where S/P is the ratio of scattered-to-primary radiation.[10]

Equation 5 states that the subject contrast of an object is greater for thicker objects, for objects that have greater linear attenuation coefficient differences with their surroundings, and when less scatter is imaged. For a given object, $\Delta\mu$ decreases with increasing kVp and for the range of kVps routinely employed in fluoroscopy [60 to 120 kVp] $\Delta\mu$ for soft tissue/fat, bone/soft tissue, and barium/soft tissue decreases by respective factors of approximately two, three, and four.

The contrast-reducing effect of scattered x-rays, a well-known phenomenon in diagnostic radiology, is illustrated in Figure 8.4, in which the fraction of possible or primary beam contrast imaged is plotted versus S/P. In abdominal fluoroscopy the ratio of S/P emerging from the patient ranges from 2 to 7 depending on field size, patient thickness, and to a lesser extent on kVp. Typically, an 8/1, 41 line/cm grid is employed to suppress scatter. Its efficiency depends on kVp due to increased scatter penetration of the lead grid septa at higher kVp. The S/P ratio imaged with such a grid varies from approximately 0.3 to 1.4 depending again on field size, patient thickness, and kVp. In reference to equation 6 or Figure 8.4, this means that only from 40 to 75 percent of the possible or primary beam contrast is imaged in fluoroscopy. The contrast imaged with a remote-controlled unit is greater because the fixed source-to-image intensifier distance allows the use of higher ratio grids.

For a mirror viewing system γ_{dis} is determined by the image intensifier, while for a TV system it depends

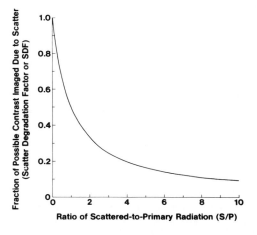

Figure 8.4. Plot of the scatter degradation factor versus ratio of scattered-to-primary radiation.

also on the camera tube and monitor setting; that is

$$\gamma_{dis} = \gamma_{int} \cdot \gamma_{cam} \cdot \gamma_{mon} \qquad (7)$$

where γ_{int}, γ_{cam}, and γ_{mon} are the contrast responses of the image intensifier, TV camera, and TV monitor, respectively. The degradation of contrast in an image intensifier is due to x-ray scatter produced in the glass entrance window, internal electron scatter, output phosphor substrate reflections, light reflections (scatter) occurring in the glass output window, and, to a lesser extent initially, internal light conduction. It is given by

$$\gamma_{int} = (R_c - 1)/R_c \qquad (8)$$

where R_c is the contrast ratio of the image intensifier.* Typically, values for γ_{int} range from 0.90 to 0.95 (ie, contrast ratios of from 10/1 to 20/1[6]). Recently introduced image intensifiers with metallic entrance windows (resulting in less scatter) and fiberoptic output windows (minimizing light reflections and flare) have slightly higher values. Also, it should be noted that this large area contrast loss depends to some extent on object size and is taken into account in determining the image intensifier's modulation transfer function (MTF).

The contrast response or gamma of a TV camera, γ_{cam}, is defined as the slope of its log signal versus log illumination plot. For a Vidicon tube camera a typical value is 0.7, while lead oxide Vidicon cameras have values closer to unity.[11] The contrast response of a TV monitor can be quite large (~ 10) and is non-linear. It depends in a complex manner on both the contrast and brightness control settings. The greatest contrast is achieved by turning up the contrast control to its highest setting and adjusting the brightness control until the undesired regions of the picture become black. The region of interest will then be displayed with the greatest possible visual contrast. In practice this results in too much contrast, and the settings are adjusted so that the full range of patient anatomical variations are displayed. However, for a given contrast setting optimal results are always obtained when the brightness control is adjusted so that the darkest parts of the picture are black. Increased image contrast is the major advantage of TV over mirror viewing systems. Other advantages are a brighter image, flexibility, unrestricted head movement and convenience (especially during catheterization), video recording capability, and the ability of more than one individual to view the fluoro-

scopic image. A mirror system, however, is simpler and is, therefore, more reliable and less expensive.

SHARPNESS

The fidelity with which patient attenuation differences are imaged is conveniently described by the imaging system's modulation transfer function (MTF). The system MTF specifies the fraction of object–subject contrast that is imaged for each spatial frequency component of an object's spectrum. This is illustrated in Figure 8.5, which shows that a greater fraction of a large object's (low spatial frequency) subject contrast is imaged than of a small object's (high spatial frequency). Resolution and sharpness are parameters that depend on the system MTF. The resolution of a system is the greatest number of line pairs/mm of a test pattern that can be resolved by the imaging system, and the sharpness of an image is the subjective impression of the distinctness or abruptness of a border. It is possible for a system to produce sharper images and have less resolution than another system. This is illustrated in Figure 8.6. System A will result in a sharper image with less resolution than an image obtained with system B. The reason for the distinction is that the eye is more sensitive to, and an object has more, lower spatial frequencies. This also is the reason why sharpness is a more important parameter than limiting resolution. That is, a system with the greatest resolution may not be the best system clinically, and it is often useful to compare system MTFs.

In fluoroscopy the system MTF depends on several factors: focal-spot size, object magnification, the image intensifier, the lens system, and the TV system. A useful property of the modulation transfer function is that the system MTF is, at each spatial frequency, the product of the component MTFs at that frequency, and for a fluoroscopic system one can write

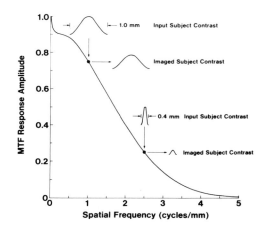

Figure 8.5. Effect of MTF on the imaged subject contrast of large and small objects.

---

*The contrast ratio of an image intensifier is defined as the luminance ratio in the center of the output phosphor without and with a centrally placed lead disk covering 10 percent of the input phosphor. It is generally measured with a 7-mm Al HVL beam quality and a 1 mR/sec input phosphor exposure rate.[6]

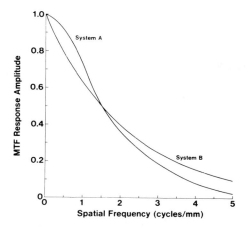

Figure 8.6. Effect of MTF on sharpness and resolution. System A has less resolution than system B, but results in a sharper image.

$$MTF_{sys} = MTF_{foc} \cdot MTF_{int} \cdot MTF_{len} \cdot MTF_{TV} \qquad (9)$$

where the subscripts sys, foc, int, len, and TV refer, respectively, to the system, focal spot, image intensifier, lens system, and TV system. Since by definition the value of the MTF at any spatial frequency is at most one and usually has a fractional value, the MTF_{sys} will always be equal to or less than the poorest component MTF at any spatial frequency. For certain exams and types of camera tubes, patient motion is important and it is necessary to include a motion component MTF in equation 9.

The component MTFs and system MTF are plotted in Figure 8.7 for a typical fluoroscopic geometry and imaging system. The image intensifier and TV are obviously the limiting component MTFs. The improvement or degradation in system MTF resulting when higher or lower line TV displays are employed is illustrated in Figure 8.8. The degradation resulting with the 525-line TV display is significant, while the system MTF incorporating the 1,023-line TV is only slightly better than that of the 875-line display. This slight improvement is usually not sufficient to offset the increased cost of the higher line TV display. The system MTF of a fluoroscope utilizing a mirror viewing system is not limited by the TV component MTF and, as illustrated in Figure 8.9, has a better MTF. It should be noted that it was assumed in Figures 8.7 to 8.8 that the horizontal TV MTF (i.e., the bandpass of the video amplifier) was matched to that of the line raster (vertical) MTF. In practice, the horizontal MTF often exceeds the vertical MTF for lower line video systems. Also, the image tube MTFs plotted in Figures 8.7 to 8.9 and in subsequent figures are for a state-of-the-art tube and, in the experience of the authors, usually exceed the performance of image intensifiers currently in clinical use.

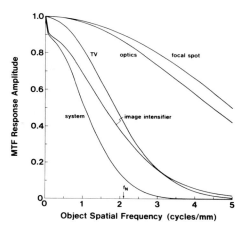

Figure 8.7. Component MTFs and system MTF of a typical fluoroscopic geometry (1.25× magnification) and imaging system (9-in image intensifier, 0.6-mm focal spot). The image intensifier MTF was experimentally measured,[12] and the optical MTF was based on experimentally measured resolution values for a tandem lens system.[13] The focal spot and TV MTFs were calculated in a standard manner.[14,15] A uniform square x-ray source of the dimension indicated was assumed for the focal spot, and a gaussian response for the TV was assumed with a 38 percent response at the line raster's Nyquist frequency, f_N.

Figure 8.10 indicates that the MTF for a TV fluoroscopic system is markedly improved when the image intensifier is operated on the magnification mode. This occurs because the TV is looking at a smaller area, and its MTF relative to objects in the image is improved; in addition, the image intensifier MTF is improved. The improved image intensifier MTF is illustrated in Figure 8.11 and occurs because, relative to the projected input phosphor dimension, the light diffusion occurring in the output phosphor is less in the magnification mode, and also because less degradation occurs in the elec-

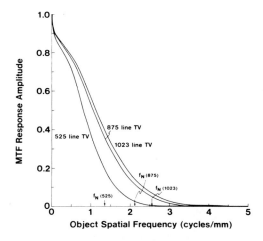

Figure 8.8. Effect of different line TV systems on fluoroscopic system MTF (9-in image intensifier, 0.6-mm focal spot, and 1.25× geometrical magnification).

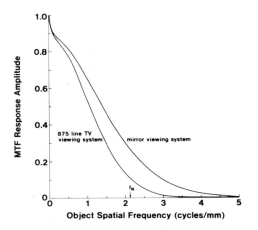

Figure 8.9. Comparison of TV and mirror viewing system MTFs (9-in image intensifier, 0.6-mm focal spot, and 1.25× geometrical magnification).

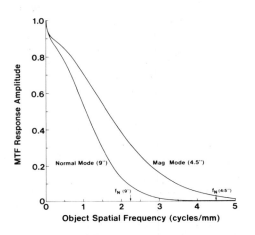

Figure 8.10. Comparison of fluoroscopic system MTFs when the image intensifier is operated in the normal and in the magnification mode (0.6-mm focal spot, 1.25× geometrical magnification and 875-line TV). The image intensifier MTFs were experimentally measured.[12]

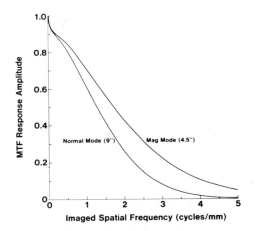

Figure 8.11. Comparison of normal and magnification mode image intensifier MTFs.[12]

tron optics.[16] As noted in the previous section, when an image intensifier is operated in the magnification mode, there is less minification gain. To achieve the same image brightness at the output phosphor, the automatic brightness control (ABC) must increase the exposure rate to the input phosphor by increasing either the kVp or mA or both. For example, when one switches to the 4.5-in mode on a 9-in image intensifier, the ABC increases the exposure rate to the input phosphor by a factor of four.

The relationship between object and image spatial frequency is illustrated in Figure 8.12. In a fluoroscopic imaging chain almost every stage either magnifies or minifies the image, and in general the component and system MTFs appropriately scaled and plotted as a function of either the displayed image or object spatial frequency. The latter convention is used in this chapter except when image receptors are compared.

By geometrically magnifying the object, the limitations of the image intensifier and TV become less important, and their responses increase as a function of object spatial frequency. These improvements have to be weighed against the decreased focal-spot MTF and also the increased patient exposure rate. System MTFs are shown in Figure 8.13 for different focal-spot sizes and geometrical magnification factors. The 2× magnification is the extreme that can occur for the conventional fluoroscopic configuration of Figure 8.1; the 1.25× factor is typical. If the 1.25× system MTF, incorporating a 0.3-mm focal spot was plotted in Fig-

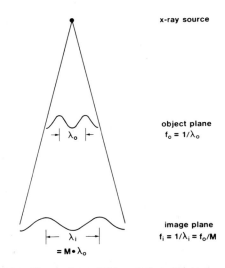

Figure 8.12. Illustration of the relationship between object and image spatial frequency. The projected or imaged wavelength, λ_i, is related to the object wavelength, λ_0, by the geometrical magnification factor, M (ie, $\lambda_i = M \cdot \lambda_0$). Since spatial frequency is the inverse of the wavelength dimension, the imaged spatial frequency, λ_i, is equal to the object spatial frequency, f_0, divided by the magnification factor (ie, $f_1 = f_0 / M$).

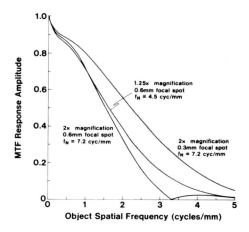

Figure 8.13. Effect of focal-spot size and geometrical magnification of fluoroscopic system MTF (image intensifier operated in the 4.5-in mag mode, 875-line TV).

ure 8.13, it would be slightly above the MTF of the 1.25×, 0.6-mm focal spot system. A gain in the system MTF of the 0.3-mm focal spot results when the magnification is increased from 1.25× to 2×; whereas, a degradation occurs with the 0.6-mm focal spot. The degradation is more pronounced with focal spots larger than 0.6 mm. In a remote-controlled geometry, due to the normally large source-to-object and source-to-image receptor distances, little geometrical magnification is possible and there is little advantage in employing a 0.3-mm focal spot.

NOISE

Noise in a fluoroscopic image is evidenced by continuously changing spatial fluctuations in image brightness. These visual contrast fluctuations in a modern fluoroscope are due mainly to quantum noise. In early TV fluoroscopic systems, appreciable noise was generated in the TV chain due to less efficient image intensifiers and poor video amplifiers.

In an intensifier tube the image energy carrier is changed several times. That is, in each stage the image consists of a pattern of discrete bundles of energy or quanta, namely, x-ray photons, light photons, electrons, and finally light photons again. However, compared to the initial stage the number of quanta comprising the image pattern in subsequent stages is large and the relative fluctuations introduced in these stages is small. The initial stage, which is the number of x-ray quanta absorbed per unit area per second in the phosphor layer, is known as the quantum bottleneck or quantum sink. It exhibits the greatest fluctuations and is the major source of quantum noise. Other factors that make the fluctuation level somewhat higher than one would anticipate from quantum fluctuations are phos-

phor light output variations due to the absorption of different x-ray photon energies and the escape of cesium and iodine K-characteristic x-rays from the phosphor.[17]

In their classic paper Sturm and Morgan established that the quantum sink in a conventional fluoroscopic system was the number of light photons absorbed in the retina of the eye.[18] This was also the case in early image-intensified systems that employed mirror viewing. However, due to the high conversion factors of modern image intensifiers this is no longer the case in current mirror systems. The quantum bottleneck is the same as that of a TV system—the number of x-ray photons absorbed in the input phosphor layer.

Visual contrast fluctuations due to quantum noise, $(\Delta L/L)_{noi}$, can be expressed as

$$(\Delta L/L)_{noi} = \gamma_{dis}/(\dot{n}_{neq} \cdot a_{eff} \cdot \tau_{eff})^{1/2} \tag{10}$$

where $\dot{n}_{neq}$ is the average noise equivalent number of x-ray quanta absorbed per unit area per second in the image intensifier phosphor layer, a_{eff} is effective area of the viewing aperture, τ_{eff} is the effective integrating time constant of the eye and display system, and γ_{dis} is as defined previously. This equation states that noise in a fluoroscopic system depends on display contrast and decreases when more x-rays per second are imaged (ie, when there is a greater input phosphor exposure rate), decreases with larger effective viewing apertures (ie, greater viewing distances or smaller display image sizes), and decreases for systems with more lag (ie, TV display systems with greater persistence). For a mirror viewing system γ_{dis} reduces to γ_{int}, and the τ_{eff} depends on the integrating time constant of the eye and, to a lesser extent, that of the image tube output phosphor.

Due to the additional factors mentioned previously the amplitude of the fluctuations in a fluoroscopic image will appear to be comprised of fewer quanta than is actually the case. This smaller number is known as the noise equivalent number of quanta[19] and is related to the absorbed or detected flux of x-ray quanta, $\dot{n}_{det}$, by

$$\dot{n}_{neq} = \xi_{neq} \cdot \dot{n}_{det} \tag{11}$$

where ξ_{neq} is defined as the noise equivalent efficiency of the phosphor. For a typical x-ray spectrum and cesium iodide (CsI) phosphor coating thickness (~200 μm), the value of ξ_{neq} is approximately 0.7.

The effective time constant of the display τ_{dis}, and eye τ_{eye}, is given to first order by

$$\tau_{eff} = (\tau_{eye}^2 + \tau_{dis}^2)^{1/2} \tag{12}$$

In a TV chain the display time constant depends mainly on the response of the camera pickup tube. For a Vidicon the time constant is comparable to that of the eye, ~0.1 to 0.2 sec, while for a Plumbicon, or lead oxide Vidicon, it is less. (Plumbicon is the Philips trade name for a lead oxide Vidicon.) This persistence of "stickiness" of a Vidicon TV chain has advantages and disadvantages. Compared to a lead oxide Vidicon system it results in an image comprised of more x-ray quanta and less noise. However, if the object being imaged moves suddenly, the system cannot respond and a blurred image results. Since this is not usually a problem in fluoroscopy, the lower noise Vidicon image is generally preferred. However, in cases when the video system is employed to record high-contrast dye studies in a rapidly moving object, such as in coronary angiography, a lead oxide Vidicon pickup tube is preferred.

For a given imaging system (and image intensifier magnification mode) the noise or visual contrast fluctuation level is determined by the input phosphor exposure rate. Recently an operator-controlled means of varying the input phosphor exposure rate and fluoroscopic noise level for a given image luminance has been developed.[20] This is accomplished by varying the efficiency (f-stop) of the lens system (see equation 1). The capability of varying the patient exposure rate (by a factor of three at a given kVp) also has been introduced recently by certain manufacturers by varying the video gain of the TV camera.

SIGNAL-TO-NOISE RATIO AND PATIENT EXPOSURE RATE

It has been established that the perception of low contrast objects in an x-ray image depends on their signal-to-noise ratio (SNR). The signal of an object is the product of its contrast as given by equation 4 and an MTF factor. As pointed out previously, for large objects the MTF factor is close to unity while for very small objects it is close to zero. The noise associated with an object is given by equation 10, but the effective imaged area of the object, A_{eff}, replaces a_{eff}. This implies that the smaller an object the greater the fluctuation level for equivalent areas in the object's vicinity. The SNR of an object imaged fluoroscopically can be increased by decreasing the kVp (and increasing the mA), employing a TV camera tube with more lag, reducing the amount of scatter, increasing the patient exposure rate, employing the image intensifier magnification mode and, with small focal spots, employing direct geometrical magnification. All of these methods except the use of a TV pickup tube with more lag result in an increase in patient exposure rate.

Following the reasoning in the preceding paragraph, the SNR and the relative probability of perceiving an imaged object in fluoroscopy is given by

$$SNR \sim SC \cdot (\text{MTF factor}) \cdot \left(\dot{n}_{neq} \cdot A_{eff} \cdot \tau_{eff} \right)^{1/2} \qquad (13)$$

Equation 13 indicates that for a given subject contrast and exposure rate (which determine $\dot{n}_{neq}$), the perceptibility of smaller objects is less for two reasons: a smaller fraction of its subject contrast is imaged (ie, the MTF factor) and fewer photons are utilized in imaging it (ie, the $\dot{n}_{neq} \cdot A_{eff} \cdot \tau_{eff}$ product). That is, in order for smaller objects to be perceived their subject contrast has to be greater than that of larger objects. How much greater depends on the system MTF. The contrast required for perception of large and small objects depends on the imaging system's ability to utilize the x-rays emerging from the patient and the amount of additional noise introduced in the process. A plot of the minimum subject contrast perceivable versus object size for a given exposure rate is known as a contrast-detail diagram. Such diagrams have been employed to determine experimentally the efficacy of different fluoroscopic imaging systems.[21]

FACTORS AFFECTING SPOT-FILM IMAGE QUALITY

CONTRAST

Detail perception in a radiographic or fluorographic spot film depends on the same factors, with the exception of brightness, as it does in fluoroscopy: contrast, sharpness, and mottle (noise). That is, a border between two densities is easier to see if the density difference is great, abrupt, and not degraded by excessive mottle. Large-area radiographic or fluorographic contrast is the difference in density, ΔD, between the object of interest and its surroundings. As in fluoroscopy it can be divided into display contrast and subject contrast,[9] or

$$\Delta D = SC \cdot (\gamma_{dis}/2.3) \qquad (14)$$

For film/screen spots γ_{dis} is equal to γ (film contrast) while for fluorographic spots it is equal to $\gamma_{int} \cdot \gamma$ where γ is the slope of the film's sensitometric curve between the densities of interest.

Equation 14 corresponds to equation 4 for fluoroscopic contrast, and all the general trends mentioned concerning fluoroscopic subject contrast (SC) can be carried over and applied to equation 14. One disadvantage of the 100-mm or 105-mm film employed for fluorography is that it has less film contrast than can be obtained with film/screen combinations. Typical average gradients* for film/screen image receptors range from 2.5 to 3.0 while for fluorographic film a value of 2.0 is typical. Also, there is a smaller selection

---

*The average slope of a film's sensitometric curve between net (above base plus fog) densities of 0.25 and 2.0.

of 100-mm or 105-mm fluorographic film available. Fluorographic spot filming, however, is more convenient, and less time elapses between pressing the exposure button and obtaining the film. That is, it is easier to capture on film what is seen during fluoroscopy with 100-mm or 105-mm fluorography than with conventional film–screen spots.

The grid employed during fluoroscopy also is employed frequently in spot filming. In certain high-contrast examinations, such as a full-column barium enema, films of diagnostic quality can be obtained for small field sizes (ie, four on one spots) without employing a grid. Shorter exposure times and reduced patient motion result. Often the decrease in patient motion associated with the shorter exposure time more than offsets the loss in contrast. Also, for certain low-contrast examinations, such as the gall bladder, improved spot films can be obtained for small field sizes without a grid by employing lower kVp techniques. For large field sizes it has been suggested for the conventional geometry of Figure 8.1 that a second linear grid with its strips positioned orthogonal to those of the fluoroscopic grid be incorporated during radiographic spot filming.[22] Such grid arrangements have been introduced recently by certain x-ray equipment manufacturers and allow the selection of a single linear grid for smaller patients and crossed grids for larger patients. The use of crossed grids results in substantial contrast improvement on larger patients. On smaller patients the improvement is less noticeable and is not usually sufficient to offset the increase in radiation exposure that results when the second grid is employed. Recently, novel and efficient scatter suppression techniques have been developed or suggested for radiography,[23-28] and one can anticipate that some of these methods will eventually be incorporated in fluoroscopic equipment.

SHARPNESS

The sharpness of a spot film depends on image receptor sharpness, focal spot size and geometry, and patient motion. Figure 8.14 compares the MTF of a relatively fast film–screen combination with fluorographic MTFs when the image intensifier is in the normal and in the magnification mode. This comparison indicates that the film–screen combination is slightly better than the fluorographic system with the state of the art image intensifier in the normal mode, while when the magnification mode is employed the fluorographic modality results in sharper images. However, this is not usually the case for fluorographic systems currently in the field and the authors have obtained superior results for static test objects with film-screen combinations. Patient motion is also an important consideration which is exam dependent.

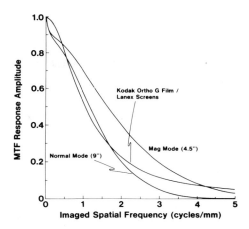

Figure 8.14. Comparison of fluorographic camera and film–screen combination MTFs. The fluorographic camera MTFs do not include the film MTF. For 100-mm or 105-mm film, neglect of this component makes little difference.

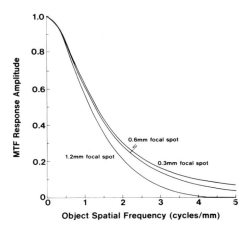

Figure 8.15. Effect of focal-spot size on radiographic system MTF (Kodak Ortho G film/Lanex screens, 1.25× magnification).

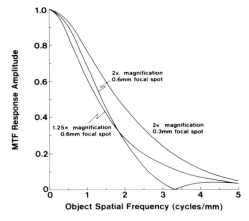

Figure 8.16. Effect of focal-spot size and magnification on radiographic system MTF (Kodak Ortho G film/Lanex screens).

When it is a problem the shorter exposure times of the normal mode fluorographic spots often result in diagnostically superior films. The effect of different size focal spots on system MTF is shown in Figure 8.15 for a typical spot radiographic geometry. The effect of $2\times$ magnification is compared for 0.3-mm and 0.6-mm focal spots in Figure 8.16. A 1.2-mm focal spot significantly degrades the spot radiographic system MTF, while, as in the fluoroscopic case discussed previously, $2\times$ magnification with a 0.3-mm focal spot results in an improved system MTF. Similar conclusions result if one analyzes the effect of focal spot size on fluorographic system MTF.

NOISE

The mottle in a radiographic or fluorographic image is the fluctuation in film density from one area to another. Film granularity and quantum mottle both contribute these fluctuations in the following manner

$$\sigma_D = \left(\sigma_G{}^2 + \sigma_Q{}^2 \right)^{1/2} \tag{15}$$

where σ_D is the standard deviation of the density fluctuations and σ_G and σ_Q are, respectively, the contributions from film granularity and quantum mottle.[29]

For many years it was believed that film granularity was a negligible contribution to the total density fluctuations. However, recent experimental evidence indicates it is responsible for 25 percent or more of the total.[30] The film granularity component can be expressed as

$$\sigma_G = \left(a_g / 2.3 \right) \cdot \left(n_g / a \right)^{1/2} \tag{16}$$

where a_g is the average developed grain area, n_g is the average number of grains per unit area at the density of interest, and a is the area of the scanning or viewing aperture. The important implication of equation 16 is that the smaller the viewing aperture, the greater the film granularity. That is, if an x-ray image is minified onto a film, as is done in fluorography, the greater the minification the greater the film granularity contribution to fluorographic mottle. The greatest image minification occurs in cine, in which film granularity can be the major factor contributing to fluorographic mottle.

The quantum noise contribution to the total noise in a spot film can be expressed as

$$\sigma_Q = \left(\gamma / 2.3 \right) / \left(n_{neq} \cdot a_{eff} \right)^{1/2} \tag{17}$$

where n_{neq} refers to the average number of noise equivalent quanta per unit area (as mentioned previously, a number somewhat smaller than the number of x-ray quanta absorbed per unit area in the phosphor) and γ

and a_{eff} are as defined previously. Equation 17 corresponds to equation 10 for quantum noise in a fluoroscopic image; a_{eff} is defined the same way in both equations and is somewhat larger than the viewing aperture, a, due to the unsharpness of the image receptor. Equation 17 indicates that the quantum mottle contribution to the total density fluctuations arises primarily from statistical fluctuations in the spatial distribution of absorbed x-ray photons and that its imaged appearance is modulated by the unsharpness of the image receptor and film contrast (γ). Also, the closer one views the image the smaller the effective viewing aperture, a_{eff}, and the greater the amount of quantum noise perceived.

SIGNAL-TO-NOISE RATIO AND PATIENT EXPOSURE

As in a fluoroscopic image the perception of low contrast objects in a spot film depends on their SNR. The signal of an imaged object is the product of its contrast ($\gamma \cdot SC / 2.3$) times an MTF factor. The noise associated with the image of the object is given by equations 15, 16, and 17, with A_{eff}, the effective (blurred) imaged object area, replacing a and a_{eff}. Making the appropriate substitutions in equation 15 one obtains

$$\sigma_D = \left(a_g^2 \cdot n_g + \gamma / n_{neq} \right)^{1/2} / \left(2.3 \cdot A_{eff}{}^{1/2} \right) \tag{18}$$

It was pointed out in the preceding section on spot film sharpness that employing direct geometrical magnification with a small focal spot improves the imaging system MTF and thus results in a larger signal. In addition, with greater geometrical magnification the imaged area and effective area of objects becomes larger, which, according to equation 18, implies less noise. That is, direct geometrical magnification with a small focal spot improves the detectability of objects by both improving their signal (if a small focal spot is employed) and reducing noise. This point is illustrated in Figure 8.17, which compares fluorographic spots of a test object taken at geometrical magnification factors of 1.0 and 2.0. The same arguments hold for fluoroscopic imaging, with which increased geometrical magnification also results in increased patient exposures.

Employment of the magnification mode when taking a fluorographic spot results in an improved MTF (Fig. 8.14) and reduced noise. The latter results because there is less image minification (less film granularity) and more x-ray photons are required to obtain the image (less quantum mottle). This can be seen by changing A_{eff} appropriately in equation 18 (a_g, n_g, and n_{neq} are the same in both the normal and magnification modes since it is assumed that the same film is used for

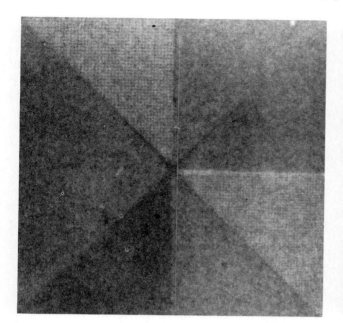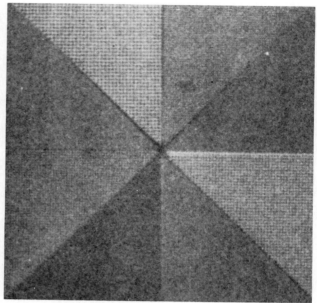

Figure 8.17. Comparison of contact (left) and 2× geometrically magnified (right) radiographs of a wire mesh test object. Kodak Ortho G film/Lanex screens, a nominal 0.3 mm focal spot, 2 mm added Cu filtration and 100 kVp (3φ) were employed for both radiographs. Photographic enlargement was employed on the contract radiograph to obtain the same image size on both prints. The geometrically magnified film has less mottle (noise). Sixty, seventy, eighty, and ninety wire mesh/inch are readily visible on the 2× radiograph compared to sixty and seventy wire mesh/inch on the contact radiograph. However, the radiation exposure of the test object in the magnified radiograph was four times that of the contact radiograph.

both). Normal and magnification mode fluorographic spots are compared in Figure 8.18. Here the superior SNR of the magnification mode is readily apparent. Accompanying this improvement, however, is a four-fold increase in exposure. Radiographic and fluorographic spot films are compared in Figure 8.19. The radiation exposure and exposure times were roughly equivalent for the two films, and the superior image quality (ie, greater SNR) of the radiographic spot film is due primarily to its better system MTF (Fig. 8.14). That is, the image tube employed to obtain Figs. 8.18–8.20 did not have the performance of the state of the art tubes plotted in Figs. 8.7–8.11 and 8.14.

In the preceding paragraphs a variety of ways to increase SNR and perceivable detail have been discussed. However, in many cases where spot films are taken the patient contrast is so great that little, if any, information is lost when the SNR of the image is reduced. This is illustrated in Figure 8.20, which compares normal and magnification mode fluorographic spot films. As pointed out above, the SNR (and patient exposure) of the magnification mode spot is substantially greater than that of the normal mode spot, yet the same amount of diagnostic information is contained in both films.

EQUIPMENT REQUIREMENTS AND CONCLUSIONS

The fluoroscopic unit selected by a radiologist will be influenced mainly by the type and imaging requirements of the examinations to be performed. The unit may be the conventional configuration of Figure 8.1 or remote controlled, depending on the preference of the operator. Examinations in which the table can be rather simple and fixed in the horizontal position are arthrography, enteroclysis, retained stone removal, and checking of the position of biopsy and diagnostic devices and tubes. Also, in peripheral, CNS, and cardiac angiographic procedures the table may remain fixed in the horizontal position. However, in these cases the table-top movement should be sufficient to allow the patient to be positioned after catheterization over the film changer or, in the case of cardiac angiography, the imaging system should have a cinefluorographic camera and be capable of angled views.

A motor-driven fluoroscopic table that can tilt 90° from the horizontal is generally adequate for conventional upper-GI and colon examinations, ERCP,*

---

*Endoscopic retrograde cholangiopancreatography.

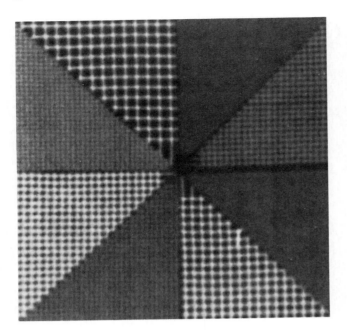 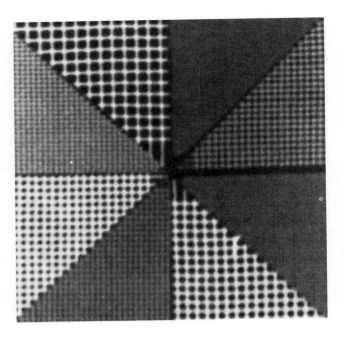

Figure 8.18. Comparison of normal or 9-inch (left) and magnification or 4.5-inch (right) mode 105 mm fluorographic spot films of a wire mesh test object. DuPont MRF-21 film, a nominal 0.6 mm focal spot, 1.25× magnification factor, 2 mm added Cu filtration, and 80 kVp (3φ) were employed for both films. Photographic enlargement was employed on the normal or 9-inch mode film to obtain the same image size on both prints. Compared to the normal mode film, the magnification mode images finer wire mesh, has noticeably less mottle, and requires four times the radiation exposure.

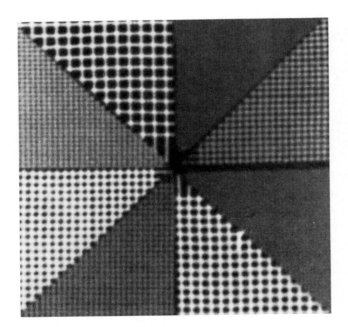 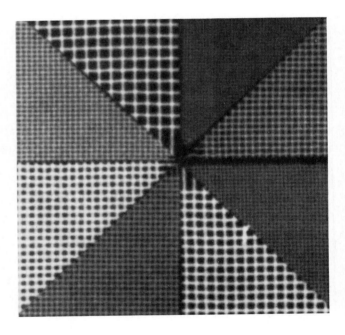

Figure 8.19. Comparison of fluorographic (left) and radiographic (right) spot films of a wire mesh test object. Both films were taken with 2 mm of added Cu filtration, 80 kVp (3φ), a nominal 0.6 mm focal spot size, 1.25× magnification, and the same field size. Essentially the same exposure time and radiation exposure were utilized for both. DuPont MRF-21 105 mm film was employed for the fluorographic film, and Kodak Ortho G film combined with Lanex screens were utilized to obtain the radiographic film.

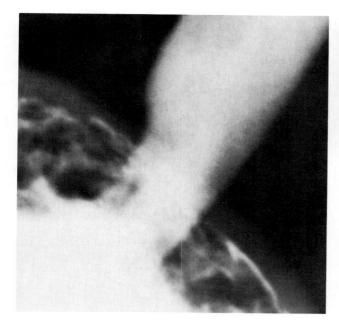
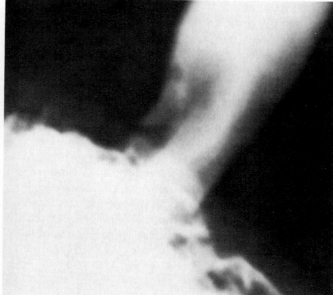

Figure 8.20. Comparison of normal or 9-inch (left) and magnification or 4.5-inch (right) mode 105 mm fluorographic spot films of the esophagogastric junction. Both spots were obtained with DuPont MRF-21 film, 100 kVp (3ϕ), a nominal 0.6 mm focal spot, and 200 mA. The respective exposure times were 25 msec (9-inch) and 104 msec (4.5-inch). Photographic enlargement was employed on the spot film taken in the normal (9-inch) mode to obtain the same image size in both prints.

T-tube cholangiography, gall bladder spot films, percutaneous cholangiography, positioning of tubes, and voiding cystourography. A table that can tilt 90° in one direction and 75° or 90° in the other is desirable for myelography, air contrast GI studies, and bronchography.

The capability for filming and fluoroscopically imaging fine detail is required for most angiographic procedures, air contrast GI examinations, arthrography, sialography, and ERCP. The capability of imaging fine detail is also desirable in cardiac and lung fluoroscopy. As shown in Figure 8.20, less detail is acceptable in some high-contrast studies. These include the full column barium enema and GI studies, myelography, cholecystography, voiding cystography, and fluoroscopic examinations to monitor tube placement and diaphragm movement.

The latter class of examinations can be accommodated by either a 6-in or 9-in single-field image intensifier (the larger field is preferred for obvious reasons), a 1.0 mm focal spot/12° target x-ray tube, and a conventional spot-film device utilizing fast or moderately fast rare-earth screens. Recently available large field (14-in and 16-in) image intensifiers[5] can also be employed for such examinations. They eliminate the need for overhead films, thereby increasing patient throughput and offsetting to some extent their greater cost. High-speed anode rotation is a desirable feature, and in GI and

ERCP exams, where patient motion can be a problem, it is essential. The image intensifier can be viewed with either a TV or mirror system, and if preferred, spot filming can be accomplished with a 100- or 105-mm camera. Such cameras use either roll film or cut film, with the latter being less wasteful.

For the fine detail class of exams, Figures 8.8 to 8.11 and 8.13 indicate that it is advisable to have a dual- or preferably triple-field image intensifier coupled with a 0.3-mm focal spot. The finest detail will be realized when the image intensifier is operated in 4.5-in magnification mode with 2× geometrical magnification. If the coupled image intensifier is viewed with a TV system, 875 lines are preferable. TV systems are more convenient than mirror-viewing systems and generally are considered essential for angiographic procedures.

High-quality radiographic films can be obtained by employing a relatively sharp, moderate speed rare-earth film–screen combination with 1.25× geometrical magnification and a 0.6-mm focal spot, or by employing a relatively fast rare-earth film–screen combination with 2× magnification and a 0.3-mm focal spot. High-quality fluorographic spot films can be obtained with a 100- or 105-mm camera and the image intensifier in the 4.5-in mode. If the patient area to be recorded is sufficiently small and motion is not a problem, fluorographic detail can be further increased by employing a

0.3-mm focal spot and greater (2×) geometrical magnification. High-speed anode rotation should be employed in both cases to reduce exposure time and patient motion.

A 50-kW three-phase generator (or 40-kW single-phase) is sufficient to handle the tube loading requirements for the focal spots discussed above. In a remote-controlled system, larger focal spots (typically a 0.6-mm/1.2-mm combination) and source-to-image receptor distances are employed and a 70-kW generator is more appropriate. As was noted previously, the large source-to-image receptor and source-to-object distances employed in remote systems limit the geometrical magnification and the capability of improving the system MTF and reducing the relative image noise that occurs with the use of a 0.3-mm focal spot and increased geometrical magnification.

REFERENCES

1. Blackwell HR: Contrast thresholds of the human eye. J Op Soc Am 36: 624–643, 1946
2. Chamberlain WE: Fluoroscopes and fluoroscopy. Radiology 38: 383–412, 1942
3. Fuchs H, Hofmann FW: An x-ray image intensifier with improved image quality—results of practical trials with the 70 mm camera. Electromedia 3: 94–97, 1971
4. Birken H, Bejczy CI: A new generation of x-ray image intensifiers—characteristics and results. Medicamundi 18: 120–127, 1973
5. Kuhl W, Schrijvers JE: A new 14 inch x-ray image intensifier tube. Medicamundi 22: 9–10, 1977
6. Morgan HT: Private communication, 1978
7. Methods of Evaluating Radiological Equipment and Materials. Washington DC, National Bureau of Standards Handbook 89, 1963, pp 3–7
8. Gebauer A, Lissner J, Schott O: Roentgen Television. New York, Grune and Stratton, 1967, p 3
9. Morgan RH: An analysis of the physical factors controlling the diagnostic quality of roentgenographic images. Part III, Contrast and the intensity distribution function of a roentgen image. Am J Roentgenol 55: 67–89, 1946
10. Barnes GT, Cleare HM, Brezovich IA: Improvement of contrast and/or reduction of patient exposure in diagnostic radiology by means of a scanning multiple slit assembly. In Carson PL, Hendee WR, Hunt DC (eds): Proceedings of the Ninth Midyear Symposium of the Health Physics Society. Denver, February 1967, pp 791–795
11. Gebauer A, Lissner J, Schott O: Roentgen Television. New York, Grune and Stratton, 1967, p 30
12. Scheid CC, Jensen GA: Private communication, 1979
13. Rich HE: Television in the Radiology Department. Milwaukee, General Electric Co, 1969, pp 29–30
14. Morgan RH: The frequency response function. A valuable means of expressing the information recording capacity of diagnostic x-ray systems. Am J Roentgenol 88: 175–186, 1962
15. Schade OH: Image Quality. A Comparison of Photographic and Television Systems. Princeton, RCA Laboratories, 1975, p 2
16. Kuhl W: Design considerations on x-ray image intensifier systems. Proc SPIE 56: 80–88, 1975
17. Swank RK: Absorption and noise in x-ray phosphors. J App Phys 44: 4199–4203, 1973
18. Sturm RE, Morgan RH: Screen intensification systems and their limitations. Am J Roentgenol 62: 617–634, 1949
19. Dainty JC, Shaw, R: Image Science. New York, Academic Press, 1974, pp 156–158
20. Rossi RP, Wesenberg RL, Hendee WR: A variable aperture fluoroscopic unit for reduced patient exposure. Radiology 129: 799–802, 1978
21. Webster EW, Wippfelder R: Contrast and detail perception in television and cine systems for medical fluoroscopy. J SMPTE 73: 617–624, 1964
22. Skucas J, Gorski J: New grid design for a fluoroscopic spot film device. Radiology 115: 732–733, 1975
23. Barnes GT, Brezovich IA, Witten DM: Scanning multiple slit assembly: a practical and efficient device to reduce scatter. Am J Roentgenol 129: 497–501, 1977
24. Brezovich IA, Barnes GT: A new type of grid. Med Phys 4: 451–453, 1977
25. Sorenson JA, Nelson JA, Niklason LT, Jacobsen SC: Rotating disc device for slit radiography of the chest. Radiology 134: 227–231, 1980
26. Rudin S: Fore-and-aft rotating wheel (RAW) device for improving radiographic contrast. Proc SPIE 173: 98–107, 1979
27. Barnes GT, Moreland RF, Yester MV, Witten DM: The scanning grid: A novel and effective Bucky movement. Radiology 135: 765–767, 1980
28. Korbuly D, Moore R, Formanek A, et al: Scanography with rotation of the radiographic tube: A new method. Radiology 135: 495–499, 1980
29. Rossmann K: Modulation transfer function of radiographic systems using fluorescent screens. J Opt Soc Am 52: 774–777, 1962
30. Holland RS: Fundamentals of radiographic noise. In Haus AG (ed): The Physics of Medical Imaging: Recording System Measurements and Techniques. New York, Am Inst of Physics, 1979, pp 152–171

CHAPTER 9

Digital Fluoroscopy

CHARLES A. MISTRETTA
ANDREW B. CRUMMY

GENERALIZED SUBTRACTION IMAGING

The success of computerized tomography has illustrated that in some imaging situations, contrast resolution is more important than spatial resolution. Among the major reasons for the increased contrast sensitivity provided by computerized tomography are the elimination of scatter and the quantitative treatment of the transmission data. Another important aspect, however, is the location of selected attenuation information. In the case of tomography, the information selected consists of the attenuation values in a particular plane. This selection of information can be considered to be a form of generalized subtraction imaging[1] in the sense that the subtraction of intensities at two closely spaced planes, transverse to a conventional radiograpic beam, would produce a differential image corresponding to the attenuation occurring in the slice between the two planes (Fig. 9.1). Since detectors may not be inserted into the patient, the isolation of attenuation information in the plane must be accomplished by nonsubtractive means, specifically by scanning in the plane and by using reconstruction algorithms. However, the net result is equivalent to the subtraction of intensities of the adjacent planes of Figure 9.1.

Since the transmitted x-ray intensity depends on x-ray energy E and time t, as well as the spatial variables, it is reasonable to hope that subtraction processes involving the time and energy variables might, by isolating a subset of relevant transmission information, provide a high degree of image contrast sensitivity.

The advantages of time-substraction angiography, in which a preinjection film is subtracted from postinjection films, are well known. However, the superposition of several pairs of films is tedious and impractical for generating displays with frame rates approaching those used in fluoroscopy. Furthermore, once the information of interest has been isolated, there is no convenient means of increasing its contrast by large factors.

COMPUTERIZED FLUOROSCOPY

Through digital electronic technology, analogous to that used in computerized tomography, several time and energy subtraction algorithms have been developed. Apparatus for this purpose (Fig. 9.2) consists of a conventional image-intensified fluoroscope, a digital image processor, a control computer, and a means for storing a sequence of subtraction images, such as a tape, disc, or kinescope recording.[2] The digital processor contains dedicated circuitry, which permits image processing at rates much higher than those allowed by standard computers. This is essential for algorithms involving dynamic subtraction displays at rates up to 60 images per second. The computer is used to preset the digital circuitry, which actually performs the chosen algorithm and generally does not operate on image information except in non-real-time postprocessing of information stored on the tape or disc.

Because the data to be processed is provided by conventional image-intensified fluoroscopic equipment and, admittedly, because the name implies that advantages as important as those achieved in computerized tomography might be achieved, this apparatus configuration has been referred to as computerized fluoroscopy. The potential remains to be determined. However, feasibility studies with animals and humans

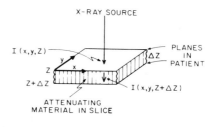

Figure 9.1. Tomography represented conceptually as a subtraction of intensity information at two nearby planes in the patient.

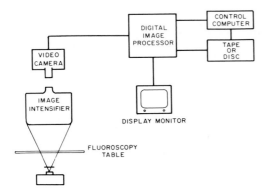

Figure 9.2. Basic apparatus for computerized fluoroscopy.

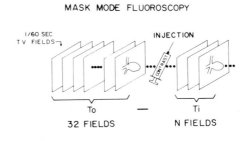

Figure 9.3. Basic elements of mask mode fluoroscopy. Preinjection information may also be integrated for 0.5 seconds. Postinjection information may also be integrated before subtraction.

have been done, and clinical evaluation is just beginning.

Although we will continue to refer to the overall approach as computerized fluoroscopy, it should be realized that several algorithms are possible, some of which occur on a time scale that would be more appropriately called computerized radiography. Most of the algorithms involve subtraction, either of images occurring at different times, or associated with different x-ray beam energies. The common characteristic of most of them is that they provide, relative to conventional fluoroscopy, an 8- to 16-fold increase in the amplitude of signals displayed from low-contrast objects.

IMAGING MODES

The primary application of the time-dependent subtraction algorithms developed thus far has been in intravenous angiography using peripherally injected iodine in boluses of 0.1 to 1 cc/kg of body mass. Several of these algorithms are illustrated below.

MASK MODE FLUOROSCOPY

This procedure is analogous to film subtraction angiography but differs in several important ways. The elements of this mode are illustrated in Figure 9.3 and include the following:

1. Logarithmic processing of the video information
2. Integration of preinjection video images over times typically on the order of 0.5 seconds
3. Use of a heavily filtered (eg, 150 mg/cm² of Samarium) x-ray beam
4. Subtraction of postinjection information at rates up to 60 images per second

Logarithmic processing of the data prior to subtraction is necessary to ensure that in the subtraction images, a given amount of iodine will produce the same residual signal independent of the local image brightness in the unsubtracted images. Integration of preinjection video images ensures that the quantum, statistical, and electrical noise in the preinjection mask are negligible. An alternative approach to provide a mask of negligible noise is to employ high current pulse of x-rays and a specialized low-noise video camera.[8,9] The latter approach yields a sharper mask in the presence of motion but requires a nonstandard video chain. There are advantages and disadvantages to sharp masks, which depend on the details of the application. For imaging coronary arteries following intravenous injection, subtraction of phase-related sharp masks may be necessary to minimize unsubtracted background.[10] However, for continuous study of cardiac chamber performance and ventricular wall motion, a time-integrated mask, though blurred, is adequate. Sharp masks have permitted subtraction images to be digitally amplified by factors of more than 10 relative to unprocessed fluoroscopic displays.

Such an application is illustrated in Figure 9.4, which shows a series of canine heart images made following injection of 20 cc of Hypaque-60 into the front leg of a 25-kg dog. Right and left heart structures are visualized sequentially during the first pass of the contrast bolus. In the 60 image/sec live display, the three major coronary arteries may be visualized due to integration of more image information than can be shown in these static images. The entrance exposure for these images was 200 mR/sec.

Adequate visualization of left ventricular wall motion can be achieved with contrast volumes as small as 2 ml. The images shown in Figure 9.5 are analogous to those of Figure 9.4 except that a 2-ml bolus and a 50 mR/sec entrance exposure were used.

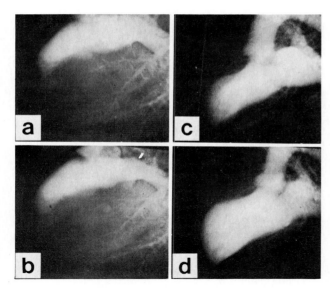

Figure 9.4. Mask mode fluoroscopy of a canine heart in LAO projection. Twenty ml of Renografin were injected into front leg vein of a 25-kg dog. The entrance exposure was 200 mR/sec. **A.** Right ventricular systole. **B.** Right ventricular diastole. **C.** Left ventricular systole. **D.** Left ventricular diastole. (Courtesy Radiology 132: 739–742, 1979.)

A similar examination of the heart of one of the authors (ABC) is illustrated in Figure 9.6. This exam was done using 60 cc of Renografin-60. It is currently felt that 30 cm^3 injections will decrease overlap of right and left heart structure without significantly decreasing the opacification of the left ventricle. The images of

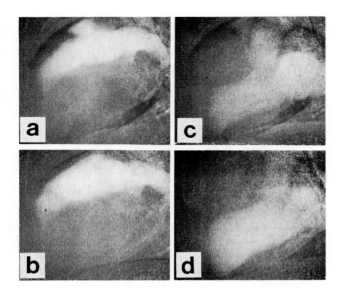

Figure 9.5. Examination similar to that of Figure 9.4 with 2 ml of contrast and 50 mR/sec entrance exposure. (Courtesy Radiology 132: 739–742, 1979.)

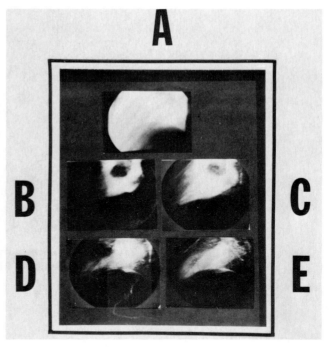

Figure 9.6. One-fifteenth of a second mask mode exposures following simultaneous injection of 30 ml of Renografin-60 into veins in each forearm of a 75-kg human. **A.** Preinjection mask. **B.** Right ventricular systole. **C.** Right ventricular diastole. **D.** Left ventricular systole. **E.** Left ventricular diastole.

Figure 9.6 contain some unsubtracted ribs due to a slight amount of patient motion. Such motion during the 10 or 15 seconds needed for this examination is an inherent limitation of the intravenous mask technique, in which substraction artifacts may be generated by images separated in time by many seconds.

Examination of the lungs using mask mode fluoroscopy should be easier because of greater iodine concentration, better x-ray transmission, and shorter examination time. This is illustrated in Figure 9.7 for the case of a 25-kg dog following a 10-cc injection of Renografin-60 into a front leg. Images such as these are being studied as a possible means of diagnosing pulmonary embolism. Mask mode fluoroscopy has been used in a preliminary attempt to visualize coronary artery bypass grafts (Fig. 9.8).

MASK MODE RADIOGRAPHY

When significant motion is absent, mask mode fluoroscopy may be replaced by a series of time separated subtraction images analogous to serial subtraction radiography. Depending on the amount of filtration used, available x-ray power, quality of the video system

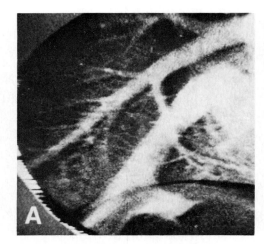
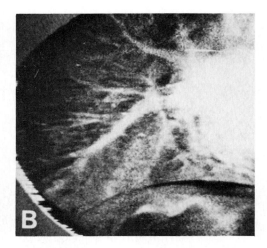

Figure 9.7. One-sixtieth of a second mask mode exposure of right lung following injection of 10 ml Renografin-60 into hind leg of 15-kg dog. **A.** Arterial phase. **B.** Venous phase.

available, and the temporal resolution required, post-injection images may be obtained by the use of short x-ray pulses and digitization of video information from a single scan of the video camera target or by integration of several (typically four) digitized fields of video information obtained with moderately short exposure rates. The former approach requires a low-noise camera with signal-to-noise ratios approaching 1,000 to 1, and provides greater spatial resolution in the presence of arterial pulsations. The latter approach, which is often adequate, permits the use of conventional fluoroscopic equipment.

Examples of mask mode radiography are shown in Figures 9.9 through 9.11. All are intravenous examinations using from 0.5 cc/kg (human carotids) to 0.8 cc/kg (dog studies).

Mask mode radiography is subject to artifacts due to any motion that may occur between the preinjection

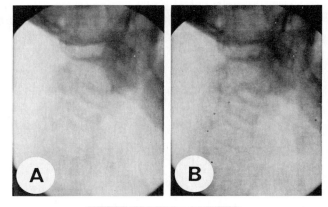
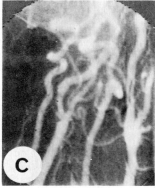

Figure 9.9. Mask mode fluoroscopy above the aortic arch of a 15-kg dog following 15-ml injection of contrast. **A.** Preinjection mask. **B.** Digitized fluoroscopic image (four TV field) taken approximately 12 seconds after injection of 40 cc of Renografin-76 at the rate of 15 cc/sec into the cephalic vein (56kVp, 300 mA, 1/15 sec exposure). **C.** Subtracted arterial phase image. (Courtesy Radiology 132: 739–742, 1979.)

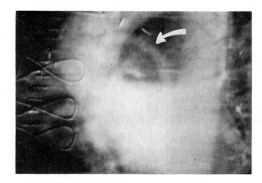

Figure 9.8. Aorta–left coronary artery bypass graft is seen following an injection into the right basilic vein.

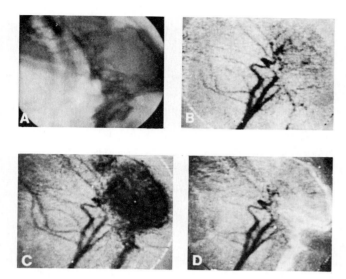

Figure 9.10. Dog head (lateral projection) following intravenous injection of 1 ml/kg of contrast. **A.** Preinjection mask. **B.** Arterial and early capillary phases. **C.** Perfused brain and mixed arterial and venous phases (long time). **D.** Separate display of arteries (black) and veins (white).

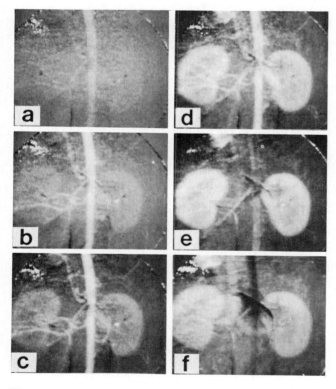

Figure 9.11. Serial mask mode radiography of canine kidneys following 0.8 cc/kg intravenous injection. **A.** through **F.** show transition from arterial to venous phase. A 256×256 image matrix was used. (Courtesy Radiology 132: 739–742, 1979.)

mask and the appearance of the bolus at the site of interest. For some examinations, such as in the kidneys, it is possible to take the mask image during the passage of the bolus through the lung in order to decrease the period in which respiration must be suspended. In addition to respiratory motion, swallowing can be a problem during imaging of the carotid arteries. During imaging of abdominal structures, the movement of the overlying bowel may need to be suppressed with drugs.

TIME INTERVAL DIFFERENCE (TID) MODE

Instead of using a preinjection mask, it is possible to subtract transmission information associated with more closely spaced time intervals, for example, intervals separated by 1/15 second. Such images display the change in x-ray transmission or, in most applications, the change in iodine pathlength in gm/cm². This mode is illustrated in Figure 9.12.

TID examinations may be obtained in real time during the first pass of iodine bolus or by reprocessing the mask mode fluoroscopy from video disc or tape. Figure 9.13 represents TID images obtained from the human mask mode data associated with images of Figure 9.6. In this mode, increases in iodine content are displayed as white signals and decreases are displayed as dark signals. Because closely spaced, 1/15 second time intervals were used, rib artifacts due to misregistration have disappeared. The TID mode is quite insensitive to respiratory motion and may be useful in extracting information from examinations in which significant patient motion has occurred.

Although the characteristics of the TID images of the heart are not well understood at the present time, it is apparent that this mode may be particularly useful for detecting dyskinetic left ventricular wall motion. Figure 9.14 shows left ventricular images during in-

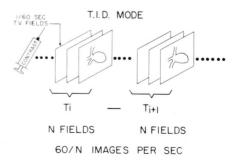

Figure 9.12. In time interval difference (TID) imaging a group of *N* video fields are subtracted from a similar group from the immediately preceding time interval. Increases in iodine appear as white. Decreases are black.

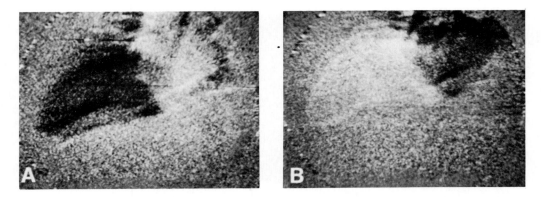

Figure 9.13. TID images of human left heart, reprocessed from data of Figure 9.6.
A. Ventricular contraction. **B.** Expansion.

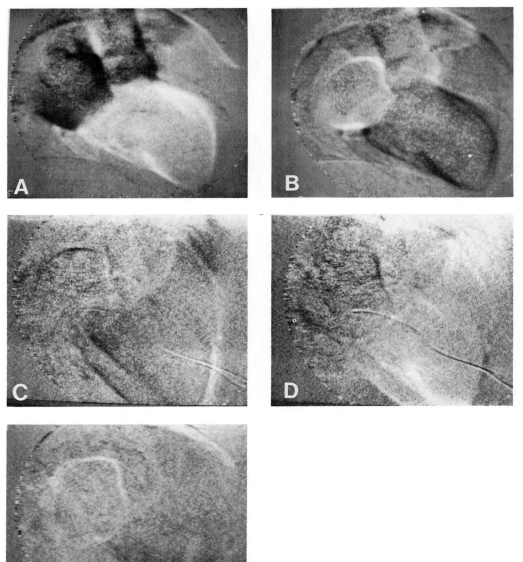

Figure 9.14. **A.** TID image of healthy canine heart in LV diastole. **B.** Systole. **C.**, **D.**, **E.** Heart of dog accidentally rendered anoxic for several minutes.

travenous examinations of a dog before and after accidental anoxia. In the healthy heart, uniform contraction (black) and expansion (white) signals were obtained. In the dyskinetic heart, these uniform signals are clearly absent.

In a more carefully controlled experiment, the circumflex coronary artery was occluded with a Gelfoam embolus. The mask mode images of the systolic and diastolic phases are shown in Figure 9.15 for examinations before, one half hour, and 18 hours following occlusion of the artery. The anomalous wall motion following occlusion differs considerably from the uniform contraction and relaxation seen prior to occlusion. The abnormal motion may be represented directly in terms of gray shade alterations in the TID mode (Fig. 9.16). The apical and posterior borders are dem-

onstrated to be out of phase with normal anterior wall. The infarcted area bulges (white signals) in systole and fails to relax in diastole.

While the same information is provided by mask mode, the TID display is much less dependent on patient cooperation. Therefore, it can often be used to salvage examinations that otherwise might have been unsuccessful because of motion artifacts.

K-EDGE FLUOROSCOPY

The TID mode displays changes in iodine content rather than the instantaneous iodine concentration and therefore requires a dynamic state. Another possibility for dynamic iodine display that is immune to respira-

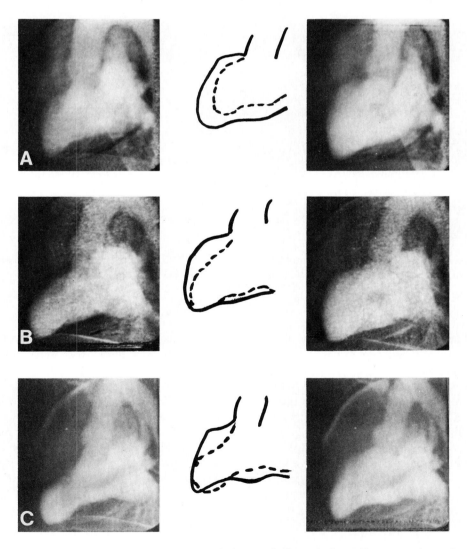

Figure 9.15. Mask mode images before and after occlusion of circumflex artery in a dog. **A.** Before occlusion (systole, outlines of systole and diastole, diastole). **B.** 30 minutes after occlusion. **C.** 18 hours after occlusion.

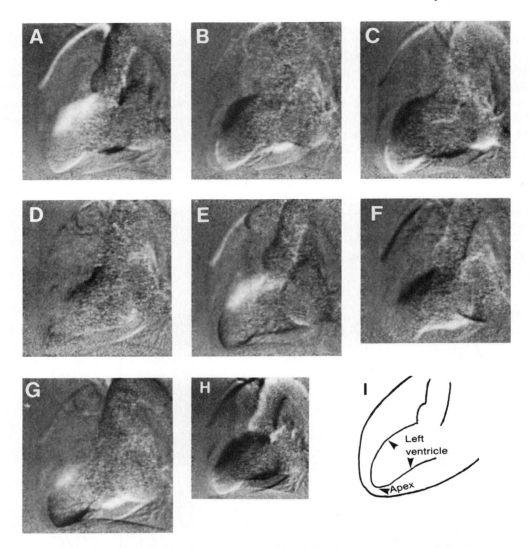

Figure 9.16. TID images of left heart shown in Figure 9.15. Note presence of simultaneous expansion and contraction signals in contrast to images 9.14.

tory artifacts utilizes the principle of energy subtraction; it is called K-edge fluoroscopy.[6] This mode relies on the abrupt increase in iodine attenuation coefficient at the 33 keV K edge shown in Figure 9.17. Quasi-monoenergetic x-ray beams are formed by filtration with cerium, which forms a beam with average energy above the iodine K edge, or by iodine, which forms a beam with average energy below the K edge. Since bone and tissue attenuation coefficients undergo a much smaller change as the beam energy is moved from below the K edge to above, a difference image using the cerium- and iodine-filtered beams will suppress these substances and isolate the iodine signal, which then can be greatly amplified.

For heart studies, the use of a single kVp near 50 kVp with 225 mg/cm^2 of cerium and 125 mg/cm^2 of iodine alternated 60 times per second (Fig. 9.18) ap-

pears adequate. So far, only canine hearts have been studied. In this case, ribs cancel well and ventricular wall motion is observed well without suspension of respiration (Fig. 9.19).

The K-edge fluoroscopy mode is presently limited to x-ray tube power requirements. Cine-pulsed operation at 60 pulses per second at 1,000 mA at 50 kVp will not provide enough input exposure for adult human hearts because of the attenuation in the iodine and cerium filters.

K-EDGE RADIOGRAPHY

For static situations in which the time distribution of iodine is too slow to permit mask mode subtraction, and in which small iodine concentrations are to be

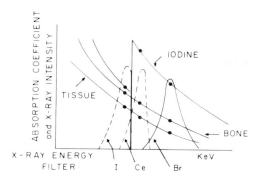

Figure 9.17. Iodine, bone, and tissue attenuation coefficients shown in relation to three quasimonoenergetic beams used for K-edge imaging. The I and Ce beams are used for K-edge fluoroscopy. The Br beam is added for K-edge radiography.

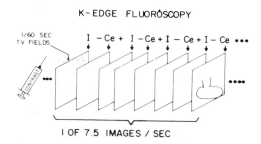

Figure 9.18. In K-edge fluoroscopy iodine and cerium filters are switched in and out of the beam at a rate of 60 per second. Eight video fields are combined to reduce quantum noise. Rapid alternation of filters reduce motion artifacts.

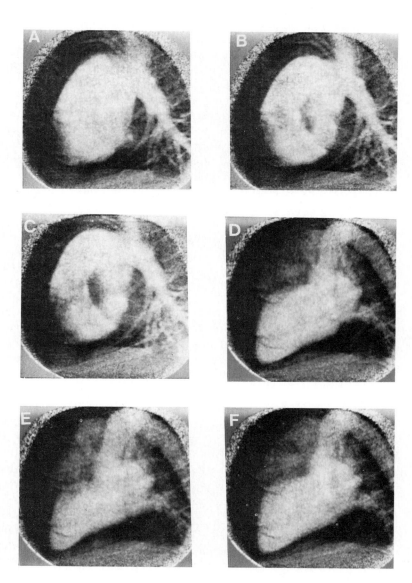

Figure 9.19. K-edge fluoroscopy of heart at 7.5 per second following 1 ml/kg iodine injection. This mode is immune to motion artifacts but is presently limited by the tube power requirements. Pediatric applications may be possible. (Courtesy Invest Radiol 14: 270, 1979.)

imaged in the presence of large bone and tissue variations, the use of three separate x-ray spectra is required, as shown in Figure 9.20. The third spectrum (see also Figure 9.17) is required for more accurate isolation of bone, tissue, and iodine. Basically, the three spectra provide the three transmission equations needed to solve for the energy-dependent attenuation contributions characteristic of iodine, Compton scattering, and the photoelectric effect. Since all noniodinated tissue can be represented as a combination of Compton and photoelectric effects, it is possible to isolate iodine and eliminate all tissue background, regardless of its exact attenuation coefficients.

Figure 9.21 shows an examination of a monkey head in lateral projection. Three ml of metrizamide were injected into the cisterna magna three hours before imaging. In the original film radiograph, the iodine signals were indistinguishable from those of bone, or were too low in contrast to be seen. In the K-edge radiograph, the subtracted cerebellar cisterns are clearly identified and the bone images are removed.

K-edge radiography does not suffer from the same limitations as K-edge fluoroscopy, since time integration, which is used in a static situation, allows the accumulation of sufficient transmission information. K-edge radiography is expected to be useful in regions where bone or large tissue variations normally limit the low contrast iodine signals to a small fraction of the dynamic range of the display system, eg, intravenous cholangiography. K-edge subtraction may also be combined with tomography to provide images in which iodine slices are isolated.[11, 12] Thus far, only phantom studies have been done using K-edge tomography.

FUNCTIONAL PHASE DISPLAY

Another algorithm used to process intravenous angiography data involves conversion of the point-by-point information regarding time of maximum opacification to a continuous gray scale display. Picture elements that opacify early are shown as black, and late elements are white. This similar algorithm was used to generate the phase display of the canine heart shown in Figure 9.22. This examination was performed without contrast material and presumably shows time of maximum opacification provided by blood flowing through the heart, with some contribution due to reorientation of overlying tissue structures. Individual cardiac chambers are not visualized. However, the general regions of the right and left atria are shown later to be filling. This image represents information during a single heart cycle. It may be possible to decrease the noise content of the image by EKG-gated integration over several heart cycles. This process is, of course, subject to irregularities in the heart rate. Further information, including delineation of individual chambers, may be achievable by using contrast infused slowly enough to ensure that the cardiac phase information rather than the phase of nonuniform contrast bolus is imaged.

OTHER STUDIES WITHOUT CONTRAST MATERIAL

Motion of the myocardial border is of interest[13] and can be readily observed with the TID mode without the use of contrast agents. TID provides excellent cancellation of anatomy even with respiratory motion. Thus it is possible to amplify signals related to differential transmission through the heart by a factor of 16 or more, which permits visualization of minor changes in border position. Furthermore, those changes may be observed around the entire border and are not limited to the portion that borders the lung. An example of this technique is shown in Figure 9.23, which show a canine myocardium in periods of contraction (black border signals) and expansion (white border signals).

Although such studies are interesting, they provide much less information than those employing contrast material. In view of the ease of intravenous contrast examinations and their relatively safe nature, it is not expected that examinations without contrast material will be as useful.

VIDEODENSITOMETRY OF INTRAVENOUS CARDIOVASCULAR STUDIES

Videodensitometry is a well known technique for studying a variety of problems in the cardiovascular system.[15] Most of these studies utilize data from catheterization procedures. However, similar techniques can be applied to intravenous studies. The high contrast resolution of computerized fluoroscopy provides images in which structures of interest are detectable in spite of the low concentrations of iodine achieved by intravenous injection (typically a factor of 30 less than with direct

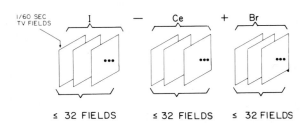

Figure 9.20. In K-edge radiography three images are integrated for about 0.5 seconds using iodine, cerium, and brass filtration. All three are needed for optimal bone and tissue subtraction.

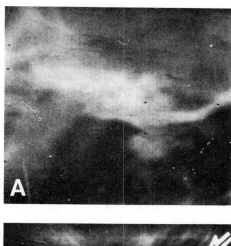

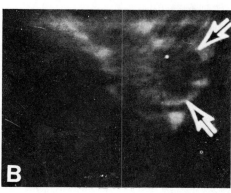

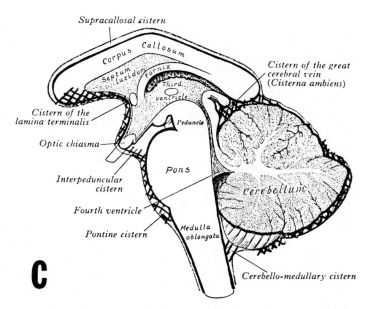

Figure 9.21. K-edge radiography of monkey head in lateral projection. **A.** Digital image (unsubtracted) three hours after injection of 3 ml of metrizamide into the cisterna magna. Iodine is indistinguishable from anatomy. **B.** K-edge subtraction image showing iodine in cisternal system with bone images removed. **C.** Corresponding human anatomy with cisterns crosshatched.

injection via catheter). Once structures are recognized, windows for videodensitometric integration of time-dependent iodine contrast can be chosen. Because these windows encompass many picture elements, the net signal-to-noise ratio after spatial integration should be sufficient for most applications in spite of the low iodine concentrations present within the window.

For videodensitometric studies, a light pen is used to designate those picture elements to be included in

the integration. These form an arbitrarily shaped integration region, which is stored in a small window memory. This memory is used to gate the integration of mask mode subtraction data. The results of the integration are stored in a small memory and may be processed further by a computer before display.

A typical application is shown in Figure 9.24, which shows an opacified canine left ventricle with a superposed integration window. Because anatomy is sub-

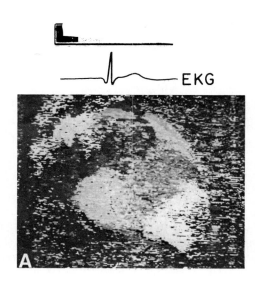

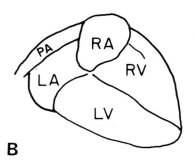

Figure 9.22. Cardiac phase display obtained without contrast injection. Individual chambers are not seen, but the general features are distinguishable.

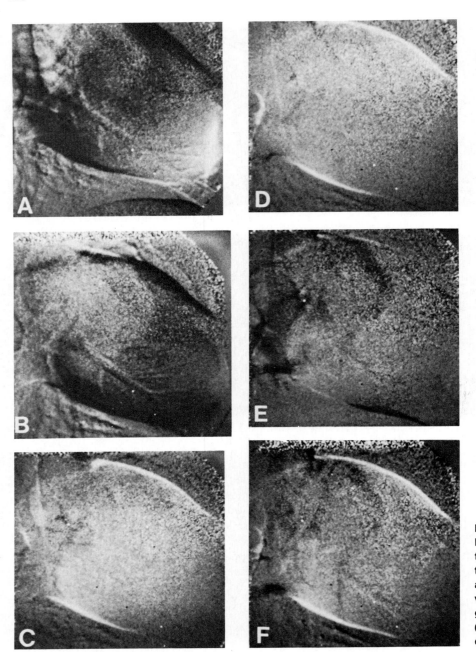

Figure 9.23. TID images in canine heart obtained without contrast injection. Expansions (white) and contractions (black) of the myocardial border are evident. Overlying pulmonary vasculature is seen in **A.** and **B.** The general shift of attenuating material (predominantly blood) is seen by comparing **A.** and **F.**

tracted, the window need not be placed exactly at the ventricular border. Except for possible overlap of residual contrast in the right heart or pulmonary structure, there is not significant iodine contribution outside the ventricular border. Some error is introduced in placement of the window in the region of the mitral and aortic valves. The estimate of ventricular iodine content obtained in this way is displayed 60 times per second in Figure 9.24. With analysis procedures analogous to those used in nuclear medicine, which include correction for overlying iodinated structures, left ventricular ejection factor and other quantities may be calculated very accurately.

Videodensitometric analysis of intravenous angiography is in its early stages but could be an important adjunct to the qualitative interpretation of the basic image display.

HYBRID VERSUS PURELY DIGITAL TECHNIQUES

Mask mode fluoroscopy and radiography may be accomplished by two separate techniques. Purely digital subtraction, in which preinjection images and post-

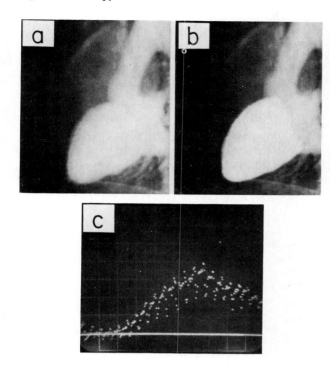

Figure 9.24. Videodensitometric determination of left ventricular iodine content. **A.** Mask mode fluoroscopic image of canine heart following intravenous injection. **B.** Left ventricle highlighted by light pen. **C.** Time display (60 integrals per second) of iodine content representing first passage of contrast bolus through the heart.

injection images are identically processed, provides the most precise cancellation of anatomy and flexibility in terms of processing options. However, in some situations, a combination of analog and digital techniques can be used to permit inexpensive implementation of the simplest computerized fluoroscopy algorithms with high resolution (Fig. 9.25).[7]

In this case, a low resolution (256×256) preinjection mask is stored digitally and reconverted to analog form to permit subtraction with postinjection un-

digitized video. The postinjection video channel should be of high resolution (eg, $1,000 \times 1,000$ picture elements) in order to display the high spatial frequency components of the injected iodine information. If the anatomical background does not contain significant high-contrast signals at high spatial frequencies, the low resolution digitally stored preinjection mask suffices to cancel the anatomy and permits a factor of 10 amplication of injected iodine signals. In this way, high-resolution iodine information may be obtained without large amounts of memory or high digitization rates.

Initial experience with the hybrid technique indicates that good images may be obtained of the heart (Figs. 9.4, 9.5), lungs, and kidneys. In the head, however, the presence of high spatial frequency information due to bones leads to unsubtracted anatomical backgrounds. Figure 9.26 shows a canine lung examination obtained using a 10-cc iodine injection into the hind leg. These images should be compared to those of Figure 9.7, which is a 256×256 digital version of a similar examination. The hybrid subtraction examination done with a conventional 525-line television system provides better detail and could be extended easily to higher resolution simply by replacing the video system with one of higher resolution (Fig. 9.26).

Figure 9.27 shows a hybrid subtraction examination of the kidney performed with an injection technique similar to that of Figure 9.11, which is purely digital. Again, greater detail is provided by the hybrid technique.

Figure 9.28 shows a hybrid examination of the head. This is analogous to the purely digital images of Figure 9.9. In this case, the spatial resolution is somewhat better than in Figure 9.9. Because of the uncancelled high spatial frequency bone shadows, however, the images are more difficult to interpret. For this reason, it is likely that purely digital subtraction will be more desirable in the head and that higher resolution, if desired, must be achieved by increased memory size.

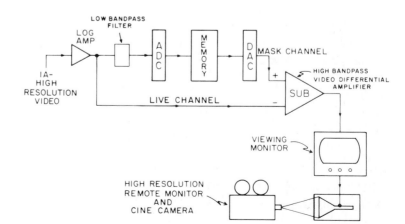

Figure 9.25. Circuitry for hybrid subtraction fluoroscopy and radiography.

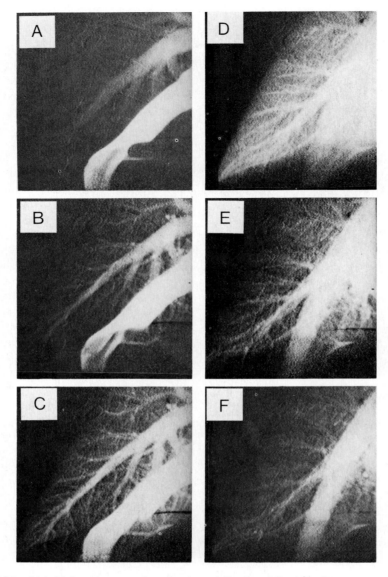

Figure 9.26. Hybrid fluoroscopy of canine lung following 0.6 ml/kg intravenous injection of contrast. Spatial resolution is twice that of Figure 9.7.

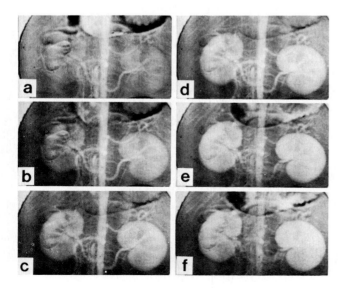

Figure 9.27. Hybrid radiography of canine kidney following 0.8 ml/kg intravenous injection. Compare with Figure 9.11. (Courtesy Radiology 132: 739–742, 1979.)

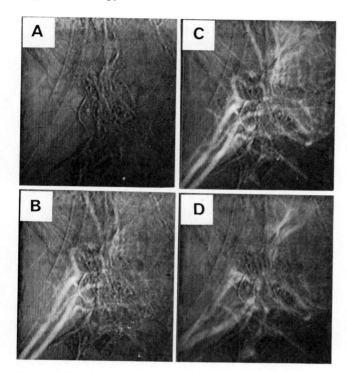

Figure 9.28. Hybrid radiography of canine head following 0.8 ml/kg intravenous injection. Compare with images of Fig. 9.9. **A.** Subtraction artifacts before arrival of contrast. These are due to mismatch of spatial resolution of digital mask and postinjection analog video images. (Courtesy Radiology: 739–742, 1979.)

X-RAY EXPOSURE IN COMPUTERIZED FLUOROSCOPY

X-ray exposures required for the imaging methods discussed above are comparable to those used in computerized tomography. In each case, the required exposure increases as spatial resolution requirements are increased and as the contrast of the subject to be imaged is decreased. Thus, for intravenous angiography, x-ray exposure is related to amount of contrast injected, to the spatial resolution of the subtraction hardware, and, as usual, to patient thickness and x-ray beam energy.

The optimal exposures for the various algorithms discussed above have not been established at this time. The exposure rates for the human left heart study (Fig. 9.6) are typical and are on the order of 200 mR per second. The duration of the exposure may vary from a few seconds, if only the left ventricle is studied, to 10 or 15 seconds if the entire course of the bolus is to be followed from the right heart to aorta.

For examinations beyond the heart, for example, of the carotid arteries or kidneys, one reduces irradiation of the patient by delaying the x-ray exposure until the time of arrival of the contrast in the area of interest. Also, in order to minimize the possibility of motion

artifacts, the patient can be instructed to suspend breathing shortly after injection rather than before. The mask image is then taken during passage of the bolus to the site of interest.

THE ROLE OF COMPUTERIZED FLUOROSCOPY

The range of applications for computerized fluoroscopic techniques has not been fully established at this time. However, a comparison of its properties with those of conventional techniques and with its tomographic counterpart may suggest areas of potential usefulness.

All x-ray transmission examinations can be characterized by their contrast resolution, spatial resolution, and characteristic imaging times. In Figure 9.29 the relative properties of several techniques are compared on the basis of their positions in a three-dimensional space defined by three orthogonal axes representing detectable object size, detectable contrast, and characterisitic imaging time.

Conventional film radiography offers the highest spatial resolution and has reasonably good temporal properties (as in rapid serial radiography) but has poor contrast resolution. Cinefluoroscopy also has good spatial resolution, excellent imaging rates, but poor contrast resolution. Computed tomography offers excellent contrast resolution, moderate spatial resolution, and except for one system presently under development,[16]

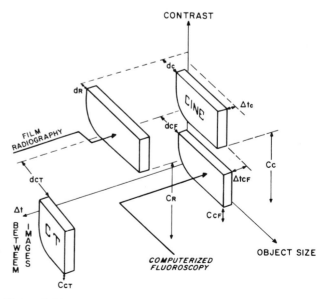

Figure 9.29. Relative properties of several imaging methods. Computerized fluoroscopy offers advantages when high contrast resolution and high imaging rates are required. (Courtesy Radiology 132: 739–742, 1979.)

poor temporal resolution (on the order of one second or more).

Computerized fluoroscopy can be expected to play an important role in clinical examinations requiring excellent contrast resolution (though less than in computerized tomography due to acceptance of additional scatter), moderate spatial resolution (that of television fluoroscopy), and excellent temporal resolution (60 images per second).

It is interesting historically to note that the development of computerized tomography preceded computerized fluoroscopy even though the algorithms required in tomography are more complicated than those used to process fluoroscopic data. Two important factors contributed to this. First, the computational problem of reconstructing two-dimensional slice images from multiangular projection data is sufficiently difficult to require a computer. Second, the fact that standard computers of reasonable price are not fast enough to process fluoroscopic data delayed the development of computerized fluoroscopy by requiring, except for simple off-line applications, the construction of special-purpose high-speed digital processors.

The evaluation of the potential utility of computerized fluoroscopy and its several distinct imaging algorithms is just beginning. Because many of these algorithms, including those which appear to be most useful, only require processing of conventional image-intensified fluoroscopy images, the apparatus needed for this technique should become readily available as an accessory item to upgrade existing fluoroscopic systems at moderate expense.

REFERENCES

1. Mistretta CA: The use of a general description of the radiological transmission image for categorizing image enhancement procedures. Optical Engineering 13 (2): 134, 1974
2. Kruger RA, Mistretta CA, Lancaster J, Houk TL, Goodsitt MM, Riederer SJ, Hicks J, Sackett J, Crummy AB, Fleming D: A digital video processor for real-time subtraction imaging. Optical Engineering 17 (6): 1978
3. Kruger RA, Mistretta CA, Crummy AB, Sackett JF, Riederer SJ, Houk TL, Goodsitt MM, Shaw CG, Flemming D: Digital K-edge subtraction radiology. Radiology 125: 243–245, 1977
4. Kruger RA, Mistretta CA, Houk TL, Riederer SJ, Shaw CG, Goodsitt MM, Crummy AB, Zwiebel W, Lancaster JC, Rowe GG, Flemming D: Computerized fluoroscopy in real time for noninvasive visualization of the cardiovascular system. Radiology 130 (1): 49–57, 1979.
5. Kruger RA, Mistretta CA, Riederer SJ, Ergun D, Shaw CG, Rowe GG: Computerized fluoroscopy techniques for noninvasive study of cardiac dynamics. Invest Radiol 14 (4): 279–287, 1979
6. Houk TL, Kruger RA, Mistretta CA, Riederer SJ, Shaw CG, Lancaster JC: Real-time digital K-edge subtraction fluoroscopy. Invest Radiol 14 (4): 270–278, 1979
7. Ergun D, Mistretta CA, Kruger RA, Riederer SJ, Shaw CG, Carbone D: A hybrid computerized fluoroscopy technique for noninvasive cardiovascular studies. Radiology 132 (3): 739–749, 1979
8. Frost MM, Fischer HP, Nudelman S, Rohrig H: Digital video acquisition system for extraction of subvisual information in diagnostic medical imaging. Proc SPIE 127: 208–215, 1977
9. Ovitt T: Noninvasive contrast angiography. Proceedings of Conference on Noninvasive Cardiovascular Measurements, Stanford University, Palo Alto, Calif., September 1978
10. Brennecke R, Brown TK, Busch J, Heintzen PH: Computerized video image preprocessing with application to cardio-angiographic roentgen—image series. In Nagel HH (ed): Digital Imaging Processing. New York, Springer, 1977, p 244
11. Riederer SJ, Mistretta CA: Selective iodine imaging using K-edge energies in computerized x-ray tomography. Med Phys 4 (6): 1977
12. Kruger RA, Riederer SJ, Mistretta CA: Comments on the relative properties of tomography, K-edge imaging, and K-edge tomography. Med Phys 4 (3): 244–249, 1977
13. Höhne KH, Böhm M, Erbe W, Miolae CC, Pielffer G, Sonne B, Bücheler E: Die Messung und Differenzierto Bildische Darstellung der Nierendurdblutung mit der Computerangiographie. RöFo, Band 129, Heft 6, Stuttgart, Dec 1978
14. Rosen L, Silverman NR, Higgins CB: Differences in the velocity-displacement relationship of systolic contraction of normal and ischemic canine myocardium. Radiology 124: 7–12, 1977
15. Heintzen PH, Bursch JH (eds): Roentgen Video Techniques for the Analysis of Structure and Function of the Heart and Circulation. Stuttgart, T Thievae, 1978
16. Ritman EL, Robb RA, Gilbert BK, Kinseg JH, Wood EH: High temporal resolution cylindrical scanning transaxial Roentgen tomography. Read before National Bureau of Standards Symposium on Real Time Radiologic Imaging: Medical and Industrial Applications. Gaithersburg, Md, May 8–10, 1978

CHAPTER 10

Image and Equipment Considerations in Conventional Tomography

CRAIG M. COULAM
JON J. ERICKSON
S. JULIAN GIBBS

The objective of conventional tomography (motion tomography, planography, or body-section radiography, as it is alternatively known) is to choose a plane of specified thickness within the body such that the image of this plane on film is in-focus while the image of objects or body parts not lying in the plane is blurred. To achieve this objective, four aspects of tomography need to be considered: (1) how is the desired image plane and its associated thickness chosen; (2) what methodology is required to blur objects lying outside (above or below) the desired plane of interest; (3) what pictorial and mechanical parameters describe or influence the image quality of the object lying in the focal plane; and (4) how does the presence of non-focal-plane artifacts distract from or diminish the pictorial information displayed. An understanding of these four aspects of tomography is essential because they delineate what pictorial features an ideal tomographic image should and should not contain, how well the various types of contemporary tomographic equipment are able to produce the ideal image, and how optimum use of different types of tomographic equipment can be utilized for a given clinical setting. This chapter will discuss tomographic image generation in general, evaluate those image features that make up the in-focus and blurred aspects of the display, and present some generalizations concerning patient irradiation.

BASIC TOMOGRAPHIC IMAGE CONSIDERATIONS

BLURRING MOVEMENTS AND FOCAL-PLANE CONCEPTS

All conventional tomography systems consist of three primary components: the x-ray tube, the object to be imaged, and the x-ray film carrier. To produce an image of a desired plane or section of the body, two of the three components of the tomographic system must move in a mechanically linked and usually, but not always, diametrically opposite fashion. That is, either the x-ray tube and body must move relative to a stationary x-ray plate (a seldom used method), the x-ray tube and x-ray plate must move relative to a stationary body (the most popular method), or the body and x-ray plate must move relative to a stationary x-ray tube (again, a seldom used method). How the component parts move with respect to each other has great bearing upon the resultant image quality. Since it is movement that produces blurring of the image of objects not lying in the focal plane, it is the relative motion that determines the uniformity or completeness of the blurring process. Conventionally, the blurring process is broken down into two major categories[1,3]: linear and complex blurring (or movement). Since almost all commercially available equipment manufacturers design around the stationary body, moving x-ray tube and plate concept, this linear and complex blurring methodology will be discussed in some depth.

Linear Blurring Movements. In this system, the x-ray tube is mounted on one side of the stationary object and the x-ray plate on the opposite side, as shown in the classical configuration of Figure 10.1.A. As the x-ray tube moves linearly from A to A', the x-ray plate moves linearly from B to B', such that the fulcrum or plane of no motion, F, lies in the body at the desired anatomical level and its image on the film always lies in focus at F'. The images of objects located above (point C) or below (point D) the focal plane are blurred between C' and C", and D' and D" by the x-ray tube and plate movement.

The pathway by which x-ray tube and plate move from points A to A' and B to B' has considerable influence on the intensity of exposure of object parts

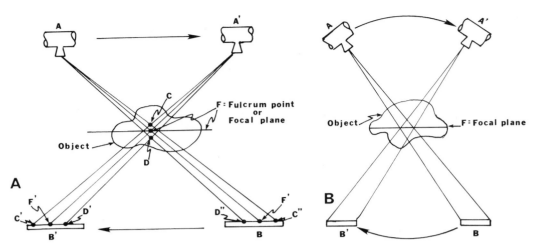

Figure 10.1. **A.** The classical tomographic system description. The x-ray tube moves from A to A′ while the x-ray plate moves from B to B′. The fulcrum point F defines the focal plane. Objects lying above (C) or below (D) of the focal plane are blurred between C′–C″ and D′–D″ respectively. **B.** The Grossman tomographic principle. The x-ray tube moves from A to A′ following a curvilinear trajectory. Likewise the x-ray cassette moves from B to B′ on a curvilinear trajectory such that the x-ray tube to cassette distance (AB) is constant.

on the x-ray plate. Figure 10.1.A shows a horizontal linear motion between A and A′, and B and B′, while Figure 10.1.B shows a curvilinear relationship. The motion of the first method has been attributed to Andrews and that of the second to Grossman[1]. Alternatively, the first method is known as the adjustable-fulcrum system and the second as the fixed-fulcrum system. With the adjustable-fulcrum system, the desired focal plane can be chosen by mechanically moving the fulcrum point up and down relative to the patient, or alternatively, by using a book cassette (ie, multiple x-ray films sandwiched together between sheets of non-x-ray opaque filler material) to make multiple tomographic images simultaneously. In either case, as can be seen in Figure 10.2 the adjustable-fulcrum system generates a slightly different amount of relative angular movement of the x-ray tube and film cassette, depending upon the chosen body sectional level and a more intense exposure of the patient and x-ray plate when the x-ray tube and plate are perpendicular to the axis of the desired image plane. As will be seen subsequently, both of these features affect the overall quality of the tomographic image.

With the fixed-fulcrum system, Figure 10.3, the desired image plane is chosen by moving the x-ray tube and film cassette up and down relative to the stationary patient, rather than moving the fulcrum point. Alternatively, the patient may be moved up and down relative to the x-ray tube and plate. Because of the curvilinear motion of the x-ray tube and plate, and because of the constant distance between them (ie, during movement from point A to A′), the intensity of the x-ray film exposure is relatively constant independent of tube

position, and the relative angular movement between points A and A′ remains fixed and equal for each focal-plane level evaluated.

Complex Blurring Movements. Alternatively available tomographic systems do not move from A to A′ linearly, but from A through A′ (and/or A″) and back to A along a complex path, such as circular (Fig.

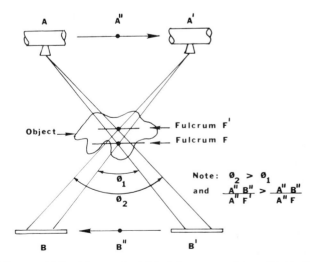

Figure 10.2. The adjustable-fulcrum system allows for changes of the focal plane by mechanical changes in the fulcrum point. Since the x-ray tube and cassette move through the same sequence, raising the fulcrum point increases the relative tomographic arc-swing angle (ie, $\phi_2 > \phi_1$) and thus decreases the sectional thickness of the focal plane and increases the image magnification factor.

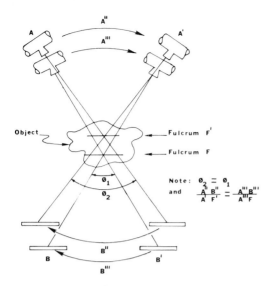

Figure 10.3. The fixed-fulcrum system allows for changes of the focal plane by either moving the x-ray tube and cassette or the patient up and down. The relative tomographic angle remains the same during the tube motion; thus the sectional focal-plane thickness and image magnification remain constant.

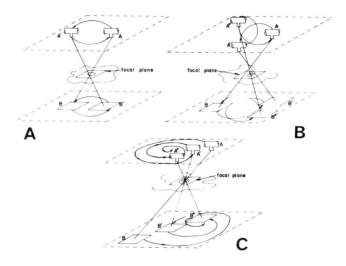

Figure 10.4. Complex blurring motions. **A.** Circular. **B.** Hypocycloidal. **C.** Trispiral. These complex motions generate a more complete blurring of non-focal-plane objects at the expense of prolonged examination time. Note in all three systems the x-ray tube never passes perpendicular to the focal plane. Furthermore, because of their geometrical pathways, hypocycloidal and trispiral motions have a continuously varying x-ray-tube-to-cassette distance and consequently nonuniform accentuation of anatomical parts on the cassette.

10.4.A), hypocycloidal (Fig. 10.4.B), or trispiral (Fig. 10.4.C). In general, complex motion machines have been designed to yield a more complete blurring of non-focal-plane objects and to overcome a variable focal-plane depth, as will be discussed below. The principle trade-off between the complex-motion tomographic system and the linear tomographic system is that the complex-motion systems produce a different non-focal-plane blur pattern and consequently produce a different form of image artifact. Because of the differing motion-related image artifact problems (or false shadows as they are also known), circular tomography and its variant, ellipsoid tomography, have not proven to be clinically popular, except as an axial tomographic system. For the remainder of this chapter, complex-motion tomography will refer to either hypocycloidal or trispiral blurring motions.

As illustrated in Figures 10.4.B and 10.4.C, the x-ray tube-to-plate distance varies during the tomographic motion because of the hypocycloidal and trispiral blurring movements. With the hypocycloidal system, a more intense patient and x-ray film exposure occurs whenever the x-ray tube and plate pass in a nearly vertical direction relative to the focal-plane axis. This happens approximately three times during a hypocycloidal exposure. Thus a nonuniform weighting of the object's image on the x-ray plate occurs, depending upon the position of the x-ray tube and film cassette. Likewise with the trispiral motion (Fig. 10.4.C), more intense patient and film exposures are obtained during

the third or inner spiral as compared to the first or peripheral spiral. This nonuniform exposure will be examined in greater depth in a subsequent section.

Additional Focal-Plane Concepts. The implication of Figures 10.1 to 10.4 is that certain geometrical relationships must exist between the focal plane in the body and the x-ray film (cassette). Conventionally we think of the orientation of the focal plane in the body and of the x-ray cassette as being parallel to each other and both parallel to the tabletop on which the patient lies. This latter relationship (parallel to the tabletop) is not necessary.[1, 4] It is sufficient that the focal plane in the body and the film cassette be parallel in order that geometrical distortion of the image does not occur (Fig. 10.5.A and 10.5.B). On the other hand, even though no geometrical distortion of the image occurs, a nonuniform x-ray exposure of the patient and film cassette does occur because of the altered proximity of the x-ray plate (and focal plane) to the x-ray tube during the blurring movement. This can be overcome, however, if need be, through use of wedge filters or through the appropriate use of the x-ray tube heel-effect. From a clinical point of view, the rule calling for relaxation of the focal-plane parallel to the tabletop is exciting as it opens up new dimensions in body section radiography. As yet, only one commercial company offers this nonparallel feature (Versagraph, Xionics Inc.).

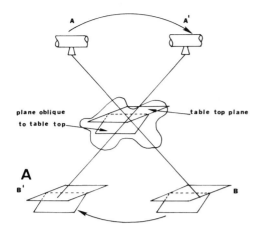

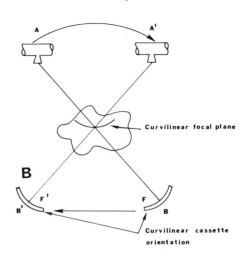

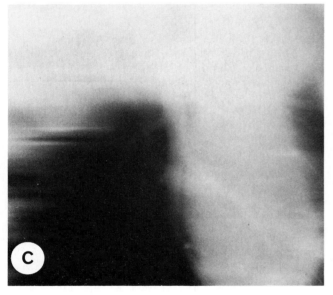

Figure 10.5. A tomographic principle is that the orientation of the x-ray cassette during the tomographic movement determines the focal plane in the object. **A.** An oblique focal plane. **B.** A curvilinear focal plane. This method could be used as a basis of pantography. Thus it is not necessary that the x-ray plate always be parallel to the tabletop. **C.** An oblique view of the entire pulmonary artery (arrows) of a dog. The dog was supine on the table and the x-ray plate was oblique. (Reproduced with permission, Carl E. Ravin, MD, Duke University Medical Center.)

FUNDAMENTAL IMAGE QUALITY CONSIDERATIONS

TOMOGRAPHIC SECTION THICKNESS

Linear Blurring Motions. The thickness of the tomographic section must be considered relative to the anatomical structure one is trying to image. For the linear blurring motion system, the section thickness will be dependent upon two things: the arc swing of the x-ray tube and cassette, and, equally important, the orientation of the anatomical structure relative to the linear motion. The smallest sectional thickness is achieved with the widest arc swing of the x-ray tube and cassette and with the anatomical structure oriented perpendicular to the linear tube motion. For convenience one should assume only that the x-ray cassette is also parallel to the table top. Section thickness can be measured by scanning an inclined wire or ruler embedded in clear plastic and oriented so that the axis of

the wire is perpendicular to (or if a ruler is used, parallel to) the linear tube motion.[1] Plotting sectional thickness against arc length (in degrees) produces Figure 10.6.A. For any arc length, the width of the blur pattern will also change depending upon the orientation of the wire relative to the tube motion. By repeating the process with the axis of the wire lying parallel to the tomographic focal plane but not perpendicular to the tube motion (say at 75°, 60°, 45°, 30°, 15°, and 0° relative to the tube motion), Figure 10.6.B is generated. From Figure 10.6.B, one can see that the apparent sectional thickness, as portrayed by the blur width, is dependent upon the orientation of the structure relative to the tube motion. Also, linear structures are more dependent upon the direction of tube motion for their correct blur pattern than are circular structures. Figure 10.7, in which the tomographic motion is parallel to the trachea and centered at the mid-thorax level, demonstrates this. Note that the image of the tracheal walls indicates an infinitely thick section (ie,

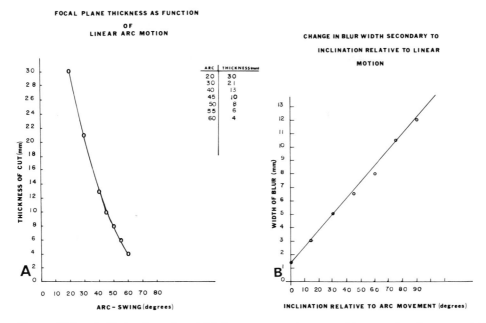

Figure 10.6. A. Plots of sectional thickness versus tomographic movement, measured in degrees of arc swing (or alternative, tube inclination angle) for a linear blurring system. **B.** The width of the blur pattern for any given arc swing is a function of the orientation of the object relative to the direction of tube movement.

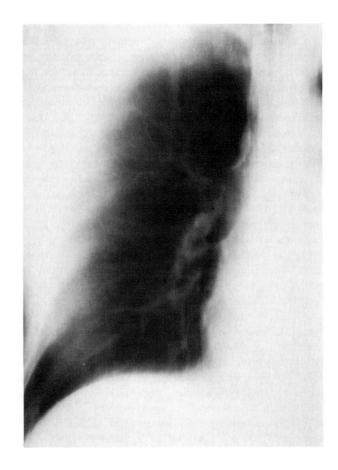

Figure 10.7. Depending upon the orientation of objects in the thorax, an infinite series of sectional thicknesses are present. Here the mid-lung structures have the smallest sectional thickness (ie, arc-swing orientation approximately 90°), the right mainstem bronchus has an intermediate thickness (ie, arc-swing orientation approximately 45°), and the tracheal wall is infinitely thick (ie, arc-swing orientation approximately 0°). If the direction of tube travel were perpendicular to the trachea, upper and lower lung structures and mediastinal structures would then lie in the smallest sectional thickness.

object axis at 0° relative to the tube motion). Similarly, the bronchi and pulmonary vessels in the extreme upper and lower lung fields indicate very thick sections (ie, object axis within 15° of tube motion). The right main-stem bronchus, on the other hand, lies approximately 45° relative to the tube motion and has a considerably thinner image sectional thickness. Finally, the pulmonary vessels and bronchi in the mid-lung regions have very thin sectional thicknesses because the axis of their orientation is approximately 90° relative to the tube motion. If the same thorax were tomographed at the same anatomical level, but with the tube motion perpendicular to the trachea, then the image of the trachea and the upper and lower lung field vessels would have the thinnest sectional thickness and the mid-lung vessels would have the greatest sectional thickness. Obviously, with linear tomography the tube motion and arc length should be perpendicular to the object to be imaged.

It is important to note that when adjustable-fulcrum systems and/or book cassettes are used, the arc swing of the x-ray tube and cassette varies as a function of distance from the tabletop (Fig. 10.2). Thus tomographic images made near the tabletop have the smallest arc swing (in degrees) and largest sectional thickness. Conversely, images made the farthest from the tabletop have the largest arc swing and smallest sectional thickness.

Complex Blurring Motion. When a complex x-ray tube and cassette movement is used, section thickness is not dependent upon the object orientation but only upon the maximum and minimum angles subtended by the x-ray tube and film cassette relative to the focal plane (Figs. 10.8.A, B). Since the sectional thickness is not dependent upon object orientation, complex-motion tube movements give an almost uniform section thickness throughout. The term "almost uniform" needs to be emphasized, because when the x-ray tube and cassette are at their largest angle of inclination relative to the focal plane, the thinnest section is being recorded. Conversely, when the x-ray tube and cassette are at their smallest angle of inclination relative to the focal plane, the thickest section is being recorded. As the angle of inclination changes from the largest to the smallest values, intermediate sectional thicknesses are produced. Thus the overall image is a composite or summation of many thicknesses. The effective or apparent thickness is primarily determined by the time spent in the movement from the greatest angle of inclination to the smallest. That is, if more time is spent at the larger inclination angle relative to the smaller inclination angle, a thinner section will be seen and vice versa. Complex-motion tomography is used clinically when the thinnest, most uniform sectional thicknesses are desired, such as of the inner ear or sella

turcica regions of the head, and when the greatest amount of non-focal-plane blurring is required, independent of object orientation.

FOCAL-PLANE IMAGE QUALITY

Spatial Resolution. The amount of blur or edge unsharpness in a tomographic image of an object lying in the focal plane is a measure of the spatial resolution of the image. This can be measured by plotting the full-width-half-maximum of a wire scanned in the focal plane (and whose axis is perpendicular to the tube movement for a linear system) against the arc swing of the tube in degrees. Or alternatively, the image of the wire of each arc swing can be subjected to a Fourier series transformation and the resulting modulation transfer functions (MTFs) plotted as a family of curves.[5,6]

It is more constructive, however, to understand why increasing arc swing tube movements produce increasing image unsharpness in the focal plane. Consider a circular object, as shown in Figure 10.9.A. As the tube and film move between endpoints b and c, to generate the focal plane, the projection of the edge of the object on the film appears to move to and fro. This results from the fact that in positions b and c the edge appears to be at a point more lateral than when the tube is in position a. This is an effect secondary to the tangential nature of the beam. In the positions between b and c the edge appears to project to corresponding intermediary positions on the film. This apparent motion of the edge results in the unsharpness of the object in the image. Furthermore, as the arc swing increases and the focal-plane thickness narrows, the spread of the edge of the object increases and its intensity (ie, film darkness) decreases. Ideally, the material composing the object should be as radiodense as possible to offset the loss of radiographic contrast in the density profile resulting from the tomographic movement. This effect is important clinically when small focal planes are chosen; objects of high inherent radiodensity give better thin section detail (eg, the bones of the inner ear) than do objects with a lower object-to-background density difference (eg, the edge of a kidney).

Besides the edge uncertainty, the focal-spot size of the x-ray tube also has an effect on the resolution. If the cross-sectional diameter of small objects lying in the focal plane begins to approximate the dimensions of the diameter of the effective focal-spot size of the anode of the x-ray tube, geometrical distortion occurs (Fig. 10.10.A–C). The smaller the object diameter, the larger the image penumbra effects and the poorer the spatial resolution. While small focal spots are necessary to better image small objects, heat loading characteristics of the x-ray tube usually dictate the smallest practical focal-spot diameter that may be used. Furthermore,

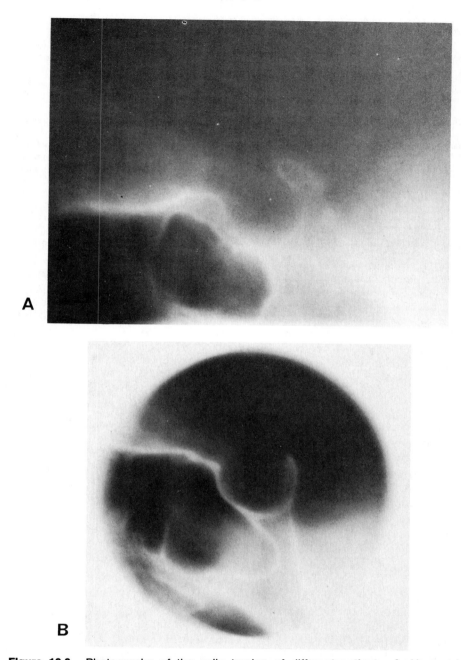

Figure 10.8. Photographs of the sella turcica of different patients. **A.** Hypocycloidal movement. **B.** Trispiral movements. Note both systems are nearly identical in minimal sectional thickness available. However, during tube movement, both systems change continuously the relative tube inclination angle and therefore the sectional thickness. The final thickness is a composite of many sectional plane thicknesses.

focal-spot size must be considered when evaluating tomographic systems because of the inherent image magnification that occurs. For fixed-fulcrum systems, this magnification is nearly constant and runs around 1.2 to 1.5, depending upon the mechanical design. For adjustable-fulcrum systems, the magnification is variable, depending only upon the chosen fulcrum level, and

runs from 1.0 to 2.0. Thus, variable magnification and varying penumbra changes secondary to magnification serve to diminish the spatial resolution of the image and increase image unsharpness.

Another major factor responsible for loss in spatial resolution is the use of intensifying screens. In general, the faster the intensifying screen, the greater the loss of

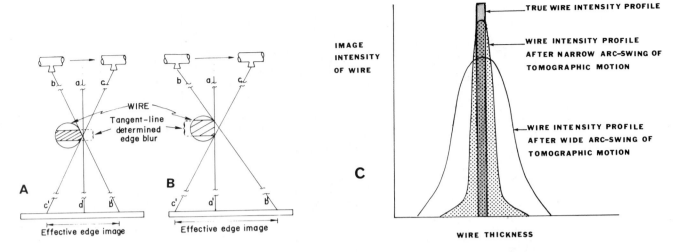

Figure 10.9. Focal-plane unsharpness arises at the edges of structures because of the increasing tangential nature of the x-ray beam during the tomographic movement. **A.** Smaller tube movements (ie, larger sectional thickness) produce less unsharpness. **B.** Larger tube movements (ie, smaller section thickness) produce more unsharpness. **C.** If a wire were the object to be measured, the resultant wire profile would be shown as a function of the tomographic arc swing. Full-width-half-maximum measurement can be made from these wire profiles, and MTFs of the system computed.

spatial resolution.[1,8] This problem is compounded when book cassettes are used with adjustable-fulcrum systems because graded screens are also employed (slower screens on top and faster screens on the bottom) in order to offset the differential absorption of x-ray photons from higher films and screens. Ironically, however, the higher screen–film combinations have wider tube arc swings. Thus the gain from the slower screen–film combination is offset by increasing edge unsharpness secondary to the tube movement and associated narrower focal planes.

Image Distortion. Image distortion of objects lying in the focal plane occurs because of nonuniform magnification of the object, depending on whether the object lies near the center of the focal plane or near its periphery. This can be seen in Figure 10.10.D. If an object lies at C in the focal plane its in-focus projection onto the x-ray cassette occurs at C′, C″, and C‴. Note, however, that the x-ray tube to object plane distance (and also the object plane to x-ray cassette distance) changes because of the use of a flat x-ray film. The change in object-to-film distance creates a spatially varying image amplification and thus object size distortion. Thus the object size has its greatest amplification at C′ or C‴ and its least amplification at C″. Littleton has measured this distortion factor and found the amplification factor to be a constant $1.75\times$ at C′ and $1.33\times$ at C″ for his fixed-fulcrum system.[1] For adjustable-fulcrum systems, the C′/C″ relationship was a function of the height of the fulcrum point above the

tabletop. At 27 cm, it was $1.75\times/1.43\times$, at 20 cm, $1.57\times/1.32\times$, at 10 cm, $1.39\times/1.19\times$, and at tabletop (0 cm), $1.23\times/1.09\times$. Thus the object's location in the focal plane influences its projection onto the x-ray film and also its spatial resolution because of a varying object amplification.

Density Resolution. Density resolution in tomography represents the system's ability to detect or resolve objects lying in the focal plane whose radiographic density is close to that of the surrounding background. Two features affect density resolution: image mottle or noise and scatter radiation, or alternatively, the image's signal (S) to noise (N) relationship (S/N ratios). Image noise or graininess comes from two sources: (a) the variation in x-ray flux arising from the x-ray tube during exposure (which is Poisson distributed with respect to time), and (b) the speed of the film–screen combination used.

Desired film blackening dictates the kVp and mA techniques the x-ray technician must use. The x-ray film–screen combinations commercially available require that one use as high a milliamperage station and as low a kilovoltage potential as possible in order to penetrate the object and produce the desired screen phosphor–photon interaction. The choice of x-ray film speed and intensifying screen speed has been the subject of considerable debate, especially now that rare-earth screens are available.[9] Several investigators have shown that, in general, both image mottle and patient irradiation can be minimized by using a fast screen and

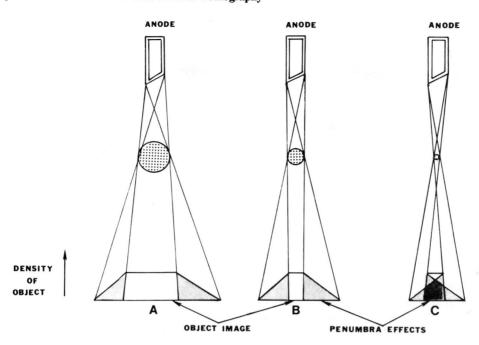

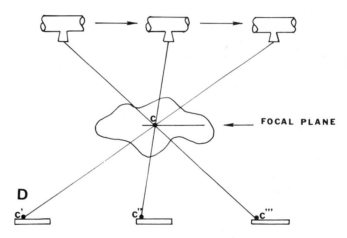

Figure 10.10. Effects of object diameter size as it approximates the effective tube anode focal-spot size. **A.** Object greater than focal spot. **B.** Object equal to focal spot. **C.** Object less than focal spot. Since magnification is inherent in all tomographic systems, the effect of the increasing penumbra size, **(A)** through **(C)**, is enhanced, and serves to further diminish object edge unsharpness. **D.** Variable object amplification occurs for objects located in the focal plane depending upon their anatomical proximity to the center of the focal plane. Objects lying near the periphery of the focal plane cast larger images onto the x-ray film than do those lying near the center of the focal plane.

slow film combination.[7,8] The logic behind this combination is that the fast screen produces a large number of light photons for each absorbed x-ray photon (permitting lower patient irradiation), while the slower film minimizes the inherent image mottle arising from the faster screen because of its reduced sensitivity to the light photons. Fast screens, however, do tend to diminish spatial resolution because of the lateral diffusion of light that occurs. Thus screens represent a trade-off between the spatial resolution and density resolution variables.

Scattered radiation affects density resolution because the scatter of nonprimary photons increases the overall blackening of the x-ray film while the primary photons forming the objective image remain essentially unchanged. Unevenness of background film darkening occurs because x-ray photons are generally scattered only through small deflection angles (less than ± 10°)

and are more intense near high radiographic density objects. Linear tomographic systems can minimize the effects of scattered radiation through the use of postpatient, prefilm grids. The grids, however, must be oriented so the grid lines are parallel to the tube movement and angled to accommodate the diverging nature of the x-ray beam (Fig. 10.11). For most tomographic systems, grids present no problem in alignment as their construction is identical to that of nontomographic systems. Degradation of the image grid effects will be most pronounced near the periphery of the image and least near the central axis of the image because of x-ray beam cutoff effects arising from improper orientation of the grid plates. Far-focus and near-focus grid effects (Fig. 10.11) become apparent depending upon the tube level above tabletop and manifest themselves near the peripheral aspects of the image. In addition to the far/near focus effects, off-centering effects of grid

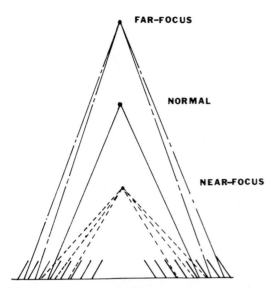

Figure 10.11. For linear and complex blurring tube motions, focused-grids may be used to diminish the effects of scatter radiation on the image and thus improve the density (contrast) resolution of the objective plane. Careful alignment of the tube must be done, however, to avoid far-focus, near-focus, and lateralizing image cut-off effects. For example, if a linear tomographic system were to be used here the direction of tube motion would have to be into and out of the plane of this figure. Complex tube motion also requires grid *rotation* to retain proper geometrical relationships.

image may be present. Both the fixed and adjustable-fulcrum systems are equally sensitive to off-center lateralizing effects of grids, whereas adjustable-fulcrum systems are only sensitive to far/near focusing effects. Complex-motion systems also use grids but require grid rotation because of the tube movement patterns. Grid rotation is necessary to maintain the direction of the grid lines pointing to and from the inclination angle of the x-ray tube. In general 10:1 to 12:1 grids work best in tomographic systems.

Other Factors Affecting Focal-Plane Image Quality. Two additional variables affect both the spatial and density resolution in the focal plane: patient motion and uniformity of exposure. Patient motion diminishes both density and spatial resolution. Tomographic systems are particularly susceptible to motion artifact because of the length of time required for the exposure. Even when breath holding minimizes the voluntary motion effects, cardiac pulsations and intestinal peristalsis will always be present to lower image quality. The quantitation of the effects of patient motion is beyond the scope of present day mathematics.

Nonuniformity of patient exposure implies that some views of the anatomy get greater x-ray flux than others during exposure, and thus the weighting of flux

effects on the film is greatest at particular tube orientations. For example, if greater x-ray flux occurs at the center of the linear tomographic sweep (because the tube is closer to the object) than at the ends of the sweep, image spatial resolution will be enhanced, but the focal-plane sectional thickness will also be the greatest (ie, we approach a conventional x-ray exposure). Thus a uniform exposure during tube motion is essential to avoid nonlinear density weighting in the image. This uniform exposure is enhanced by using a constant tube-to-film and patient-to-film distance. In a similar manner, constant velocity during the tube movement is essential to maintain uniformity of exposure. These equipment-related features will be discussed in greater detail later.

NON-FOCAL-PLANE BLURRING: IMAGE QUALITY VERSUS ARTIFACT PRODUCTION

Part of the quality in the tomographic image is the uniformity of blurring of the objects not lying in the focal plane. The blurring is directly related to the tube motion involved (ie, linear or complex) and the extent of the tube inclination angle present. Figures 10.12.A–D illustrate the blurring patterns of a large paper clip lying off the focal plane for the linear, circular, hypocycloidal, and trispiral movements. When examining these images, attention should be paid to (a) the uniformity of the blur pattern relative to the tube motion, (b) the width of the blur pattern relative to the tube motion, and (c) any tendency for the blur patterns to superimpose and thus add visually so as to produce artifactual images (sometimes referred to as false shadows).

The human eye, in evaluating a tomographic image, places everything which is in focus in the focal-plane and everything blurred or out of focus outside the focal plane. Thus if the blurring pattern is either nonuniform (eg, the edges of the blur pattern for the circular tube motion) or certain object configurations or periodicity result in superimposition of the blur patterns such that the overlapped shadows appear to be in focus, an inherent propensity is present for generating false shadows in the resultant image. Figures 10.12.A–D demonstrate that the complex tube motions generate the greatest uniformity of the blurring pattern and have the least tendency to form artifactual images. The trade-off is that a longer time interval is required to complete the complex tube movement (thus giving a greater chance for patient-motion induced artifacts to occur) and greater patient irradiation occurs because of the longer exposure and increased patient thickness (oblique views) necessitated by tomographic blurring motion.

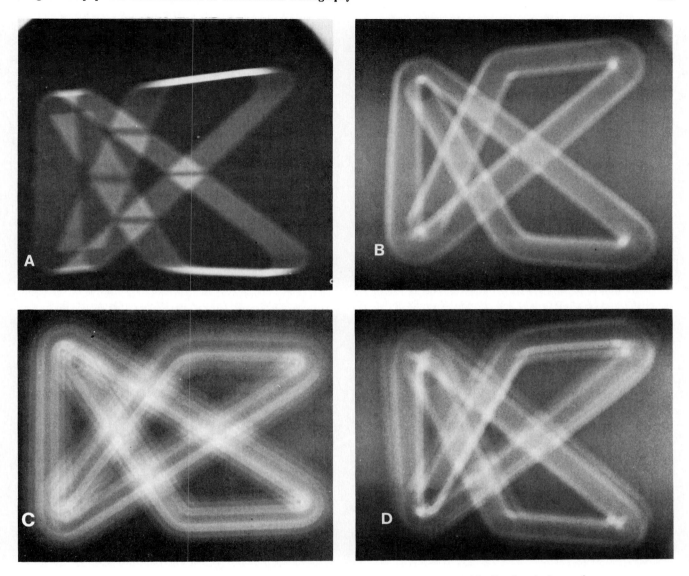

Figure 10.12. Blurring patterns of a paper clip located 1.5 cm outside the focal plane of the tomographic system. **A.** Linear blurring patterns. **B.** Circular blurring patterns. **C.** Hypocycloidal blurring patterns. **D.** Trispiral blurring patterns. The edge enhancement on the circular blurring pattern is considered a form of false shadow because it may be interpreted as lying in the focal plane. Furthermore, superposition of blurring shadows can add so as to create false shadows. This occurs primarily when multiple objects lie outside the focal plane and/or have similar anatomical orientations as is many times the rule in human anatomy, eg, the ribcage or pulmonary vascular markings.

TOMOGRAPHIC EQUIPMENT CONSIDERATIONS

TYPES OF EQUIPMENT COMMERCIALLY AVAILABLE

Contemporary tomographic systems fall into one of four categories: (a) adjustable fulcrum, (b) fixed fulcrum, (c) axial transverse, and (d) pantographic. Since adjustable- and fixed-fulcrum systems have al-

ready been discussed in some detail, attention is now directed to the axial transverse and pantographic equipment.

Transverse axial tomography (TAT) systems are presently manufactured by Toshiba, Inc., and Xionics, Inc., but were originally discovered and patented by a British technologist named W. Watson in 1937.[10] The Toshiba device is similar in operation to the British instrument in that the x-ray tube is stationary while both the patient and the x-ray cassette move (Fig.

10.13.A). The versagraph is more conventional in design in that the patient is stationary and the x-ray tube and cassette move (Fig. 10.13.B). In either case, the principle is the same: The sectional plane imaged on the film is parallel to that of the x-ray cassette, and the blurring movement optimally encompasses approximately 360° for complete blurring of all non-focal-plane objects. The angle between the axial body dimension and the line drawn between the x-ray tube and center of the x-ray cassette (angle ϕ, Fig. 10.13) is optimal at 20° because smaller angles (ie, $\phi < 20°$) create too much unsharpness in the focal plane (ie, loss of spatial resolution), and angles greater than 20° (ie, $\phi > 20°$) require too long an oblique pathway through the patient, resulting in greater patient irradiation and increased x-ray scattering effects with loss of density resolution (ie, diminished S/N ratio). Variation in the incident angle ϕ, however, does allow for changes in focal-plane sectional thickness. In general, the smaller the angle ϕ, the smaller the sectional thickness, and vice versa. Image quality is fairly easily understood when one realizes that TAT is really just circular tomography except the inclination angle is $90° - \phi$. Thus off-focal-plane blur patterns are similar to circular tomographic blur patterns.[11] In some cases however, incomplete blur patterns may emerge if 360° blurring is not used (eg, Versagraph, Xionics, Inc., uses a 220° blur pattern).

been developed principally by the dental profession to provide a radiographic image of the entire mouth and jaws on a single film. Because of the panoramic nature of the image, the method has been termed pantomography. It was first proposed in 1929, and films were produced in 1933. Practical development of the method, initially for arcs of cylindrical sections, was started by

Paatero in 1949.[12] The first American machine was developed by Hudson, Kumpula, and Dickson.[13] Unlike conventional flat-plane tomography, pantomography uses a moving-slit x-ray beam, with motion of the film synchronized appropriately for imaging the desired layer with the subject. The moving-slit method can also be used for flat-plane tomography, but for curved planes, its use is essentially obligatory.[14]

Geometry of curved-plane tomography, in simplified form, is shown in Figure 10.14. In this example, the sectional thickness (referred to as the focal trough in the dental literature) is an arc of a cylindrical section. Note that the axis of rotation is not contained within the focal trough. For complex arcs, such as the human jaws, a single axis of rotation is inadequate; therefore, multiple or moving axes of rotation must be provided.[15] Mathematical analyses of the method have been published.[12, 13, 15]

Approximately 20 different pantomographic machines are now commercially available. Image size for most is 6 in × 12 in; a few use 5 in × 12 in. Many use curved cassettes to minimize the physical size of the film carrier. Some cassettes are flexible, and are wrapped around a metal drum carrier in the machine. Most require that the patient be erect; in some, the patient must be seated in a chair that is an integral part of the machine.

Because of the complex nature of the tube-head–film movement, the focal trough (sectional thickness) for most machines is fixed. Therefore, patient positioning must be precise. The various manufacturers have provided ingenious means for ensuring correct patient positioning, but each in his own way. Some utilize chin rests, some bite blocks, and a few use light pencils as positioning aids. Most provide head restraints to dis-

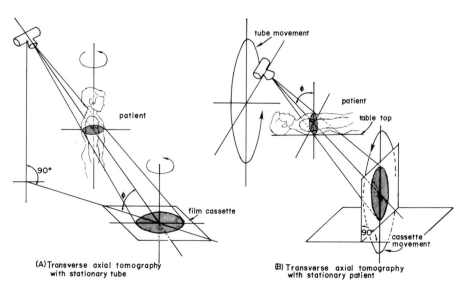

(A) Transverse axial tomography with stationary tube

(B) Transverse axial tomography with stationary patient

Figure 10.13. A. Transverse axial tomography (TAT) can be accomplished by one's holding the tube stationary and rotating synchronously the patient and x-ray cassette. **B.** It can also be accomplished by one's holding the patient stationary and rotating the x-ray tube and cassette. The optimal angle between the x-ray tube and cassette, ϕ, occurs at approximately 20°. Variations in this angle increase or decrease sectional thickness, but trade-offs between image spatial and density resolution do occur.

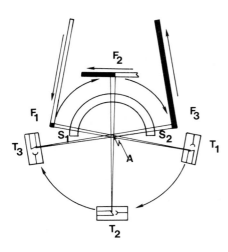

Figure 10.14. Diagramatic illustrations of a pantographic system that uses a curved-plane, moving-slit beam and arc of a cylindrical surface. Tubehead (T) and film carrier (F) revolve about a single axis (A), from initial positions T_1 and S_1 to final positions at T_3 and S_3. The focal trough is a cylindrical arc S_1 to S_2. As the film carrier revolves (curved arrows), the film translates (straight arrows) along an axis perpendicular to the slit beam, at a velocity such that the focal trough is relatively motionless to the film during the brief time that the particular region is being exposed. The blackened portion of the film carrier indicates exposed portion of film. For clarity, only a portion of the film and carrier is shown at the intermediate position, F_2.

courage patient movement during exposure. Sudden, brief patient movement during exposure can lead to unusual artifacts on the image, since motion artifacts will be present only on the part of the film that was exposed during patient movement. Sometimes, these artifacts appear as discontinuities in anatomical structures, resembling fractures. Exposure time for most machines, for a complete pantomographic projection, is on the order of 15 seconds. Reproducible geometry provided by the precise positioning requirement may be an advantage in longitudinal or follow-up studies.

At least one machine currently available has facilities for adjustment of the dimensions of the sectional thickness to fit the size of the patient being examined. Several machines provide a second focal trough setting, generally designed for curved-plane tomography of the mid-facial region. One newer machine is designed for use with supine patients. It permits selection of several focal troughs, to provide for curved-plane tomography of virtually any section of the head.

The pantomographic technique has gained widespread acceptance in dentistry as a supplement to conventional intraoral dental radiography. Use of the method is increasing in hospital settings, for a variety of purposes. For example, the technique has recently been documented as extremely useful in the diagnosis of facial fractures.[17]

MEASUREMENT TECHNIQUES: MACHINE-TO-IMAGE RELATIONSHIPS

As indicated earlier, certain machine design considerations influence image quality in the form of spatial resolution, density resolution, and blurring motion. Some of the more important relationships are (a) constant tube-to-film and patient-to-film distance during exposure, (b) uniform patient exposure throughout the tomographic movement, (c) accurate centering of x-ray tube with respect to the x-ray grid alignment, and (d) accurate orientation and geometric pathways of tube–cassette movement (ie, a presumed circular blurring movement is performed using a circular tube–cassette movement and not an elliptical one).

The above relationships can all be measured using a pinhole phantom, with the pinhole *not* centered in the focal plane (Fig.10.15.A–C). Mechanical instability (constant tube-to-patient and patient-to-film distances) can be detected by curvilinear changes of the image of the pathway. These curvilinear changes usually show up as a wobble, flattening of an arc of a circle, variations in intensity of exposure, etc. Nonuniformity of exposure arising from changes in x-ray photon flux appears as variations in intensity of exposure somewhat like changes in tube-to-cassette distances, but generally more pronounced. The variations may also have a beaded appearance secondary to using single-phase rather than three-phase voltage regulators. Changes in off-centering grid alignment show up as unilateral and/or bilateral fading of the exposure near the peripheral aspects of the film. Finally, orientation and type of geometric blurring motion are automatically registered during the x-ray exposure. By this means, orientation of the various types of blurring motions (ie, the linear blurring movement should parallel the long axis of the tabletop and not be slightly oblique to it) may be checked, especially if the tube movement is expected to be critical in certain clinical situations or individual patient positioning configurations.

QUALITY CONTROL

Quality control should consist of two features: (a) routine preventive maintenance of mechanical parts to ensure as friction-free smooth-movement of the x-ray tube, x-ray cassette, grids, and tabletop as possible; and (b) routine, periodic calibration and documentation of the x-ray tube kVp exposure and focal-section thickness using the pinhole and incline-wire (or ruler) phantoms.

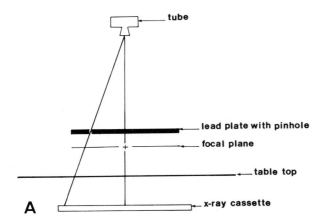

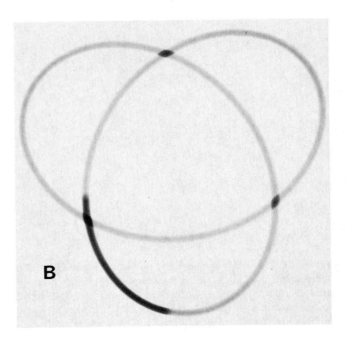

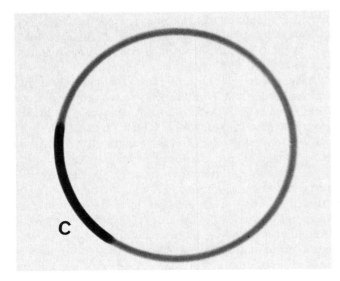

Figure 10.15. Pinhole phantom results and setup. **A.** Pinhole lead sheet mounted above focal plane. **B.** Hypocycloidal motion showing uniform exposure throughout the tube movement as manifested by the uniform blur pattern. **C.** Circular tube movement with no effects of wobble in blur pattern, indicating a true linear tube/cassette orientation during movement. The double exposure area indicates a delayed turning off of the x-ray tube upon completion of the tube mechanical motion. Pinhole phantoms should be an integral part of a routine preventive maintenance program.

CLINICAL CONSIDERATIONS IN TOMOGRAPHY

PATIENT IRRADIATION

Tomography studies generally deliver an increased irradiation dose to a patient in comparison with conventional radiographic techniques. Patient irradiation is increased because (a) multiple exposures are generally made since multiple focal planes must be examined, and (b) increased irradiation occurs during each focal plane exposure because oblique x-ray pathways must be compensated for.

The number of tomographic sections required to study adequately a section of body anatomy is a function of (a) the appropriate plane thickness relative to the size of the structure and the distance between cuts; (b) the orientation of the anatomy, since multiple structures generally will not all lie perpendicular to the tube movement and thus will have different sectional thicknesses (assuming here a linear blurring movement); and (c) those situations where overlapping sectional thick-

ness must be employed in order to ensure complete coverage of minute pathology. Most radiologists unknowingly use an overlapping technique of body sectioning because of incomplete knowledge of the relationship between tube inclination angle and sectional thickness. While this unintentional overlapping methodology does tend to guarantee adequate studies relative to criteria (a) and (c) above, criteria (b) is *not* solved unless a complex motion tube movement is also employed. For linear blurring movements, the direction of travel of the tube relative to the patient must be altered so that the orientation of most of the anatomy of interest is as perpendicular to the direction of tube movement as is possible. Since the patient always pays for mistakes in the form of absorbed x-radiation, taking the minimal number of nonoverlapped, correctly oriented images goes a long way toward lowering patient dose and improving image quality.

Increased patient irradiation does occur during the making of a tomographic exposure, when compared to a conventional, nontomographic exposure, if the amount of film darkening is to remain the same for both imaging techniques. Because the x-ray photons must pass through greater lengths of anatomy secondary to the obliquity of the x-ray tube-to-patient orientation necessitated during the tomographic movements, the overall *average* thickness of a patient is greater for tomographic studies than for conventional x-ray studies. This in turn calls for increases in the operating kilovoltage and/or milliamperage stations used by the technologist relative to conventional x-ray studies. In general, each tomographic exposure is approximately 1.3 times greater than the standard, non-tomographic image of the same body part.[1,2]

When book cassettes are used, exposure factors and techniques are increased even further in order to compensate for the differing intensifying screen speeds, the increased thickness of the book cassette, and the associated spacer material. In general, the kVp and mA stations are chosen to accommodate the slowest intensifying screen speed, which is usually the topmost screen. Use of rare-earth screens and appropriate x-ray films can help considerably to lower patient dosage.

PATIENT POSITIONING GUIDES

The ability to set up quickly the appropriate focal-plane locations and/or adjust prepatient collimators to allow for irradiation only of a limited anatomical area is extremely advantageous. Furthermore, it can result in increased patient throughput in a busy hospital setting; the increased throughput will usually offset the additional costs required to purchase some of these optional set-up aids. These positioning guide features usually consist of a radiograph of the anatomy perpendicular to the desired tomographic sections (Fig. 10.16), and/or a minifluoroscopic system that views the anatomy end-on, as the tomogram would be taken.

The set-up radiograph made perpendicular to the sectional planes of interest (eg, if A-P tomograms are desired, a cross-table lateral x-ray is obtained) generally has marker lines indicated on the exposed radiograph, where the marker center is fixed relative to the fixed fulcrum of the system. Measurements made on the lateral radiograph can then be programmed directly into the system (eg, with a micrometer dial — Versagraph, Xionics, Inc.) for automatic and proper patient focal-plane sections. Since the patient's position does not change between the set-up radiograph and the making of the tomographic sections, gravity-induced organ displacement is minimal.

Minifluoroscopic systems materially aid in performing tomographic studies when small anatomical parts must be imaged precisely using a highly collimated x-ray source (eg, inner ear or sella turcica studies). The high collimation requirement minimizes scatter radiation effects and improves image density resolution.

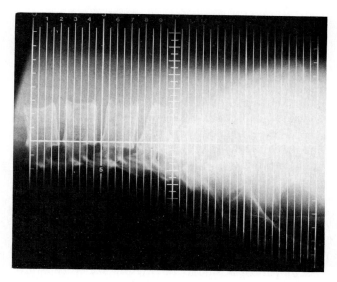

Figure 10.16. Set-up radiograph perpendicular to desired tomographic plane. Center of cross hairs indicates fulcrum point. Desired focal planes above or below (or even angulated) can be measured from horizontal lines and entered into the system using micrometer dials on the table for automatic patient positioning. This particular set-up radiograph was made in preparation for a TAT study of the lumbar spine. (Courtesy of Xionics, Inc.)

Thus exact orientations of the anatomy, relative to the x-ray cassette axis, need to be achieved quickly in order to increase patient throughput. When repeat studies are indicated for following changes in subtle pathological processes, nearly exact patient repositioning can be obtained using either or both the minifluoroscopic or perpendicular-radiograph system.

FILM/SCREEN COMBINATIONS

As mentioned above, certain x-ray film and intensifying screen combinations appear better suited for tomography than other combinations in order to minimize image noise or graininess. Under this consideration, fast-speed screens and slow-speed films seem to be better.[8] Another consideration relates to attempts to improve tissue-to-background contrast through the use of high-contrast film and/or screen combinations. This subject has been examined in some depth by others.[7,9] In general, as high a film contrast gradient as possible (3.0 to 4.0) should be used whenever possible along with slow film speed (1.0 to 1.9 relative speed) in order to maximize density (contrast) resolution. When high inherent image contrast is already present (eg, bones of middle ear or sella turcica), medium-speed screens are recommended over fast, unsharp screens to preserve spatial resolutions.[9]

FUTURE CONSIDERATIONS IN TOMOGRAPHY

STANDARD TOMOGRAPHIC SYSTEMS

Clinical indications and competitive devices should continue to control the types of tomographic systems manufactured. Relative to the standard tomographic systems available today, greater demand and development is expected to occur along lines of improved patient positioning aids, such as the perpendicular view and C-arm tomographic assembly recently introduced by Xionics, Inc. In addition, further clinical studies need to be initiated to understand better the "rediscovered" principle of using obliquely oriented x-ray cassettes (relative to the tabletop) in order to better examine body anatomy not lying parallel to the tabletop and/or to avoid uncomfortable or dangerous (posttrauma) patient positions. Finally the use of transverse axial tomography is expected to become more prevalent for vertebra and spinal cord work because of the continuing tight economic controls placed upon competitive computed tomography scanner installations by the certificate-of-need laws and the third-party payer doctrine.

COMPETITIVE EQUIPMENT

Competition among equipment systems involves mostly CT scanners (Chapters 14 and 15) and possibly nuclear medicine tomographic devices (Chapters 16 and 18).[18,19,20] In many areas of the body, CT images will continue to encroach upon domains that were previously considered conventional tomography. For example, CT of the pulmonary parenchyma and thoracic mediastinum has already been shown to be more sensitive to disease detection than standard linear chest tomograms,[19] and work emerging on the use of CT for detecting pituitary microadenomas appears very promising.[20] Clinical and economical efficacy studies must continue to be done, however, before third-party payers will unconditionally accept these competitive imaging procedures. Thus these efficacy analyses will slow any complete takeover by competitive equipment, should it prove more efficacious.

FUTURE TOMOGRAPHIC SCANNERS

With the improvement in solid-state and gaseous x-ray detector technology following on the heels of CT scanning, and with the widening clinical acceptance of computer-produced images, it is not unreasonable to conceive of situations in which multiple standard tomograms could be assembled by computers using only one tomographic sweep motion, thereby minimizing patient irradiation, avoiding the need for repeat views, and allowing for computer-enhanced feature analysis (such as edge enhancement, smoothing, highlighting, and in-

teractive image manipulation). Such a system is simply conceived in Figure 10.17. Here the x-ray cassette is replaced with a flat surface of solid-state detector cells (in matrix arrangement), and each cell connects to computer memory through analog-to-digital converter circuits following appropriate signal amplification. For each location (or firing) of the x-ray tube as it swings through its tomographic movement (linear or complex), the individual images are stored in computer memory in an ordered fashion. After the tube movement is over, the operator chooses one or more fulcrum positions (corresponding to desired anatomical focal planes) for image assembly, and the computer uses the chosen fulcrum level to dictate how the individual images must be assembled into one composite image. Once assembled, the image(s) is (are) displayed on a cathode-ray tube (CRT) like the present CT images and "hard copies" are obtained using multiformat cameras, before or after additional computer manipulation. Thus, the operator's choice of the fulcrum point is the key to how the computer will assemble the multiple standard images into one tomographic image, and the "windowing" capabilities of the CRT determine the final image pictorial information content.

SUMMARY

Tomographic imaging systems are unique in that the x-ray tube and cassette movements allow focal planes to be created as sharp, in-focus images of variable thickness, while non-focal-plane objects have their effects blurred so they become nondistracting. The image quality varies due to a complex interdependence of several factors, such as geometric unsharpness, patient motion, mechanical vibration and stability, angulation and complexity of the arc swing of the x-ray tube relative to the x-ray cassette, orientation of the x-ray cassette relative to the tabletop, inherent object-to-background contrast, film–screen combination used, scatter radiation effects, image amplification, and the presence or absence of false blurring shadows. It is only through a thorough knowledge of how the tomographic image is assembled or created on the film and how the different image variables affect the final image that the clinical situation will be correctly evaluated and high quality, diagnostic images obtained with minimal patient exposure. A continuous monitoring of the performance of tomographic equipment using appropriate phantom material and periodic preventive maintenance is necessary to keep the equipment in prime condition. Finally, an awareness of future tomographic designs allows competitive equipment and innovative new tomographic ideas to be incorporated into any radiology department's diagnostic armamentarium at equipment replacement or upgrade times.

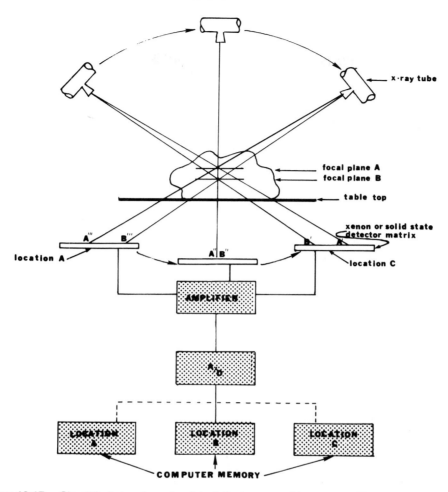

Figure 10.17. Simplified drawing of a futuristic tomographic system. The x-ray cassette has been replaced with a matrix arrangement of xenon or solid-state detectors, which enter their image information directly into digital computer memory following appropriate signal amplification and analog-to-digital (A-D) conversion. For each position of the x-ray tube during its tomographic movement, the detector matrix is entered into memory. Individual focal-plane images are assembled by the computer by adding appropriate image matrix values together to form a composite image. For example, a point in focal plane A is assembled by adding data from matrix locations A', A", and A'''. Likewise, a point in focal plane B comes from matrix locations B', B", and B'''.

REFERENCES

1. Littleton JT: Tomography: Physical principles and clinical applications. In Robbins LR (ed): Golden's Diagnostic Radiology, Sec 17. Baltimore, Williams and Wilkins Co, 1976
2. Christensen EE, Curry TS III, Dowdey JE: An Introduction to the Physics of Diagnostic Radiology, ed 2. Philadelphia, Lea and Febiger, 1978
3. Meredith WJ, Massey JB: Fundamental Physics of Radiology, ed 3. Chicago, John Wright and Sons, 1977
4. Watson W: British Patent 508381, 1937
5. Orphanoudakis SC, Strohboehm, JW, Metz CE: Linearizing mechanisms in conventional tomographic imaging. Med Phys 5(1): 1–7, 1978

6. Orphanoudakis SC, Strohbehn JW: Mathematical model of conventional tomography. Med Phys 3(4): 224–231, 1976
7. Cohen G, Barnes JO, Pena PM: The effects of the film–screen combination on tomographic image quality. Radiology 129: 515–520, 1978
8. Barnes GT, Witten DM: Film–screen considerations in tomography. Radiology 113: 477–479, 1974
9. Rao GUV, Fatouros P: The relationship between resolution and speed of x-ray intensifying screens. Med Phys 5(3): 205–208, 1978
10. Watson W: Axial transverse tomography. Radiology 28: 179, 1962
11. Harding G, Butram U, Weiss H: Towards optimum blurring in spiral tomography. Med Phys 5(4): 280–284, 1978

140

The Physical Basis of Medical Imaging

12. Paatero YV: A new tomographical method for curved outer surfaces. Acta Radiol 32: 177–184, 1949

13. Hudson DC, Kumpula JW, Dickson G: A panoramic dental x-ray machine. US Armed Forces Med J 8: 46, 1957

14. Wuehrmann AH, Manson-Hing LR: Dental Radiology, ed 3. St Louis, CV Mosby, 1973, pp 157–169

15. Manson-Hing LR: Panoramic Dental Radiography. Springfield, Ill., CC Thomas, 1976

16. Welander U: A mathematical model of narrow beam rotation methods. Acta Radiol 15: 305–317, 1974

17. Noikura T, Shinoda K, Ando S: Image visibility of maxillo-facial fractures in conventional and panoramic radiography. Dento-Maxillo Facial Radiol 7: 35–42, 1978

18. Amtey SR, Read ME: General theory of motion tomography. In Freedman GS (ed): Tomographic Imaging in Nuclear Medicine. New York, Society of Nuclear Medicine, Inc, 1973

19. Muhm JR, Brown LR, Crowe JK, Sheedy PF, Hattery RR, Stephens DH: Comparison of whole lung tomography and computed tomography for detecting pulmonary nodules. Am J Roentgenol 131: 981–984, 1978

20. Haughton VM, Williams AL, Cosick JF, Syverstsen A, Eldevik OP: CT diagnosis of pituitary microadenomas, abstracted. Proceedings of Scientific Program, Radiological Society of North America, 1978, p 183

CHAPTER 11

Angiography

AMIL J. GERLOCK, JR.
MALCOLM SLOAN

Angiographic imaging requires a knowledge of some of the most sophisticated biomedical equipment used in medicine today. Since much of the basic physics and engineering aspects of this equipment has been explained in other chapters of this text, no attempts will be made to describe them further. Instead, emphasis will be placed on broad concepts concerning the design and utilization of the angiographic room and its components.

ANGIOGRAPHIC ROOM

The angiographic room must be large enough to accommodate the following equipment: angiographic table, film changers, image intensifiers, television monitors, radiographic tube housings, instrument trays, cabinets, an anesthesia machine, a contrast pressure injector, and physiologic monitoring devices. In spite of all this equipment, adequate space must be provided so that the patient can be readily approached from either side or end of the angiographic table. To accomplish this, the room must be at least 20 ft × 20 ft.[12] A design for an angiographic room and its components is shown in Figure 11.1. There should be at least three entrances into the angiographic room. One of these entrances must be large enough to admit stretchers and hospital beds with ease, while the other two entrances need only to be large enough to allow passage of the operating personnel. The room should be brightly illuminated with a rheostat control so that the overhead lights can be dimmed in conjunction with the use of the image intensification equipment. All electrical wiring must be concealed under the floor or in the walls and the radiographic tubes, television monitors, and image intensifiers must be suspended on overhead tracks to keep the floor area free of unnecessary equipment. The personnel can then move freely about the room, and the floor and walls can be readily cleaned. Cabinets are provided in the room for immediate availability of all catheters and materials used during the examinations.

In order to provide adequate space around the patient, the angiographic table should be placed in the center of the room. In addition to the main angiographic room, space should be allocated for use as personnel scrubbing areas, for storage of sterile and nonsterile equipment, for cleaning of instruments, and for a control panel area (Fig. 11.2). Since all the film-changer programming and radiographic exposures generally originate from the control room, it must contain a large viewing window affording a complete view of the patient and monitoring equipment at all times. The locating of automatic film processing units and radiographic view boxes close to the angiographic room is essential.

RADIOGRAPHIC GENERATORS

In angiography, images of contrast medium flowing rapidly through a pulsating vascular system must be obtained with high spatial and contrast resolution. This

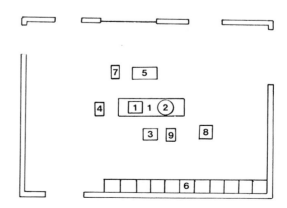

Figure 11.1. Design of an angiographic room and its components. (1) Angiographic table and film changer, (2) image intensifier, (3) television monitor, (4) radiographic tube, (5) instrument tray, (6) cabinets, (7) pressure injector, (8) anesthesia machine, (9) physiologic monitoring device.

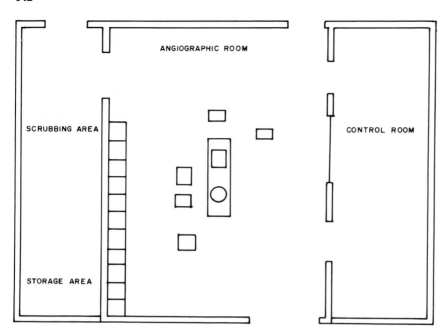

Figure 11.2. Design of the angiographic room scrubbing area, storage area, and control room.

requires the use of very short exposures and high tube currents. Because of this, single-phase 500 milliamperage (mA) generators are not suitable for angiography. These generators are only capable of delivering 50 mAs exposures in one-tenth of a second (500 mA × 0.1 sec = 50 mAs). In general, the one-tenth of a second exposure is too long, because the angiographic image appears unsharp due to the pulsating motion of the vessels. For abdominal angiography exposure times of 40 milliseconds (msec) or less are necessary, and for pulmonary angiography exposure times of 20 msec or less are required. Image contrast is also less with a 500 mA generator because it requires a high kVp in order to offset x-ray photon limitations arising from the limited mA generator capacity. This is a major disadvantage in angiography, since a high-contrast differentiation between the contrast medium in the blood vessels and the surrounding tissues is essential. To enhance image contrast in angiography, exposures should be made in the range of 70 to 80 kVp.[3] However, with a single-phase 500 mA generator, exposures in the range of 90 to 100 kVp are often required in order to maintain the proper film density. All of these problems have been solved, to a great extent, by the introduction of the 1,000 to 1,500 mA, three-phase generators. Generators of this type are ideal for angiography because they allow 100 to 150 mAs exposures to be made over times of 40 msec or less. In addition, the increased mAs generated by these units allows exposures to be made at the optimum 70 kVp range ensuring images of good contrast even with muscular or obese patients. These generators operate from a three-phase power line and, depending on the manu-

facturer and model, may produce a pattern of 6 or 12 pulses per cycle. With a 12-pulse generator, peak and average kilovoltage are almost identical (3 to 4 percent ripple) and are referred to as constant potential generators. Cine and spot-film cameras are readily adaptable to these generators as dependence on line frequency for exposure times and filming rates is eliminated.

Because of the above considerations, if a room is to be dedicated to the performance of angiographic procedures it should include at least one 1,000 to 1,500 mA constant potential generator from the beginning. Installing a 500 mA generator will undoubtedly place serious limitations on the room's productivity. Cine and spot-film cameras may not be readily adaptable to the 500 mA generator. If these are required in the future because of a slight change or expansion in service, a new generator may have to be purchased. Since the generator is expensive, it is less likely to be updated in the future, and the one that is installed initially most likely is going to have to remain in place throughout the duration of the use of the room.

RADIOGRAPHIC TUBES

Angiographic tubes are distinctly different from those used in general diagnostic radiology. The general diagnostic tube can sustain complete heat loading of the anode with a single exposure as there is usually time for the anode to cool between exposures. In angiography, numerous exposures are made within a short time, and there is virtually no time for anode cooling between exposures. Each angiographic exposure series, then, must be considered as a single exposure with regard to its anode heat loading and cooling characteristics. Maximum heat loading of the anode is referred to in kilowatt-seconds (kWs) and is calculated by multiplying kV by mA by time. Every angiographic tube has a maximum kWs rating, which must not be exceeded for any given exposure. In order to prevent exceeding of the maximum kWs rating, each tube is provided with a tube rating chart. These charts are based on the specific construction of the tube and on the specific design of the generator used to power it. A tube with a 0.3-mm focal spot, 12° target angle with an anode rotation of 10,000 rpms, and powered by a three-phase 12-pulsed generator must be correlated with the tube rating chart for these characteristics. The tube rating chart should then be carefully examined when there is any doubt about the maximum number of exposures that can be made at a given milliamperage, time, and kilovoltage. In practice a simplified chart may be used to establish quickly the maximum filming rates and total exposures that can be made at a given kVp and mA (Table 11.1). The more recently introduced generators, however, now employ more computer logic circuits to do these calculations for the technician and/or radiologist. Such microprocessors are preprogrammed with the individual tubes kWs maximum ratings and automatically compute the kWs based upon the chosen kVp and mA settings. If an overload condition is present, the technician is warned through visual displays, the filming sequence aborted, and, on some units, alternative settings suggested. More sophisticated use of microprocessor logic in generator control can be anticipated in the near future.

A large number of x-ray tube focal-spot sizes are now available, and much effort has gone into their evaluation.[4,5,6,7] Careful consideration must be given to any focal spot-size selected because it not only affects the image but also the tube kWs ratings and field-size coverage as well. The major advantage of a small focal spot is that the spatial resolution is increased (Table 11.2). This resolution is increased irrespective of the object film distance and explains why a small focal spot of 0.3 mm or less is essential in magnification radiography. Unfortunately, with small focal-spot tubes, the permissible heat loading of the anode decreases. Consequently, the kVp and mAs per exposure, as well as the total number of exposures, are limited, rendering them unacceptable for use in routine angiographic examinations. Small focal spots are constructed by decreasing the incident angle of the anode (line-focus principle, see Chapter 5) as illustrated in Figure 11.3. As the incident angle decreases, the heel effect becomes a major factor affecting uniform field density and the size of the field coverage must be reduced to have acceptably uniform density. This is a major problem in routine angiographic examinations but offers no obstacle in magnification radiography as small fields coned to the area of interest are used. For routine angiographic studies, radiographic tubes with 0.6 mm to 1.2 mm focal spots are satisfactory, while in magnification radiography a 0.3 mm focal spot is required.

ANGIOGRAPHIC FILM CHANGERS

Film changers provide the means by which rapid serial images are obtained during the angiographic examination. These film changers are designed to use cut film or roll film. Each has certain advantages and disadvantages that must be weighed in choosing one type of design for a specific angiographic installation. Whichever type is chosen, the field size must be 14 by 14 inches whenever cardiac and visceral studies are to be performed.

Cut film changers are generally preferred because of the ease with which each individual film can be viewed following the exposure of an angiographic series and can be filed in regular film jackets. Roll film, on the other hand, has to be cut before it can be filed or stored in boxes in roll form. Two types of cut film

TABLE 11.1. **Tube Rating Chart, Three Phase Full-wave Rectification**

Maximum Load (kWs per exposure)		

Exposures per sec	2 exposures	5 exposures	10 exposures
1	6800	5000	3700
2	4200	3200	2500

Focal spot size 0.3 mm
Target angle 12 degrees
High speed anode rotation

TABLE 11.2. **Compromises between Magnification and Nonmagnification Focal Spots**

Effects	Magnification Focal Spot	Nonmagnification Focal Spot
Penumbra	Decreased	Increased
Unsharpness	Decreased	Increased
Resolution	Increased	Decreased
Tube ratings	Decreased	Increased
Anode rotation speed	Increased	Decreased
Target angle	Decreased	Increased
Field coverage	Decreased	Increased
Stop motion sharpness	Decreased	Increased
Exposure time	Increased	Decreased

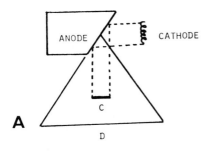

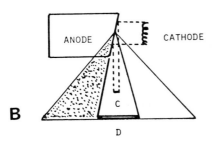

Figure 11.3. Accentuated diagram of angled anodes showing the decrease of apparent focal-spot size due to the anode heel effect. **A.** The large angled anode has a large apparent focal spot (C) and a large field (D) not affected by the anode heel effect. **B.** The small angled anode has a small apparent focal spot (C) but the field (D) is decreased due to the anode heel affect. The stippling indicates the portion of the x-ray beam affected by the anode heel affect.

changers are available. They are known as the cassette and cassetteless types. In the cassette type each film is placed into its own cassette before it is loaded into the changer, while in the cassetteless type the films are placed into loading magazines without cassettes before they are placed into the changer. The placing of each film into its designated slot in the loading magazine can be a tedious process. However, the darkroom technicians generally prefer this method to the time consuming process of unloading and loading each film into cassettes. Cassette film changers do offer better screen–film contact than noncassette changers. This is particularly true when vacuum-packed cardboard cassettes are used instead of non-vacuum-packed metal cassettes.[8] The metal cassettes are also heavier to carry than the cardboard cassettes. Replacing or updating the screens in either of these cassette systems is expensive as each screen in each cassette has to be purchased.

Cassetteless cut film changers contain a light-tight compartment through which the film moves. This eliminates the need for cassettes. The light-tight compartment also contains one set of screens, eliminating the need for a separate screen for each film. Screen–film contact is not as good with these changers as it is with

the cassette changers. Monthly screen–film contact tests are necessary to assure the optimal screen–film contact. Replacing or updating the screens in this system can be done frequently and inexpensively as only one set of screens has to be replaced. Transport of the films to and from the darkroom requires only the use of the loading and receiving magazines, eliminating the need to carry multiple cassettes.

Roll film changers are attractive because of their fast film transport mechanisms. This allows films to be exposed at a maximum rate of 12 per second. Exposure rates of this speed are important in angiocardiography, especially in pediatric disease, but have little use in visceral or neuroradiography. The main problems with roll film changers involve the handling, viewing, and filing of the rolls. To solve this problem, roll film changers are now being developed that cut the roll into 14-in by 14-in sections after the exposures are made. Both cut and roll film changers are now being developed with built-in image intensifiers. Traditionally, the image intensifier has been placed overhead and its fluorographic tube built underneath the angiographic table (Fig. 11.4). Film exposures are made with a separate radiographic tube placed over the top of the angiographic table. By building the image intensifier into the film changer under the table, the fluorographic tube can be eliminated from the system (Fig. 11.5). The overhead radiographic tube is then used for both fluoroscopy and filming of the angiographic series. These systems are called see-through film changers because during exposures the x-ray beam passes completely through the film changer, simultaneously exposing the films and activating the image intensifier. This allows the exposures of the angiographic series to be stored on video disc for instant replay and/or to be viewed on a television monitor at the same time they are recorded on film. If the injection is incorrect, it can be corrected immediately without having to wait for the films to be developed, or if the injection is correct, the catheter tip can be moved to a new location. Another advantage of the see-through film changer system is that the patient does not have to be moved between fluoroscopy and filming.

The major disadvantage of this system is the large amount of scatter radiation received by the examiner from using the overhead tube in fluoroscopy. This results in several times the radiation dose to the examiner than would be received with the traditional under-the-table fluoroscopy units unless a pulsed-type of fluoroscopic mode is used. Pulsed-mode fluoroscopy decreases the patient and radiologist irradiation burden at the expense of having a noncontinuous visual monitor of the catheter tip during catheter manipulation. However, independent of whether a pulsed or continuous mode of fluoroscopy is used, patient-produced

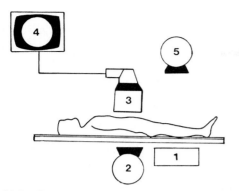

Figure 11.4. Diagram of the traditional image-intensifier radiographic system. (1) Film changer, (2) fluoroscopic tube, (3) image intensifier, (4) television monitor, (5) overhead radiographic tube.

x-ray scatter will still be present. Most of this scatter radiation can be removed with leaded-glass shields and lead aprons. Also, in order to keep the patient's radiation exposure to reasonable levels, it is important to remove the radiographic screens from the x-ray beam during fluoroscopy or to use the individual film cassette changers. The advantages and disadvantages of the see-through film changer system must be weighed carefully when comparing it to the traditional systems.

Most cut and roll film changers can be placed in the vertical position for cross-table lateral filming and biplane angiography. Biplane angiography in the frontal and lateral projections requires the use of two film changers to eliminate the need for separate injections with repositioning of the patient or the film changer. In order to eliminate the radiation cross-scatter inherent in biplane exposures, cut film changers are preferred over roll film changers. The reason for this is that the

films in a cut film changer can be alternately loaded. For example, the loading magazine of the frontal changer is loaded 1, 3, 5, and so forth, while the lateral changer is loaded 2, 4, 6, and so on. When the frontal exposure is made, the film in the lateral changer has not yet moved into position so it cannot become fogged from cross-scatter radiation and vice versa. With alternating loading techniques, the maximum exposure rates are 3 per second when the programmer is set for 6 per second. Alternating film techniques are impossible with roll film changers since a continuous roll of film is used. To achieve alternate filming with these changers would require the exposure of every other film. This would be impractical and result in a great waste of film. Crosshatched grids are used to reduce cross-scatter when biplane angiography is performed on these changers. These grids are also used with cut film changers when exposure rates greater than 3 per second are required since the films cannot be loaded alternatively but must be loaded in sequence.

Specially designed film changers are available for serial imaging of the abdominal aorta, pelvic vessels, and vasculature of both lower extremities with one injection of the contrast media. In order to include all this information in one angiographic series, these changers are equipped with four to six cassettes with inner measurements of 14×51 in. Because of the mechanics involved in the transport of these large cassettes, film exposures are limited to a maximum of 1 per second, and the total number of exposures available is less than with conventional film changers. These are not serious limitations because rapid filming techniques with numerous exposures are not required in peripheral angiography. In order to include the wide field of coverage required for these cassettes an additional radiographic tube must be installed with a source-to-image distance of 79 inches. Smaller cassettes (14×36 inches) can be obtained that allow the tube to be placed at a shorter source-to-image distance of 65 inches. These tubes are generally placed on ceiling mountings. Before this film changer is obtained, the angiographic room must be surveyed to make sure that it can accommodate such a large piece of equipment. Ideally, the changer should be stored in its functioning position at the foot of the angiographic table when not in use. This eliminates its repositioning underneath the ceiling mounted tube each time an extremity angiographic procedure is performed. If the room cannot comfortably accommodate this large cassette film changer, then these examinations will have to be done using a standard 14 in $\times$ 14 in film changer. By using standard film changers, extremities can be radiographed on tabletops that are programmed to move preset distances during the exposure sequence. This technique is less preferable than the long cassette film

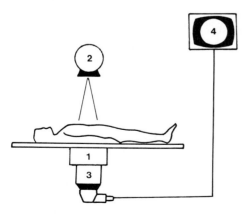

Figure 11.5. Diagram of the see-through changer film system. (1) Film changer, (2) overhead tube used for fluoroscopy and radiography, (3) image intensifier, (4) television monitor.

changer for peripheral angiography unless the ability to estimate the rate of flow of the contrast media through diseased vessels can be built into the tabletop movement. An advantage of this technique, however, is that film exposure can be programmed for each tabletop location to compensate for changes in x-ray attenuation between different body parts, such as between the pelvis and the extremities.

A recent innovative addition to the film changer panel has been computer microprocessor logic circuits. Not only do these computer circuits allow for variable combinations of film exposures (eg, 1/sec×2 sec, 3/sec ×2 sec) in an operator selectable mode, but many different programs can be stored simultaneously for single-button access. Thus, programs for aortic arch studies, abdominal aortic studies, pulmonary artery studies, etc, can be preprogrammed into the microprocessor's memory and then retrieved randomly without reprogramming.

ANGIOGRAPHIC TABLES

Tables with specially designed tops and pedestal bases are available for use in angiographic suites. Like most radiographic tables their tops are made of radiolucent prestressed plastic-foam. There is, however, a new trend toward constructing these tops from carbon-fiber reinforced plastic. Tops constructed from this material are attractive because they are stronger and have less attenuation of the x-ray beam than the plastic-foam tops. Carbon-fiber reinforced plastic tops have an attenuation coefficient equivalent to 0.6 mm of A1 at 100 kVp while plastic-foam tops have an attenuation coefficient equivalent to 1.2 mm of A1 at 100 kVp. This is an important feature as all of the fluoroscopic positioning of the catheter and most of the radiographic exposures are carried out with the x-ray beam traversing the tabletop. Another important consideration is the surface of the tabletop. It can be either flat or concave. Elderly patients may find the concave tops difficult to negotiate when moving from the stretcher onto the table due to its concavity. The flat top eliminates this difficulty. Regardless which type of top is used, it is essential that it be freely movable in either direction and contain a good set of locks. Most tables are equipped with a cantilevered four-way floating tabletop motion. This allows the top to be moved from side to side within a range of 10 to 11 inches from the center line. Longitudinal movement is generally 50 to 59 inches toward the head or foot end of the table, as measured from the center of the table base. A panning handle with a push button lock release attached to the side of the tabletop affords the examiner good control of the tabletop movement. The examiner or assistant can then readily move the top in any direction under the fluoroscope

during catheterizations and lock the top into position over the film changer when an angiographic film series is to be obtained. In addition to the lock-release button it is also convenient for the panning handle to contain the fluoroscopic shutter controls. The sides and head of the table should be readily adaptable for the attachment of accessories. These include arm boards, headrest extensions, compression devices, restraining handles, high-intensity lights, IV poles, transducer holders, and even the contrast injector (for moving-table injection programs).

The entire tabletop assembly is supported by the base or pedestal. Elevating mechanisms, for use in magnification angiography, are located in the table base. This allows the tabletop to be moved up or down 33 to 51 inches above the floor. Manufacturers specify this by stating that the table has a 7 or 18 inch elevating base.

Another advantage of the elevating base is that it facilitates movement of the patient on and off a stretcher as the tabletop can always be adjusted to the level of the stretcher. It can also be adjusted to provide optimal tabletop film changer distance and examiner comfort. Fluoroscopy can be carried out with the table partially elevated at the fluoroscopic tube, and the collimator is raised and lowered automatically with the top; thus the distance between the fluoroscopic tube and image intensifier remains constant.

Optionally available with the table base is the Bucky tray. It should be constructed so that it does not restrict the vertical clearance of the film changer below the table or obstruct horizontal fluoroscopic viewing.

Table bases are also available that contain oxygen and suction outlets. These are preferred to wall-mounted oxygen and suction outlets because connecting tubes are not stretched across the room thus limiting access to the table.

Newer table mountings are being developed that eliminate the table base completely. The angiographic table is suspended from the ceiling by an overhead bridge. The table is virtually suspended in midair by a single support arm mounted on the overhead bridge. Total body suspension tables of this type are suited for use with the advanced C- or U-arm imaging systems.

IMAGE INTENSIFIERS

The image intensifier converts the x-ray beam into a visual image (Fig. 11.6; see also Chapter 7). To accomplish this the x-ray beam is first changed into light photons by a fluorescent screen. Screens made of cesium iodide are considerably better than those made of zinc cadmium because they convert a higher percentage of incident x-ray quanta into light.[9] The light emanating from the cesium iodide screen is then changed into

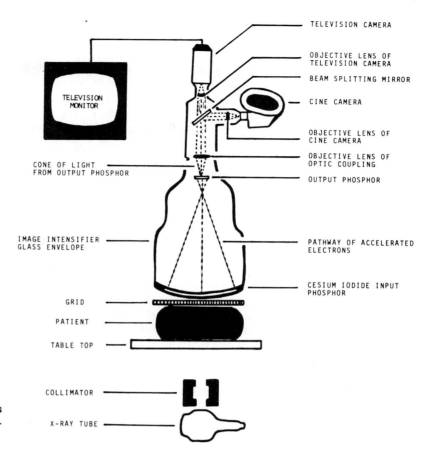

TELEVISION CAMERA

OBJECTIVE LENS OF
TELEVISION CAMERA

BEAM SPLITTING MIRROR

CINE CAMERA

OBJECTIVE LENS OF
CINE CAMERA

OBJECTIVE LENS OF
OPTIC COUPLING

OUTPUT PHOSPHOR

TELEVISION
MONITOR

CONE OF LIGHT
FROM OUTPUT PHOSPHOR

IMAGE INTENSIFIER
GLASS ENVELOPE

PATHWAY OF ACCELERATED
ELECTRONS

CESIUM IODIDE INPUT
PHOSPHOR

GRID

PATIENT

TABLE TOP

COLLIMATOR

X-RAY TUBE

Figure 11.6. Diagram showing the various components of a closed-circuit television system.

electrons, which are accelerated through a high-voltage field and strike a smaller output screen. Once the electrons strike the output screen they are converted back into light to produce an amplified light image. This light image can be viewed on a closed circuit television system or recorded on video tapes or discs, cine cameras, and 70 to 105 mm spot-film devices. A mirror system can also be used. It has a higher resolution than any of the amplified television viewing systems because the mirror views the light image directly from the image intensifier. Manipulating a catheter at a patient's groin while trying to look into a mirror centered over the patient's upper abdomen is awkward. It is also important for the assistants to be able to view the fluoroscopic image with the examiner so that the catheter placement can be marked and the catheter correctly positioned over the film changer for the angiographic film series. For these reasons, the closed-circuit television system is preferred to the mirror system even though there is some degradation of resolution with its use. With the closed-circuit television system, the amplified light image on the image intensifier output screen is focused onto a television camera pickup tube (Fig. 11.6). The lead monoxide Vidicon television camera pickup tube should be used. It has a short lag time and produces sharp images of rapidly

moving objects without any significant loss of contrast. A pleasing picture is also obtained on the television monitor because the lead monoxide Vidicon tube has a low level of scintillation noise. Other types of television camera pickup tubes are available, but they are either not as good as or have no advantage over the lead monoxide Vidicon tube. They are the standard high-resolution Vidicon tube and the Orthicon tube. The standard high resolution Vidicon tube has a prolonged lag time, which causes blurring of the image. This can be a problem in examinations of fast-moving objects such as the heart. Although the Orthicon is much more sensitive than the Vidicon it has an increased signal to noise ratio.[9] This electronic noise appears as snow on the television monitor. For this reason, the Orthicon cannot be operated at its full potential and its functional sensitivity is equal to that of the lead monoxide Vidicon tube.

Linking the television camera pickup tube to a television monitor completes the closed-circuit television component of the image intensifier. In selecting a television monitor, its size (diagonal length), line rate, and band width should be considered. A 14 inch monitor is adequate for most angiographic installations. Larger monitors require greater viewing distances than are usually available in most angiographic rooms. Line rates are important because they form the vertical resolution of the monitor. Television monitors are available with 525, 625, and 875 or more lines per frame. Band width is related to the horizontal detail of the monitor (see Chapter 7). Most biomedical television monitors use a band width of at least 5 MHz. For a cesium iodide image intensifier with a lead monoxide Vidicon tube, a 14 inch monitor with an 875-line rate and a band width of 15 MHz would produce high-detail images. Adequate images can also be obtained with this system using a monitor with a 525 line rate and a 5 MHz band width.

Two controls, one for brightness and one for contrast, should be provided on the monitor. All other controls should be adjusted only by the service representative.

Some image intensifiers and x-ray tubes are mounted on specially designed C- or U-arm assemblies so any conceivable view of the patient's anatomy can be imaged simply by maneuvering the arm assembly and not the patient. These x-ray tube–intensifier assemblies are especially useful in neuroradiology, cardiac radiology, and emergency vascular radiology procedures where precise imaging positions are mandatory or patient movement must be minimized. The disadvantage of this equipment is that considerably higher scatter radiation dose can be given to the radiologist and/or technician because the variable locations of the tube and intensifier relative to the patient make shielding of scattered x-rays difficult. One solution to this problem appears to lie in the pulsed fluoroscopy modes of operation. Such equipment is available with pulse modes of 5, 7.5, 10, 15, 20, and 30 pulses per sec. Thus, if catheter tip position location is critical, such as during catheter manipulation, the 20 to 30 pulses/sec modes can be used; otherwise, the 5 to 10 pulses/sec modes would be used in order to minimize the intensity of the scattered x-rays.

Once the image intensifier is installed in the angiographic room it can be used to provide images for various recording systems. These include spot-film cameras, cine cameras, and video tape or disc recording systems. The spot-film camera and the cine camera record the image from the output screen of the image intensifier while the video recordings are obtained from the output of the television camera tube.

Spot-film cameras that use either roll film or cut film with 70, 90, 100, or 105 mm film sizes are available. Film magazines are available with capacities of 150 to 430 exposures. These films can be exposed at rates up to 12 frames per second. Because of this rapid film rate, some medical centers are filming angiographic procedures with spot-film cameras. This provides a great savings in film cost, but the image detail with spot-film cameras is not as good as it is with direct radiography since the image must be recorded from the image intensifier. For this reason, a standard film changer with direct radiography is preferred for most angiographic procedures. As the resolving power of the image intensifiers improves, more angiography will be done with spot-film cameras. Another disadvantage of the spot-film camera is the difficulty in processing the film. Most film processors are designed to handle 14 × 14 in cut film. It is an added inconvenience to have to bother with a film format size that is different from the rest of the films used in a radiology department. Film processors designed specifically for the processing of camera film are available.

Cine cameras that use either a 16 mm or 35 mm film size are available. For the most part, 16 mm film is less expensive and easier to handle than the 35 mm film. More information can be recorded on the 35 mm frame since it has four times the area of a 16 mm frame. This increased filming area produces images with higher resolution than the 16 mm film. Both high-resolution images and the ability to project these images before a large audience can be achieved by an initial recording of the image on 35 mm film and transfer of it onto a 16 mm fine-grain copy film for projection. Cine cameras can obtain filming rates up to 150 frames per second. To accomplish this, cine cameras must be operated in conjunction with three-phase, 12-pulse, constant potential generators. These generators must also have rapid switching capabilities so that the x-rays can be synchronized with the shutter speed of the cine camera. This prevents the patient from being continuously irradiated regardless of whether the cine camera shutter is opened or closed. Modern cine cameras switch the generator on only when their shutters are open. This requires extremely rapid switching of the x-ray beam on and off during a filming series. Such rapid switching causes the x-rays to occur in pulses controlled by either the constant potential generator or grid-controlled x-ray tubes. The wave from the generator must be constant so that each frame of the cine film is exposed with the same density. Since the cine camera records its information from the output screen of the image intensifier, its resolution is not as good as that obtained by direct radiography. This loss in image resolution is compensated for in cine angiography by the fact that the image quality of cine film is improved by the integration power of the human eye when the projected cine film is viewed at fast film rates. Field sizes and magnification factors can be controlled in cinefluorography by changing the ratio of the focal length of cine camera lens.

Since cine cameras are most useful for studying the dynamic flow of contrast media through the heart, they are used extensively in cardiac angiography. Cine cameras with a frame speed of 250 frames per second are of particular use in pediatric cardiac angiography.

Spot-film cameras, cine cameras, and video recorders can be mounted on the output screen of the image intensifiers for simultaneous viewing and recording of the image. This is an important advantage when see-through film changers are used, as it ensures that the desired field of interest is being recorded during the injection process. To accomplish simultaneous viewing and recording, the light image from the output screen of the image intensifier is split into two parts by a reflective mirror. Ten percent goes to the television camera pickup tube while 90 percent goes to either the spot film camera, cine camera, or video recorder.

Video tapes and discs offer another means of recording an image from the image intensifier by recording the video signal of the television camera pickup. The major advantage of video recorders can be put to practical use by simultaneously video-taping a cine recording. The need to process the cine film to see if the right image has been obtained is then eliminated as an instant replay of the cine recording is available on the video tape. The examiner can study the video image immediately to make sure the proper projection, injection, and field of view were included on the higher resolution cine film. Instant replays provided by the video tapes and discs also allow the examiner to study more carefully the fast events that were recorded during the cine filming without being concerned about operating the fluoroscopic equipment.

Video tape recorders or tape decks are available with recording widths of 1/2, 3/4, 1, or 2 inches. The magnetic tapes can be supplied in the reel-to-reel or cassette formats. The resolution of video tape decks is improved with wider recording tapes since more information can be recorded in the larger area. Resolution is also dependent upon the tape speed and the size of the gap in the record or replay heads. Since it is impractical to move the tape at rapid speeds, this is compensated for by moving the heads at rapid speeds. The tape usually moves at 10 cm per second while the recording head moves at 30 meters per second. A narrow gap in the recording or replay head also produces an image with higher resolution. In order to use a recording or replay head with a narrow gap, a higher band width from the video signal of the television camera pickup tube is required. Before any video recorder is obtained it is important to remember that the band width of the recorder must correspond with the band width of the television pickup tube and of the television monitor used in the image intensifier system.

If a video recorder is to be obtained for single frame image display rather than motion image display, a disc recorder is preferred over the tape recorder. The disc recorder can produce single-frame images with higher quality than the tape recorder. A previous disadvantage of older video disc recording systems was that only a few images could be recorded. Video disc that will allow for the recording of up to 500 images can now be purchased.

After reviewing all the different available types of image recording systems, it is important to understand how they can be coupled to the image intensifier. This should be done so that the recorder receives the light image from the output phosphor of the image intensifier with as little loss in quality and intensity as possible. Currently, two coupling systems are available for angiography: the optical and fiberoptic coupling systems. The optical system must be used if simultaneous viewing and recording are required. If the image intensifier is to be used only for fluoroscopy, then the fiberoptic coupling system may be preferred.

The optical system consists of an objective lens that takes the cone of light from the output phosphor of the image intensifier and converts it into a parallel light beam. This parallel beam is necessary so that a reflecting mirror can be inserted to split the beam into two parts. The reflecting mirror is called a beam splitter. It is used to reflect the light image from the image intensifier output phosphor onto the objective lenses of the television camera and a spot-film or a cine camera simultaneously. This allows the image to be viewed on the television monitor at the same time it is being recorded on the spot-film or cine camera. Although simultaneous viewing and recording are obtained, some intensity of the light image is lost due to the presence of the lenses in the optical system. The optical system does not interfere with the image resolution as long as the lenses are kept in focus. Resolution is limited by the image intensifier and not the optical system. A good optical system can resolve approximately 8–9 line pairs per millimeter while an image intensifier can only resolve 4–5 line pairs per millimeter.

The other method of coupling utilizes fiberoptic bundles. These are capable of transmitting light with a minimal loss of intensity. Fiberoptic couplings are small and lighter than optical couplings. Their use can reduce the height of an image intensifier by 16 cm and make it easier to use. The main disadvantage of a fiberoptic coupling system is that a beam splitter cannot be used. So simultaneous viewing and imaging cannot be performed without the use of the video signal. This limits the resolution of the fiberoptic system and makes it a poor choice for use with spot-film or cine cameras. It is, however, ideal for use with the television camera.

Spot-film cameras, cine cameras, video recorders, television camera pickup tubes, television monitors, and their coupling systems were included in this section on image intensifiers because they all must function together as a unit (Fig. 11.6). Of all the components in the system the image intensifier is the most important.

It would be superfluous to obtain the finest components available and link them to a poor functioning image intensifier. This is why it is extremely important to obtain a cesium iodide image intensifier from the beginning. The average resolving power of a good cesium iodide image intensifier tube is about four line pairs per millimeter. This means that the total system cannot resolve anything greater than four line pairs per millimeter on film. An image intensifier with less resolving power would degrade the entire system.

GRIDS

Grids, like collimators, are used to enhance image quality by decreasing the amount of scatter radiation that reaches the film or image intensifier. To accomplish this, they are placed in front of the input phosphor of the image intensifier and on the surface of the film changer.

For direct radiography with a film changer, a focused grid with 50 to 80 lines per inch and a ratio of 8:1 may be used. Focused grids are necessary because of the short focal film distances used in angiography. The lead strips in these grids are angled slightly so that grid cutoff does not occur from the accentuated divergence of the x-ray beam that results when the focal film distance is decreased. Since most of the exposures are made with a focal film distance of 40 inches, a grid with a 40-inch focal distance is used. In practice this does not necessarily mean that the grid has to be used at exactly 40 inches but can be used within the focusing range of the grid. This focusing range is indicated on the grid. A good working focusing range is 30 to 60 inches for a 40-inch focused grid with a ratio of 8:1.

The grid ratio is defined as the ratio of the height of the lead strips to the distance between them. The higher the ratio, the more radiation the grid will absorb and, therefore, more radiation will be required to penetrate through the grid to the film. It has been shown that above the ratio of 8:1 there is little additional cleanup of scatter and more x-ray technique (increased patient dose) is required to achieve the desired film density. These grids are also suitable for 70 kVp used in angiography. Above 90 kVp, 12:1 grids are preferred.

Lines per inch indicates the number of lead strips per inch of the grid. In practice, when grids are constructed with many lines per inch, both the thickness and height of the lead strips are decreased. These grids are thinner, and improve contrast less than grids of comparable ratios with fewer lines per inch. For comparison, a 103 line 10:1 grid improves contrast about the same as an 80 line 8:1 grid.

Crosshatched grids have two layers of lead strips with one set at right angles to the other. These grids provide better absorption than linear grids, but also require higher radiation levels. For these reasons they are used mainly in neuroradiology for performing simultaneous biplane angiography.

For fluoroscopy a low-dose 6:1 80 line grid is used.

ANGIOGRAPHIC INJECTORS

An angiographic injector is used to deliver the volume of contrast media needed to make the vasculature radiopaque. The injector should produce flow-rate injections, use disposable syringes, and be electrically grounded, mobile, simple to operate, and triggered by a remote device.

The injector head contains a screw rotated by an electric motor (Fig. 11.7). Rotating the screw in a forward direction injects the contrast media while reverse rotations allows the injecting syringe to be filled with contrast media. The injector head is operated and programmed by the circuitry and switches on the control panel of the injector (Fig. 11.7). Two methods of injection are available: pressure-controlled and flow-rate injections. On a flow-rate injector the switches can be set so that a precise volume of contrast media is injected in a precise length of time within the pressure capabilities of the injector. Most flow-rate mechanical injectors are capable of producing pressures up to 1,200 pounds per square inch.

Pressure-limiting switches are provided on the control panel so that the pressure can be limited to obtain the desired flow rates. If the pressure-limiting switch is set for a pressure lower than that needed for a desired flow rate, a flow rate below that desired will be obtained. When the pressure-limiting switch is set for a pressure higher than needed for a desired flow rate, only the pressure needed to obtain the desired flow rate will be used by the injector. Setting the pressure-limiting switch at a level than higher necessary is spoken of as setting the backup pressure. This maneuver is used to ensure that the injector is programmed with enough pressure to obtain the desired flow rate. Injectors operated by these means are called constant-flow injectors because as long as they have the pressure capability they will keep the flow constant. They are also called flow-rate injectors because a constant flow in cubic centimeters can be programmed to occur in specified lengths of time.

Since in angiography the injection of contrast media must be done rapidly, the time used is one second. The flow rate can be increased by injecting a higher volume

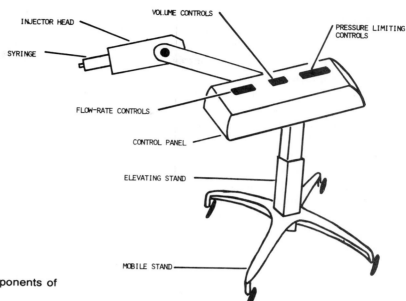

Figure 11.7. Diagram showing the various components of an angiographic injector.

per second or decreased by injecting a lower volume per second. With a flow-rate injector a total volume of contrast can be delivered in numerous ways. For example, a total volume of 40 cc can be injected at 40 cc/sec for 1 second, 20 cc/sec for 2 seconds, or 10 cc/sec for 4 seconds. The disadvantage of this system is that the maximum flow rate in cc/sec must be known for each type of catheter and contrast media used. It is also just as important to know the equivalent pressure in PSI (pounds per square inch) necessary to obtain these flow rates. Exceeding the maximum flow rate or PSI tolerated by a catheter results in its rupture.

Charts providing this information for each catheter can be kept in the angiographic room. An example is shown in Table 11.3. To demonstrate its use suppose an injector is set to deliver 40 cc/sec of contrast media (X) through a 6.5 French polyethylene pigtail catheter 100 cm long with an end hole and 12 side holes, at a pressure limit of 1,000 pounds per square inch. As programmed this injector would be allowed to use 1,000 PSI to keep the flow rate constant at 40 cc/sec. The catheter probably would rupture as its maximum flow rate is 23 cc/sec and maximum PSI is 650. Consulting the chart before using the injector would have

prevented this mishap since the 7.1 French size catheter would have been used. From Table 11.3 it can be seen that the 7.1 French size polyethylene pigtail catheter can withstand a maximum flow rate of 43 cc/sec at an equivalent pressure of 1,025 PSI. One way of preventing the 6.5 French catheter from bursting would have been to decrease the limit of pressure to 600 PSI. Although this would have prevented the catheter from bursting, it only would have injected a flow rate of approximately 20 cc/sec. This amount is considerably less than that desired by the examiner and probably would not have produced a satisfactory image. Under these circumstances it is good to have a flow-rate meter built into the injector so that the examiner can immediately determine the problem. This will eliminate unnecessary inspections of the other angiographic components for the source of the unsatisfactory image.

A flow-rate injector is also available with a rate/pressure computer. The computer is used before the injector to predict what pressure is needed to achieve the selected flow rate. This requires programming the computer with information about the catheter and contrast media before each injection is made. If the catheter specifications and desired flow-rate combination re-

TABLE 11.3. **Catheter Flow Rate Chart**

Type Catheter	French Size	Length (cm)	No. Side Holes	Maximum flow rate (cc/sec)	Equivalent Pressure (PSI)
Polyethylene pigtail	6.5	100	12	23	650
Polyethylene pigtail	7.1	100	12	43	1025

quire a pressure greater than that selected, an amber light flashes to warn the examiner that the desired flow rate will not be achieved. A different catheter or higher pressure may then be used to obtain the flow-rate desired. The injector can be used with or without the computer assistance, and injections can be made according to any pressure set on the control panel.

The pressure-control mode of injection is quite different from the constant flow-rate mode. A rotating screw drive is also used to power the injector head, but instead of the power being adjusted to keep the flow rate constant it is adjusted to keep the pressure at the back of the injecting syringe constant. Circuitry and switches on the control panel are then used to control the pressure and not the flow rate. The disadvantage of these injectors is that the relationship between the pressure at the back of the injecting syringe and pressure and flow at the catheter tip varies with the catheter and contrast media. To determine flow rates requires meticulous calibrations of each catheter used. Since numerous catheters and flow rates are employed in angiography, these calibrations have become too numerous to perform, thus making pressure-controlled injectors impractical.

Since the angiographic injection is in a good position to conduct electricity through the contrast media filled catheter to the patient, it must be properly grounded. Therefore the manufacturer's instructions must be understood and followed carefully before any examinations are undertaken.

In order to move the injector freely about the room, the injector should be supported on a mobile stand. If magnification angiography is to be done, the stand should be able to raise and lower the injector head so that it is always above the tabletop. Alternatively, the injector must be affixed to the tabletop so it can move with it.

Clear syringes should be used with the injector so that the examiner at all times can see the amount of contrast media and any air or air bubbles present in the syringe. Disposable plastic syringes are preferred over nondisposable glass syringes because the need to clean and maintain them is eliminated.

A remote-control hand switch is necessary for triggering the injection from the control room and out of the immediate area of radiation exposure. The hand switch should operate so that when the button is pressed the injection starts and when it is released the injection is stopped. Programmers that trigger the injector should be equipped with a system for stopping an injection once it has begun. A practical application for the examiner-controlled injection is that if the catheter ruptures at the beginning of an injection, it can be terminated immediately. This prevents the remainder of the contrast media from being disseminated about the room. If a patient moves a great deal at the begin-

ning of an injection, the injection can be terminated immediately before the entire volume of contrast media has been injected.

Before an injector is purchased, care should be taken to note if it will interface properly with film changers, x-ray generators, spot-film and cine cameras. This interfacing is important and permits automatic control of all events in an injection program. By synchronizing the injector with the film-changer programmer and x-ray generator one can obtain the best diagnostic results and reduce the human error factor to a minimum.

PREVENTIVE MAINTENANCE

After the angiographic equipment has been installed and checked by the company representatives, the radiologists, and the hospital or departmental radiation physicist, the hospital or department can officially accept the equipment for clinical use. During the first few weeks of operation, most parts and service are under warranty by the manufacturer. During this time, it is important for the radiologist, technicians, and the physicist to become familiar with the intricacies of the equipment's operation and to set up a program of quality control and preventive maintenance. In general, the x-ray generators and tabletop need to be serviced every three to four months to prevent potential drifting of the operating kVp settings and lubricated to prevent wear on bearings or other moving parts. The film changers need to have their screens checked and cleaned weekly with an antistatic solution and replaced every six to twelve months, depending upon use (see Chapter 20). The contrast-media injector should be cleaned daily and also covered by a service contract so breakdown time can be minimized and new injector components added as they are developed. Finally, continuous surveillance for degradation of image quality needs to be conducted by the radiologist weekly or monthly with an anthropomorphic phantom. Careful maintenance in general will make for better equipment reliability and a happier angiographic team.

REFERENCES

1. Bierman HR: Selective arterial catherization. Springfield, Ill., Charles C Thomas, 1969, p 68
2. Brinker RA, Skucas J: Radiology special procedure room. Baltimore, University Park Press, 1973, p 3
3. Reuter SR, Redman HC: Gastrointestinal Angiography, 2 ed. Philadelphia, W B Saunders Company, 1977, p 359
4. Bookstein JJ, Voegeli E: A critical analysis of magnification radiology. Laboratory Investigation. Radiology 98: 23-30, 1971

5. Mattson O: Focal spot variations with exposure data-important factors in daily routine. Acta Radiol Diagn (Stockholm) 7:161, 1968

6. Milne ENC: The role and performance of minute focal spots in roentgenology, with special reference to magnification. CRC Crit Rev Radiol Sci 2:269-310, 1971

7. Rao GUV, Soong A: Physical characteristics of modern microfocus x-ray tubes. AM J Roentgenol Radium Ther Nucl Med 119:626-634, 1973

8. Tenner MS, Wood EH: Evaluation of the vacuum cassette in neuroradiologic diagnosis. Acta Radiol (diag), 9:77-82, 1969

9. Thompson TT: A practical Approach to Modern X-ray Equipment, 1 ed. Boston, Little Brown and Co, 1978, p 83

10. Christensen EE, Curry TS III, Dowdey JE: An Introduction to the Physics of Diagnostic Radiology, 2 ed. Philadelphia, Lea and Febiger, 1978, p 104

CHAPTER 12

Ultrasound: Basic Principles

RONALD R. PRICE
THOMAS JONES
ARTHUR C. FLEISCHER
A. EVERETTE JAMES, JR.

Ultrasound is defined as acoustical waves that have frequencies greater than 20,000 cycles/sec, which represents the upper limit of perception by the human ear. Unlike electromagnetic waves which can propagate through a vacuum, ultrasound is a mechanical wave phenomenon and, as such, requires a medium for its propagation. The velocity of sound depends upon the physical characteristics of the medium, specifically, the density and compressibility. The formation of images of internal body structures is based upon the SONAR (Sound Navigation and Ranging) principle that was developed by the military during World War II to detect underwater objects (Fig. 12.1).

The SONAR technique is used to determine the location of an object within a medium by measuring the time interval between the production of an ultrasonic pulse and the detection of its echo resulting from the reflections from the object's surface. By measuring the time interval (t) between the transmitted and detected pulse, we can calculate the distance (S) between the transmitter and the object by the following equation:

$$S = V \cdot t/2 \tag{1}$$

where V is the velocity of the sound in the medium. The factor of 2 arises because the pulse must travel to the object and return. In medical imaging, the medium is soft tissue and the reflecting objects are the internal organs. The velocity of sound is not equal in all soft tissues (Table 12.1). All commercial instruments, however, assume a constant velocity of 1540 meters per second in order that the SONAR equation may be solved. This value represents the average velocity of sound in soft tissue.

Ultrasonic pulses are referred to as waves. A wave implies any phenomenon that has a cyclic variation. A sound wave consists of alternating regions of high pressure (compression) and low pressure (rarefaction) that travel outward through a medium from the sonic source. At any point in the medium, the pressure will exhibit a cyclic variation (wave) (Fig. 12.2).

Any wave motion may be described by three parameters: (1) wavelength: the physical distance between any two similar points on the wave (eg, distance between two rarefaction minima or two compression maxima); (2) frequency: the number of complete cyclic variations that occur per second at a given point; and (3) velocity; the speed at which the wave propagates through the medium.

Mathematically:

$$V = f \cdot \lambda \tag{2}$$

where V = velocity (meters/sec), f = frequency (cycles /sec, Hertz = 1 cycle/sec), and λ = wavelength (meter).

GENERATION AND DETECTION OF ULTRASOUND

The device that is used to generate and detect ultrasound is commonly referred to as a transducer. The most important component of the transducer is a thin

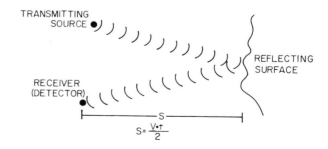

Figure 12.1. Illustration of SONAR principle. The distance between the source of ultrasound and a reflecting surface can be calculated if the time (t) required for a pulse to travel from the transmitting source to the surface and then back to the receiver is measured. The SONAR principle assumes a constant velocity of propagation (V).

TABLE 12.1.   Ultrasound Velocities in Different Human Tissues

Tissue	Velocity (m/sec)
Water (20°C)	1480
Blood	1580
Bone	2240
Brain	1540
Fat	1450
Kidney	1560
Liver	1550
Muscle	1580
Soft tissue (average)	1540

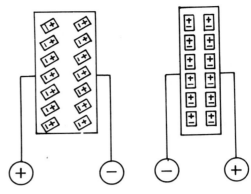

Figure 12.3. A piezoelectric crystal is composed of dipoles that are firmly bound in a crystalline matrix. When an electric field is applied across the surfaces of the crystal, the dipoles rotate under the applied force causing the crystal thickness to change.

(less than 1 mm thick) piezoelectric crystal, which is made up of dipoles (a molecule that appears to have one end positively charged and the other negatively charged) that are firmly bound in a crystaline structure (Fig. 12.3). The dipoles are arranged in an orderly symmetric manner such that when an electric field is placed across the crystal the dipoles will realign and thus change the physical dimensions of the crystal. If an electric field (voltage) is suddenly applied across the crystal faces and then quickly removed, the crystal will vibrate. The vibrating crystal, when coupled to tissue, gives rise to a sonic wave which propagates into the body.

The echoes that return from reflecting surfaces within the body are detected by the reverse of the piezoelectric effect. When the crystal is placed in the path of an acoustic wave, the surfaces of the crystal will be forced to vibrate. The physical movement of the crystal surfaces causes a small measurable voltage to appear across the surfaces.

Some naturally occurring materials exhibit piezoelectric properties; for example, quartz and Rochell salt. Most of the crystals used in medical transducers today are man-made crystals consisting of some form of barium titanate and lead zirconate titanate (PZT).

The thickness of the piezoelectric crystal determines its operating frequency (f). The crystal is constructed to have a thickness equal to one-half wavelength as determined by the wave equation where the velocity is taken equal to the velocity of the crystal.

In medical sonography, the crystal is made to vibrate at its natural frequency by a single voltage pulse. The time interval between the initiation of the wave and the cessation of all vibrations is called the ring-down time. Because the transducer serves as both a transmitter and a receiver, a very long ring-down time is unsatisfactory for ultrasonic imaging. Because the transducer cannot send and receive at the same time, the vibrations are damped to a few wavelengths by a backing block that is attached to the crystal. Backing blocks are made of combinations of tungsten and rubber powder in an epoxy resin. Typically in medical imaging systems (pulse-echo), the transducer is pulsed approximately once every millisecond.

The pulse length is typically only 1 to 10 microseconds long (Fig. 12.4). Therefore, the crystal is generating waves only a small fraction of the time and thus is available for detecting returning echoes most of the time.

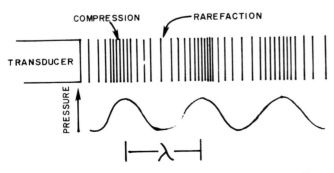

Figure 12.2. A sound wave propagating through a medium. Tissue consists of alternating regions of high pressure (compression) and low pressure (rarefaction). The wavelength (λ) is the distance between corresponding points on the wave.

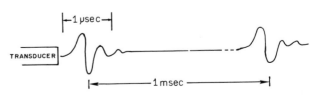

Figure 12.4. The transducer is pulsed approximately one thousand times a second (every msec). However, the pulse length is only about one millionth of a second long (1 μsec). Therefore, the transducer is busy producing sound only a small fraction of the time. The rest of the time it can "listen" for returning echoes.

INTERACTION WITH MATTER

When an ultrasonic beam is incident upon a boundary between two tissue interfaces, part of the beam is reflected and part is transmitted into the second medium (Fig. 12.5). If within the second medium another interface is encountered, the same processes will also apply. The fraction of the incident beam intensity that is reflected depends upon the acoustic impedances of the two tissues. Acoustic impedance is a fundamental property of matter. For longitudinal ultrasonic waves (vibrational motion in the same direction as the wave propagates) acoustic impedance (Z) is equal to the product of the material density and the velocity of sound in the material.

$$Z = \rho \cdot V \qquad (3)$$

where Z = acoustic impedance (Rayls), ρ = density (gm/cm^3), and V = velocity of sound (cm/sec). For practical purposes, all ultrasonic propagation in soft tissue is via longitudinal waves. Transverse wave propagation (vibration perpendicular to propagation) may exist to some degree in bone.

It can be shown that the fraction (R) of the incident beam intensity that is reflected at an interface between two tissues is given by:

$$R = (Z_1 - Z_2 / Z_1 + Z_2)^2 \qquad (4)$$

where Z_1 and Z_2 are the acoustic impedances of the two tissues. This relationship shows that the greater the difference between Z_1 and Z_2, the greater will be the reflected intensity. Table 12.2 shows the percent reflectance for a number of tissue interfaces encountered within the body.

Any interface involving air as one of the components will be an impenetrable barrier for the ultra-

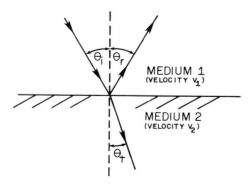

Figure 12.5. An ultrasonic beam incident upon a surface at angle θ_i will result in a fraction of the beam intensity being reflected at an angle θ_r ($\theta_r = \theta_i$) and a fraction transmitted into medium 2 at an angle θ_t. V_1 and V_2 are the velocities of propagation of the sound in medium 1 and medium 2, respectively. Since $\theta_i \neq \theta_t$ in general, the wave front will appear to be bent, ie, refracted.

TABLE 12.2. Ultrasound Reflected Energy Properties of Human Tissue

Interface	Reflected Energy
	(%)
Blood/muscle	0.07
Kidney/fat	0.64
Muscle/fat	1.08
Muscle/bone	41.23
Air/soft tissue	99.99

sound. For this reason, the transducer is carefully coupled to the skin via mineral oil or gel in a manner that will eliminate all air bubbles.

The fraction of the ultrasonic beam that remains after reflection is transmitted into the second medium (Fig. 12.5). The transmitted beam will in general deviate from its original direction. The degree of deviation depends upon the relative velocity of sound in the two media. Similar to light, the direction of the transmitted beam is given by Snell's Law:

$$\sin\theta_t / \sin\theta_i = V_2 / V_1 \qquad (5)$$

where V_1 is the velocity in medium 1, V_2 the velocity in medium 2, and θ_i and θ_t are the incident angle and transmitted angle, respectively, of the beam as defined in Figure 12.5.

When an ultrasonic beam passes through tissue, the beam is attenuated by absorption and scattering. The vibrational motion imparted to the particles making up the tissues is ultimately dissipated in the form of random molecular motion (heat). A small rise in tissue temperature may result. The amount of beam attenuation depends upon the thickness of tissue traversed and the viscosity of the tissue. Attenuation has been found to exhibit an exponential behavior. Expressed mathematically:

$$I_x = I_o e^{-\mu x} \qquad (6)$$

where I_o is the initial beam intensity, I_x is the intensity at tissue depth x and μ is called the attenuation coefficient. It has been found that μ varies in proportion to frequency, ie, the higher the frequency the greater the attenuation. For this reason, the upper limit on the medically useful frequency is about 20 mHz.

When comparing the relative intensities of two ultrasonic beams (incident to reflected or incident to transmitted) the decibel notation is most frequently used.

The ratio of two beam intensities (I_1, I_2) is expressed in decibel (dB) notation by the following relationship:

$$dB = 10\log_{10}(I_2/I_1). \qquad (7)$$

TABLE 12.3.   Relationship Between Decibels and Ultrasound Density Ratios

dB	Intensity ratio
$(10 \log_{10}[I_2/I_1])$	(I_2/I_1)
0.0	1.00
0.5	1.12
1.0	1.26
5.0	3.16
10.0	10.00
20.0	100.00
30.0	1000.00

The decibel value will be negative when I_2 is less than I_1, eg, absorption of initial beam intensity. The correspondence between direct intensity ratios and the same ratios expressed in terms of decibels is found in Table 12.3.

TRANSDUCER CHARACTERISTICS

There are a number of ultrasonic transducer performance parameters that affect diagnostic image quality. These include frequency, axial resolution, beam pattern, and sensitivity. These parameters are interrelated and not independent.

Frequency primarily determines the penetrating ability of the ultrasonic beam. When the frequency is higher, the penetration is less. As will be discussed later the transducer frequency also helps determine both its axial and lateral resolution. If all other parameters are kept constant, the higher the frequency, the better the axial (ie, along the beam) resolution. In addition, for a given transducer diameter, higher frequency beams have less divergence resulting in better lateral resolution.

When a transducer is delivered, the manufacturer provides a number that is the frequency of the transducer. This number is actually the average or most dominant frequency because the pulse from an ultrasonic transducer exhibits a spectrum of frequencies rather than a single frequency.

The bandwidth of the transducer is defined as the range of frequencies contained within the ultrasonic pulse. Short pulses contain a large range of frequencies (large bandwidth). The pulse length is the primary factor that affects axial resolution.

Short pulse lengths (in both time and space) are achieved by damping the vibrations of the transducer after its excitation by an electrical impulse. In a pulse-echo system, rapid damping is important; if the transducer is still vibrating, then it will not be sensitive to returning echoes from the body.

Ring-down is a measure of the length of time required for a transducer to damp its vibrations. Ring-down is frequently measured in terms of the number of half-cycles required for the oscillations to decay to 10 percent of the maximum peak amplitude. The spatial pulse length is determined by the ring-down time. If, for example, it takes 2μ seconds for the pulse to be damped to 10 percent, at a velocity of 1500 meters per second, the pulse would be 3 mm long.

Axial resolution can be defined as the ability to distinguish two closely adjacent reflecting structures. The minimum separation at which the surfaces can be recognized as being separate is termed the axial resolution. This parameter is illustrated in Figure 12.6.

Both the frequency and spatial pulse length affect axial resolution. From the example, a 3-mm spatial pulse length implies not only that echoes from the first 3 mm of tissue will not be detected but also (and more important) reflecting structures within the body separated by less than 3 mm will be difficult to resolve.

The lateral resolution is affected primarily by the transducer beam pattern. The most important components of this beam pattern are the beam width, which depends upon the size of the transducer, the frequency of the transducer, beam focusing, and the distance from the transducer face. Beam width is usually defined as the diameter of the ultrasonic beam measured at the 50 percent amplitude point.

A diagram illustrating the shape of the ultrasonic beam from an unfocused transducer is shown in Figure 12.7. The region where the beam is approximately

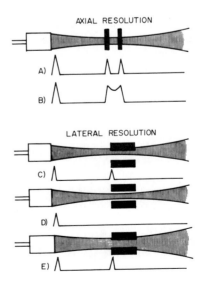

Figure 12.6. Illustration of a system response with good axial resolution (**A**) and poor axial resolution (**B**). Response of a system with good lateral resolution (**C**) and (**D**), and poor lateral resolution (**E**). Lateral resolution is dependent upon beam width. In response (**E**), the beam is wider than the separation between the two reflectors.

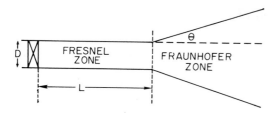

Figure 12.7. The shape of an ultrasonic beam from an unfocused transducer is approximately cylindrical for a distance L (Fresnel zone). Beyond the Fresnel zone the beam diverges (Fraunhofer zone). The divergence angle θ is given by the following: $\sin \theta = 1.22 \lambda / D$, where λ is the wavelength and D is the diameter of the transducer.

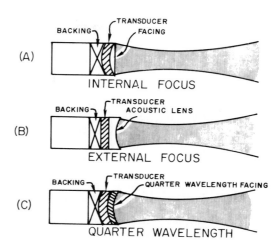

Figure 12.8. Transducer focusing techniques. **A.** Internal focusing implies that the piezoelectric crystal has a curved face that will result in beam focusing. **B.** External focusing implies that an acoustic lens has been placed in front of a parallel face transducer. **C.** Quarter wavelength transducers have a layer of facing material one-quarter wavelength thick with an acoustic impedance that is intermediate between the transducer crystal and tissue, ie, matched impedance.

cylindrical in shape is called the *near-field* or *Fresnel zone*. The region exhibiting divergence is called the *far-field* or *Fraunhofer zone*.

The length of the near-field is given by:

$$L = D^2/4\lambda \qquad (8)$$

where D is the effective diameter of the transducer and λ is the wavelength. This equation shows that large transducers will yield longer near-fields if operated at the same frequency. In general, scanning the near-field in the transition area between the two fields yields the best lateral resolution. Similarly, from the equation, for equal sized transducers, a higher frequency (shorter λ) results in a longer near-field.

Thus far we have assumed cylindrical transducer elements that produce near-fields that are circular in cross-section. Linear and phased array real-time units contain transducers that are rectangular in shape. Rectangular elements tend to produce more elliptical beam cross-sections, which implies a lateral resolution that varies depending upon the plane of the beam.

The purpose of focusing an ultrasonic beam is to minimize the width of the beam with an associated increase in sensitivity at a specified depth. The transducer may be focused either internally or externally (Fig. 12.8). Focusing can only be accomplished in the near-field. Internal focusing is accomplished by forming the piezoelectric crystal with an appropriate radius of curvature. The radius of curvature and frequency combine to determine the location of the focal point. The resulting concave surface is usually filled in with a facing material to produce a flat surface for better patient contact. In external focusing, the crystal is flat and a concave acoustic lens facing is bonded to the crystal. Transducers with external focusing will have concave faces. Very high frequency transducers (7 to 15 MHz) are generally very thin and fragile. Because of this, high frequency transducers are usually focused externally.

The sensitivity of a transducer is enhanced by

focusing, which increases the intensity of the beam at a specified depth. This results in an increased sensitivity about the focal zone. The sensitivity will fall off on either side of the focal zone.

One of the most important recent technologic advances that has affected transducer sensitivity is the development of "quarter wavelength" technology. The difference between quarter wavelength transducers and standard transducers is a precision quarter wavelength thick facing. The quarter wavelength thickness is chosen to take advantage of constructive interference of reflected waves from the skin/transducer interface to increase the amount of energy that actually passes through the interface. The facing is not only carefully chosen to be one-quarter wavelength thick, but it is also chosen so that its acoustic impedance matches body tissues. The end result is increased transducer efficiency for transmitting energy into the body as well as an increased efficiency for detecting reflected waves.

A-MODE INSTRUMENTATION

The "A" in A-mode stands for amplitude. An A-scan is an echo amplitude modulated tracing on a cathode ray tube (CRT) (Fig. 12.9). The tracing is controlled by horizontal and vertical deflection plates. An internal circuit called a "sweep circuit" controls the horizontal deflection plates. It is designed to move the beam horizontally across the CRT at a constant speed. In pulse-echo systems a pulser is used to excite the

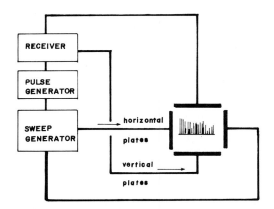

Figure 12.9. Schematic of cathode ray tube (CRT) instrumentation used to produce an A-mode scan.

transducer with an electrical impulse approximately 1000 times per second. This is known as pulse-repetition rate. The sweep circuit of the CRT is synchronized with the pulser that drives the transducer. The pulse-repetition rate of 1000 pulses per second allows the eye to perceive these horizontal motions as a steady horizontal line on the CRT face. By adjusting the speed of horizontal deflection of the CRT, various scales of distance can be displayed along the horizontal axis as a function of time. In order to display 1 cm within the body as 1 cm along the horizontal axis of the CRT, the time for the horizontal deflection on the CRT to move 1 cm must equal the time the echo takes to travel 2 cm in the patient. In the patient, the echo must travel 1 cm and return 1 cm to the transducer for detection. Since the speed of the echo in tissue is 1.54 mm per μsec it takes 13 μsec for the sound pulse to travel 20 mm (2 cm) in the patient. Therefore, the horizontal deflection of the CRT should travel 1 cm per 13 microseconds. This would then allow 1 cm on the CRT display to represent 1 cm in the patient.

Because the face of the CRT is usually only 10 cm in length, only 10 cm of the patient can be displayed upon the oscilloscope at any given time. Therefore, the horizontal speed of the CRT can be varied to travel one-third as fast, which would yield 1 cm on the CRT to a distance of 3 cm in the patient. This is scanning at a three-to-one ratio or on a three-to-one scale. By varying the time of the CRT horizontal trace, various ratios such as four-to-one, two-to-one, or one-to-one can be obtained.

The voltage from the returning echo is used to drive the vertical deflection plates of the CRT. This provides a vertical spike on the oscilloscope face perpendicular to the horizontal baseline. The amplitude of the vertical deflection is directly proportional to the amplitude of the echo causing the deflection. Therefore, amplitude mode or A-mode is echo-modulated

vertical deflections plotted against a horizontal baseline representing time (Fig. 12.10). Scale markers can then be added to the A-mode trace so that depth distances can be measured from the CRT. For example, in a one-to-one mode, a scale marker would be added every 13 μsec corresponding to a distance of 1 cm in the patient. The timing of the scale marker is then varied with respect to the scale used.

A-MODE ARTIFACTS

When the sound beam passes from one medium to another, its frequency will remain constant, but its wavelength will change to accommodate a different velocity in the second medium. This change in wavelength may cause a change in direction known as refraction. Refraction does not occur when the interface is perpendicular to the sound beam, but it becomes important when the interface is not perpendicular to the beam. Refraction increases when the propagation velocity changes are large. Refraction artifacts are generally manifested as a real structure that has been displayed in the wrong location.

Highly reflective interfaces can cause reverberations. Reverberation artifacts are recurring echoes that are placed at locations at fixed distances from the original interface. Because of the regular occurrence, it causes them to be spread along the horizontal axis of the A-mode trace. Because the time is used as an indicator of distance, these reverberation artifacts appear to show interfaces where interfaces do not exist.

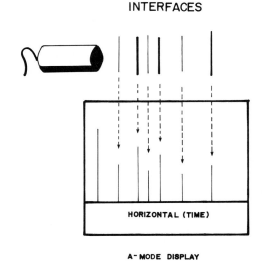

Figure 12.10. Relationship between the location of tissue interfaces relative to the transducer face and the A-mode display. Interfaces that result in large echoes are displayed as a large vertical deflection on the A-mode display.

Certain strong reflectors when properly oriented can cause multiple paths for echoes to return to the transducer. This again causes an erroneous display on the CRT. Likewise, a curved irregular surface may yield multiple reflections from a single interface.

Errors in depth can occur when structures have significantly different velocities. For example, scanning through a water-filled structure causes the back wall to appear farther away than it actually is, due to the slower velocity of sound in water.

B-MODE INSTRUMENTATION

The designation "B" in B-mode is chosen because it represents brightness. The returning echo is displayed on the CRT as a light dot; the brightness of the dot varies directly as the intensity of the returning echo. The transducer is mounted on an arm that is hinged and allows motion in only one plane. This hinged arm contains several position sensors. The signals from the sensors are processed electronically and then a dot, representing the echo, is placed in the appropriate x, y coordinate on the CRT display (Fig. 12.11). Since the brightness of the dot varies with the amplitude of the echo, this display is frequently referred to as gray-scale imaging.

As with A-mode, the transducer is pulsed by a pulse generator. The pulse generator is synchronized with other components within the system, such as the time gain compensation (TGC) and display sweep. The returning echoes are converted to electrical signals by the piezoelectric transducer. The signal is amplified by a high frequency amplifier (sometimes referred to as the radiofrequency or RF amplifier because of the frequency content of the signal) and then rectified and demodulated before amplification by the video amplifier. Demodulation provides wave envelopes that are proportional to the amplitude of the original echo amplitude. These signals are then sent to the video amplifier for further amplification and display.

Bistable B-mode displays were the earliest form of B-mode. Although these particular displays are B-mode, they contain no facility for gray-scale. In this display mode, an operator determines the echo amplitude threshold before beginning the scan. Returning echoes below this threshold are not displayed while all those above the threshold are displayed with the same intensity. Thus, only two data components are available in this system. Bistable has been supplanted in modern instruments by gray-scale equipment that allows some quantitative recording.

Gray-scale displays allow the varying degrees of brightness to be displayed on the oscilloscope in the appropriate position given by the x, y coordinates from

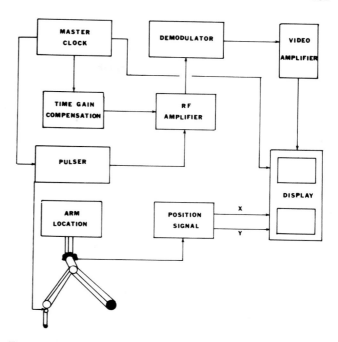

Figure 12.11. Schematic representation of the components needed to produce a B-mode image.

the positional sensors. The number of gray shades displayed depends upon the type of "scan converter" that translates the pressure change to electrical impulses. In an analog system, scan converter tubes are used to store information electronically. Once an image has been stored, the scan converter tube is "read" and these results are displayed on a video monitor. The intensity of each picture element of the stored image varies with the applied voltage. This allows a relatively "infinite" gray-scale without definite fixed steps or levels that produce an esthetically pleasing image. Because of tracking errors and noise, however, the scan converter tube has limitations in resolution. Scan converter tubes need periodic alignment and have also been found to be very temperature sensitive. Systems utilizing analog scan converters generally require long warm-up periods for the equipment to perform properly and frequently drift during use. This drift is subtle and difficult to detect before it becomes clinically significant. Newer instruments for B-mode imaging use "digital scan converters." In these systems, the voltage levels that correspond to the returning echo amplitudes are converted from an electronic signal to digital numbers. These numbers are then stored in the digital memory of the recording device. The memory is then interrogated and the image displayed upon a television monitor. The brightness of the television signal representing each picture element is controlled by the value stored in the corresponding digital word. The number of shades of gray available is determined by the length of the digital word. Three bit words provide the capacity for displaying eight shades of gray, four bits provide sixteen shades of gray, and five bits provides thirty-two shades of gray. These shades of gray are discreet. The discreetness of the gray-scale shades provides an image that is not as "smooth" as the analog image. The appearance of the image will be different and the margin between data points (picture elements) will be more definite than with analog displays. However, the digital system is more stable and less sensitive to heat, which eliminates long start-up time, and allows one to institute pre- and postdigital image processing. The clinical role of pre- and postprocessing as yet has not been defined. In the near future, digital data from B-scanners may be further analyzed by computer for quick and accurate area and volume determinations.

B-MODE ARTIFACTS

Many of the artifacts previously described in A-mode scanning are also observed in B-mode scanning; reverberation artifacts are often present (Fig. 12.12.A). When an acoustic signal encounters a highly reflective surface, reverberations may occur. Only the original echo represents a real interface. The remainder of

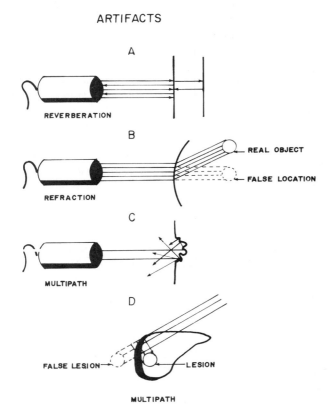

Figure 12.12. Ultrasound artifacts. **A.** Reverberation. **B.** Refraction. **C, D.** Artifacts resulting from multiple return paths for the echoes.

echoes will be displayed in the image in multiples of the distance from the transducer to the reverberating surface. Therefore, they will occur at regular intervals. Reverberations will decrease in intensity because of attenuation from the tissue and thus will have a characteristic appearance. Specular reflectors located at right angles to the sound beam are more likely to cause reverberations. As might be expected, the higher the gain setting on the imaging device, the more likely that reverberation artifacts will be seen. Soft tissue/air interfaces create a significant number of reverberations because of the almost total reflection of the sound beam at the interface. The signal is then returned rapidly and almost undiminished to the transducer.

Shadowing is the term used to describe the phenomenon of sound beam absorption distal to a structure or interface. Shadowing posterior to a rib or posterior to a fetus is a commonly encountered artifact. The shadowing caused by ribs may create diagnostic problems when evaluating underlying structures by adding confusing areas of lack of echoes perceived as lucencies.

Refractive artifacts also occur in B-scanning. Refraction may cause an object to appear in a false position (Fig. 12.12.B). Multiple path artifacts are also common in B-scanning (Fig. 12.12.C). It is possible for lesions within the upper portion of the liver to appear to be projected into the lung due to multiple path error (Fig. 12.12.D).

Artifacts can cause a significant clinical problem in diagnostic ultrasound at the present time. The significance is amplified because of the large number of individuals entering the discipline without training or experience, the rapid development of instrumentation without standardization, and the changing display formats. Documentation of the causes of artifacts, increasing user awareness, and appreciation of their characteristic appearances are as crucial to the advancement of ultrasound presently as the description of the patterns associated with a particular disease entity.

REAL-TIME INSTRUMENTATION

The term *real-time* in this context refers to the visualization of a structure or, more importantly, an event in reasonable temporal relationship to the time in which the reflection of sound occurs. No other area of diagnostic ultrasonic instrumentation has experienced greater technologic advances in recent years than has the area of real-time imaging. Slow manual movement of the transducer in standard B-scan systems precludes its use for imaging the motion of internal body structures. B-scan image formation requires from 15 to 30 seconds for its generation while real-time systems, on the other hand, form 15 to 60 images per second. Until recently, real-time imaging applications have been limited because of the relatively poor spatial resolution, restricted echo dynamic range, and limited field of view. Current real-time instrumentation offers resolution and gray scale rivaling state-of-the-art B-scanners. The field of view of modern real-time units, however, is still smaller than that of B-scanners.

Real-time instruments may be classified on the basis of whether the transducer crystal or element remains stationary or moves during the imaging procedure.

STATIONARY CONFIGURATIONS

Included in this category are linear phased arrays, multielement linear arrays, and multielement annular arrays. Through the proper phasing of the transmit-receive timing of the transducers that are used to fabricate the arrays, a composite sound beam can be created. In this manner, the beam can be focused and steered electronically. Fundamental to electronic focusing is the fact that each element of the array generates a sound or energy that has a definite phase relationship with the waves from the other elements. The waves generated by each element can be superimposed in a precise manner to create the effect of a single wave front.

The linear phased array is frequently termed an electronic-sector scanner since the resulting field is pie-shaped with the field diverging as the distance from the transducers is increased. The outside transducers are activated first and the inner transducers are delayed in time. The central transducer has the greater delay to yield a wave axis perpendicular to the plane of the transducer (Fig. 12.13). By varying the order of the delay, the wave front can be scanned into a sector of 60 to 90 degrees.

Multielement linear scanning arrays are pulsed so as to produce a wavefront that moves normal to the transducer face thus yielding a rectangular field (see Fig. 13.4.A). The length of the transducer array may vary with frequency, but at 3.5 MHz most transducers are on the order of 10-cm long. The sequencing of transducer activation may be chosen and can occur in groups.

The transducer array is usually composed of many small crystals (M) arranged in a row. Because the field from a single, small, crystal element diverges very rapidly, several elements (N) are driven simultaneously and electronic focusing is used. As described previously in the phased array discussion, in the subgroup of N crystals the outer crystals may be pulsed first with the inner crystals delayed. In this circumstance, the field from the N elements will be focused at a depth depending upon the magnitude of the delays. By changing the magnitudes of the delays, the focal zone can be con-

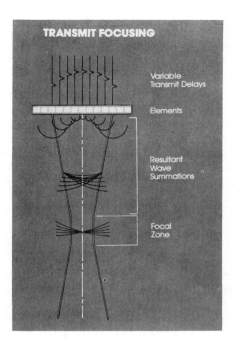

Figure 12.13. Electronic focusing of a phased linear array. Beam steering is produced in the same manner by using transmit delay patterns in which one side of the array is activated before the other in systematic pattern of increasing delays. The direction of the resultant wave summation will as a result be "steered" from one side of the array to the other in a "pie"-shaped pattern. (Courtesy of EMI Medical Inc., 4000 Commercial Drive, Northbrook, Illinois)

tinuously scanned through a specified range of depths. The elements may also be designed so as to be sensitive to the returning waves in a manner determined by the same delay factors used in transmission, thus constituting a focusing effect on the returning signals, ie, "double focusing." A single scan line in the real-time image is formed in this manner. The next adjacent scan line is generated by utilizing another group of N crystals formed by shifting from the previous N crystals, one crystal position along the transducer array. The same transmit-receive pattern is then repeated for this set of N crystals and subsequently for all other sets of N crystals along the array in a cyclic manner. The technique as described ignores the ends of the array and yields M scan lines. That is, the same number of scan lines as there are transducers in the array. Focusing not only improves lateral resolution but it also improves sensitivity by increasing the amount of energy in the focal zone (constructive interference).

In order to achieve a higher scan line density, one may decrease the size of the individual crystals and use more crystals (technically difficult and expensive), rescan using a smaller subgroup, or use electronic steering to sample between previous scan lines. The third technique is the most commonly used. Using the combined techniques of "double-focusing" and beam steering to increase line density, current real-time systems are capable of lateral resolution on the order of 1.5 to 2 mm.

MOVING CONFIGURATIONS

The term moving configurations describes imaging systems in which there is mechanical motion of either the transducer itself or of a reflecting mirror (Fig. 12.14, see also Fig. 13.4.B). The mirror can be used to direct the ultrasonic beam to a specified distance. By rotating the mirror or the transducer, the beam can be scanned through the volume of interest to form the image. In order to assure good ultrasonic coupling, moving configurations most frequently employ a "water path" geometry. The water path implies that the transducers and mirror, if present, are housed entirely within a water-filled chamber. The chamber is fitted with a flexible membrane that forms an "ultrasonic window." It is this window that makes direct contact with the patient. The image-framing rate of mechanical scanning systems is governed by the speed of mechanical motion, ie., either transducer or mirror. This allows a rapid acquisition rate without complex electronics.

There are a number of different designs of mechanical systems that are in use today (Fig. 12.15). These include rotating single or multiple element scanners, "wobbling" single or multiple element scanners, and oscillating element scanners. The rotating or wobbling transducer scanners generally form a sector-shaped field of view. The opening angle of the wobbler sector scanner can be varied from 15 to 60 degrees. The framing rate (wobbling rate) is most commonly 15 to 30 per second. The image rate is faster for the smaller opening angles that provide the basis for compromise considerations in transducer design. The sector-shaped

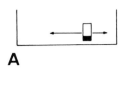

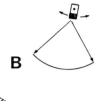

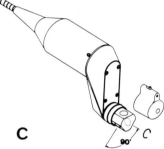

Figure 12.15. Ultrasonic scanners with moving transducer configurations: **A.** Single element scanner with an oscillating transducer produces a rectangular field-of-view. **B.** Wobbling transducers produce a pie-shaped or sector field-of-view. **C.** Rotating three-element scanner produces a sector shaped field-of-view with opening angles 60 to 90 degrees. (Courtesy of ATL Corporation.)

fields have been found to be well-suited for cardiac examinations. In a circumstance where the field of view increases with depth, scanning between ribs is possible. Systems with combinations of wobbling transducers are designed to provide larger fields of view by superimposing the fields of the individual transducers or, alternatively, to use a single transducer when the application dictates. These considerations require an appreciation of the merits and limitations of choosing the transducer complexity and the physical arrangements.

Rotating transducer systems can be designed either in combination with a reflecting mirror or without. Systems with multiple transducers on a rotating wheel generate a sector-shaped field similar to wobblers; however, the opening angle may be as wide as 90 degrees. This has been employed successfully by several manufacturers.

QUALITY CONTROL

The purpose of a quality assurance program is to ensure that the diagnostic information provided by the images is maintained at the maximum attainable level for that instrument and technology. Part of this program must include monitoring procedures that will

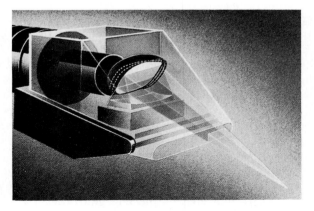

Figure 12.14. Water path configuration utilizing an oscillating mirror with a stationary transducer. (Courtesy of BioDynamics Corporation, Indianapolis, Indiana)

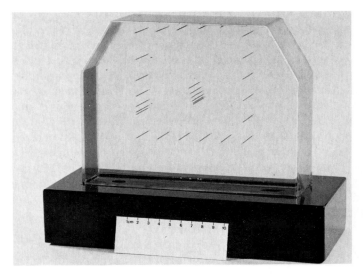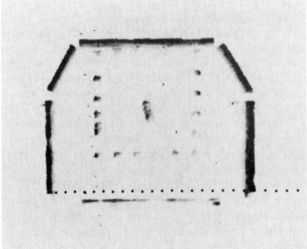

Figure 12.16. Photograph of AIUM Standard 100 mm Test Object (left). Ultrasonic scan of AIUM Test Object (right).

ensure the proper and consistent operation of all equipment. Acceptance tests must be performed upon the delivery of all new equipment and repeated whenever major equipment repairs are made. Quality control tests should be performed on a routine basis to detect deviations from the baseline acceptance tests. Quality assurance is a joint responsibility of the physician, technologist, and service support personnel.

There are numerous test objects and instruments that are now available for assessing the performance of ultrasonic equipment. A number of documents are also available that contain detailed protocols for establishing a quality assurance program.[1-5] Probably the single most versatile and complete test object that can be used in these studies is the AIUM Standard 100 mm Test Object (Fig. 12.16).

A minimal quality control program should include routine monitoring of the performance of the gray-scale photography, image sensitivity, axial resolution, accuracy and linearity of distance markers, and B-mode registration. Aside from the evaluation of the gray-scale photography, the AIUM Test Object may be used to partially assess each of the other system parameters. The minimal quality control program provides relative parameter values. Relative values are useful for detecting early changes in image system characteristics. Absolute measurements of system parameters are more difficult and may require additional test objects and equipment.

Of equal importance to the actual performance testing is the documentation of the test results. These recorded data are essential for accurate monitoring of equipment performance and are useful to both the equipment service personnel and the equipment manufacturer. It is also an incumbent possibility that this will be required by government regulatory and certifying agencies in the near future.

The initial camera settings and/or scan converter output controls depend largely upon individual points of reference. Once a baseline has been established, a daily evaluation should be made to assure that the

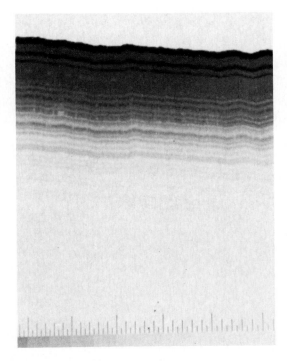

Figure 12.17. Quality assurance test for the stability of gray-scale imaging devices. Scan was created by coupling a coin with gel directly to the surface of the transducer face.

same range of echo amplitudes can be seen as was present on previous test exposures.

Most systems now generate gray-scale bars that are displayed on one side or at the bottom of the image. This bar should be examined daily for consistency of step distribution and display. This comparison can be made either by visual inspection or with the aid of a densitometer which is more quantitative.

In addition to the gray-bar evaluation, the range of gray shades present in the recorded image arising from echoes that have been processed through the transducer electronics should be evaluated independently. This can be facilitated by creating a B-scan image from a stable source of echoes. This source may be a sophisticated electronic device called a *logarithmic tone-burst generator*, which replaces the transducer in the circuit, or simply a coin coupled with gel directly to the surface of the transducer face (Fig. 12.17). In either instance,

the A-mode display should be adjusted to provide echoes ranging continuously from the maximum to that at the threshold of being discernible. B-scans created in this manner should be performed routinely and internally referenced for consistency. In most current digital machines, it is possible to perform a more quantitative test of gray-scale performance by simply monitoring the range of voltage levels present in the video output of the scan converter. Figure 12.18 shows photographs of oscilloscope tracings from two digital machines, each of which were designed to produce 12 shades of gray. In the imaging device that is functioning properly, one can discern 12 distinct voltage levels in the video image by inspection. As few as 8 levels will be delineated with the malfunctioning instrument.

A simple quality control test for A-mode and B-mode sensitivity stability can be performed with the aid of the AIUM phantom. After carefully positioning the

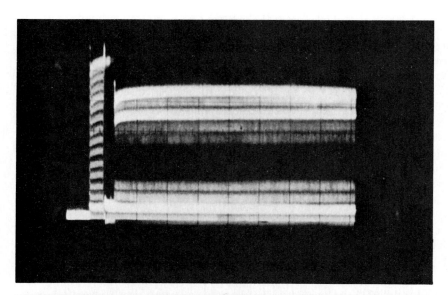

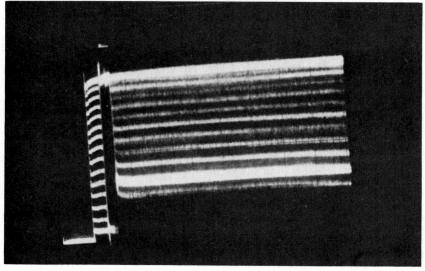

Figure 12.18. Oscilloscope tracings of video output signals from a digital scanner with 12 shades of gray in the image. The shades of gray are represented by the distinct voltage levels on the oscilloscope trace. The narrow vertical levels at the left is the internally generated gray bar test and contains 16 distinct levels. **Top.** Malfunctioning machine that exhibits only 8 to 9 gray levels in the image with missing levels in the middle of the range. **Bottom.** Tracing from a machine that is functioning properly.

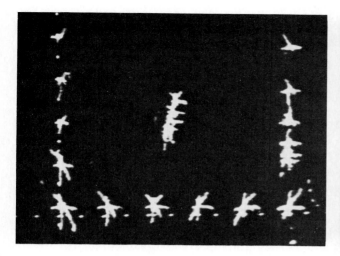 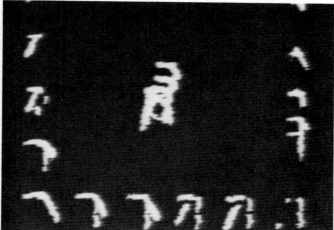

Figure 12.19. **A.** Scan of AIUM Test Object illustrating acceptable registration errors. All scan lines should intersect ideally at their centers. Note system generated distance markers along the bottom of the scan near the group of wires that are known to be separated by 2 cm. The distance markers are separated by 1 cm. A comparison of the two separations provides a measure of the accuracy of the generated markers. **B.** Scan of AIUM Test Object that illustrates unacceptable registration errors.

scanning arm and transducer directly above the reference wires that are spaced 2 cm apart (making sure the transducer face is flat against the phantom surface), the system gain (attenuation or output) settings should be adjusted to display a one division echo from the most distant wire. These gain settings should not change on subsequent recordings. Similarly, the minimum gain settings required to yield a discernible echo in the B-mode should not change with time. By this method, the stability of the instrumentation over time can be determined. Since the AIUM phantom exhibits relatively low attenuation, sensitivity measurements may be more meaningful if made with a more highly attenuating "tissue-equivalent" phantom.

A single pass B-mode image of the AIUM phantom will provide data on axial resolution as well as the accuracy and linearity of the distance markers. Axial resolution is assessed from the minimum resolvable spacing in the set of diagonal wires at the center of the phantom. Within this set, wire spacings range from 5 mm to 1 mm. Most imaging systems should exhibit the ability to resolve 2-mm wire spacings, and this value should remain constant over time.

The accuracy and linearity of the system-generated distance markers can be evaluated by a direct measurement of the distances of the vertical and horizontal wires from a B-mode image. The distance between the uppermost and bottom wires in the 2-cm spaced group is actually 10 cm, and this distance, as estimated by the markers, should not differ by more than 2 mm.

By performing a compound scan of the AIUM phantom, one can assess the degree of registration errors that may be present (Fig. 12.19). Ideally, a compound scan created by scanning along each of the five sides of the phantom should exhibit, at the location of each wire, five lines all intersecting at their centers. Lines that do not cross at their centers indicate the presence of registration errors. These errors result from uncertainties in arm angle determination either from mechanical failure or malfunction of the potentiometers.

Each of the above mentioned parameters should be determined routinely and the results documented. Although no formal decision as to the proper period between monitoring procedures has been published, many laboratories and physicians working in this area have chosen to make these relative measurements twice weekly.

The information contained in Chapter 12 has been provided as a basis for a more practical discussion of the principles in Chapter 13. The reader may wish to refer to this basic chapter to enhance the value of the discussions in Chapter 13.

REFERENCES

1. Stewart HF, Harris GR, Frost HM: Development of principles and concepts for specifications of ultrasonic diagonistic equipment performance. In White DN, Brown RF (eds): Ultrasound in Medicine, New York, Plenum Press, 1977, pp 2115–2142

2. The AIUM 100 mm Test Object and recommended procedures for its use. Reflections 1 (2): 74–91, 1975

3. Carson PL: Standardization, calibration and performance evaluation. In Holmes JH III (ed): Diagnostic Ultrasound, 1974, pp 271–311

4. Recommendations for Quality Assurance for Diagnostic Ultrasound. ACR Committee on Physics, American College of Radiology Publication, August, 1979.

5. Goldstein A: A routine procedure for monitoring ultrasound equipment. JCU 3: 267–271, 1975

6. James AE Jr, Goddard J, Price RR, et al: Advances in instrument design and image recording. Radiol Clin North Am 18(1): 3–20, 1980.

7. Price RR, Jones TB, Goddard J, James AE Jr: Basic concepts of ultrasonic tissue characterization. Radiol Clin North Am 18 (1): 21–30, 1980

CHAPTER 13

Ultrasound: Certain Considerations of Equipment Usage

A. EVERETTE JAMES, JR.
ARTHUR C. FLEISCHER
THOMAS JONES
RAY POWIS
DONALD BAKER
KENNETH J. W. TAYLOR
JOHN GODDARD
RONALD R. PRICE

Certain aspects of ultrasonic instrumentation usage will be emphasized to include certain fundamental features of machine adjustments, instrument design, and image display. The developments in instrumentation, at present, are so widespread and are occurring so rapidly that the approach to specific guidelines will be a generic one. Certain basic principles of user techniques that will prove germane to future advances as well as to present day instruments will be stressed. In the more fundamental considerations in Chapter 12, the basic physics of ultrasound, as well as the generation and interactions of this energy form are considered. In this chapter, the appropriate application of these principles will be discussed.

TYPES OF IMAGING DEVICES

The basic principles of ultrasound generation, tissue interaction, and operation of static articulated arm and real-time B-mode ultrasonic scanners have been described in Chapter 12. In the practical aspects of the use of such scanners, the effect of various scanner control settings and image display and recording formats on the overall image quality will be emphasized. One of the primary considerations in establishing an ultrasonic facility is the selection of one or more suitable ultrasonic instruments. This topic will be considered on the basis of the virtues and limitations of each type of imaging device.

Ultrasonic scanners are fabricated in several basic designs, some of which are general purpose instruments while others are intended for specific uses. The selection of instrument design will, therefore, be largely influenced by the population of referred patients and to a great extent by the type or types of examination to be performed.

There are a myriad of companies that offer a variety of ultrasonic scanning instrumentation and accessory items. Because of this, the selection of a satisfactory imaging system can often be difficult and time consuming. While there are no definitive guidelines in the selection of a scanner there are some general considerations that might be helpful.

The majority of imaging procedures can be performed with a general purpose real-time or static B-mode scanner. The general design of a static B-mode scanner has been described in Chapter 12 but should be repeated for emphasis. Such a scanner will typically be composed of (1) the mechanical scanning assembly plus a set of transducers; (2) an electronic signal processing unit with controls to vary the power output of the transducer and the TGC setting; (3) a gray-scale display unit for observing the imaging during scanning, and which is equipped with controls for varying the image brightness and contrast; (4) a display for observing A-mode trace and the TGC curve; and (5) an image display unit with a Polaroid, 35 mm, 70 mm, or multiformat camera attachment for permanent recording of the images. A character generator for superimposing patient identification data and other information on the image is a useful option that is offered in a number of imaging systems. Some instruments have an optional time-motion (T/M) unit that allows one to perform echocardiographic studies. There are also several echocardiography T/M systems available that are designed specifically to perform T/M studies only, and obviate the need for a mechanical scanning assembly and expensive gray-scale image display. These systems are less expensive than general purpose static B-mode scanners with T/M option. Consequently, this instrumentation type is used most frequently in cardiology studies. Since the most static B-mode scanners are equipped with an A-mode display, they can be used as a conventional A-mode scanner that may continue to have utility in certain measurements, in tissue characterization, and in cyst evaluation. Although static B-mode scanners can be adapted for ocular imaging, there are several less expensive instruments that are specifically designed for this purpose and have some advantages.

The scan conversion unit of a general purpose static B-mode scanner will be either analog or digital based. As late as 1977, nearly all of the scanners had analog scan converters, but at present most of manufacturers offer only digital based units. Some instrument companies also provide an upgrade of analog systems to state-of-the-art digital systems.

At present, there is only rudimentary objective clinical evidence that the scan quality obtained with a digital unit is superior to that obtained with a well-tuned relatively new analog unit. This is partly because the digital units have not been in use long enough to permit a thorough evaluation and there is currently no generally accepted method of objectively evaluating ultrasonic scan quality. Therefore, any comparative evaluations are likely to be subjective in nature. One of the major difficulties with units emphasizing analog scan converters has been their tendency to drift, resulting in less than optimum scan quality and requiring frequent servicing. To compound this problem, the drift is often subtle and the type of image degradation that occurs is difficult to detect without a rigorous quality control program (see Chapter 12). Drifting of an analog scan conversion unit can produce a blurring or defocusing effect on the image as well as an alteration in the echo amplitude to gray-level assignment.

Digital scan conversion units, by the nature of their basic mode of operation, are drift-free. Another fundamental difference between analog and digital scan conversion units is the echo amplitude versus gray-level transfer curve. The shape of such a transfer curve determines the gray level that will be displayed in the image for a particular amplitude value of ultrasonic echo. The shape of the curve will not, in general, be linear because of the requirement to record a 60-dB range of echo amplitudes in the same display format as that used with a 20-dB range. A certain amount of dynamic range compression, therefore, is inevitable to preserve the full range of the echo amplitude data.

Development of a wider range of decibel displays is an expected future development.

In an analog scan converter unit, the transfer curve is calibrated and set at the time of manufacture and a characteristic shape of the curve is determined to display low-, mid-, and high-range echo amplitudes. In a digital scan converter unit, several transfer curve shapes may be stored in the system. This will allow the operator to select a suitable one immediately prior to performing a scan. This ability to select one of several transfer curve shapes is sometimes referred to as "tissue texture preprocessing" and "tissue texture postprocessing." The advantage of this capability is that it permits operator selection that may allow discrimination between two similar yet different echo amplitudes that otherwise would appear at the same gray level in an analog system (Fig. 13.1). Figure 13.2 is an example of the effect of several tissue texture preprocessing and postprocessing schemes. The clinical importance of tissue texture preprocessing and postprocessing has yet to be realized and further research is required to optimize the various techniques to the various normal and pathological tissue states.

ULTRASONIC TISSUE CHARACTERIZATION

When ultrasonic fields interact with tissue, the characteristics of the field will be affected in a manner that depends upon the acoustic properties of the tissue. Experimental observations indicate that the changes in the ultrasonic field may prove to be a unique signature of the isonified tissue.[1,2] There are many modes whereby ultrasonic energy may interact with tissue. The effect of these interactions on the ultrasonic field may be measured in terms of basic acoustic parameters of the tissue, probably the most important of these being attenuation (absorption and scattering), velocity, and impedance.[3] Although significant advances have been made in recent years to improve the gray-scale imaging technology employed in clinical ultrasonic imaging devices, these instruments make use of only a small fraction of the potentially available tissue parameter information, ie, the 180 degree (backscatter) scattered echo amplitudes. In spite of this apparent paucity of information, physicians have been able to visualize the image texture of the backscattered echoes from internal tissue structure and have been able to relate the texture to tissue pathology.

Acoustic parameters of tissue are in general dependent upon frequency and other physical variables such as temperature. In order for these acoustic parameters to provide a unique signature of a specific tissue type, the parameters must be determined in such a manner as to ensure that they are independent of the apparatus employed to make the measurements. This in

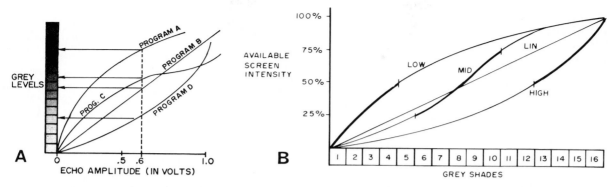

Figure 13.1. A. Preprocessing curve. This figure shows the relation between gray-scale levels and echo amplitude for the different processing programs. Program A is low level enhancement; program B is linear arrangement; program C is midlevel; program D is high-level enhancement. These allow varied gray-scale assignments for emphasis of certain echo amplitudes. (Courtesy of Picker Corporation, Miner Road, Cleveland, Ohio.) **B.** Postprocessing curves. This technique allows varied gray-scale assignments but permits one to return to the original data. Unlike the preprocessing curve technique, the postprocessing technique retains the original data in a linear fashion.

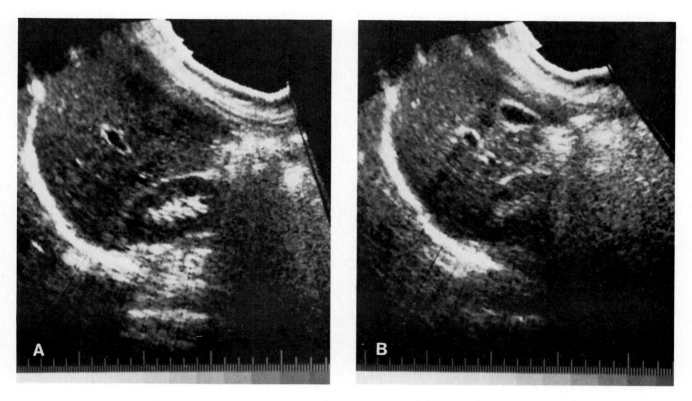

Figure 13.2. A. Longitudinal view of the right lobe of the liver. Original image of linear amplitude display. **B.** Low-level emphasis preprocessing, linear postprocessing (*cont'd.*).

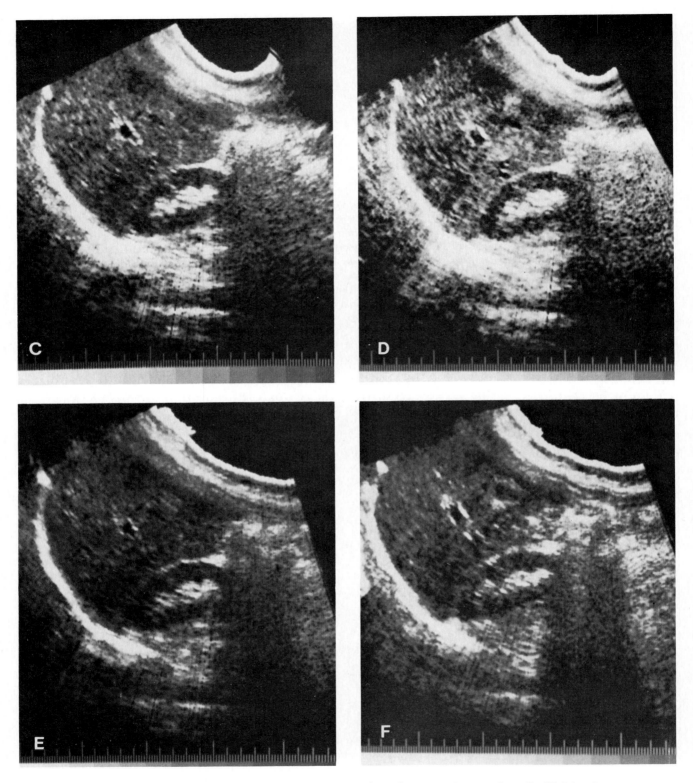

Figure 13.2. C. Mid-level emphasis preprocessing, linear postprocessing. **D.** High-level emphasis preprocessing, linear postprocessing. **E.** Linear preprocessing, low-level emphasis postprocessing. **F.** Linear preprocessing, mid-level emphasis postprocessing (*cont'd.*).

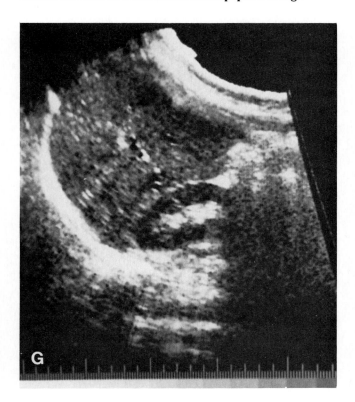

Figure 13.2. G. Linear preprocessing, high-level emphasis postprocessing.

itself is a rather formidable undertaking.

Values for attenuation, velocity, and impedance as a function of frequency have been measured for many body organs and tissues.[4] Generally, it has been found that attenuation and velocity increase in proportion to the relative content of protein and collagen. These properties decrease in proportion to the water content. Numerous research protocols are now being directed toward the diagnosis of many tissue abnormalities, with special interest directed toward the development of techniques for the early detection of cancer and the classification of tissue as either benign or malignant.

A brief review of recent literature will cover many of the present clinical uses of tissue characterization. Kobayashi[5] has been able to characterize malignant and benign tissue in the breast. Wells et al[6] have used Doppler techniques to detect increased vascularization in the breast, which is associated with malignancy among other causes. Lizzi et al[7] using spectrum analysis techniques have been able to distinguish hemorrhage, fat, melanoma, and glioma within the eye. Fry[8] has employed signal processing techniques to assist in the diagnosis of breast cancer. Levi and Keuivez[9] have used differential attenuation measurements to distinguish pelvic tumors. Lele et al[10] and O'Donnell et al[11] have utilized ultrasonic parameters to differentiate infarcted myocardium from normal tissue. It is suggested that attenuation decreases immediately after infarction. Hepatic fibrosis is characterized by an in-

creased number of sound waves backscattered from the fine parenchymal structures of the liver; however, the pattern is not sufficiently distinctive always to separate this disease from several others.[12]

The precise scattering mechanism that occurs in the liver is not yet completely understood. Fields and Dunn[13] have stated that variations in elasticity largely account for the observed echoes from the gross soft tissue structures. Furthermore, the collagenous fibers have a higher elastic modulus compared to that of other soft tissues. Therefore, the amount of collagen may be the dominant factor in determining ultrasonic visualization. Cirrhosis of the liver can be associated with a threefold increase in collagen content compared to normal. Ultrasonic visualization in this disease characteristically depicts a pattern of interlacing prominent echoes in the interior of the liver, which normally exhibits little internal structure. Basically, the echoes are dense and many of the usual interfaces such as veins, arteries, and biliary ducts are not well seen.

In a more detailed analysis of ultrasonic backscatter from human liver tissue in vitro, Freese and Lyons[14] found a significant correlation of the backscatter levels with the protein content in normal livers and with the lipid content in abnormal fatty livers. Their results suggested that in normal liver inherent differences in the protein content may result in the average envelope backscatter coefficient varying as much as 9 dB. Taking the protein content into account, they found that the effective scattering contributions by the protein and lipid were roughly comparable on a percentage weight basis. The fact that their ultrasonic measurements on the liver samples were conducted, however, with two exceptions, within 1 to 3 days postmortem, is a source of criticism since Bamber et al[15] have shown that backscatter parameters vary significantly with the time after excision.

Most of the knowledge that has been assembled regarding these parameters is based upon empirical approaches. At this time, little progress has been made in establishing a good theoretical description of the interaction in biologic tissues.[16] Most descriptions of acoustic interactions assume an ideal, linear, homogeneous liquid medium that may not apply directly to inhomogeneous biologic tissues. In an ideal elastic medium, the free-field velocity of propagation (V) of a longitudinal sound wave is

$$V = \sqrt{\frac{B}{\rho_o}} \tag{1}$$

where B is the elastic bulk modulus of the medium and ρ_o is the mean density.

The quantity $\rho_o V$ is the characteristic impedance of the medium (Z_o):

$$Z_o = \rho_o V = (\rho_o B)^{1/2} \tag{2}$$

The specific acoustic impedance, which is defined as the ratio of the imposed acoustic pressure to the velocity of the tissue particles, is numerically equal to Z_o for plane traveling waves. When an acoustic wave propagates through tissue, energy from the sound beam is transferred to the particles of the medium in vibrations. The vibrational energy is then dissipated as random molecular motion or molecular excitation. The exact mechanisms of absorption in tissues are complex and are not completely established at present.

The intensity and amplitude of the acoustic wave is attenuated (losses by both absorption and scattering) in an exponential fashion:

$$I_x = I_o e^{-\mu x} \tag{3}$$

where I_o is the initial acoustic intensity, I_x is the intensity at the tissue depth x, and μ is the total attenuation coefficient per unit distance. The corresponding "amplitude" attenuation coefficient is equal to $\mu/2$. For water, the classical attenuation coefficient is proportional to the square of the frequency, while temperature dependence is proportional to the viscosity of the liquid. These dependencies do not apply for biologic materials and in the case of soft tissue, the attenuation coefficient is approximately linear with frequency, ie, as the frequency becomes greater, the attenuation increases. A description of the observed attenuation of biologic materials, therefore, must include relaxation processes. These phenomena reflect mechanisms within the tissues that require a finite time interval for the energy to be transferred. Since a single relaxation process is usually inadequate to describe observed absorption spectra, one must consider the observed spectra to represent the sum of a number of such processes.

Frequency analysis is basic to many of the techniques used by investigators to arrive at a tissue signature. Frequency analysis provides a different method of viewing conventional A- and B-scans. For example, by means of a Fourier transformation, one can utilize the echo amplitude versus time plot of the A-scan or the echo amplitude versus position information of the B-scan and convert to an amplitude versus frequency presentation. Fourier analysis is based on the fact that any arbitrary mathematical function (eg, A-scan or B-scan profile) can be decomposed into a finite sum of other elementary functions. The Fourier analysis technique decomposes the arbitrary function into a finite sum of sine and cosine functions.[17] The component sine and cosine functions will in general have different amplitudes, phases, and frequencies. Very rapidly changing amplitude/time (A-scan) or amplitude/position (B-scan) functions require high frequency sine and cosine functions to constitute the function. By employing a Fourier decomposition of an acoustic waveform before and after the wave interacts with a tissue specimen, the effects of the tissue interaction at each frequency present in the beam can be determined.

When carrying out spectral determinations, it is important that these be made with the most faithful representation of the reflected or transmitted waveform. In most commercial instruments, the viewed waveform undergoes a number of nonlinear electronic processes (rectification and filtering) before it is displayed on the A-mode display. This processing removes most of the high-frequency information that was present in the original waveform. The waveform must be monitored and recorded as near to the transducer as possible, therefore, before any electronic signal processing has taken place.

The dependence of the various acoustic parameters on frequency has also been used to characterize tissue. The most popular method uses the frequency spectrum (broadband) emitted from a damped stationary transducer operated in the pulse-echo mode.[10] In this technique, the frequency content of the beam is analyzed before and after passage through a specimen; the entire frequency-attenuation characteristic can be obtained with a single measurement.

A second approach to spectral analysis is to use a variable frequency-transmitting transducer and an opposed receiving transducer. Measurements are made with and without a specimen placed between the transducers. The attenuation resulting from the specimen for each frequency is then determined.

In addition to frequency-dependent parameters, the degree of acoustic scattering from a specimen as a function of scattering angle has been found to yield information on the internal organization of the tissue similar to the Bragg effect that is observed when x-rays are scattered from crystalline structures.

B-SCAN IMAGE ANALYSIS AND PATTERN RECOGNITION

The routine use of digital ultrasonic equipment has now made practical a number of approaches to the quantitative characterization of B-mode images using digital image analysis techniques. Image enhancement and sophisticated pattern recognition techniques developed by the military and NASA programs can now be applied to ultrasonic images. This approach is also in its infancy, but encouraging results have been obtained by some investigators. Mountford and Wells[18] used a manual technique to quantify the A-mode display and were able to differentiate normal from cirrhotic liver tissues using a measure of the mean A-mode echo amplitude.

Quantitative data is most easily extracted from the ultrasonic signals by means of a digital computer. The signal must first undergo an analog-to-digital conversion, however, the number of bits of an analog-to-digital converter (ADC) specifies the number of discrete levels into which the range of the analog signal will be divided. This number is equal to two raised to the power equal to the number of bits. Current commercial units provide images that have been digitized to 5 bits or 32 shades of gray that corresponds to a 30 dB echo amplitude range. This range is inadequate to capture the approximately 100 dB echo amplitude range that is present in the unprocessed signals in our current ultrasonic imaging devices. In addition, sampling theory requires that a signal must be sampled in time at a rate at least twice as fast as the highest frequency present in the signal if all of the available information is to be recovered. Neither of these criteria are met by present commercial ultrasonic units. For this reason, special high-speed ADCs (transient recorders) are often required for tissue characterization. The instruments commonly utilize acoustic waveform analysis.

The spatial distribution and texture of echoes in a gray-scale image can experimentally distinguish tissue types, but the clinical reliability of this approach is still being tested. Preliminary investigations have attempted to characterize tissues by evaluating parameters of the frequency histogram of reflected echo amplitudes from specific regions of interest identified on the B-scan image. These parameters have included the mean echo amplitude, the spread of the echoes about the mean (standard deviation), and the asymmetry of the distribution (skewness). This technique has been applied to the classification of cirrhotic liver disease.[19] Parameters of image texture such as echo gradients that reflect the degree of roughness and autocorrelation analysis, which is a measure of periodic spacing, are also under study. At this time, most of the techniques being used to characterize tissue are in their infancy. These methods will have to undergo further development and are not immediately applicable to clinical practice. Linzer and Wells[20] have proposed that mass screening for breast cancer is one clinical problem area that might be solved by ultrasonic tissue characterization.

There are numerous opportunities in ultrasonic tissue characterization. These include the development of realistic tissue models and theories and the measurement and cataloging of data on tissue velocities, attenuation, scattering, and impedance. New techniques utilizing computed tomography and digital-image processing and pattern recognition techniques appear very promising. Complete and definitive clinical validation of these techniques should be forthcoming. This discipline will be one of great emphasis and will lead to successful application of physics and biomedical engineering techniques to diagnostic imaging.

INSTRUMENTATION ADVANCES

Although it has not yet been conclusively demonstrated that digital articulated arm B-mode scanners are superior in clinical diagnostic abilities to analog systems, they do not appear to be in any way inferior. Because significant technical advances in digital scanners can be expected in the future, it is prudent to ensure that a current generation of an analog or digital scanner is capable of being upgraded to a more modern and improved version. Digital scan conversion appears to be the direction the discipline is moving.

Many of the recent technical advances in diagnostic ultrasound have been made in the area of real-time imaging. There are currently four basic types of real-time scanners available: (1) the linear sequenced array, (2) the linear phased array, (3) the annular phased array, and (4) the mechanical sector scan types. Each of these designs has very definite advantages and each possesses certain limitations. Differences among the instrument types arise from differences in the design of the transducer.

To be utilized for cardiac imaging, a transducer should be physically small enough to fit between the ribs or to be angled under the rib cage. Many instruments employ either the linear phased array or the mechanical sector scan transducer. Real-time imaging can also be applied to the rest of the body. One of the advantages of real-time imaging is that this methodology permits a large region to be studied rapidly. This allows a rapid determination of optimum scan planes. This is particularly important, for example, in fetal scanning where it is crucial to determine the correct plane through the fetal abdomen for diameter measurements. Because the image is viewed continuously and instantaneously, linear structures such as blood vessels can be followed and their three-dimensional nature reconstructed. With real-time imaging, there is little need for the patient to remain immobile or to suspend respiration during the study. Thus, infants, children, and patients whose physical conditions render them uncooperative may be studied with less difficulty than with conventional static B-mode scanners. Because study and viewing angles are rapidly achieved, structures can be evaluated and their size, shape, and internal consistency determined quickly. There is less dependence on the skill of the ultrasonographer. Thus, unlike static B-mode scanning, artifacts such as those produced by image overwriting are avoided. Within limits, the image quality is independent of the speed at which the transducer is moved over the body. In real-time abdominal and pelvic scanning in adults, the transducer size requirements are less rigid than those demanded in cardiac scanning. As large a field of view as possible must be produced to permit easy identification of anatomic landmarks and to simplify image interpretation.

Real-time instrumentation has introduced the practice of using the water enema to determine relative anatomic orientation (Fig. 13.3.A). In addition, air bubbles in the liquid provide a sonographic "contrast media," not unlike that obtained in radiographic fluoroscopy. Another technique involves the patient ingesting decanted or water mixed with methyl cellulose to

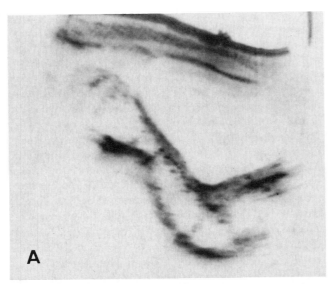

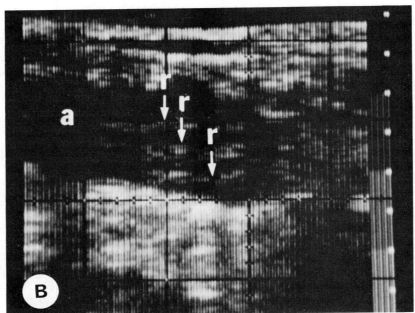

Figure 13.3. A. Longitudinal view of the pelvis with filled bladder technique. The water has been instilled into the rectum and sigmoid colon. Prior to installation, there was the appearance of a sonolucency which is shown by the water enema to represent fluid-filled bowel. The anatomic relationships between the bowel and the bladder are noted. This patient had a hysterectomy and on the scan prior to water enema, the bowel had assumed the position and appearance of the uterus. The water enema was clinically significant in delineating that this did, indeed, contain large bowel filled with fluid and debris. The vaginal cuff that was left following the hysterectomy is delineated. **B.** The fluid-filled stomach and antrum (a) serves as an acoustic window (r = rugae).

create an "acoustic window" through the stomach and duodenum. This latter technique is illustrated in Figure 13.3.B.

The two types of real-time instruments that have been designed specifically for body scanning have large transducers. They are the linear sequenced array transducer and the annular phased array transducer

(Fig. 13.4). Phased array and mechanical sector scan transducers give rise to sector-shaped images with an apex angle typically between 60 and 90 degrees (Fig. 13.5). While this format presents no significant problem in cardiac imaging, the restricted field of view in the apex of the sector is inconvenient for imaging superficial structures and organs during body scanning. In

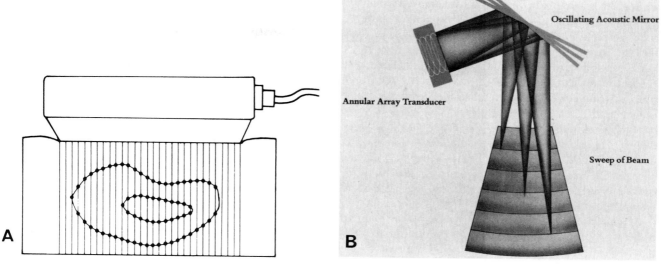

Figure 13.4. A. Linear sequenced array transducer. (Courtesy of Advanced Diagnostic Research, Tempe, Arizona.) **B.** An annular phased array. (Courtesy of Xerox Corporation, Pasadena, Calif.)

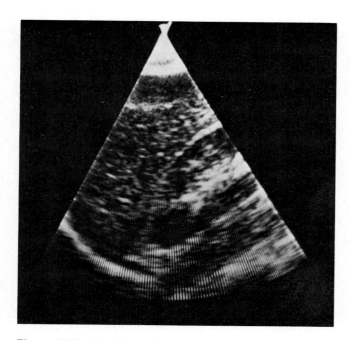

Figure 13.5. Real-time sector scanner. The so-called pie-shaped images are produced. The apex angles are between 60 and 90 degrees. In certain instances, this may provide some difficulty with image distortion. (Courtesy of Picker Corporation, North Haven, Conn.)

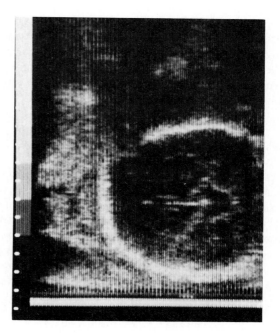

Figure 13.6. Rectangular image produced by a linear sequenced array. (Courtesy of Advanced Diagnostic Research, Tempe, Arizona.)

comparison, linear sequenced array and the annular phased array transducer type instruments yield a rectangular image format that is much more suited to body imaging (Fig. 13.6).

One of the important determinants of real-time scan quality is the echo dynamic range discernible on the display.[21] For x-y oscilloscopes, which are usually employed in analog based real-time scanners, the echo dynamic range is very restricted. Clinically, such analog scanners can display only a limited amount of echo amplitude information. Usually this only includes the stronger echoes that originate from specular reflections at gross tissue interfaces and not tissue texture. Thus, while such analog instruments are adequate in displaying the heart and its valves, as well as fetal structures, they are often inadequate in displaying the echoes from the fine parenchymal structures that make up the internal composition of organs such as the liver, spleen, and placenta. In contrast, the displays of digital based real-time instruments have a much wider echo dynamic range, and gross tissue interfaces as well as fine parenchymal details can be discerned. As discussed earlier, the ability to "tissue characterize" is a goal in ultrasound that is gradually being achieved. Certain changes in texture of specific organs at present, however, are sufficiently characteristic to suggest certain diagnoses.

Real-time instrumentation appears to be a direction of progress for ultrasound. At present, some controversy exists regarding the wisdom of having a real-time or a static B-mode instrument as the only ultrasonic imaging device in a single department. The authors believe that these types of imaging instruments offer such different capabilities that in most laboratories both are necessary. There is a need for physiologic evaluation and monitoring, which can only be achieved by real-time. Of equal importance is the ability to record images that have the same resolution as those created during the actual performance of the studies. Many observers believe that only articulated arm B-mode instruments offer this capability at present. Improvements in static recording from real-time studies will be accomplished in the near future.

DOPPLER TECHNIQUES

At present, no practical ultrasonic method has been developed for the noninvasive determination of volumetric blood flow. To appreciate the difficulty of this measurement, one needs to understand the concept of volumetric blood flow and measurements that are required to derive it. No directly calibrated single step measurement of volumetric blood flow seems possible using noninvasive methodology at this time. Volumetric blood flow, while having the units of liters per minute, actually is derived from two independent measurements when determined ultrasonically. These include the vessel lumen cross-sectional area (cm^2) and the average flow velocity (cm/sec) over that area. Determining the average velocity is a dual measurement since the angle between the sound beam and the blood flow direction or axis (θ) must also be determined. This can be expressed as:

$$Q = \vec{V} A \qquad (4)$$

where Q = Volumetric flow rate in liters/min or

cm^3/sec; $\overline{V}$ = Average velocity in cm/sec moving along the vessel axis at 90 degrees to the plane of the cross-sectional area. $\overline{V}$ is a vector having both direction and magnitude. A = blood vessel lumen area in cm^2.

Medical ultrasonic Doppler techniques have concentrated almost entirely on only one aspect of this problem; that is, the detection and measurement of flow velocity. Vessel area (A) and sound beam angle (θ) are potentially measurable using recent developments in instrumentation. Before discussing these, blood flow variables as clinical parameters should be considered in detail. Because volumetric flow measurement is technically difficult, other more readily derived parameters stemming from velocity measurements have evolved and are being evaluated:

1. Average velocity over the vessel lumen presented as an analog waveform. This method is used in peripheral vascular disease diagnosis.
2. Velocity distribution within sample volume or point located within the vessel or heart and displayed as a frequency spectrum. This is the primary detection and display mode used in cardiac and some vascular applications.
3. Velocity at a point within the vessel or intracardiac structure presented as an analog waveform. This particular technique has been employed by some in analysis of cardiac vascular disease.
4. Velocity distribution summed across the lumen of a blood vessel and displayed as a frequency spectrum.
5. Two-dimensional flow images of the blood vessel lumen either in long axis or cross-section depending upon the type of Doppler instrument employed and whether it is pulsed or continuous wave. This technique is utilized almost exclusively in peripheral vascular disease evaluation.

At present, none of these parameters is routinely calibrated to give the true flow velocity or spectra. Blood flow images are "semi-calibrated" but usually appear larger than actual size because of sound beam distortion and resolution effects. Since calibration for quantitation is difficult to accomplish clinically at the present time, most of the Doppler blood flow applications are qualitative and subjective. Physician observation currently serves as the best processing system to evaluate normal and abnormal blood flow signals.

Accurate use of Doppler blood flow detection techniques requires a thorough understanding of fluid dynamics in a biologic setting in addition to appropriate knowledge and appreciation of the Doppler principal and the interaction of ultrasound with moving blood.[6] The simplest Doppler instrument transmits a continuous beam of ultrasound at frequencies in the range of 3 to 10 MHz. The sound intensities will vary from less than 100 milliwatts per square centimeter (mW/cm^2)

to several hundred mW/cm^2 on some commercial units. The sound beam dimensions, including lateral width and position of the focal zone, will depend on the size of the transducer element and whether a lens is fixed to the crystal face. Beam widths as narrow as 1 mm or less can be achieved at frequency of 10 MHz with a sharply focused transducer. In a continuous wave Doppler, the appropriate resolution specification of interest clinically depend on the lateral width of the sound beam.

As stated in Chapter 12, when the sound leaves the transducer face and propagates through the tissue, it will undergo several effects. First, it will be absorbed to reduce the sound intensity at each point along the beam. This decrease is about 1 dB/cm/MHz. For a 4-MHz wave traveling 10 cm through the tissue, the loss will be 40 dB or a factor of 100. Twenty decibels corresponds to a loss factor of 10 and 60 decibels corresponds to a loss factor of 1000. Sound will be reflected at each point along the beam that the acoustic impedance changes according to the relation as expressed in $Z_a = PC$, where P = tissue density and C = velocity of sound in tissue, about 1540 meters per second. If the structure is stationary, the frequency of the reflected wave will be identical to the impinging wave. A moving structure will cause the back-scattered signal frequency to be shifted up or down by an amount proportional to the interface velocity acting along the sound beam axis. This shift is given by the following equation:

$$\pm \Delta f = \frac{2\overline{V}f_o}{c}\cos\theta \qquad (5)$$

where Δf = Doppler shift in Hertz (Hz), $\overline{V}$ = vector velocity in interface cm/sec, f_o = frequency of impinging sound beam Hz, c = velocity of sound in tissue media cm/sec, and θ = angle in degrees between sound beam axis and velocity vector. The actual received frequency (f_r) from a moving structure will be:

$$f_r = f_o \pm \Delta f \qquad (6)$$

Therefore

$$\pm \Delta f = f_o - f_r \qquad (7)$$

When the impinging sound beam passes through a blood vessel, scattering occurs. In this process, small amounts of sound energy are absorbed by each red cell and reradiated in all directions. If the red cell is moving with respect to the sound source, the back-scattered energy returning to the receiving transducer will be shifted in frequency; the magnitude and direction is proportional to the velocity of the respective cell. If the sound beam is considered to fill the entire lumen of a blood vessel, then the back-scattered signal will consist of all the Doppler shifts produced by the red cells

moving through the sound beam. Because there will always be a range of velocities present, from zero at the vessel wall to a peak value near the center, a spectrum of Doppler shift frequencies will always be present. This spectrum will become significantly complex with pulsating blood flow and vessel wall motion.

Blood flow disturbances from anatomic defects, eg, vessel wall irregularity or ulcerated plaques, narrowed or partially occluded vessels, and stenotic heart valves, can be readily detected by noting differences in the frequency spectrum of the Doppler signal. Usually, these can be detected by listening to the Doppler difference frequency (Δf). For ultrasonic frequencies in the range of 3 to 10 MHz, Δf will range from zero to approximately 10 KHz for velocities from zero to 100 cm/sec. A partial occlusion will, for example, cause a region of high-flow velocity to exist in the narrowed area. This high velocity can be readily detected from the Doppler signal by the high-pitched frequencies present. Another effect occurs as a result of the vessel narrowing that also facilitates detection. The moving blood will gain kinetic energy as it accelerates through the narrowed vessel or valve opening. Once it passes this point into a region of larger caliber, the velocity must decrease. At this point, the stored kinetic energy is given up in the form of blood flow disturbances or turbulence. Although true engineering turbulence may not exist, the flow will be disturbed to produce eddies and vortices. The flow velocity vectors are, therefore, rotated like a ball or wave in all directions like an oscillating string. Doppler instruments are very sensitive to this kind of flow. The output will contain a wide spectrum of Doppler shift frequencies caused by the rapidly changing wide range of velocities present in disturbed flow. Disturbed blood flow has a characteristic harsh sound to it, compared to smooth flow, which has a smooth or tonal quality.

A variety of simple continuous wave Doppler flow detectors are available for evaluating the peripheral circulation. They detect sites of high velocity or disturbed flow because of partially occluded vessels. These flow detection devices are useful if one is familiar with the method and interpretation of the signals. Both arterial and venous flow in the lower extremities can be assessed by these devices and methods.

In the continuous wave (CW) Doppler instruments, the transmitted and received signals are continuously being mixed or compared by the receiving transducer. Because sound is constantly being radiated into the tissue in this circumstance, there is an abundance of non-Doppler-shifted signals present from the many stationary interfaces occurring along the sound beam. These large amplitude, overriding, nonshifted signals mix with the very low amplitude Doppler return from moving blood in vessels within the same beam. Following this inherent mixing process, the Doppler difference frequency can be determined by using the amplitude modulation (AM) detection methods of radio communications.

For many clinicians, the complexity of the Doppler blood flow signal has been an obstacle. There are no images to view; flow waveforms and frequency spectrum plots seem remote from the disease process, even when the user has a thorough understanding of the physics. A number of imaging schemes have been devised to provide some orientation to the vessel anatomy and to indicate the site of blood flow detection. The simplest of these uses a continuous wave (CW) Doppler transducer fixed to a mechanical arm (Spencer). As the transducer moves back and forth over a vessel of interest, an image is produced on a storage oscilloscope corresponding to each site. The various deficiencies of the simple continuous wave (CW) Doppler instruments cause them to fall far short of providing a basis for quantitative blood flow measurements. More sophisticated methods and devices are needed to achieve the goals of calibration of the blood flow through specific vessels.

The most practical means to add depth resolution to a Doppler instrument is to pulse the source and add a range gate to the receiver. The pulsed Doppler is an implementation of this idea. It is similar to a pulse-echo instrument in that bursts of ultrasound are emitted at a regular repetition rate into tissue. A new pulse is not transmitted until the echoes from the previous pulse have subsided. The depth of a pulse can be determined by noting the time of its flight to an interface and return. Relatively short bursts 0.5 to 1.0 μsec in duration can be used to give high axial resolution for detection of the location and separation of interfaces to within 1 mm or less.

With the caveat that both employ sound energy, the principal of the pulsed Doppler is quite different from a pulse-echo instrument. To determine the Doppler shift of an echo at a particular depth or at many depths simultaneously the operator has to know the precise frequency of the original transmitted burst. This is best accomplished by exciting the transmitting transducer at a precise and known frequency. Further, when the echoes return one must be able to compare their frequency with the original transmitted burst to determine the difference or Doppler shift. Each transmitted burst excitation is derived from a master oscillator (MO) which operates in a continuous mode, eg, 5 MHz. Initially this technique will divide the continuous frequency 5 MHz down to, eg, 12.5 KHz. This low frequency is precisely related to the 5 MHz and becomes the pulse repetition frequency (PRF) of the transmitted bursts. This PRF signal is used to sample or time gate the 1.0 μsec long burst (5 cycles at 5 MHz) from the 5 MHz MO which are precisely spaced 80 μsec apart. When oriented in this manner, each trans-

mitted burst will be exactly in step with the master oscillator frequency. This signal is amplified and applied to the transmitting transducer crystal. The fact that there is an 80 μsec space or time between each transmitted burst means that, for this example, it will be possible ultimately to detect flow signals from vessels as deep as 6 cm, based on a calibration of 13 μsec of transmission time from the tissue for each centimeter of depth. If the PRF is lowered, evaluation at greater depth is possible, and, if increased, the examination is limited to more superficial depths in soft tissue. It is believed that pulse Doppler techniques will provide a future avenue of tremendous clinical growth of ultrasonic use.

IMAGE RECORDING AND DISPLAY

The development of gray-scale imaging represents a very significant development in ultrasound. This technique of using the CRT dot intensity to reflect signal strength has provided a measurable increase in sonographic capability.

The acceptance of this imaging modality has been greatly enhanced by gray-scale presentation. Equipment manufacturers now offer various weighting functions (gray-level assignment in relation to signal intensity) to relate the cathode ray intensity to the gray-scale signal level into a more clinically useful form. The manner in which this conversion is to be performed depends to some extent upon what is intended by the study, and the preferences and expectations of the interpreting physician.

It is, of course, recognized that the final data transfer of any imaging process is through recording properties of the human eye. Despite sophisticated considerations and techniques of electronic signal-weighting, the human eye and its physiology remain the limiting process for data transfer to the brain. Thus, a most important consideration is the amount of data that can be processed through the human eye—not just the recording aspect but the cognitive relationship as well.

A gray-bar generator producing 32 signal levels for an ultrasonic image can impose 32 perceptable shades of gray on the display. By the use of eye movement, most individuals can view the generated levels and distinctly perceive all 32 shades. Despite this fact, there is a widely held belief that the human eye can only differentiate approximately a dozen shades of gray. Physiologic data of the response characteristics of human and mammalian eyes support the concept that gray-scale discrimination is much greater than 10 to 12 shades of gray.

The concept that the human eye functions like a simple camera is an inaccurate oversimplification. Although both the eye and a camera have a lens and iris, once the image is formed on the retina the visual perception process becomes much more complex than mere recording. From this point onward, the similarities between the eye and a camera rapidly diminish. Studies show that the configuration of data points formed on the human retina is not mapped as an unaltered image upon the brain. Instead, the image is separated into bits formed by responses of individual receptors. Afterwards, it is shaped, enhanced, coded, and transmitted through pathways to the brain where this process is repeated. These data then seem to converge on one or a few cells in the upper cortex of the brain. This encoding and enhancement response appears to allow very accurate perception of the lighted world.

Perception through the human eye involves subtle cues that are as much psychologic as physiologic. Appropriate testing procedures are necessary to separate the purely physiologic responses from those characterized as psychologic or emotional. Optical illusions clearly indicate that our visual system can be deceived and these constructed illusions also provide understanding of how the visual system operates. From measurements of cellular events, optical illusions, and anatomic studies, a great deal is known regarding the organization and function of the human eye.

Information on visual recordings and the perception thereof is incomplete. Much remains to be discovered by controlled experiments and simulations. Although many of the events that will be described here are measurable, much of our understanding about higher ordered image integration is based on circumstantial evidence and inference. These extrapolations, nonetheless, represent the best explanation of experimental results regarding gray-scale image perception observed and recorded over the past 100 years. During the middle-to-late nineteenth century, a number of fundamental experiments were performed to determine certain aspects regarding the eye function. These experiments generally evaluated the difference between the data or signal presented to the eye and that transmitted to the brain. Mach[22] published observations on bands that appeared in nonlinear gray-scale fields that were a product of visual processing, which have been described as Mach bands or lines. Konig and Brodhun investigated the relationship between the change of luminance and the background luminance. They demonstrated that with a bright level of luminance, the eye can see an intensity change of less than 0.025 of the background level. They also showed that the general ability of the eye to see a change in intensity is increased as the background level of light is increased.

A series of optical illusions was created that demonstrated additional eye functions. One of the classic illusions involved the ability of the eye to record white data points on a black background versus black on white.[23] A white square placed on a black ground appears larger than a black square of equal size viewed against a white background. These experiments demonstrate that the eye does not see white on black the same as black on white. Hubel and Wiesel demonstrated that the basic mechanisms that are part of the physiologic function of the eye correlate with the phenomena fundamental to the observations of Mach and Konig.[22]

The relationship between shape and function is important in consideration of neurologic systems such as the eye in which the interconnection of cells determines their collective function. The basic organization of the retina is the receptor rods and cones arrangement. These cells function as energy transducers; they change light energy to electrical. The responses of the rods and cones are connected to ganglions through bipolar cells. This connection is complicated because of the lateral connection of synapses through horizontal cells. The lateral, receptor, and bipolar cells respond with a potential that is graded to the intensity of the simulus. In the ganglion cells, light information is transformed from an analog, graded potential response to a digital format of frequency-modulated action potentials.

The ganglion cells are an appropriate area of inquiry for studying retinal responses to various stimuli. To understand the neutral processing of visual data, one must have an understanding of the concept of "visual field." The visual field of any cell is the portion of the retina that will produce a response when appropriately illuminated. A visual field can also be thought of as the region of adequate simulus, that is, a region where the proper stimulus must be applied for maximum cell reaction. Any light pattern that does not illuminate the visual field appropriately, therefore, will produce less than a maximum response from the cell. One then should consider visual field for a ganglion cell. Many of these cells respond maximally when a light pattern is placed on the retina that has an illuminated or "on" center and a shaded or "off" surround.[22] When the receptive field is flooded with light, the cell manifests a response and when the receptive field is flooded with a dark segment the cell does not respond at all.

Based on this visual field response, one should consider the anticipated physiologic change of the retina to the presentation of a light-dark boundary. The receptive fields with both center and surround flooded with light will have a small response, whereas receptive fields in the dark segment will respond minimally or not at all. Only at the boundary where the center is illuminated and a segment of the surround darkened will the cells respond maximally. The eye will manifest, therefore, a better response to a contrast boundary and will physiologically function to enhance the contrast boundary to form the Mach bands at that location. One can observe these phenomena in the gray-bar test pattern presented on many scan converters. Two fields with different intensities will seem to change in intensity close to the boundary; the lighter field gets lighter and the darker field appears to become darker.

The eye is not as facile in recording absolute intensity differences as it is contrast boundaries. These light and dark bands seen as sharp changes in intensity are the same bands observed by Mach who correctly predicted that these bands would be found to originate from a contrast enhancement process of the eye.[24] This was an astute interpretation considering the absence of the supporting single-cell data confirmation at that time.

In addition to the contrast processes, the mammalian eye is very sensitive to motion.[22] Various cells in the cerebral cortex are dedicated not only to responding to distinct positions of light-dark boundaries, but also to the direction in which the boundary is traveling. The human eye utilizes moving boundaries so well that should a boundary be stationary, the brain will move the eye over the boundary in a series of small rapid eye movements. This is part of the explanation for the phenomenon that real-time images appear to contain more information while moving than "frozen" for observation or for recording.

As we have previously commented, one can demonstrate through optical illusions that the eye senses white data on a black background differently than black on white. Whole organ measurements have shown that the brighter the background level, the more sensitive the eye becomes to small intensity changes that can occur on the single cell level. This is evidenced by the cells in the lateral geniculate nucleus that will change firing rate with increments and decrements in light level around an adapting level.[25] As the adaptive light level decreases in intensity, so will the dynamic range of the geniculate cells.

We know that contrast boundaries are a stimulus for the eye and the eye responds quite actively to moving boundaries. Additionally, the eye will enhance contrast at a boundary and sees white on black in a different manner than black on white. These properties can be related to perception in ultrasonic imaging. As was previously stated, the eye can record and perceive more than a dozen shades of gray provided the background adapting level is sufficiently bright. From data that has been presented, if one wishes to utilize the widest dynamic range of the eye to interrogate the gray scale of an image, a black-on-white format would seem preferable. This statement conforms to observations that the eye can see smaller changes in intensity when the background is brightly illuminated. In practical terms, if an observer is interested in low-level echoes such as tissue texture patterns or organ parenchymal changes, a permanent recording format of "dark" data points on a "light" background should provide the maximum opportunity for perception. Conversely, when organ boundaries and linear structures are of primary interest, a white-on-black format would seem to be most appropriate. In this image-recording format, the eye is operating over a shallower dynamic range and boundaries will appear both larger and more distinct.

Most current diagnostic ultrasonic instruments have a video inversion switch that can be employed for this change. A true "reversal" does not always occur, however, as a result of differences in film response. If one wishes to have both presentations in a single study, some adjustment of the camera lens may be necessary. From these discussions, it is apparent that perception of the data contained in ultrasonic images is a complex process. The choice of recording format can more appropriately be made if these phenomena are understood, however. Certain practical considerations exist in choosing the type of display for permanent image recording. With conventional B-mode gray-scale images, the choices are generally those of Polaroid 35-, 70-, or 105-mm film in single frames, or a film emulsion multiformat with an 8- or 16-image capacity for each film. Other types of image recording are under development and may achieve general clinical application. Real-time instrumentation offers the same operator choices along with videotape display and voice-sensing devices.

Polaroid photography has distinct advantages and disadvantages to the user. The gray-scale capabilities are compressed into a small number of levels of contrast that can be visually separated. Operation of the camera itself is simple and images are immediately available for viewing. No specific quality assurance testing or processing apparatus is required. The films are individually separate and must either be mounted or affixed to a flat surface such as cardboard or placed in a film packet of some type. Arrangement of these individual views for conferences, consultation with clinical colleagues, as well as for teaching and tutorial sessions can sometimes prove difficult. Polaroid imaging is expensive when one considers the cost of an individual view and is a consideration that must be weighed against the expenditure for processing equipment and the volume of studies to be performed by a laboratory. Preparation of 35-mm slides for presentation and prints for publication is easily facilitated by Polaroid imaging, which has enhanced the use in ultrasonic departments engaged in teaching and research.

Single frame imaging in 35-, 70-, or 105-mm format has been successfully utilized in other types of diagnostic imaging. The film can be processed in the regular automatic film processors of a medical imaging department and is relatively inexpensive. Once the series of views are developed, however, some permanent form of arrangement is necessary for viewing, consultation, or retention for the laboratory archives. Many gastrointestinal radiology sections use this type of format so that it may be widely available in many radiology departments.

Multiformat film has received rather widespread acceptance in both computerized axial tomography and ultrasonography. This type of imaging system has become sufficiently utilized so that companies that do not sell the usual imaging instrument will sell multiformat recording systems. This type of image presentation is the most uniform if regarded as a part of the overall imaging department and has distinct advantages for consultation, correlation, and storage. Radiologists and other physicians who have had previous experience with radiographs are familiar with type of presentation and viewbox demonstration. Film manufacturers have developed a number of special types of films for ultrasonic recording. In choosing an appropriate film, one should be particularly attentive to the stability of response and reproducibility of density. This is especially of concern in recording low-level "texture" echoes. Manufacturers in producing multiformat images that are compatible with the many B-mode scanners available have not always utilized appropriate coupling screens or lens systems of sufficient quality. Some manufacturers, therefore, are considering or have begun to produce their own multiformat cameras.

In recording real-time studies, cine, videotape, and motion picture film have been used. These, however, are often difficult and cumbersome for individual physician consultation. The ability to have a permanent image in the same format as conventional B-mode recorders has increased physician acceptance of the value of real-time studies. Recording a part of the study for later reviews, however, may be very worthwhile for consultation, teaching, and hard-copy static recording of the most significant image.

BIOLOGIC BURDEN IMPLICATIONS

Practicing physicians wish to be assured of the complete safety of diagnostic ultrasound. This is not possible given the present state of knowledge regarding this energy source, or, for that matter, other types of diagnostic and therapeutic medical procedures. Difficulty exists in assessing the relevance of the multiple fragmentary studies obtained with experimental machines on animal tissues to the possible effects of diagnostic sonographic studies. With some degree of assurity, we can make the following statements:

1. The vast majority of the ultrasonic diagnostic examinations involve a technique in which two-dimensional echo images are produced by emitting very short pulses of microsecond duration that are repeated at a rate of up to 1000 times per second. For 99.9 percent of the study time, therefore, the target is not insonated and the transducer is used to "listen" for the returning echoes.
2. No deleterious effects have been reported in humans subsequent to insonation with machines using such short pulse-echo techniques.[26]
3. Isolated reports have shown no confirmation of deleterious effects to animal models from B-mode equipment used in clinical practice. There are now a number of unconfirmed reports on such effects from Doppler devices in clinical use.

The most important aspect of diagnostic ultrasound is the extreme brevity of the pulses and the relatively long intervals between them. This relatively long interval implies that the actual insonation time will be only one-thousandth the total time required for the clinical scan. Clinically significant bioeffects appear to be theoretically unlikely unless summation occurs. The interest in biologic effects has increased with the advent and wide clinical use of real-time equipment with linear or phased arrays. For dynamic (real-time) presentation, rapid data acquisition is at a premium, and one means for achieving this is to increase the pulse repetition rate to at least 3000 pulses per second. This results in a definite increase in dose to the patient, which may be compensated by decreased examination time. Linear arrays, in particular, employ very low ultrasonic intensity, so that their use may not cause undue concern.

The possible physical and biologic effects of ultrasound and the parameters of insonation required for their production will be considered in a rather summary fashion.

PHYSICAL EFFECTS OF ULTRASOUND

HEAT

There is a low average intensity involved in the SONAR technique (less than 20 mW/cm^2). Thus, no significant degree of heating occurs. Doppler devices used for fetal monitoring should have an output of less that 20 mW/cm^{-2} and similarly should also be free of adverse heating effects. Other Doppler devices, used particularly for arterial studies, employ intensities that may produce significant heating, and these should be labeled as being unsuitable for fetal investigation. At these intensities, adverse bioeffects have been described.

CAVITATION

Cavitation refers to a complex phenomenon in which gas-filled bubbles grow in a sound field. It is not known whether these bubbles are already present prior to insonation, or if they develop during insonation from gaseous "nuclei" of smaller (characteristically invisible) size.[27] At high-sound levels, these bubbles may collapse suddenly and violently in the positive phase of the sound cycle, causing large but localized temperature rises, the thermal decomposition of water, and release of free radicals. This phenomena has been termed *transient cavitation*. At lower sound levels, the gas bubbles may pulsate over an indefinite period of time, enlarging during the negative phase of the sound cycle and reducing during the positive phase. This is described as *stable cavitation*.[28] Stable gas bubbles that are caused to vibrate by ultrasound can, even at low sound levels, generate shearing stresses that can affect the structure as well as presumably the behavior of cells in their locality.[29] The threshold intensity for cavitation varies with the frequency. Recent studies suggest that cavitation can be produced in suspension of cells in tissue culture fluid by intensities of 500 mW/cm² and, presumably, by lower intensities at lower frequencies.[30]

Hill et al[31] have shown that the threshold for cavitation varies with the pulse length and that the threshold is lowest when the pulse length is in the range of 1 to 30 msec. The occurrence of cavitation is facilitated by the cumulative effects of multiple sound wave cycles. The converse is also true: The threshold intensity for pulses of microseconds duration has not yet been established. Findings so far indicate, however, that it is high. The brevity of the pulses used in clinical ultrasonography probably prevent the occurrence of cavitation at the intensities used for diagnostic purposes.

The continuous nature of insonation inherent in Doppler diagnostic devices implies that the peak intensity should be retained below the cavitation threshold. Thus, in addition to avoiding the thermal changes, Doppler devices for obstetric purposes should be of very low output to avoid cavitation. Clinically, peak intensities of less than 20 mW/cm^{-2} suffice for diagnostic purposes. These intensities appear to be below all known thresholds of damage or for the production of other biologic effects.[32]

Many bioeffects of ultrasound have been reported, some of which are deleterious. These deleterious effects can neither be explained by heat nor attributed to cavitation. These forces involved are well recognized, but to date it appears to be more difficult to ascribe a specific bioeffect to one particular energy effect. When an acoustic wave is transmitted through a medium, the particles are subjected to oscillatory variations in pressure, velocity, acceleration, and temperature. Because these primary forces act upon a nonhomogeneous medium, they give rise to time averaged forces and do not self-reciprocate. These forces include streaming, shear force, and Bernoulli and Oseen forces.

Change in Transport Across Membranes. Changes in the permeability of membranes have been reported.[33,34] One possible mechanism for this change is the movement of particles away from the origin of a sound beam (streaming). Changes in permeability are reflected in the ultrastructural appearance of irradiated liver cells which show swelling of the endoplasmic reticulum as well as the mitochondrial changes.[35]

Recent theoretical considerations on possible thresholds for significant stresses induced by microstreaming provide no cause for complacency.[36] Data derived from the KHz region was extrapolated to the MHz region, and a number of assumptions had to be made in the theoretical analysis. Stresses associated with microstreaming are facilitated by the presence of resonant cavities (diameter of 3 μM at a frequency of 1 MHz). Under these conditions, it has been calculated that significant stress could be induced by intensities as low as 0.5 mW/cm². This is lower than that found for any reported bioeffects, and it seems unlikely that such cavities exist in most animal tissues.

Alteration of Mitochondria. Swelling of the mitochondria and disruption of the cristae have been reported.[37,38] This may be a direct effect on the mitochondria or part of a more widespread change resulting from changes in plasma membrane permeability.

Lysosomal Changes. Insonation of the liver of rodents was reported to result in damage to the lysomal membrane. The normal small dense bodies were replaced by myelin figures. Ultrastructural examination after insonation showed evidence of partial digestion of mitochondria.[35] Partial digestion of nuclear material could result in serious consequences for the progeny of any cell that survived this insult if the genome were altered.

The parameters of insonation in these experiments have been considerably greater than those involved in the typical diagnostic SONAR examination. For the production of lysosomal damage for example, peak intensities were in the region of 25 W/cm^{-2}. Pulse lengths of 10 msec were used, separated by intervals of 90 msec for five minutes. Thus, the pulse lengths were 10,000 times longer than those used in diagnostic ultrasound.

Lysomal damage has recently been reported at lower intensities.[39] These authors noted that the permeability of epidermal lysosomes was increased in skin irradiated in vivo with therapeutic levels of ultrasound (intensity 0.5 W/cm^{-2}; frequency 3 MHz; pulsed 2 msec on, 8 msec off for 5 minutes). Permeability was assessed by means of the lysosome fragility test and gave a positive reaction to the test from 5 to 15 minutes earlier than did those of the control, mock-insonated epidermis, indicating that the irradiated lysosomes were more permeable and more "fragile." Ultrastructural studies also suggested that the permeability of various membranes of the cells had been affected by isonization.[40] Increase in lysosomal membrane permeability is not necessarily harmful,[41] however, and may even stimulate reparative processes indirectly by increasing the availability of the low molecular weight precursors needed as raw materials for repair. Siegel et al have shown that attachment (the ability of cultured cells to adhere to surfaces) is decreased by sonication at levels approaching diagnostic inputs.

Production of Centrilobular Necrosis of the Liver.
Centrilobular necrosis subsequent to insonation at 1 MHz appeared to be frequency dependent, and higher frequencies were less effective.[42,43] The dosage parameters were greater than those used for diagnostic processes.

Production of Paraplegia.
The production of paraplegia can be used as a dramatic end-point of ultrasonic damage. The dose-response curve has been elucidated.[44] By extrapolation from this curve, we can compute that the threshold intensity required for paraplegia by a single pulse of microsecond duration is in the range of 10^4 W/cm^2. The use of repetitive pulses for a longer duration (10 msec), however, showed that hemorrhage into the spinal cord and paraplegia could be produced by peak intensities in the region of only 25 W/cm^2. It was also found that the insonation time for production of hemorrhage increased with increasing frequency to 5 MHz, at which frequency hemorrhage and paraplegia no longer occurred. This damage factor appeared to be inversely related to thermal changes.

The production of hemorrhage and paraplegia was also used to investigate whether hypoxia increased the sensitivity of tissue to ultrasonic insult. Reducing the arterial oxygen tension to 50 mm Hg while retaining a normal partial pressure of carbon dioxide markedly decreased the insonation time required for hemorrhage. It appeared that the physiologic state of the tissue affected its sensitivity to insonation, which is not surprising.

This series of experiments on the production of paraplegia and hemorrhage into the spinal cord of rats also produced evidence of dose accumulation. When the intervals between adjacent pulses were increased, the onset of damage was dependent only on the integrated dose-time. By extrapolating these data to the diagnostic parameters of dosage, one finds that many hours of continued insonation would be required to produce damage, even allowing for hypoxia in the fetus. Evidence from this and other experimental studies indicated that shorter pulses, however, more similar

to those used diagnostically, were safer than the pulse lengths used in these studies.

Production of Fetal Anomalies.
Pulsed insonation of a large series of pregnant mice using various parameters and peak intensities up to 490 W/cm^2 failed to demonstrate any difference in mortality or congenital anomalies between the insonated and control groups.[45] Insonation of chick embryos at a frequency of 1 MHz using various pulsing techniques including pulses of 20 μsec duration with an interval of 180 μsec between demonstrated that when the embryos were insonated after only 18 hours of incubation and during the period of active organogenesis, a significant increase in incidence of congenital abnormalities at intensities of 25 W/cm^2 and above occurred.[46,47] The defects noted included malformation of the central nervous system and main embryologic axis. It should be noted that the pulse length used in these experiments was 20 times that used diagnostically and the pulse repetition rate was 5 times greater. Additionally, the method of insonation resulted in whole-body irradiation compared with localized irradiation for most clinical examinations.

The experiments were then repeated at a later stage of development, after organogenesis was complete and corresponding to about 6 weeks of human development. At this stage of maturity, insonation at the parameters previously employed did not produce any evidence of congenital anomalies. When the intensities were increased to a peak intensity of 100 W/cm^2 and pulse lengths were increased to 10 msec on and 90 msec off for 5 minutes, there was no apparent damage to the embryo. These experiments showed that embryos could be damaged early during gestation and, therefore, insonation in the early stages of pregnancy may involve an element of risk. After organogenesis is complete, there is evidence that the fetus becomes more resistant to ultrasonic damage.

Stimulation of Regeneration and Wound Healing.
Low-intensity pulsed ultrasound has been shown to stimulate tissue regeneration and skin repair in experimental animals and the healing of pressure sores and varicose ulcers in man.[48-52] In a tissue regeneration study, the most effective dosage was 0.5 W/cm^2 at 3 MHz, pulsed 2 msec on, 8 msec off for 5 minutes, 3 times weekly.[48] At this time and other dose levels, a characteristic pattern of response was noted. Peak stimulation occurred at 21 days when cell proliferation is normally high in this system. There was a temporary decrease between 28 and 35 days when electron microscopic investigations suggest that collagen fiber maturation is occurring. Evidence obtained by autoradiography and electron microscopy showed that cell

proliferation was stimulated and collagen fiber maturation inhibited at therapeutic dose levels.

Work on fibroblasts in vitro suggests that, although fiber maturation is retarded by ultrasound, the production of fiber precursors is stimulated.[53] Pretreatment of the cells with cortisone, a lysosomal-membrane-stabilizing agent, blocked stimulation. This suggests some form of lysosomal involvement in the process. Treatment with therapeutic levels of ultrasound (3 MHz, space-time peak intensities of 2, 1, or 0.5 W/cm², pulsed 2 msec on, 8 msec off for 20 minutes) increases the motility of sparse populations of human fibroblasts insonated while attached to plastic substrates. This increase in total displacement from a fixed point in a given time is not due to an increase in cell velocity but to an increase in cell directionality. Thus, treated cells are more likely to move in a constant direction than are mock-insonated cells. Should a similar increase in directionality occur when fibroblasts are insonated in vivo after local injury, then their speed of arrival at the wound site would increase stimulating tissue repair. The effect reported above is of a temporary nature; by 24 hours after insonation, the directionality of fibroblasts treated in vitro has generally returned to normal.

DOPPLER SONOCATION

Continuous wave is often used for Doppler investigations, which usually involve a transient insonation of the fetus to establish fetal life. The use of the Doppler principle to monitor the fetal heart rate in labor could give cause for concern unless the incident intensity was maintained very low.

A number of recent reports have indicated fetal anomalies or morbidity following exposure to low-dose continuous insonation. An increased incidence of congenital abnormalities in mice after exposure to a commercially available Doppler device has been reported.[54] An increased incidence in perinatal morbidity after a 3-minute insonation of 125 mW/cm^{-2} has been seen.[55] O'Brien[56] reported decreased fetal weight in mice insonated at intensities of 500 mW/cm^{-2} for 5 minutes.

There are conflicting reports on whether insonation produces chromosomal aberrations. McIntosh and Davey[57,58] reported that commercial Doppler devices produced an increased incidence of chromosomal aberrations but all attempts made by other workers to repeat this observation failed. Subsequently, McIntosh himself failed to reproduce his own initial results. Unfortunately, the first positive report obtained more widespread publicity than the subsequent retraction.

Dyson et al[59] observed that ultrasound in a standing wave field could produce complete, but generally reversible, red cell stasis in the chick embryo and that prolonged stasis could result in vascular occlusion following endothelial damage. The intensity threshold for this phenomenon is approximately 500 mW/cm². More recently, terHaars[60] has demonstrated red cell banding and temporary stasis in the uterine vessels of the mouse. To produce this effect, it is essential that the vessel lie between the transducer and an adequate reflecting surface.

The Bioeffects Committee of the American Institute of Ultrasound in Medicine released its Statement on Mammalian In Vivo Ultrasonic Bioeffects in August 1976. It is reviewed annually, and, at the present time, is still deemed to be operative and essentially correct:

> In the low megahertz frequency range, there have been (as of this date) no demonstrated significant biological effect in mammalian tissue exposed to intensities* below 100 mW/cm². Furthermore, for ultrasonic exposure times† less than 500 seconds and greater than 1 second, such effects have not been demonstrated even at higher intensities, when the product of intensity* and exposure time† is less than 50 joules/cm².

Deficiencies still exist in our knowledge of the bioeffects of ultrasound, but the justification for its use is overwhelming. Nevertheless, it should only be used appropriately, minimizing the exposure to that required for the acquisition of important medical data. Clinicians and patients should be encouraged by the apparent innocuous nature of ultrasonic examination.

REFERENCES

1. Ultrasonic Tissue Characterization. NBS Special Publication 453. Washington, D.C., US Government Printing Office, 1976
2. Ultrasonic Tissue Characterization II. NBS Special Publication 525. Washington, D.C., US Government Printing Office, 1979
3. Dunn F: Ultrasonic attenuation, absorption, and velocity in tissues and organs. NBS Special Publication 453: 21–28, 1976
4. Parry RJ, Chivers RC: Data on the velocity and attenuation of ultrasound in mammalian tissues—a survey. NBS Special Publication 525: 343–360, 1979
5. Kohayashi T: Correlation of attenuation and absorption in breast cancer with connective tissue content. NBS Special Publication 525: 93–99, 1976
6. Wells PNT, Halliwell M, Mountford RA, et al: Tumor

*Spatial peak, temporal average as measured in a free field in water.
†Total time; this includes off-time as well as on-time for a repeated-pulse regime.

detection by ultrasonic doppler blood-flow signals. NBS Special Publication 525: 173–176, 1979

7. Lizzi FL, Elbaum ME: Clinical spectrum analysis technique for tissue characterization. NBS Special Publication 525: 111–119, 1979

8. Fry EK, Sanghui NT, Fry FJ, et al: Frequency dependent attenuation of malignant breast tumors studied by the fast Fourier technique. NBS Special Publication 525: 85–91, 1979

9. Levi S, Kenrvez J: Tissue characterization *in vivo* by differential attenuation measurements. NBS Special Publication 525: 121–124, 1979

10. Lele PP, Mansfield AB, Murphy AI, et al: Tissue characterization by ultrasonic frequency-dependent attenuation and scattering. NBS Special Publication 453: 167–196, 1976

11. O'Donnell M, Mimbs JW, Sobel BE, et al: Ultrasonic attenuation in normal and ischemic myocardium. NBS Special Publication 525: 63–71, 1979

12. Albertson KW, Leopold GR: Liver. In Goldberg B (ed): Abdominal Grey Scale Ultrasound. New York, Academic Press, 1977

13. Fields S, Dunn F: Correlation of echographic visualizability of tissue with biological composition and physiological state. J Acoust Soc Am 54: 809–812, 1973

14. Frese M, Lyons EA: Ultrasonic backscatter from human liver tissue: Its dependence on frequency and protein/lipid composition. JCU 5: 307–312, 1977

15. Bamber JC, Fry MJ, Hill CR, Dunn F: Ultrasonic attenuation and backscattering by mammalian organs as a function of time after excision. Ultrasound Med Biol 3: 15–20, 1977

16. Chivers RC: Review: The scattering of ultrasound in human tissues—some theoretical models. In Ultrasound in Medicine and Biology, Vol 3. New York, Pergamon Press, 1977, pp 1–13

17. Rose JL, Goldberg BB: Frequency analysis. In Basic Physics in Diagnostic Ultrasound. New York, Wiley, 1979, pp 98–105

18. Mountford RA, Wells PNT: Ultrasonic liver scanning: The A-scan in the normal and cirrhosis. Phys Med Biol 17: 261–269, 1972

19. Goddard J, James AE, Price RR, et al: Quantitative computer analysis of ultrasound B-scans. Proceedings of the 23rd Annual Meeting of the American Institute of Ultrasound in Medicine, San Diego, Calif., 1: 107, 1979

20. Linzer M, Wells PNT: Report on the symposium. NBS Special Publication 525, 3–9, 1979

21. Carson PL: Grey-scale ultrasound: Understanding an innovation in imaging to speed realization of its potential. Appl Radiol 6(3): 185–189, 1977

22. Hubel DH, Wiesel TN: Receptive fields, binocular interaction and functional architecture in the cat's visual cortex. J Physiol 160: 106–154, 1962

23. Graham CH: Fundamental data. In Graham CH (ed): Vision and Visual Perception. New York, Wiley, 1965, pp 68–80

24. Graham CH: Visual form perception. In Graham CH (ed): Vision and Visual Perception. New York, Wiley, 1965, pp 648–574

25. Jacobs GH: Effects of adaptation on the lateral genicu-late response to light increment and decrement. J Optic Soc America 55: 51–58, 1965

26. Hellman LM, Dufus GM, Donald I, Sunden B: Safety of diagnostic ultrasound in obstetrics. Lancet 1: 1133, 1970

27. Gershoy A, Miller DL, Nyborg WL: Intercellular gas: Its role in sonated plant tissue. In White D, Barnes R (eds): Ultrasound in Medicine, Vol 2. New York, Plenum Press, 1976, pp 501–511

28. Flynn HG: Physics of acoustic cavitation in liquids. In Mason WP (ed): Physical Acoustics. New York, ACAD, 1B, 1964, p 57

29. Nyborg WL: Cavitation in biological systems. In Bjorno L (ed): Finite-amplitude Wave Effects in Fluids. Guildford, England: IPC Science and Technology Press, 1974, pp 245–251

30. Webster DF, Pond JB, Dyson M, Harvey W: The role of cavitation in the 'in vitro' stimulation of protein synthesis in human fibroblasts by ultrasound. In White DN (ed): Ultrasound in Medicine and Biology. England: Pergamon Press (in press).

31. Hill CR, Clark PR, Crowe MR, Hammick JW: Biophysical effects of cavitation in a MHz ultrasonic beam. In Crawford A (ed): Ultrasonics for Industry Conference Papers. Guildford, England: Illife Scientific, 1969, p 26

32. Wells PNT: The possibility of harmful biological effects in ultrasonic diagnosis. In Reneman RS (ed): Cardiovascular Applications of Ultrasound. London: Elsevier, 1974

33. Schnitzler RM: PhD dissertation. Burlington, University of Vermont, 1971 (Abstract appears in IEEE Trans Biomed Eng BME 18: 309, 1971)

34. Mummery CL: The effect of ultrasound on fibroblasts 'in vitro.' PhD Thesis. London, England, London University, 1978

35. Taylor KJW, Pond JB: Primary sites of ultrasonic damage on cell systems. In Reid JM, Sikov MR (eds): Interaction of Ultrasound and Biological Tissues. Workshop Proceedings, Session 2: 8. Washington, D.C.: DHEW Publication (FDA), 1972, pp 87–92

36. Nyborg WL: Physical mechanisms for biological effects of ultrasound. Bureau of Radiological Health, HEW Publication 78-8062, 1978, p 41

37. Bernstine RL, Dickson LG: Study of effects of ultrasound as determined by electron microscopy. In Reid JM, Sikov MR (eds): Interaction of Ultrasound and Biological Tissues. Workshop Proceedings, Session 2: 6. Washington, D.C., DHEW Publication (FDA), 1972, pp 77–81

38. Taylor KJW, Pond JB: A study of the production of haemmorrhagic injury and paraplegia in rat spinal cord by pulsed ultrasound of low megahertz frequencies in the context of the safety of clinical usage. Br J Radiol 45: 343–353, 1972

39. Dyson M, Godsland J, Smith S, Pond JB: (unpublished data)

40. Aikman AA, Wills ED: Studies on lysosomes after irradiation. I: A quantitative histochemical method for the study of lysosomal membrane permeability and acid phosphatase activity. Rad Res 57: 403–415, 1974

41. Szego CM: The lysosome as a mediator of hormone action. Recent Prog Hormone Res 30: 171–233, 1974

42. Curtis JC: Action of intense ultrasound on intact mouse

liver. In Kelly E (ed): Ultrasonic Energy. Urbana, Ill., Univ of Illinois Press, 1965, pp 85–116

43. Taylor KJW, Pond JB: The effects of ultrasound of varying frequencies on rat liver. J Pathol 100 (4): 287–293, 1970

44. Fry FJ, Dunn F: Interaction of ultrasound and tissue. In Reid JM, Sikov MR (eds): Interaction of Ultrasound and Biological Tissues. Workshop Proceedings, Session 3: 1. Washington, D.C., DHEW Publication (FDA), 1972, pp 109–114

45. Woodward B, Pond JB, Warwick R: How safe is sonar? Br J Radiol 43: 719, 1970

46. Taylor KJW, Dyson M: Possible hazards of diagnostic ultrasound. Br J Hosp Med 10: 571–577, 1972

47. Taylor KJW, Dyson M: Toxicity studies on the interaction of ultrasound on embryonic and adult tissue. Proceedings of the Second World Congress on Ultrasonics in Medicine. Rotterdam, 1973, pp 353–359

48. Dyson M, Pond JB, Joseph JJ, Warwick R: Stimulation of tissue regeneration by pulsed plane-wave ultrasound. IEEE Trans Sonics and Ultrasonics SU-17: 133–140, 1970

49. Drastichova V, Samohyl A, Slavetinska A: Strengthening of sutured skin wound with ultrasonic in experiments on animals. ACTA Chir Plast 15: 114–119, 1973

50. Paul BJ, LaFratta CW, Dawson R, et al: Use of ultrasound in the treatment of pressure sores in patients with spinal cord injury. Arch Phys Med Rehabil 41: 438–440, 1960

51. Dyson M, Franks CR, Suckling J: Stimulation of healing of varicose ulcers by ultrasound. Ultrasonics 14 (5): 232–236, 1976

52. Dyson M, Suckling J: Stimulation of tissue repair by ultrasound: A survey of the mechanisms involved. Physiotherapy (London) 64: 105–108, 1978

53. Dyson M, Pond JB, Grahame W: The *in vitro* stimulation of protein synthesis in human fibroblasts by therapeutic levels of ultrasound. Proceedings of the 2nd European Congress on Ultrasonics in Medicine. Excerpta Medica International Cong Series 363: 10–21, 1975

54. Shoji R, Momma E, Shimizu T, Matsuda S: An experimental study on the effect of low-intensity ultrasound on developing mouse embryos. J Faculty Sci, Hokkaido Univ, Series VI; Zoology 18 (1): 51–56, 1971

55. Curto KA: Early postpartum mortality following ultrasound radiation. In White DN (ed): Proceedings of the American Institute of Ultrasound in Medicine. New York, Plenum Press, 1976

56. O'Brien WD, Christman CL, Yarrow S: Ultrasonic biological effect exposure system. New York, Ultrasonics Symposium Proceedings, IEEE Cat 74, CHO 896 ISU, 1974

57. McIntosh ICC, Davey DA: Chromosome aberrations induced by an ultrasonic fetal pulse detector. Br Med J 4: 92, 1970

58. McIntosh ICC, Davey DA: Relationship between intensity of ultrasound and induction of chromosome aberrations. Br J Radiol 45: 320, 1972

59. Dyson M, Pond JB, Woodward B: Flow of red blood cells stopped by ultrasound. Nature 232: 572–573, 1971

60. terHaar G: The effect of ultrasonic standing wave fields on the flow of particles, with special reference to biological media. PhD Thesis. London, England, London University, 1977

CHAPTER 14

Image Considerations in Computed Tomography

CRAIG M. COULAM
JON J. ERICKSON

The production of computed tomographic (CT) images represents a unique and different interplay between conventional x-ray producing and detecting equipment and a digital computer. Because the images are computed or "reconstructed," certain image features may be considered as ideal and thus serve as the theoretically optimum characteristics or qualities that are to be generated or found in the images. While it is not always possible to separate the synergistic dependency of equipment and images, the physics of the pictorial aspects of CT images will be discussed in this chapter using only general terms that may be considered more or less independent of the different types of scanners presently available for producing them. The potential of the images for displaying anatomic and pathologic structures will be discussed, as well as their sensitivity to the presence or types of anatomy that can be only marginally imaged or resolved. The inherent advantages and disadvantages of CT imaging and the sensitivity of the CT image to artifact contamination will also be covered. In the following chapter, CT equipment will be described, along with how different machine designs can and do influence image quality and information content.

GENERAL CONSIDERATIONS

A CT image is a pictorial display of a thin slice or section of anatomy, somewhat similar to the focal-plane image generated by a conventional linear- or complex-motion tomographic scanner. Where conventional tomography creates an image of the thin anatomic section by blurring out the information from unwanted regions, however, the CT image is constructed mathematically by a computer so as to eliminate completely the pictorial information contained in the unwanted areas. To do this, the production of the CT image requires a different methodology for gathering the x-ray attenuation profiles that are needed to reconstruct the image.[1,2] This methodology limits the CT tomograms to cross-sectional displays of the anatomy that are oriented perpendicular (or near so, eg, within ± 20 degrees) to the axial (longitudinal) dimension of the body as shown in Figure 14.1.

Each CT picture consists of thousands of computed picture elements (pixels) arranged in rows and columns (ie, a matrix) where each pixel represents the x-ray attenuating properties of a small volume (voxel) of tissue. The conversion of the matrix of numbers into a picture represents a display of internal body anatomy based upon an individual organ's capacity to absorb radiation. The conversion of the numeric matrix into picture form is accomplished by using a cathode ray tube (CRT) whose electron beam is moved over the phosphor face of the CRT as if it were sweeping across the rows of the matrix successively. At each matrix location (ie, at each X, Y location), the electron beam is attenuated in proportion to the value of the matrix element. Large matrix values attenuate the electron beam very little and produce bright pixel intensities. Conversely, low matrix values attenuate the beam greatly, and produce darkened or diminished pixel intensities. In this manner, the matrix is converted into an image having varying shades of gray. A "hard copy" of the CRT image is produced either by using a Polaroid camera to photograph the phosphor face or by using a video converter to change the CRT electronic signal into a television signal (video) format so it can "drive" any one of a number of multiformat image display cameras.[3] The end result in either case is an image on film having shades of gray that represent in pictorial form the attenuation properties of the anatomy of interest (Figs. 14.2.A, B).

CT IMAGE PICTURE QUALITY CONSIDERATIONS

Optimum picture quality is derived from several image characteristics, all of which are equipment design variables and can be designated by numeric parameters.

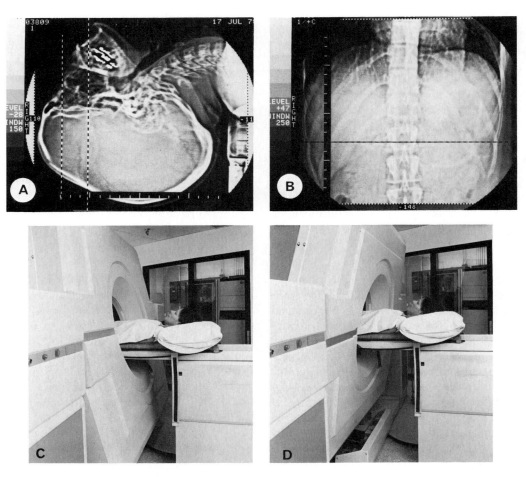

Figure 14.1. CT scanner generated lateral images of the head (**A**) and AP view of the body (**B**) showing where cross-sectional images will be made. The angulation of the image relative to the longitudinal (axial) dimension can be controlled by angulating the scanner gantry, which contains the x-ray tube and detector (**C, D**). An automated patient positioning and gantry control system can be purchased from almost every CT scanner manufacturer as an "optional item."

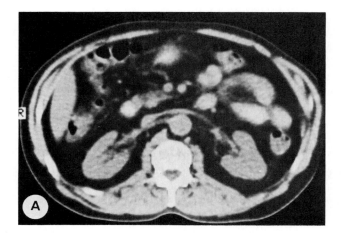

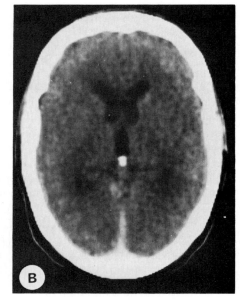

Figure 14.2. Example of CT images of the body (**A**) and head (**B**) generated on a multiformat camera. The display matrix used was 256×256 elements in size. Each pixel forming the head image represents a $1 \times 1 \times 10$ mm voxel of anatomy. Each pixel forming the body image represents a $2 \times 2 \times 10$ mm voxel of anatomy. The display relationship between pixels and voxels is generally a programming (software) variable and is controlled by the technician. The left-hand image (**A**) is viewed as if the body were sectioned in half, the bottom half removed, and one was looking up at the top half. The right-hand image (**B**) is viewed from above, downward.

These picture qualities are: (1) spatial resolution, or how well the image displays small structures or sharp tissue interfaces; (2) density resolution, or how well the image differentiates between adjacent organs or tissues with nearly identical x-ray attenuation capacity; and (3) slice sensitivity profiles, or how uniformly the image portrays tissue lying within the tomographic slice or section.

IMAGE SPATIAL RESOLUTION

Spatial resolution is a measure of the accuracy by which a CT scanner depicts minute anatomic structures. The two interrelated parameters that describe how well the scanner does this are the full-width-half-maximum (FWHM) and the line pairs per centimeter (lp/cm) values. Both of these parameters are a measure of one image property, ie, the point source response of the scanner producing the image. The FWHM is a measurement whose value is specified in the spatial domain using mm as the units, while the lp/cm parameter is a measure of the same image parameter specified in the frequency domain and describes the harmonic content of the image. Spatial domain and frequency domain concepts discussed elsewhere are related through the mathematical operations known as Fourier transforms.[1,2] To understand FWHM concepts as they apply to CT scanners, one should consider the image of a point source (ie, a minute hole in dense plastic or a thin wire on end in water) as produced by a CT scanner. The resulting image has a bright dot for a center and a progressively fading periphery, as opposed to the ideal image of a bright dot on a uniformly black background. A plot of the CT numbers on the horizontal line passing through the point source center shows the image of the hole or wire to have a bell-shaped or Gaussian-like numeric representation (distribution) as shown in Figure 14.3.A. The height of the curve represents the maximum measured CT number and the width represents the uncertainty in the measurement of the exact spatial position of the point source. The FWHM is the width of the curve at the point where the CT values are 50 percent of the peak CT value. Figure 14.3.B shows the Fourier transform of the point source response. This is also known as the modulation transfer function (MTF) of the scanner. The lp/cm value on the curve where the amplitude of the harmonic components reach 1/10 the maximum value is generally quoted as the cut-off lp/cm of the scanner's MTF.

Spatial resolution measurements are usually made using a phantom as shown in Figure 14.4.C and D, consisting of a series of slits in a bar of plastic or alternatively as a line of air-filled holes drilled in a bar of plastic, such that the diameter of each slit or hole gets progressively smaller. A typical size range is from 5 mm down to 0.5 mm. The distance between slits or holes is always equal to the diameter of the slit or hole. A scan made of the plastic bar will show that the slits can be imaged (resolved) only down to a certain diameter, beyond which the slits cannot be individually depicted. The diameter of the smallest slit that can be clearly separated from adjacent slits is quoted as the spatial resolution of the scanner. Typical scanner values would be 0.7 to 1.5 mm FWHM and would correspond to an MTF cut-off of 9 to 5 lp/cm. Note the inverse relationship that exists between the just detectable slit diameters and lp/cm values.

A number of different scanner design parameters actually determine the spatial resolution of any individual scanner:

1. The aperture opening of the x-ray detector and how closely the detector cells are spaced (or alternatively, the aperture opening of the detector and how many overlapped data measurements are made)
2. The number of projection profiles (ie, the number of circumferential transmission measurements or angles of view) made around the object
3. The high-frequency response of the convolution algorithm used in the image reconstruction process
4. The matrix (pixel) size (ie, the number of points) used in the image display
5. The object-to-background contrast
6. The thickness of the tomographic slice
7. The location of the object relative to the center of rotation of the scanner

The first three parameters are far and away the most important. The computed matrix size, while also of considerable importance, is not of major concern on any scanner using a matrix size of 160×160 to 256×256 or larger. (For exceptions to this rule see the section on zoom reconstruction.) The object-to-background contrast is very important in the clinical setting and will be discussed in much greater detail later. For now, its influence will be eliminated from the discussion by considering only high contrast (ie, greater than 12 percent) object-to-background relationships. The remaining two items (6 and 7) are of only minor importance and are not essential to the understanding of spatial resolution. Therefore, their influence will be eliminated from the discussion by considering only very thin tomographic slices (ie, 3 mm or less) with uniform sensitivity profiles, and objects located near, but not necessarily at, the center of scan rotation.

DETECTOR APERTURE OPENING CONSIDERATIONS

All present-day scanners generally fall into three basic categories: (1) translate-rotate, in which a scanning

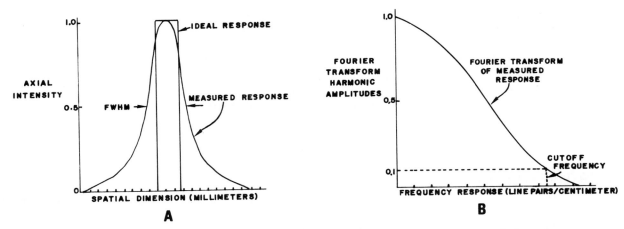

Figure 14.3. The point-source response of a CT scanner appears as a bell-shaped distribution when the matrix numbers are plotted as a graph (**A**). The FWHM is a measure of the ability of the scanner to resolve small, high-contrast objects. The Fourier transform of the bell-shaped distribution is a plot of the harmonic content of the point-source response (**B**). Where the amplitude of the harmonics drops to 10 percent of its peak value, this represents the quoted line pairs per centimeter (lp/cm) of the scanner's cut-off frequency response of its MTF.

motion is coupled with an indexing rotary motion; (2) rotate-only, moving-detectors in which a detector array rotates in opposition to a fan-beam x-ray source; and (3) moving-source, fixed-detector, in which a large number of detectors are positioned stationary about the periphery of the scanning field and only the fan-beam x-ray source rotates.

The translate-rotate and fixed-detector scanners have crystal x-ray detectors (eg, either sodium iodide, bismuth germanium oxide, or cesium iodide) with aperture openings of 1.8 to 5 mm and relatively large inter-detector spacing (eg, 0.5 to 5 mm). Data sampling is all done using an overlapped sampling technique. The rotate-only, moving-detector scanners use gas (eg, xenon) x-ray detectors and have aperture openings of 0.8 to 1.5 mm or less. The gas x-ray detector cells are mounted very closely spaced to one another so that the dead space (ie, space between detectors) is 0.1 mm or less. These scanners use a nonoverlapped method of data sampling. As stated above, the crystal detector systems utilize a method of taking overlapped data samples in order to compensate for the larger detector apertures while the gas detectors do not require the overlapped data sampling methods. To understand the differences between the overlapped and nonoverlapped measurement processes, see Figure 14.5, where both the rotate-only, moving-detector, and fixed-detector scanners are depicted. In the moving-detector system, the width of the aperture opening is crucial to the spatial resolution quality, because the width of the opening determines the width of the data-ring that characterizes the attenuation profile and, therefore, the

total radial extent of the sampling aperture information used in the reconstruction process. If the data-ring is 1 mm thick, resolution of objects less than 1 mm is difficult, primarily because the object occupies only a fraction of the space that the detector "sees." When a larger detector aperture opening is used, overlapped attenuation measurements are required in order to obtain the resolution required to visualize small objects. Overlapped measurements provide data that can be mathematically separated in order to generate many closely spaced, nonoverlapped-equivalent measurements. The ultimate resolution of the scanners using an overlapped measurement process is determined by the amount of data overlap that is allowed to occur (ie, overlap of 25 percent, 50 percent, 75 percent, etc), because the greater the amount of the overlap the smaller the nonoverlapped-equivalent measurements will be. Most commercially available scanners using data overlap measurement methods have about 0.5 to 2 mm of nonoverlapping area (ie, approximately 90 to 50 percent overlap for a 4 mm detector aperture).

ANGULAR SAMPLING CONSIDERATIONS

The number of measurements made around the periphery of the object influences the circumferential component of the spatial resolution as opposed to the radial aspect of the resolution which is determined by the x-ray detector aperture opening discussed above. As can be seen from Figure 14.6, the more closely spaced the angular measurements are made, the smaller will be

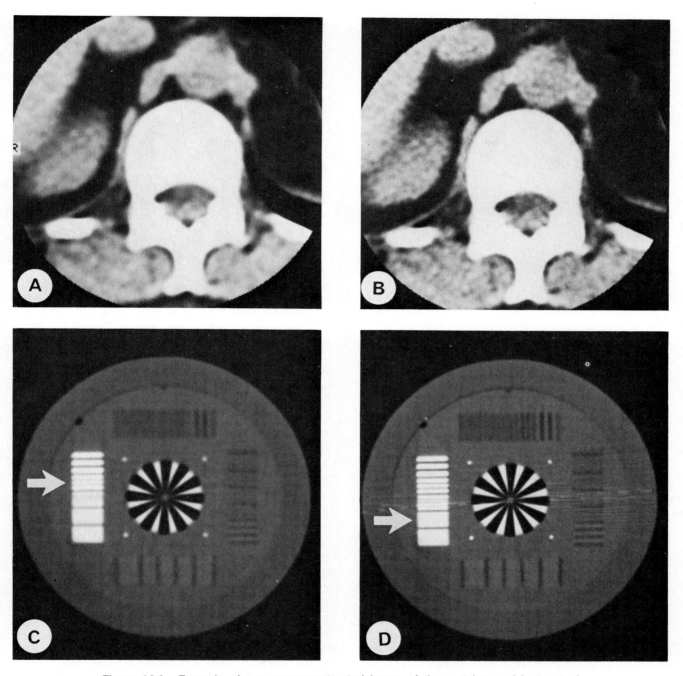

Figure 14.4. Example of a zoom-reconstructed image of the vertebra and juxtaposed structures using a low (**A**) and high (**B**) frequency convolution filter. Note increasing sharpness of edge detail with the high frequency filter *and* the more prominent image mottle (noise) pattern. The influence of the convolution filter on the resolution of the reconstructed image is shown by the phantom data where low-pass (**C**) and high-pass (**D**) filters were used in the reconstructed process. The bar thickness and spacing is, top to bottom, 3.0 mm, 2.0 mm, 1.5 mm, 1.0 mm, and 0.75 mm, respectively; 540 angles of view (measurement angles) were used in the reconstruction of both **C** and **D** images. The arrows indicate the limiting resolution.

SPATIAL RESOLUTION CONSIDERATIONS

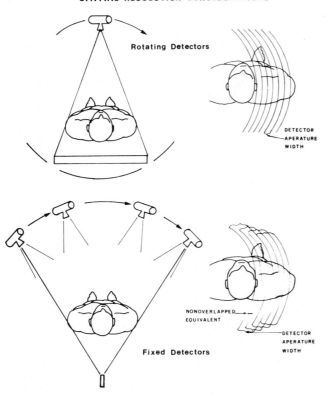

Figure 14.5. Theoretical considerations in x-ray attenuation profiles gathered from nonoverlapped (upper) and overlapped (lower) measurements. Mathematics assume uniform slice sensitivity profiles. By special mathematical techniques, the overlapped data can be rearranged into comparable nonoverlapped data.

the data-ring sector that each x-ray detector is responsible for at each measurement angle. Fixed-detector scanners, where the detector cells are mounted stationary around the patient, have the number of views limited to the number of detectors; whereas the rotate-only scanners, where the detectors rotate around the patient, are limited only by the number of views the scanner is programmed to take. Theoretically at least, rotate-only scanners can take any number of measurements about the circumference, but electronic timing considerations generally place an upper limit on this number. Most rotate-only scanners available today employ anywhere from 270 (ie, every 1.33 degrees) to 1080 (ie, every 0.33 degree) angular measurements. Fixed-detector scanners commercially available have 600, 720, or 1088 detectors (and therefore measurement angles), depending upon the particular machine.

The obvious question that needs to be asked is: How many measurement angles are required to optimize image quality? This has been analyzed by several investigators using the conditions of minimizing image

Image Spatial Resolution

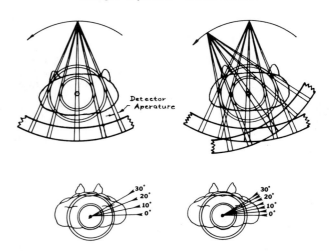

Figure 14.6. Theoretical considerations of the influence of the number of views made by the scanner around the periphery of object. The number of views determines the circumferential aspect of the data-ring sector for which each x-ray detector is responsible. The greater the number of views, the smaller the data-ring sector one achieves. Optimally, the number of views is approximately 1.5 times the number of linear samples taken (or number of detectors for moving detector-rotate only scanners).

noise and maximizing spatial resolution.[4,5] These investigators have shown that the number of adjacent data measurements (either measured directly or following the unfolding of the overlapped measurements) should be at least two measurements per spatial interval deemed to be the desired spatial resolution of the image (ie, every 1.0 mm for a FWHM of 2.0 mm). This is approximately equivalent to twice the highest-frequency sampling specified by electronic sampling theory. Correspondingly, the number of measurement angles needs to be equal to $\pi/2$ times the number of data measurements taken per linear translation or per x-ray firing for fan-beam x-ray sources. (For example, to image an object 50 cm in diameter with a spatial resolution of 2.0 mm requires the number of measurements to be approximately 50 cm $\times$ 10 mm/cm $\times$ 1 sample/mm = 500 samples and the number of angles of view be $\pi/2 \times [500] = 785$ angles.) These theoretical calculations can be shown to agree very closely with actual scanner results made on any of the contemporary machine designs and thus tend to reflect the spatial resolution quality in the CT image. Therefore, the product of the number of nonoverlapped equivalent samples and the number of projection angles can be used as a theoretically optimum figure-of-merit for CT scanners. If a greater number of either angular or linear measurements are made, this "extra" data may be considered redundant and as such, can be used to further reduce image noise and improve the image density resolution.

ALGORITHM FILTERING CONSIDERATIONS

The spatial frequency response of the convolution filter plays a major role in the spatial frequencies that are to be included in the reconstructed image. As will be shown in Chapter 15, the purpose of the convolution filter is to remove the image blurring created in the picture by the back projection process. The amount of image blurring allowed to remain in the image is controlled by the amount of accentuation applied to the high-spatial frequency (MTF) components found in the raw-data attenuation measurements. As one emphasizes the high-spatial frequency information, edges become sharper, FWHM values become smaller, and the image becomes "crisper." The trade-off, however, is that the image noise (mottle) also increases and the density resolution diminishes as shown in Figure 14.7. Thus, the choice of which convolution filter to use represents a trade-off between image "crispness," image noise, and image density resolution qualities. Ideally the radiologist should have a choice between two or more different convolution filters so the image can be tailor-made to the clinical situation and to the type of pictorial information required (Fig. 4.4).

IMAGE DENSITY RESOLUTION

Image density or contrast resolution is a parameter describing the scanner's ability to measure statistically significant differences in adjacent image pixel values. Since the computation of any one pixel value contains error in the form of statistical variation, it is this variation that describes the amount of image noise inherent in the picture. The technical parameter which describes the image noise is known as sigma, σ, and is computed, as the standard deviation of two or more pixel values made from a scan of uniform substance, such as water. That is, a scan of a water bath is made and the mean value of the pixel elements, $\overline{\mu(CT)}$, covering some finite region of the image, is computed according to the formula:

$$\overline{\mu(CT)} = \sum_{i=1}^{N} CT\#_i / N \qquad (1)$$

where $CT\#_i$ indicates the sum of the N pixel values and $\overline{\mu(CT)}$ is their average value. The noise or standard deviation of the values is given by,

$$\sigma^2(n) = \sum_{i=1}^{N} \left[CT\#_i - \overline{\mu(CT)} \right]^2 / (N-1)^2 \qquad (2)$$

Since $\sigma(n)$ is generally expressed in percentages, rela-

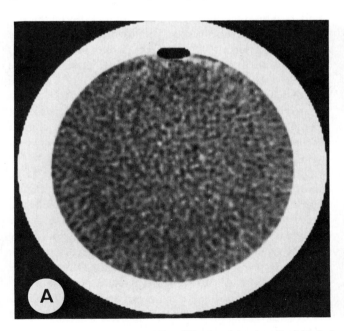
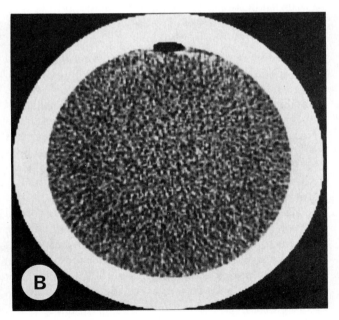

Figure 14.7. Effects of trade-off of high frequency spatial resolution information versus low frequency density resolution. The more high frequencies included in the image reconstruction, the larger the number of lp/cm that can be resolved, but at a higher image mottle (noise) level. The lp/cm and noise standard deviation for **A** and **B**, are 3 lp/cm, 0.3% and 5 lp/cm, 0.7% respectively. Scan parameters are 10 sec, 540 views, 504 measurements/view, 130 kVp, and 30 mA.

tive to the measurement scale, $\sigma(n)$ is divided by the range of the numeric scale. For example, a value of $\sigma(n) = 5$ on a scale of $\pm 1,000$ indicates a noise value of:

$$\sigma\% = (5 \times 100)/1,000 = \pm 0.5\% \qquad (3)$$

Since 0.5 percent is the "accepted or quoted" norm for the CT industry (as established by the original EMI scanner), differences in CT numbers are only considered to be statistically significant if they exceed one standard deviation or 5H (ie, Hounsfield units, H, are the standard CT unit and are based upon a scale running from -1000 [air] to 0 [water] to $+1000$ [bone]). In other words, if one pixel value is 7 and a second pixel value is 10, they cannot be considered significantly different because their difference is not greater than 5 (ie, is not greater than one standard deviation apart). Contemporary scanners have values better than 0.5 percent, generally around 0.2 to 0.4 percent, for the water bath scan and thus yield slightly better density resolution image qualities than some of the earlier scanner models.

Since noise is the ultimate limitation in the accuracy of density resolution, the image/machine parameters that affect or induce noise need to be understood. These parameters are:

1. X-ray photon flux
2. X-ray scatter rejection capacity of the detectors
3. Low-frequency response of the convolution filter
4. Computation induced
5. Machine round-off error.

The first two parameters, plus computation-induced error (parameter 4), are the main contributors to the image noise. These are discussed below. Item 3, the convolution algorithm low-frequency response, has already been discussed relative to spatial resolution requirements. To reduce image noise, the image is reconstructed with less emphasis on high-frequency information and more emphasis on low-frequency information. This means, for example, spatial frequency information above some value, say 3 lp/cm, is not included in the image reconstruction. Thus edges tend to have a somewhat rounded appearance and the image appears somewhat blurred, but the image mottle content is reduced. Machine round-off error (parameter 5) is generally not considered as a significant contributor to image noise and, therefore, can be neglected in this discussion.

PHOTON FLUX CONSIDERATIONS

X-ray photon flux refers to the number of x-ray photons impinging upon an x-ray detector cell per unit of time. While we conventionally think in terms of x-ray

flux emanating from an x-ray tube, it is the x-ray flux which reaches the detector, after passing through the object, that determines the image noise. To better understand this, consider the following: The variation in photon flux leaving the x-ray tube behaves mathematically according to the Poisson distribution; that is, the variation in photon flux is equal to the square root of the average number of photons generated. After passage through the patient, many of the original photons are absorbed or scattered and the number of photons impinging on the detector per unit of time is diminished. Since the variation in photon flux is still Poisson in distribution, the diminished flux recorded at the detector means a larger signal variation. In practice, because each set of raw-projection data occurs during a different instant of time, low photon count rates result in large raw-projection data variation and subsequently generate a graininess pattern in the reconstructed image. Thus the count variation in the image is the variation found at the detector, which in turn is dependent upon the original photon flux at the tube and the size and/or density of the object. Large patients or material of high x-ray attenuation coefficients thus decrease the intensity of the detected x-ray beam and, therefore, increase the uncertainty in the measurement. A further analysis of the image noise content also reveals that two components of photon variation are present. One component results from the overall photon flux variations generated in the x-ray source. This component is considered random or uncorrelated noise and is found uniformly throughout the image. The second component is the photon count variation attributable to object size or density changes and therefore is dependent upon the object's internal consistency variations.[6] This latter noise is called correlated image noise, and represents that noise which is most prevalent near high-density regions (eg, in or near bones, contrast-filled bladder, etc).

The second aspect of image noise is related to the size of the image matrix to be computed and the aperture opening of the x-ray detector cell. If the aperture opening of the x-ray detector is made smaller in order to improve spatial resolution, or if the thickness of the tomographic slice is made smaller to minimize partial volume effects and improve upon nonuniform sensitivity profiles (as will be discussed below) then the amount of image noise will increase because fewer photons pass into the detector per unit time. The relationship between these two parameters and the image noise can be expressed by equation 4, which also considers the dose to the patient.[7] Thus

$$\sigma(\mu) = k/(hw^3 D)^{1/2} \qquad (4)$$

where $\sigma(\mu) =$ image noise in Hounsfield units, $h =$ slice thickness in mm, $w =$ detector aperture in mm, and

D = dose in rads. Here k is a constant related to patient thickness, detector utilization efficiency, and scanner geometry. Equation 4 implies that if the x-ray detector aperture opening is decreased in size by 50 percent (ie, w is set equal to $0.5w$) the dose to the patient would have to be increased 8 times in order to keep the noise level constant.[7] Since many CT scanner designs make the pixel size of the image equal to the scanner's spatial resolution (ie, where w equals the FWHM), equation 4, therefore, also describes the effect of matrix size on the image.

Overall image noise (u), is related through equation 5, and serves to combine the effects of both components of photon $\sigma(p)$ and matrix $\sigma(\mu)$ induced image variation. Thus

$$\sigma_T(\mu) = \left[\sigma^2(p) + \sigma^2(\mu) \right]^{1/2} \qquad (5)$$

Here the photon noise, $\sigma(p)$, is the standard deviation generated from the x-ray flux Poisson distribution discussed above. Theoretically at least, the measured noise term $\sigma(n)$ (equation 2) should equal the anticipated noise term $\sigma_T(\mu)$ (equation 5).[6]

COMPUTATION-INDUCED ERROR OR NOISE

This effect applies to those scanners which utilize an overlapped method of data sampling (ie, translate-rotate and fixed-detector scanners). Since the nonoverlapped equivalent data samples must be derived from the overlapped measurements, error is introduced mathematically at this point. For example, assume a very simplified situation where one data sample x is measured from an anatomic area composed of two adjacent parts, a and b. The signal variation present on the measurement x is assumed to be Poisson in distribution and is given by $\sqrt{x}$. In a similar manner a measurement y is made from an anatomic area composed of b and c. The corresponding variation in y is also assumed Poisson in distribution and is given by $\sqrt{y}$. For a first approximation (assuming the signal contribution from area c is negligible) the signal that would have been measured from anatomic area a alone is the difference between the x and y measurements:

$$a = x - y = (a+b) - (b+c) \qquad (6)$$

The variation in the derived signal measurement a is given by $\sigma(a)$ and is equal to:

$$\sigma(a) = \left(\sqrt{x}^2 + \sqrt{y}^2 \right)^{1/2} = (x+y)^{1/2} \qquad (7)$$

Thus the variation in the individual data measurements

add rather than subtract. In the special case where the "anatomic area" measured is a water bath, $x = y$ and $\sigma(a) = (x+x)^{1/2} = 1.414\sqrt{x}$. Thus image noise is enhanced secondary to the mathematical manipulation of the overlapped data in order to obtain nonoverlapped equivalent data. In general, as the amount of data overlap increases (ie, approaches 75 percent, 90 percent, etc), so does the computation-induced noise. Most commercial scanners do not overlap data measurements more than 75 percent. In actual practice, commercial vendors do not unpack the overlapped data in exactly the same way depicted above. The computation induced noise effects, however, remain the same.

SCATTERED X-RAY DETECTION CONSIDERATIONS

The detection of scattered x-ray photons by detectors not in a direct line (or alternatively, the detection of nonprimary photons) degrades the images. This is because any one detector cannot differentiate between a primary, nondeflected photon and that deflected x-ray photon following a Compton collision within the object (Fig. 14.8), simply because no energy discrimination is used with the continuous x-ray spectra measurement. Because most scattered photons are deflected through only small angles (ie, less than ± 10 degrees), their effect is to alter the x-ray attenuation measurements recorded by immediately adjacent detectors.[8] The effect is one of adding unwanted, scattered photons to the nonprimary detectors and subtracting photons from the primary detector. This results in the effect of altering the signal (primary photons) to noise (scattered photons) ratio (S/N) by increasing the noise component in adjacent detectors. The reduction in S/N ratio effectively serves to diminish the difference in juxtaposed raw-data attenuation readings, which in turn is carried over into the pixel values in the reconstructed image.[9] Thus scattered photons serve to decrease the statistically resolvable density values in adjacent pixels and diminish the sharp interfaces between tissues of different density (eg, bone/brain interface).

Scattered x-ray photons can be controlled or their effects minimized through the use of predetector collimation or grids. CT scanners, in which a fixed relationship exists between the x-ray source and detector, as in translate-rotate or rotate-only, moving-detector scanners, can effectively use predetector collimation in order to diminish the scattered x-ray photons by limiting the angle of entry of x-ray photons into the detector cell. CT scanners that utilize a stationary detector system in general cannot effectively employ a predetector collimation system, because each detector must view the x-ray source over a wide angle of view and thus must tolerate a relatively wide angle of entry of the

Random Noise

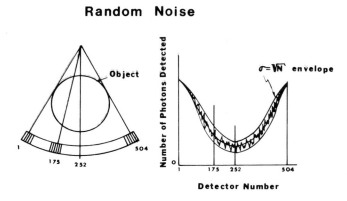

Scatter Noise

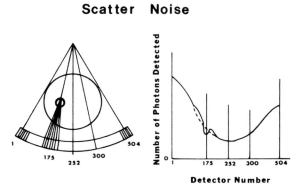

Figure 14.8. Effect of Compton scattering on the signal-to-noise ratio (S/N). Scattered x-ray decreases the S/N ratio by effectively increasing N. Therefore, the resultant density resolution in adjacent and/or nearby pixels in the reconstructed image is diminished.

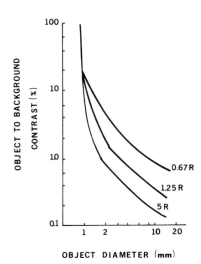

Figure 14.9. Representation of the measured relationship between object-to-background contrast difference to object size for a rotate-only detector scanning system. Note that as the object diameter decreases, the object-to-background contrast must increase or more patient irradiation be given in order to image the object. Above about 12 percent object-to-background contrast, the scanner's spatial resolution limit is reached, independent of dose delivered.

x-ray photon into the detector system. Some relief from the scattered x-ray effect is achieved by increasing the patient to detector distance, thereby giving the scattered photons a greater chance to miss the linear array of detectors. Stationary detector systems, while satisfying the 0.5 percent "industrial norm," theoretically at least, should not have density resolution capabilities as good as rotate-only, moving-detector scanners because of the resulting S/N ratio changes. In practice, however, even though the scatter rejection capacity in the two scanner designs has been found to be experimentally present, it has not yet been shown to be clinically significant.

The discussion of spatial and density resolution cannot be considered complete unless the perspective is gained that spatial and density resolution measurements are made at opposite ends of one spectrum of image quality. For example, to measure spatial resolution, only high contrast objects are used so that the density difference between the object-to-be resolved is approximately 12 percent or greater than the ambient background density. In this way, the effects of image

noise or mottle do not interfere with the FWHM measurement. As the density difference between the object and the background diminishes (toward 0.5 percent or less) the minimum size of the object that can be resolved increases. This can be understood best by considering plots of object size versus object-to-background density difference and/or plots of spatial resolution, image noise, and dose delivered. When considering object size versus object-to-background density difference, a plot similar to Figure 14.9 is used.[10, 11] The curvilinear nature of this line shows that the trade-off between spatial resolution and density resolution is not linear, but rather is more-or-less exponential. The family of curvilinear lines shows the relationship is definitely dose-dependent. Another way of viewing the spatial resolution, contrast resolution and dose relationship is to modify equation 4 as:

$$\text{Dose} = \frac{K}{\left(\dfrac{\text{spatial}}{\text{resolution}}\right)^3 \cdot \left(\dfrac{\text{slice}}{\text{thickness}}\right) \cdot \left(\dfrac{\text{density}}{\text{resolution}}\right)^2} \quad (8)$$

where K is a constant relating to the particular scanner being used. Equation 8 can be plotted as shown in Figure 14.10, and again demonstrates the nonlinear relationship between dose, spatial resolution, and density resolution. Since most soft tissues do not differ widely in x-ray attenuation values (eg, all are around 0.5 to 3 percent in value), the spatial resolution values of a scanner that are applicable to imaging anatomic

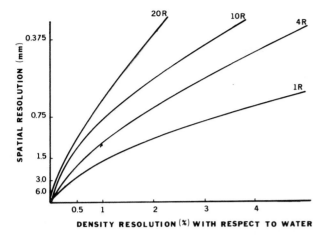

Figure 14.10. Simulations on the trade-offs between image spatial resolution and density resolution, as generated from equation 8. As the difference in object-to-background density diminishes, the size of the resolvable object increases. Clinically, most tissue differences lie between 0.5 and 3.0 percent, and spatial resolution is generally around 2 to 4 mm FWHM.

structures in a clinical setting are generally larger than the "quoted scanner values" which have been measured during a phantom analysis. Thus, the phantom data represents the best the scanner can do under optimal conditions and reflects on the esthetic quality of the image. Clinical conditions reflect more on the practical considerations of the image and dictate a "usable" spatial resolution of 2 mm to 2 cm and a usable density resolution of 0.5 to 3 percent.

CT IMAGE SENSITIVITY PROFILE

The CT image sensitivity profile refers to how uniformly the specified tomographic slice thickness is irradiated, and, therefore, how uniformly the tissues composing the slice cross-section are represented in the image. For example, if a 5-mm lesion lies in the top 5 mm of a 13-mm tomographic slice, it should have the same density and spatial representation as a similar 5-mm lesion lying in the middle of the slice or in the bottom 5 mm of the slice. In general, this is not true because the number of x-ray photons passing through the top and bottom of the slice is not the same as that number of photons passing through the center of the slice. The reason for this is the divergence of the x-ray beam. In the axial dimension, the diverging x-ray beam has a smaller cross-sectional area where it enters the object than where it exits from the object (Fig. 14.11). As the x-ray source rotates around the object, obtaining the multiple data profiles required for the image reconstruction, a biconcave cross-sectional slice irradiation pattern emerges as shown in Figure 14.12. Thus, lesions lying in the midportion of the cross-sectional slice thickness will have a more exact representation in the final image than those lesions lying near the top or bottom of the tomographic slice. Conceptually, peripherally lying objects may not even be seen if they lie near the top or bottom of the slice and near the center of rotation. This latter phenomena has been documented on the original EMI scanner where an above and below detector arrangement is used.[12]

To prevent nonuniform sensitivity profiles requires that the x-ray beam be made parallel (ie, nondiverging)

Slice Sensitivity Profile Considerations

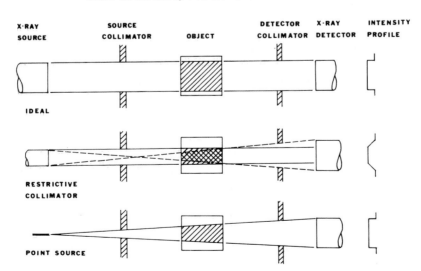

Figure 14.11. Slice thickness profiles of x-ray beams originating from small focal spot and long anode tubes. The effect is to create entrance and exit irradiation pathways with differing thicknesses secondary to the diverging nature of the beam.

SLICE SENSITIVITY PROFILE CONSIDERATIONS

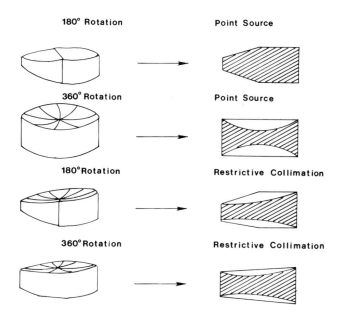

Figure 14.12. Simulated x-ray slice sensitivity profiles resulting from reconstructing x-ray attenuation patterns having the diverging beam characteristics shown in Figure 14.11. More intense weighting of tissue x-ray attenuation properties occur in center of "slice" relative to the upper or lower boundaries of the slice where fewer x-ray photons pass.

with respect to its thickness profile. This requires either a long narrow x-ray focal spot (eg, 2 mm × 13 mm) and special preobject beam-sandwiching collimators to "shape" the beam into parallel form and to minimize any inherent penumbra effects, or else a large tube-to-patient distance. Preobject sandwich collimators can be very effective in shaping the beam into a parallel form, but they also reduce the photon flux available for the x-ray attenuation measurements. Thus either more powerful x-ray tubes are required (usually at the expense of doing away with the rotating anode air-cooled tube and using a fixed-anode, water/oil-cooled tube) or a longer scanning time must be used.

The measurement of sensitivity profiles is done using a phantom containing an inclined plastic bar surrounded by water as shown in Figure 14.13.A. A cross-sectional CT image of this bar made through the center of the phantom would create a uniformly dense band extending only part way from one side of the image to the other, while a plot of the CT numbers perpendicular to the band would produce a square distribution (ie, the theoretically optimum image and distribution). Adjacent cross-sectional scans above or below the centermost scan would result in juxtaposed square distributions on the CT number plot. In practice, square distributions are not produced because of

the slice sensitivity profile limitations in the image; rather, Gaussian-like distributions are found.[13] Juxtaposed cross-sectional slices show overlap of the Gaussian distributions (Fig. 14.13.B). Furthermore, Gaussian distributions made from the top of the image band (upper part of the CT slice) should look like the Gaussian distributions made from the middle (center of the CT slice) and bottom (lower part of the CT slice) of the image bands. Differences, therefore, in the Gaussian shapes and heights tend to reflect sensitivity profile changes resulting from nonuniform plastic bar irradiation from the top of the cross-sectional image to the bottom. In general, scanners gathering their raw data profiles over 360 degrees yield more symmetrical sensitivity profiles from top to bottom of the cross-sectional slice than do scanners gathering data over 180 degree rotations. Finally, be aware that CT manufacturers generally quote only the FWHM of the Gaussian-like distributions made at the center of the CT slice, and not the top and bottom FWHM values.

CT IMAGE ARTIFACT

Image artifact arises from many causes and it is important to try to understand the source of the artifact whenever possible so its effects can be either eliminated or minimized. This knowledge also results in artifacts being correctly recognized as such and not erroneously interpreted as real pathology in the image. Artifacts can be broadly broken down into equipment-related and patient-related categories. Equipment-related artifact is caused by some electrical or mechanical part of the scanner behaving differently than presumed by the computer algorithms during the gathering of the raw-projection data. The component parts responsible may lie in (1) the x-ray tube, (2) the x-ray detectors, (3) the x-ray tube or detector alignment, (4) the scanner-to-computer information transfer, or (5) any computer logic misfunction. Because each of these problems is a subject unto itself, each will only be simply described and, where possible, the type of artifact expected from each will be illustrated.

If the x-ray tube changes its anode voltage potential (kVp) or its cathode milliamperage (mA) output over a short period of time during data collection, the x-ray detectors during that brief period would receive a different number of photons for that specific angle of measurement. The altered number of photons would be interpreted by the scanner as resulting from a variation in the radiodensity of that portion of the object. The false numerical value would in turn be back-projected during image reconstruction and thus a wedge-shaped artifact would be created for the rotate-only, moving detector scanners or a streak artifact would occur for

SLICE SENSITIVITY PROFILES

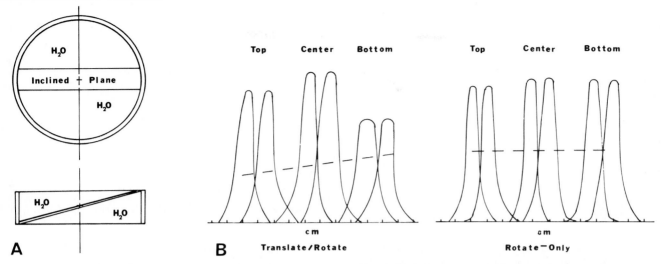

Figure 14.13. **A.** Line drawing of the inclined plastic bar phantom used to measure slice sensitivity profiles. **B.** Examples of plots of CT numbers taken from the CT images of the phantoms. The Gaussian-like distributions reflect the changing sensitivity of the scanner by its location in the upper, middle, or lower parts of the cross-sectional slice. Scanners having 360 degrees rotation during raw-data accumulation yield more symmetrical sensitivity profiles than scanners using 180 degree rotation patterns.

translate-rotate or fixed-detector scanners. This kVp or mA effect is minimized in commercial scanners by using a reference detector to "sample" the x-ray photon flux continuously during the image-making process. Should this detector, however, become "uncalibrated," erroneous data may be used in the reconstruction process and the above artifacts produced.

If any single x-ray detector changes its sensitivity to incoming photons during data collection (or during one measurement), eg, because of either a time-variant or energy-dependent calibration error, a change in the detector reference voltage, a noncompensated detector scintillation after-glow phenomena, etc, the computer would assume that the change in the detector response represented a diminished (or increased) number of x-ray photons secondary to the beam having passed through a radiodense (or radiolucent) portion of the object. This projection would, in turn, be folded back into the image through the back-projection/convolution process with a resultant streak artifact being apparent on translate-rotate scanners, a ring on rotate-only, moving-detector scanners, or a wedge on the fixed-detector scanners (Fig. 14.14). Careful prescan or during-scan detector calibrations tend to minimize these errors.

If the x-ray source and detector system are misaligned, the x-ray source and detector system are effectively (as far as the back-projection algorithm is concerned) rotating about a center of rotation which is different from the center of rotation of the gantry.

Because the back-projection algorithm assumes that the gantry-designated center of rotation is the correct one, it back-projects the attenuation profiles onto the image matrix in a place where they were not measured. Pictorially, this error may not be detectable on the image at all; it may subtly alter the correct shades of gray of the tissue representations, or it may result in ring-artifact or streak-artifact. Preventive maintenance and quality control checks (using an appropriate phantom) designed to evaluate the scanner center-of-rotation alignments can detect this error.

Abnormal data transfer from the scanner to the computer may constitute anything from incorrect analog-to-digital signal conversion, because of a faulty microprocessor board, to incorrect angle of view measurement information transmitted by faulty timing graticules. If a data measurement transmission error occurs, the back-projection algorithm thus assumes that the measurement was made at one location when in fact the measurement was made somewhere else. Errors of this type generally occur because of faults in the electronic timing or mechanical marker systems, resulting in the attenuation profiles being incorrectly back-projected, with resultant alteration in image pixel values, or blurring of tissue margins (ie, changes in density and spatial resolution) (Fig. 14.14.B). Careful and precise mechanical design and quality control checks are required to minimize these errors.

Should the computer malfunction, anything may happen to the image. Suffice it to say, if the microcom-

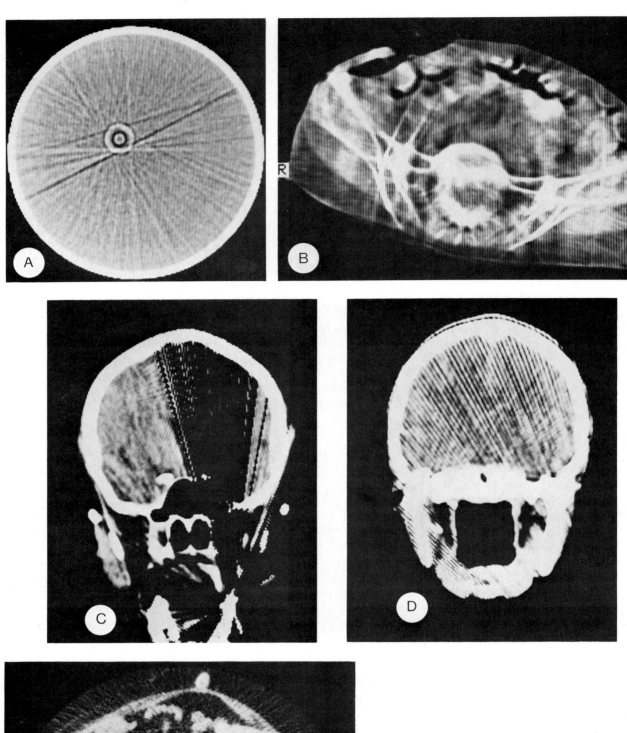

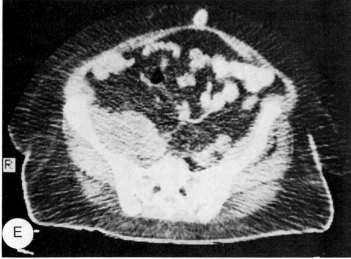

Figure 14.14. Examples of image artifact created by changes in calibrations in the x-ray detector (**A,B**), photon attenuation from passing through high density areas within (**C**) and outside the patient (**D**), and photon starvation images resulting from excessive photon attenuation resulting from the x-ray beam passing through an extremely obese individual (**E**). All scans were made on a rotate-only (third generation) scanner.

puter logic in the memory or array processors (eg, the back-projector or convolution algorithm boards) goes askew, any type of streak, wedge, ring, or "star burst" artifact may appear. It should be apparent that any kind of streak or circular artifact may occur on any type of scanner and that good preventive and corrective maintenance is very important in maintaining good clinical images.

Patient-related artifact is primarily of four forms: motion induced, high Z or density induced, partial-volume related, or beam-hardening induced. Motion-induced artifact results in streak artifact or the so-called star-burst artifact arising from high-density/low-density interfaces in the field of view. Generally this occurs because the surgical clips or air–fluid levels move during the measurement process so different angles of view find the clip or fluid interface in slightly different places. During the back-projection process each back-projection summation effect does not accentuate or attenuate previous back-projection data generated from the different angles of view. Thus, there is incomplete cancellation and accentuation of the data near the clip or fluid interface and the familiar star-burst or streak pattern occurs. It should be noted, however, that other causes of the star-burst pattern may be attributed to algorithm-related overshoot in the reconstruction process or to the operation of the detector in its nonlinear response regions.[14] Patient motion effects may be minimized using faster scanners (ie, shorter scanning times) and/or the use of glucagon for diminishing bowel peristalsis.

Objects having material of exceptionally high or low absorption capacity, which lie along the pathway traversed by the x-ray photons, create artifact by forcing the x-ray detectors to operate in their nonlinear response regions (Fig. 14.14.C and D). This means tissue or other material absorption responses may be over- or underestimated during the measurement process.[15] Because this over- or underestimation response is dependent upon the direction of the pathway through the object, streaks are generated in the resultant image because of incomplete cancellation of the superimposing data during the back-projection process. Scatter radiation effects can also result in detector operation in nonlinear regions and produce streak or ring artifacts (Fig. 14.15.A).[9]

Partial volume error arises because of tissue averaging effects that occur when materials of high and low x-ray absorption capacity both partially occupy a voxel of the cross-sectional slice (Fig. 14.15.B). For example, if lung tissue of CT# = −500H occupies 1/4 of a slice thickness and diaphragmatic tissue of CT# = +30H occupies 3/4 of the slice thickness, the resultant (averaged CT# of −120.5H) results and implies a tissue having fat consistency when in fact no fat is present. Partial volume error is further enhanced when very nonuniform slice sensitivity profiles are present (ie, deeply biconcave profiles, see previous section) because this leads to nonlinear weighting of the material in the superior, middle, or inferior portions of the cross-sectional slice.[13]

Beam-hardening artifact manifests itself as a "cupping-effect" around the inside of the calvarium (Fig. 14.16.A), as streak densities between the petrous pyramids (Fig. 14.16.B), between the iliac bones in the pelvis (Fig. 14.16.A), off the internal occipital protuberance of the skull, as "lucent shadows" beneath the ribs in the abdomen, or as "dense shadows" in mediastinal structures (Fig. 14.16). The reasons for this artifact are described in depth in Chapter 15. Briefly, however, the artifact is related to the polychromaticity of the x-ray beam used in CT scanning.[16,17] Since the x-ray detector averages all of the energy emerging from the patient into one value (ie, the effective energy), any selective attenuation of low x-ray photons by the tissue along the x-ray beam's pathway can shift the effective energy from a lower to a higher energy value (Fig. 14.17). The computer image reconstruction algorithms, however, assume that a monochromatic x-ray source exists and any change in the beam intensity is the result of a change in tissue composition and not from differing tissue attenuation characteristics secondary to an effective energy shift.[18,19] The interpretation error on the part of the algorithm means it assigns attenuation capacity values to each voxel that are slightly in error, either too big (for a lower effective energy shift) or too small (for a higher effective energy shift), relative to the standard reference effective energy found from a water-bath measurement. The beam-hardening effects thus are most pronounced around material of high attenuation capacity, such as bone (eg, the lucent artifact beneath ribs or between the pelvis iliac bones), or low attenuation capacity, such as lung (eg, dense artifact in the mediastinal structures), but in reality do occur throughout any cross-sectional view of an object. Beam-hardening, therefore, generates quantitative measurement errors that may or may not be obvious in the qualitative pictorial assessment.[20,21]

DIGITAL DISPLAY OF CT IMAGES

The process of making the computed CT matrix into an image (picture) was briefly described earlier under the general considerations section, and is done by assigning each numerical matrix value an x, y location on the CRT screen, corresponding to its row and column matrix location. The intensity of the electron-beam hitting the CRT phosphor at the designated x, y location is controlled by the actual value of the matrix element; this is referred to as Z axis modulation. In this manner, the matrix of numbers is converted into a picture composed of varying shades of gray.

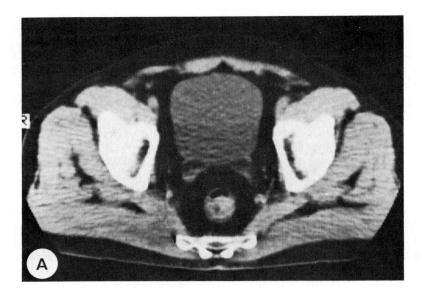

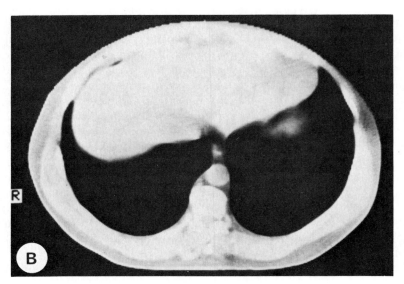

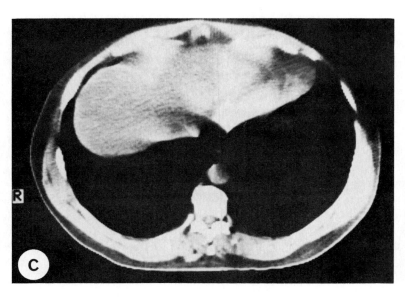

Figure 14.15. **A**. Nonuniform image effects resulting from nonlinear detector response and beam-hardening. Note in the bladder the change in image quality of urine at the level of the pelvic girdle and the presence of ring-artifact arising from detector imbalance. **B**, **C**. Partial volume effects showing the diaphragm to appear different in size because of different window settings allow partial volume effects to become manifest and lead to inaccurate object size measurements.

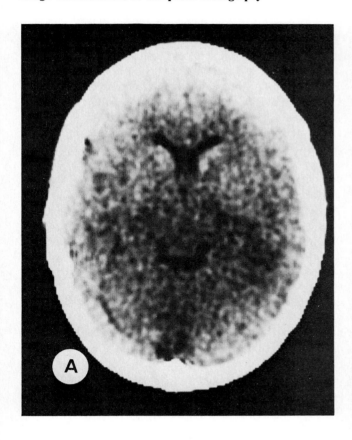

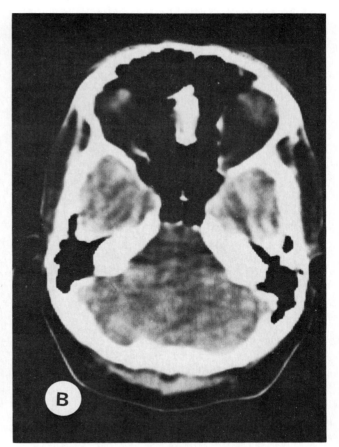

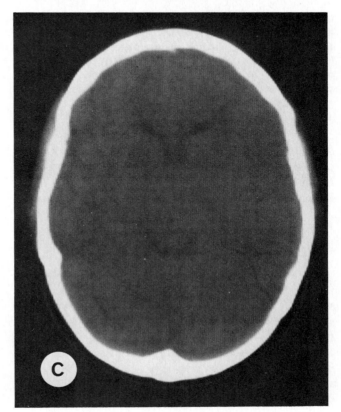

Figure 14.16. **A**. Beam-hardening artifact resulting in ''cupping'' phenomena (the tapering of light to darker density from periphery of brain toward the center). **B**. Streaks between petrous pyramids. These artifacts were recorded on a rotate-only scanner, but could be found on scanners having any type of mechanical motion. **C**. The true thickness of the calvarium is shown.

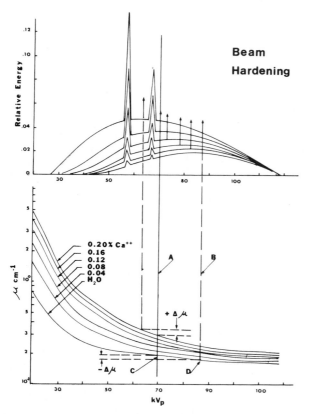

Figure 14.17. Theoretical considerations that tend to account for beam-hardening artifact arising from shifts in the effective x-ray kVp energy when the x-ray beam passes through tissue having high or low attenuation properties. As the mean kVp value changes from line A to line B because of greater x-ray attenuation of the lower kVp photons, the intercept point on the tissue attenuation curve changes from point C to point D. The recording error, $\Delta\mu$, is the difference between the C and D intercept readings on the ordinate axis of μ versus kVp.

Several limitations inherent in the matrix-to-image conversion process need to be understood in order to be able to interact with the CT image correctly. These limitations are: (1) pixel value-to-shade-of-gray conversion relationships, (2) matching of scanner and display spatial resolution capabilities, and (3) image distortion phenomena.

The assignment of a shade of gray to all of the numeric values of the matrix is both impossible and unwise. Most CT image matrix values are arbitrarily scaled to between $+1000$ and -1000, with water assigned the value 0. No oscilloscope has yet been built that can display the 2000 shades of gray necessary for a one-to-one conversion process, and furthermore, the human eye would not begin to appreciate these 2000 shades of gray, even if the conversion could be accomplished. Consequently, most CRTs display 64 to 256 shades of gray and this is generally more than sufficient

for excellent and esthetically pleasing images. To display this many shades of gray requires either (1) any successive 256 numbers be assigned shades of gray on a one-to-one basis (ie, a window width of 256) and have a variable pointer as to which 256 numbers will be assigned the gray scale (ie, a variable window center); or (2) multiples of numbers be assigned one shade of gray, such as on a two-to-one, three-to-one, etc, (ie, a window width of 512, 748, etc, respectively), and again with a variable window pointer. Because the one-to-one conversion effectively results in a short gray scale and the two-to-one or three-to-one conversion results in a long gray scale, the contrast between different anatomic regions can be varied according to the pictorial whim of the operator or the clinical situation. (It is nearly impossible, for example, to display both lung-field detail and mediastinal detail using one window width and center setting). Furthermore, short gray scales tend to emphasize image noise or mottle patterns, while long gray scales tend to minimize these effects. (For example, compare Fig. 16.16.A with Fig.16.16.C.) In general, an optimal window conversion scale is one that minimizes the image noise and maximizes the tissue contrast differences in regions of interest. This windowing conversion process also must vary from image to image, radiologist to radiologist, and study to study, thus making alteration of the window width and center a dynamic radiologist-to-image process of interpretation.

It is not readily appreciated that a major image-degrading event can occur when displaying matrix data if care is not paid to matching the spatial resolution of the scanner to the spatial resolution of the CRT. For example, if a 1 cm thick, 50 cm diameter object is to be represented (such as the body) using a 250×250 mm size matrix, each pixel element is displaying a $2 \times 2 \times 10$ mm sectional volume (eg, a voxel of tissue). If the FWHM spatial resolution of the scanner is less than 2 mm, each pixel value can and will contain independent image information. On the other hand, if a 25 cm field-of-view is reconstructed (such as of the head or zoom-type enlargement of a portion of the body) using a 250×250 mm matrix, each pixel element will only represent a $1 \times 1 \times 10$ mm voxel size. This in turn requires that the scanners spatial resolution be 1 mm or less for independent pixel information display. If a reconstruction is now attempted, say of a 12.5 cm object size (ie, each pixel represents $0.5 \times 0.5 \times 10$ mm), a scanner FWHM of 0.5 mm or less is needed for independent pixel display. This is below the spatial resolution of any known scanner on the market today. Thus, the back-projection/convolution process, in making the 12.5 diameter image, will put nearly similar data in each of four juxtaposed pixels, so that the cross-sectional CRT display area will equal the scanners spatial resolution FWHM value (assuming here a scanner FWHM of 1 mm). The important point is, that as greater and greater use is made of the zoom mode of feature display (ie, ×2, ×4, ×8, etc), no new pictorial information can be generated in the image beyond the scanners spatial resolution FWHM capacity, and the sharpness of visceral boundaries will necessarily have to become progressively blurred (Fig. 14.18).

Image distortion can occur in the digital image in two ways: (1) by the lateral diffusion of light originating from the CRT electron/phosphor interaction; and (2) by pin-cushion distortion of the displayed image occurring secondary to the curvilinear surface of the CRT face.

The lateral diffusion of light created on the phosphor by the bombarding electrons during the display will account for the loss of stepwise changes seen on curvilinear organ boundaries such as the calvarium, if the matrix size is sufficiently large (or alternatively, the pixel size is sufficiently small). If one could generate

multiple matrices of diminishing pixel size, it would appear obvious that once the stepwise loss begins to occur, the spatial resolution of the CRT display has been exceeded and that any additional pixel resolution generated through smaller pixel computation would be wasted. Thus, above certain matrix sizes, the CRT is performing an image-smoothing or filtering function. The spatial resolution of most oscilloscopes used to display CT data is such that a 512×512 image matrix contains more information than can be adequately displayed and that a 320×320 matrix contains slightly less information than what is considered optimal in the CRT display resolution capabilities. In practice, however, matrix sizes of either 320×320 or 512×512 seem to give esthetically good displays because the CT scanner is operating near the point where the spatial resolution of the scanner is comparable to the spatial resolution of the CRT. Whether a 320×320 or a 512× 512 matrix is used should be based upon whether the

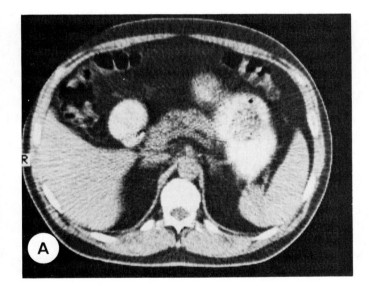

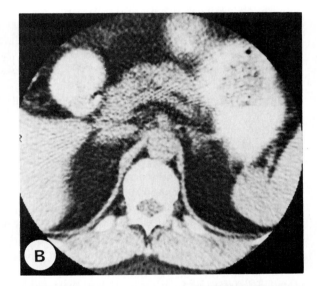

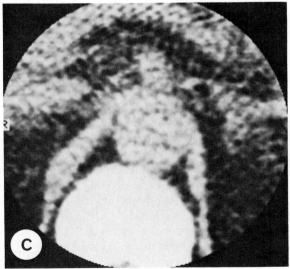

Figure 14.18. **A**. Effects of zoom reconstruction. When the spatial resolution of the scanner is greater than that of display, sharp images and organ boundaries occur. **B**. When the spatial resolution of the scanner is equal to that of the display, each pixel contains independent spatial information and boundaries are optimally sharp. **C**. When the spatial resolution of the scanner is less than that of the display, the boundaries become somewhat blurred and the noise pattern becomes more coarse because independent pixel information is not available for forming the image.

radiologist wants to be limited by the spatial resolution of the CRT and have sharp, crisp organ boundaries (ie, through the use of 512×512 matrices), or be limited by the spatial resolution of the CT scanner (such as through use of zoom features) and have slightly to moderately blurred organ boundaries (ie, use of 256×256 or 320×320 sized matrices). The main advantages of the 256×256 display is that more effective use of the zoom feature is possible before the spatial resolution of the scanner is surpassed and shorter matrix computation times are required by the computer.

Pin-cushion distortion generated by a curvilinear oscilloscope face makes an image take on a somewhat "bowed" appearance. This is not a serious qualitative image degrading event on CRT displays unless some astigmatism is also present in the CRT face. When this happens, pin-cushion and astigmatism combination will result in a nonsymmetrical form of image distortion. Pin-cushion and/or astigmatism distortion are best visualized when "hard-copy" (ie, Polaroid or x-ray film) images are made of a wire grid. Here, the wires would not be displayed parallel but have a curvilinear appearance. This nonuniform spacing between adjacent pixel values in practice does not lead to a loss of image quality subjectively, but does result in frank measurement error if quantitative size or distance measurements are taken from the hard copy image by ruler.

CT-IMAGE MANIPULATION

Almost all CT scanners today have some form of radiologist–image interactive device. This may consist of a region-of-interest (ROI) cursor or some other form of special image visual effect aid. The ROI cursor generally consists of a "joy-stick" or "track-ball" device which allows the radiologist to position a "cursor marker" (such as a small square or "x") anywhere on the CRT face. The radiologist can then enlarge the "cursor-marker" from a point to a square, to a rectangle, to a circle, to an oval, etc, in order to analyze or direct attention to specific subsections of the image. Alternatively, the radiologist can "draw" a line around any group of pixels or picture area using a nongeometric design or can measure the distance between any two selectable points on the image. If area measurements are made, besides being able to quantitate the amount of image area contained within the ROI boundaries, one can also find the average value and standard deviation of the pixel values contained inside the cursor designated area. These cursor-aided measurements have generally been found to be useful in the day-to-day interpretation of the image.

Some special image visual effect aids consist of CRT highlighting and image-inversion. Highlighting refers to designating a certain range of numbers (eg, all pixels having values between say 20 and 25 H) as being special, and thus displaying those pixels with a maximum light intensity. Thus, all pixels of a specified range can be easily visualized as shown in Figure 14.19.A. Highlighting can also be used for creating contours on the images as also shown in Figure 14.19.B. This highlight mode is a useful maneuver when trying to identify very nearly the same image density changes. Highlighting however also enhances image noise. Image inversion consists of displaying the image as black-on-white rather than the conventional white-on-black format (Figs. 14.19.C, D). Because of the nonlinear relationship in the human eye, ambient background changes affect considerably our ability to perceive shades of gray. Most physiologists recognize that the shading of images made on a white background are better appreciated than shades of gray on a black background. On the other hand, edge definition is better appreciated on a black background than on a white background. From a more empirical point of view, our own experience indicates that fine structural detail such as the trabecular pattern in bone or vascular markings in the lungs can be better appreciated on the white background image and images of the soft tissues of the abdomen are best appreciated on the black background. In either case, a video display with a video inverter control may be useful in some situations. Dual windowing capabilities can be created using an end-level black control (Fig. 14.19.D). This feature has only limited clinical application, but may be deemed useful when displaying lung and mediastinal detail on one image.

FUTURE CT-IMAGE DIRECTIONS

Most research related to improving the CT image is proceeding along one of three lines: (1) improvement in scanner spatial resolution so more effective use of zoom reconstructions can take place[25]; (2) external triggering of the x-ray measurement process so dynamic physiologic events (ie, cardiac-gating) can be studied[22]; and (3) improvement in scanner density resolution so quantitative, error-free measurements can be obtained.[23,24]

Improvements in scanner spatial resolution will come about by detector design changes whereby smaller detector cell apertures are present and overlapped data measurements are taken. Both of these will be required if spatial resolutions of 0.25 to 0.5 mm FWHM are to be obtained. Other factors (ie, the number of available detectors and their associated amplifiers) will have to be carefully considered in order to minimize scanner costs.

Another factor or technique will be to perform selected region scanning; that is, rescanning of body parts with attention limited to specific anatomic re-

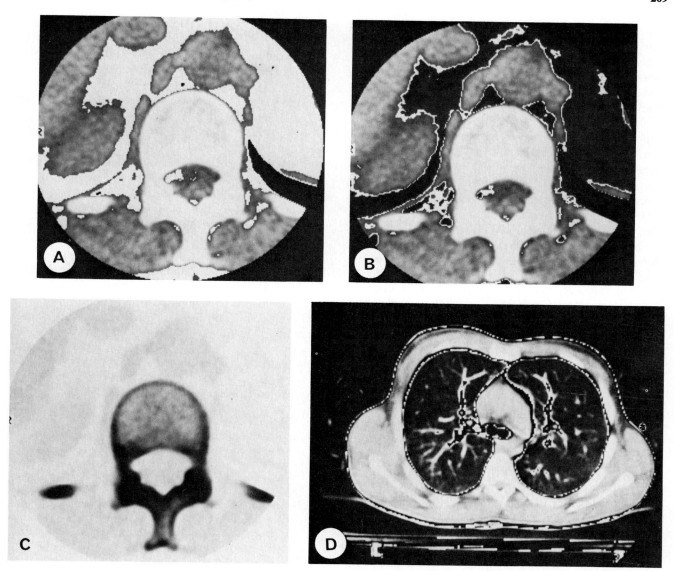

Figure 14.19. Effects of image highlighting. **A.** All pixel values falling in the range of −60 and −174 are given maximum brightness on the display, creating a banding or filling in appearance. **B.** Contouring effects can be generated through the use of the highlighting mode by narrowing the width of the highlight number range. **C.** Reversal of the image display (ie, black-on-white rather than white-on-black) is useful for evaluating high Z tissue characteristics such as bone trabecula. **D.** End-level black images can be used to create dual window images. The boundary highlight arises from tissue partial volume effects.

gions, eg, the vertebra or sella turcica. Because the attenuation of the x-ray beam is also a function of body tissues lying outside the field of view (eg, outside the vertebra), research into how this "extra" attenuation information will affect the field-of-view image reconstruction process needs to be done.[25] It is conceivable and technically possible to achieve zoom images of amplification of ×8 or ×10 without serious image degradation using only slight modifications of contemporary commercial scanners.

External gating of timing signals controlling the x-ray attenuation measurements are an attempt to make an image of one phase or instant of a cyclic event by using information gathered over multiple events, where each measurement is obtained at an identical instant in the cycle for the reconstruction process. For example, one wishes to make a cross-sectional display of the heart by using the cardiac electrical activity to trigger the measurement process precisely at end-diastole. If 360 views of attenuation data are required, end-diastole of 360 heart beats will be recorded with one heart beat at each angle of view. The fundamental underlying assumption with this methodology is that cardiac motion and electrical activity are exactly synchronous in time and space, ie, every heart beat is exactly the same. Since the heart has its own feedback control for rate and stroke volume, depending upon the demands of the body, minute changes in each heart beat do occur, even in the "resting heart." How large these minute changes can be before measurement error (both density and spatial resolution) makes the image unusable (eg, for detecting myocardial ischemia or paradoxical wall motion) is not entirely known. Furthermore, regular heart rates only can be tolerated, eliminating those patients who have arrhythmias and thus, probably need the study the most. In all probability, the future of CT cardiac imaging lies in those multiple source, multiple detector scanners that gather all their attenuation profiles in one cardiac cycle, especially if physiologic relationships between cardiac electric and mechanical activity are to be studied.[26]

Quantitative CT-density resolution measurements are attempts to make tissue characterization practical using CT scanners or alternatively to allow physiologic models to be created so as to understand better those physiologic processes that are reflected in radiographic density.[23,24] The major problem in both of these areas relates to beam-hardening considerations.[20,21] The fundamental question is whether the use of corrections for shifts in effective energy arising from use of polychromatic x-radiation is comparable to using a monochromatic x-ray source for the attenuation profile measurement information. Because monochromatic isotopic sources are not available with the photon flux which is needed for CT image spatial and density resolution requirements, the concept of effective energy correction is mandatory for quantitative measurements. This, however, assumes all tissue to be photoelectric and Compton attenuation processes also to behave in such a way that measurements of effective energy can be adequately described by the molecular makeup of the tissue. Unfortunately, either multiple different effective energy measurements must be made in order to describe the photoelectric/Compton molecular cross-sections or some assumptions must be made about the shape of the x-ray spectra as a function of energy when the molecular composition is not known. Whether the use of measurements of effective energy will be accurate enough for quantitative measurements remains to be seen.

SUMMARY

The CT image is a cross-sectional display of body parts oriented perpendicular or slightly oblique to the axial dimension of the body. In this sense, the image is comparable to that of transverse ultrasonic images,

except where visceral x-ray attenuation patterns are displayed rather than ultrasonic reflective properties. The images are very sensitive to both the display of radiographic "soft-tissue" and to "hard-tissues" (ie, bone) x-ray attenuation because of the use of highly sensitive crystal or gas x-ray detectors and windowing capabilities of the the CRT display. The spatial resolution on most commercially available scanners is between 1.0 to 2.0 mm FWHM, and the density resolution limits are around 0.3 to 0.5 percent. Image quality compromise, in the form of image noise, is related to the radiation dose delivered to the patient and by the size of the image display matrix computed. After the image has been generated, all available scanners have some form of interactive imaging device that allows the radiologist to manipulate or alter the image on the CRT in a predictable manner for the purpose of extracting additional image information, such as quantitative measurements of tissue attenuation or organ size, or to aid in the initial patient positioning/set-up protocol.

REFERENCES

1. Gordon R, Herman GT: Three dimensional reconstruction from projections: a review of algorithms. Int Rev Cytol 38: 111–151, 1974
2. Brooks RA, DiChiro G: Theory of image reconstruction in computed tomography. Radiology 117: 561–572, 1975
3. Christenson EE, Curry TS III, Dowdey JE: An Introduction to the Physics of Diagnostic Radiology; 2nd ed. Philadelphia, Lea & Febiger, 1978, pp 234–244
4. Huesman RH: The effects of a finite number of projection angles and finite lateral sampling of projections on the propagation of statistical errors in transverse section reconstruction. Phys Med Biol 22(3): 511–521, 1977
5. Synder DL, Cox JR, Jr: An overview of reconstructive tomography and limitations imposed by a finite number of projections. In Ter-Pogossian M, Phelps ME, Brownell GL, et al (eds): In Reconstruction Tomography in Diagnostic Radiology and Nuclear Medicine Baltimore, University Park Press, 1977, pp 3–32
6. Riederer SJ, Pelc NJ, Chesler DA: The noise power spectrum in computed x-ray tomography. Phys Med Biol 23(3): 446–454, 1978
7. Brooks RA, DiChiro G: Statistical limitations in x-ray reconstructive tomography. Med Phys 3(4): 237–240, 1976
8. Battista JJ, Santon LW, Bronshill MJ: Compton scatter imaging of transverse sections: Corrections for multiple scatter and attenuations. Phys Med Biol 22(2): 229–244, 1977
9. Sonestrom JP, Macovski A: Scatter considerations in fan beam computerized tomographic systems. IEEE Trans Nucl Sci 23(5): 1453–1458, 1976
10. Cohen G: Contrast-detail-dose analysis of computed tomographic scanners (Submitted)
11. CT/T Technology Continuum: Technical Performance of the CT/T System. General Electric Corporation,

Medical Systems Division, Milwaukee, Wis., 1977

12. Goodenough DJ, Weaver KE, Davis DO: Potential artifacts associated with the scanning pattern of the EMI scanner. Radiology 117: 615–619, 1975

13. Brooks RA, DiChiro G: Slice geometry in computer assisted tomography. J Comput Assist Tomog 1(2): 191–199, 1977

14. Shepp LA, Stein LA: Simulated reconstruction artifacts in computerized tomography. In Ter-Pogossian MM, Phelps ME, Brownell GL, et al (eds): Reconstruction Tomography in Diagnostic Radiology and Nuclear Medicine. Baltimore, University Park Press 1977, pp 33–48

15. Phelps ME, Gado MH, Hoffman EJ: Correlation of effective atomic number and electron density with attenuation coefficients measured with polychromatic x-rays. Radiology 117: 585–588, 1975

16. Zatz LM: The effect of kVp level on EMI values. Radiology 119: 683–688, 1976

17. Tsai CM, Cho ZH: Physics of contrast mechanism and averaging effect of linear attenuation coefficients in a computerized transverse axial tomography (CTAT) transmission scanner. Phys Med Biol 21(4): 544–559, 1976

18. Phelps MD, Hoffman EJ, Ter-Pogossian MM: Attenuation coefficients of various body tissues, fluids and lesions at photon energies of 18–136 keV. Radiology 117: 573–583, 1975

19. Rao PS, Gregg FC: Attenuation of monoenergetic gamma rays in tissues. AJR 123(3): 631–637, 1975

20. McDavid WD, Waggener RC, Dennis MJ, et al: Estimation of chemical composition and density from computed tomography carried out at a number of energies. Invest Radiol 2(12): 189–194, 1977

21. McDavid WD, Waggener RD, Payne WH, Dennis MJ: Correction for spectral artifacts in cross-sectional reconstruction from x-rays. Med Phys 4(1): 54–57, 1977

22. Alfidi RJ, Haaga JR, MacIntyre WJ, et al: Gated computed tomography of the heart. Compt Axial Tomogr 1(1): 51–57, 1977

23. Brooks RA, DiChiro G: Split-detection computed tomography: a preliminary report. Radiology 126: 255–257, 1978

24. Fenster A: Split xenon detector for tomochemistry in computed tomography. J Comput Assist Tomogr 2: 243–252, 1978

25. Abele M, Erdos J, Chase NE: Image artifacts generated by non-linear detection characteristics in computerized tomography. (Abstract) Association of University Radiologists, 26th Annual Meeting San Antonio, Tex., April 30–May 4, 1978, p 65

26. Wood EH: New vistas for the study of structural and functional dynamics of the heart, lungs and circulation by non-invasive numerical tomographic vivisection. Circulation 56(4):506–520, 1977

CHAPTER 15

Equipment Considerations in Computed Tomography

CRAIG M. COULAM
JON J. ERICKSON

Since their introduction in the 1960s, computed tomographic (CT) scanners have been, and are continuing to be, designed along three more or less general lines[1,2]: (1) scanners where the x-ray tube and detector cells utilize a translate-and-rotate type of mechanical motion; (2) scanners that employ an x-ray tube having a rotate-only motion and with detector cells either rotating synchronously with the tube or with the cells mounted stationary around the periphery of the scanner; and (3) scanners that utilize "electronic motion" between the multiple x-ray tubes and detectors.[3] In all of these designs, the primary engineering criteria has been to create the most accurate cross-sectional image possible, utilizing the shortest feasible scanning time. Early engineering and production prototype scanners were exceptionally instrumental in demonstrating that a definite dependency effect existed among the various engineering variables in the form of interrelationships between scan time, x-ray photon flux, image matrix size, cross-sectional slice thickness, etc. Following this realization, the designers of the different scanners began to optimize-on or trade-off between the different image qualities inherent in the scanners' mechanical (or lack of) motions. Therefore, the understanding of the CT equipment design does require a composite understanding of: (1) the fundamental physical and mathematical principles of CT; (2) the interrelationships of the different scanner technical parameters, such as gantry motions, x-ray tube and detector relationships, x-ray detector cell design, etc; and (3) the effects on the image of the various inherent mathematical algorithm trade-off options. Some of these relationships were discussed in Chapter 14; the others will be discussed in this chapter.

COMPUTER FUNCTIONS:
PHYSICS OF IMAGE RECONSTRUCTION

During the x-ray beam's passage through the object, some x-ray photons are absorbed and some pass through the object with no change in their energy or direction. For a homogeneous medium making up the object, the number of x-ray photons recorded at the x-ray detector is called the ray-sum and given by I:

$$I = I_0 e^{-\mu l} \tag{1}$$

where I_0 is the initial number of photons generated, μ is the linear attenuation coefficient of the medium, and l is the path length through the medium.

Taking the natural logarithm of both sides of equation 1 and rearranging yields:

$$\mu l = \ln(I_0 / I) \tag{2}$$

If the object is not composed of a homogeneous medium but an admixture of N homogeneous mediums, each having a different path length and linear attenuation coefficient, equation 2 is rewritten as:

$$\sum_{i=1}^{N} \mu_i l_i = \ln R \tag{3}$$

where R is the raw-data value or ray-sum recorded by the scanner and associated electronics. Because R is known, (or more accurately, $R(j, a)$ where j represents the jth detector in the ath angular position of the x-ray tube), it is possible to reverse the mathematics given in equation 3 and compute the individual μ's. This is done by rewriting the equation into the form:

$$\sum_{\substack{i=1 \\ k=1}}^{N} \mu_{i,k} l_{i,k} = R(j, a) \tag{4}$$

where the subscripts i and k refer to a particular image element in the x, y matrix and l refers to the path length through the particular i, k matrix element. Equation 4 is of fundamental importance because it is the equation by which all CT images are reconstructed.

At last count, at least 15 different solutions to equation 4 have been proposed; however, almost all manufacturers have presently settled on the convolution and back-projection solution method, primarily because this allows the most accurate solution to equation 4 in the shortest possible computational time, ie, reconstruction time. It is, therefore, essential that one understands the basic principles underlying these two mathematical routines.

To understand descriptively how convolution and back-projection are used in the formation of an image, it is necessary to begin with the concept of back-projection (Fig. 15.1). Because a ray-sum represents the summation of the effects of media on the x-ray photons as they traverse a specific pathway through the object, back-projection represents the mathematical equivalent of "un-doing" the summation process. That is, the value of the ray-sum is divided by the number of matrix elements that represent the tissue equivalent of the path length of the x-ray beam through the object. This quantity is computed for each matrix element and is stored in the computer. This division and summation process is repeated for each ray-sum at each ray-projection until all ray-sums have been divided by the appropriate path lengths and added to the appropriate matrix elements. With respect to the mathematics given in equation 4, this amounts to dividing out the $l_{i,k}$ term from the $R(j, a)$ reading on a pixel-by-pixel basis.

Expanding on this terminology, a ray-projection is defined as that collection of ray-sums made during one linear translation of the scanner, at one projection angle, or alternatively, that collection of ray-sums made at one x-ray tube position when multiple detectors gather the data simultaneously.

If the back-projection algorithm only were performed on all the ray-sums and ray-projections, the final image would not be sharp and crisp in detail but rather very blurred or unsharp (Fig. 15.2). The unsharpness is a natural consequence of the back-projection process and is related to the assumption that beam attenuation occurs uniformly over the entire path length. The unsharpness, however, may be removed from the image by altering the ray-sums prior to their back-projection by using a mathematical operation known as convolution.

The purpose of the convolution operation (or algorithm) is to modify or reshape the raw-projection data in such a way that some of the ray-sums take on negative values so that when the back-projection is performed some of the negative ray-sums and the positive ray-sums will cancel each others' effect in the regions where the unsharpness occurs. In so doing, the final image produced will be sharp and crisp. The application of the convolution algorithm in turn requires that one knows the equation of, or at least the shape of, a specific mathematical function that can be used to remove the image unsharpness. This "filtering" function is known by many names, the most common of which are the back-projection filter function, the convolution "kernel," and the convolution transfer function.[4-6]

The filter function is quite complex in equation form and need *not* be memorized, but for the sake of completeness is:

$$f(r) = \frac{a/d}{2\left[1 - \cos\left(\frac{\pi a}{2d}\right)\right]} \int_0^\pi J_0\left(\frac{rx}{d}\right) \sin\left(\frac{ax}{2d}\right) \frac{\sin\left(\frac{xA}{2d}\right)}{\left(\frac{xA}{2d}\right)} dx$$

(5)

In this equation, a is the detector aperture size opening, A is the x-ray tube focal spot size, d the sampling interval, J_0 is the zero-order Bessel function, and r is the distance between samples in mm. It is not necessary to understand this equation in order to understand the convolution algorithm. It is only necessary to realize that the filter function is a complex equation or wave form that is dependent upon the x-ray tube and detector characteristics and requires a digital computer or, alternatively, a dedicated, limited-function computer, ie, a hardware convolver, for its application. The general shape of the filter function should be remembered, however, and so is shown pictorially in Figure 15.3. The actual process of convolution is illustrated in Figure 15.4.

In practice, the convolution algorithm is performed on each ray-projection and the convolved ray-sums are then back-projected onto the image matrix as described

BACK-PROJECTION   RECONSTRUCTION

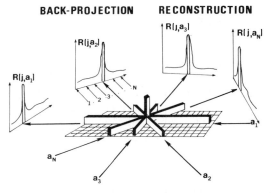

Figure 15.1. Back-projection represents the "undoing" of the ray-sum effect by dispersing each ray-sum value uniformly over the image matrix elements at the particular angle that the tube/detector gantry was when it recorded the data. Obviously, error is generated if the angle of back-projection does not coincide exactly with where the gantry was at the time of the ray-sum recording and by the assumption of uniform dispersion of the back-projection data.

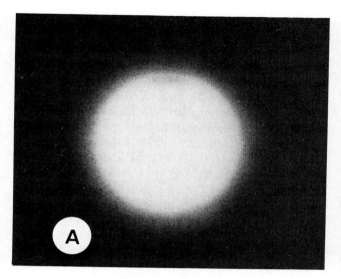
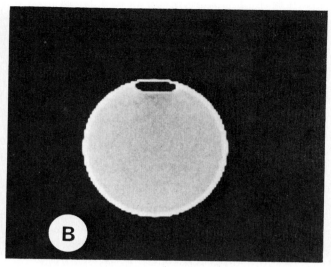

Figure 15.2. **A**. Back-projection results in a blurred, unsharp image when performed without prior use of the "filter function," as illustrated here. The reason for the blurring is secondary to the "undoing" of the ray-sum effect through the use of the average value approach. Here the assumption is made that each anatomic subregion along the course of any one ray-sum path contributes equally to the attenuation of the x-ray beam, when in reality, some regions generate a greater effect than others. **B**. When the raw data is convolved with the appropriate filter function prior to back-projection, the blurring effect may be removed.

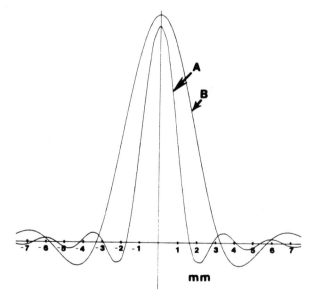
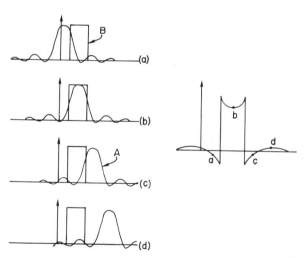

Figure 15.3. Plots of two different convolution filter functions required to remove the "blurred edges" from the raw-data prior to back-projection. Curve A was generated from equation 5 with $a=d=1$ mm and $A=0.6$ mm. This curve accentuates edge detail and increases image noise content. Curve B was also generated from equation 5 in Chapter 15 but with $a=d=2$ mm and $A=0.6$ mm. This curve diminishes image noise content, but does not provide maximal spatial resolution. The choice of the filter function to be used should depend upon whether spatial or density resolution criteria are the most imperative in answering the clinical problem.

Figure 15.4. The process of convolution consists of sliding the filter function past the raw data (shown here as a square wave function) in incremental steps. For each incremental shift, the resulting "output value" (eg, a, b, c, or d) is equal to the product of the area of the portions of the raw data and filter function curves that overlap. When the filter function drops "below the line" (ie, takes on negative values), the resultant area product value is also negative; when the filter function is "above the line," the area product is positive. The "overshooting" of the edges (ie, the "negative values") on the output or convolved raw data curve (right-hand image) are needed to offset the blurring process arising during the back-projection process.

above. Because programmable computers are, in general, too slow to perform all the mathematical operations in acceptable time, they are usually done by special purpose logic circuits called microprocessors (or alternatively hardwired convolvers and back-projectors). Since the shape of the filter function can be changed to allow as much, or as little, image unsharpness to remain in the picture as desired, different filter functions can be chosen to emphasize image edge detail or image density changes respectively. Edge enhancement also accentuates image graininess or noise content while density enhancement minimizes image graininess and diminishes the amount of edge sharpness. Thus, different "filters" should find optimal applications in different clinical studies such as imaging different parts of the body.

X-RAY TUBE EFFECTS: POLYCHROMATIC ENERGY CONSIDERATIONS

The above discussion of CT treated the attenuation coefficient as though it were a single fixed value for any given material, independent of x-ray beam energy. This, in fact, is far from accurate, as indicated in Chapter 9.[8] The attenuation coefficient of any material depends strongly on the energy of the photons irradiating it and, in general, has a roughly exponential shape over the range of energies found in the spectrum of x-rays used for CT scanners, as illustrated in Figure 15.5. This disparity between the actual physical properties of the attenuation coefficient and those that are assumed by the theory for the sake of mathematical facility does not prevent the practical implementation of the theory. It does, however, become a source of artifact and quantitative inaccuracy in the resultant images. The problem lies in a phenomena called beam-hardening. Because of the shape of the attenuation versus energy curve, a polyenergetic x-ray beam passing through any absorber undergoes preferential absorption of the lower energy (or softer) photons. This causes the relative percentage of higher energy (or harder) photons to increase resulting in what is called a harder beam. Note that this phenomena is *not* CT specific, but is present in all uses of polychromatic x-ray sources.

In order to understand the effect of beam hardening in CT, the concept of an effective energy is necessary. When a polychromatic x-ray beam passes through an absorber, some energy is removed from the beam and deposited in the absorber. This results in the exit beam having less energy than the entrance beam. The exact amount of energy reduction is a function of the shape of the attenuation curve of the absorber *and* the energy distribution of the x-ray beam. The effective

energy is that photon energy of a monoenergetic photon beam which, if passed through the same absorber, would result in the same loss in energy content in the beam. All CT scanners presently measure the total energy content of the beam both before and after it has passed through the patient and do not take into account the fact that the energy distribution and therefore the effective energy have changed. In Figure 15.5, curve A shows a typical polychromatic x-ray profile which describes the input x-ray spectrum, that is, the number of x-ray photons present at each x-ray photon energy. The line AA at 60 keV represents the effective energy that is measured by the x-ray detector during the "detection" process if no beam attenuation had occured. If the polychromatic x-ray beam passes through an object having the characteristics of curve B, the energy profile of the beam emerging from the object would have the shape of curve C. Because of the selective absorption of the lower energy photons by the material, the effective x-ray energy detected would be shifted to approximately 70 keV (line CC). In the CT image reconstruction algorithms, the assumption of a monoenergetic beam is made. This assumes that the energy AA is identical to the energy CC and that only the amplitude of the x-ray spectrum has changed. The end result of using equation 4 in solving for μ is to compute

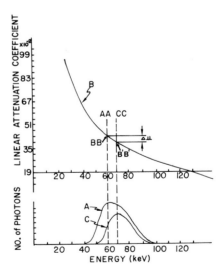

Figure 15.5. Beam-hardening effects in the CT image arise because a greater attenuation of lower energy x-ray photons occurs relative to the higher energy photons. This alters the shape of the output energy spectrum relative to the input energy spectrum and shifts the recorded effective energy to a higher value. Because of the curvilinear shape of the linear attenuation curve of the material, a lower μ value is computed than should be secondary to the added attenuation arising from the shift of the energy spectrum in addition to the inherent tissue attenuation effect.

point B'B' on curve B rather than point BB and thus to generate an error of $\Delta\mu$. Thus, $\Delta\mu$ represents the computational error arising from the shift of the x-ray profile to a higher x-ray energy value because of the beam hardening which has occurred as the x-ray beam traversed the object.

Qualitatively, the error $\Delta\mu$ does not create a large disturbance in the overall subjective image quality, except where a great deal of hardening occurs such as when the x-ray beam passes through bone. As indicated in Chapter 14, beam-hardening in the head produces a cupping-artifact. In the abdomen or thorax, where the amount of bone encountered by the x-ray beam is minimal, subjective image quality is not noticeably diminished. Quantitatively however, the error is not acceptable and must be corrected by using special beam hardening correction algorithms.[9,10] These are generally implemented as options by various scanner manufacturers and usually add to the image reconstruction time. Image-wise, the beam hardening correction produces a sharp and discrete interface between the calvarium and brain, or reduces the "shadow artifact" in a liver image beneath adjacent ribs.

X-RAY TUBE EFFECTS: OPTICS CONSIDERATIONS

Some discussion is necessary as to the difference between continuously-on and pulsed x-ray sources, even though no clinically apparent difference in image quality has yet been noticed. Pulsed systems (ie, GE CT/7800, GE CT/8800, and Varian 360-3 scanners) turn the x-ray source on at discrete time intervals during gantry rotation; milliseconds later, the x-ray source is turned off. During the on-time, very-high milliamperage stations (ie, 300 to 600 mA) are used to develop an intense, pulsed x-ray profile. Nonpulsed systems (or alternatively, continuously-on systems) leave the x-ray tube on during the entire translate/rotate or rotate-only tube movements (ie, all other CT scanners, except GE, Siemens, and Varian), but use lower milliamperage operating stations (ie, 10 to 30 mA). Assuming uniform beam filtration, the usually employed milliamperage-time product (mAs) is roughly the same for all systems (eg, 600 mA $\times$ 1.1 msec/view $\times$ 576 view = 380 mAs [GE CT/8800] compared with 30 mA $\times$ 10 sec = 300 mAs [EMI 6000]; typical head scan values), although many different combinations of mA, msec, and/or number of views can make this mAs value vary considerably.

For small focal spot tubes (ie, rotating anode) or long, narrow focal spot tubes (ie, stationary anode) beam divergence occurs both in the axial plane (slice sensitivity profile considerations) and in the coronal

plane (a in equation 5). Pulsed x-ray sources thus have a narrower tissue irradiation area on the fore side of the patient than on the aft side because of the diverging nature of the beam (Fig. 15.6, right). Thus, the attenuation of the beam by any minute volume of tissue within the patient and in the direction of the x-ray beam varies according to whether the volume lies toward the fore or aft side of the patient as the beam passes through the tissue. Thus nonuniform weighting of the attenuation of the beam can occur on the basis of tissue volume changes alone, independent of the tissue composing the volume. These erroneous attenuation changes are minimized in pulsed x-ray systems by combining the attenuation readings made 180 degrees apart. Continuously-on systems have x-ray beam profile patterns that do not show fore and aft side changes (Fig. 15.6, left). Because the beam is on during the measurement process, the entrance beam profile is "smeared" relative to the exit beam profile. If one assumes that only the proper amount of smearing occurs (a potential source of image error if the smearing is not considered in the reconstruction algorithms), then the beam profile through the patient will be parallel and of finite width. This leads to beam attenuation patterns that do not show a volume dependence rela-

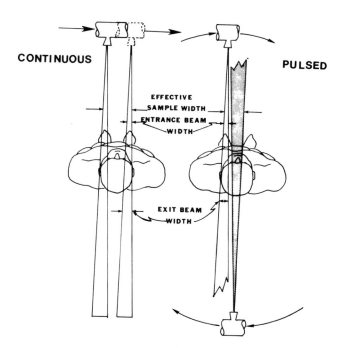

Figure 15.6. Effect of beam divergence upon tissue sampling using pulsed x-ray systems (right) or continuously-on x-ray systems (left). Continuously-on systems "smear" the x-ray beam to achieve parallel sampling profiles of finite width. Pulsed systems average the data obtained from beam profiles obtained 180 degrees apart to achieve the same effect.

tive to the traversal of the x-ray beam through the patient. Nevertheless, one must always be aware that unless a large enough number of angular samples (ray-projections) are taken, relative to the width of the x-ray beam and the cross-sectional diameter of the patient, some tissue may not be measured (ie, seen) by the scanner.[11]

X-RAY TUBE EFFECTS: PATIENT–DOSE CONSIDERATIONS

The amount of irradiation a patient receives during a CT examination, while considerably influencing the image quality obtained, needs to be looked at. Patient dosage is a function of the proximity of the patient to the x-ray tube (inverse square radiation law), scanner motion (ie, translate/rotate versus rotate-only), range of scanning (ie, 180 degrees, 360 degrees, etc), pulsed versus continuous x-ray tube operation, and the contiguity of adjacent x-ray slice profiles (ie, overlapped, nonoverlapped, and juxtaposed, or nonoverlapped and separated). The skin entrance irradiation profiles can thus vary considerably from scanner to scanner and vary with the image quality required clinically. Some overall dose can be made, however. To begin with, one should recall that tissue irradiation is defined in terms of ergs/gm/cm². This means that if no x-ray beam profile overlap occurs from slice to slice and no internal x-ray photon scattering is present, the irradiation received by the patient would be independent of the number of slices made and dependent only upon the dose delivered during *one* scan. Because x-ray beam profile overlap and photon scattering do occur, patient irradiation is somewhat higher for multiple slice studies than for a one slice study. The increase ranges from 20 to 90 percent for juxtaposed, nonoverlapped-slice scanning techniques, depending upon which scanner is employed.[7]

The two factors that influence patient irradiation the most (given identical mAs, kVp stations, and different scanners) are the proximity of the patient to the x-ray source and whether 180 degrees or 360 degrees tube motion is used. Because the intensity of the x-ray beam falls off inversely proportional to the square of the distance between the x-ray tube and the patient, it becomes important to know whether the patient is centered relative to the center of rotation. Obviously, when the tube rotation only goes 180 degrees around the patient, an asymmetrical patient irradiation profile will occur. Asymmetrical profiles will occur even on 360 degrees tube motions when the patient is not centered relative to the axis of rotation. This occurs often during head studies in order to tilt the head forward and obtain slice profiles 20 to 25 degrees

relative to the orbital-mental line. In general, however, 360-degree tube motion does produce a more uniform, lower dose profile because the x-ray energy is distributed over a greater circumferential area.

McCullough and Payne[12] have recently reviewed the irradiation profiles of different scanners using single- and multiple-slice scanning techniques. For single-scan profiles on rotate/translate scanners, the maximum skin dose for an average CT head study ran from a low of 2.0 rads to a high of 6.5 rads, and up to 19.5 rads for images obtained in the "high-accuracy" mode. Single-scan maximum skin dosage recorded on rotate-only scanners using average mAs and kVp settings ran from a low of 0.5 rads to a high of 6.5 rads, and up to 12.0 rads for the high-accuracy modes. When multiple, nonoverlapped contiguous slices were made, as is the customary clinical practice, a multiplication factor ranging from 1.2 to 1.9 had to be employed. If IV contrast studies are employed, an additional multiplication factor of 2.0 is required. Thus, it is possible in the evaluation of intracranial pathology to obtain the information with a low skin irradiation value of 2.4 rads. On the other hand, up to 74.1 rads may be given to the patient when using IV contrast, multiple slices, high-accuracy modes, and translate/rotate scanners. Obviously physician prudence needs to be exercised in order to obtain the greatest amount of clinical information at the lowest possible irradiation levels.

PRESENT-DAY INSTRUMENTATION

TRANSLATE/ROTATE SCANNERS

This mechanical motion was used in the pioneering CT efforts of Geoffry Hounsfield when he designed and perfected the EMI CT 1000 scanner (Fig. 15.7).[1,2] With this operation, the x-ray tube emits an x-ray beam that is collimated into a "knife-like" shape (sometimes called "pencil-beam" shape) having dimensions of roughly 2×13 mm. The intensity of the beam is monitored by a small x-ray detector cell prior to the beam's passing through the object to be imaged. In passing through the object, some x-ray photons are absorbed or deflected from the beam by the material while some photons pass through unattenuated. Those photons that are not absorbed by the object are "detected" by a sodium iodide (NaI) crystal mounted opposite the x-ray tube. This NaI crystal, in turn, emits a light proportional to the amount of x-ray energy deposited in the crystal lattice. The emitted light, in turn, is converted by a photomultiplier tube (PM tube) into an electrical signal proportional to the detected light, amplified by electronic circuits, and sent into a digital computer using an ADC. During the scanning process, the x-ray

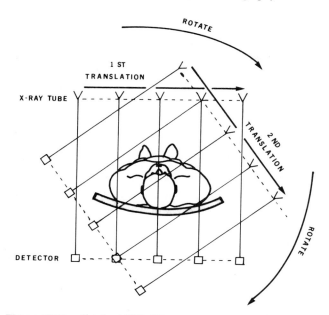

Figure 15.7. Original EMI CT scanner concept (first generation) where x-ray photons are generated from a single source, are collimated into a pencil-beam shape, pass through the patient, and are detected by a single x-ray NaI detector. The x-ray tube and detector *translate* linearly across the patient obtaining multiple readings of object's x-ray absorption. The x-ray tube/detector system then *rotates* a fixed increment (usually about one degree) and a second translation process is performed; 180 degrees of rotation are generally made around the patient.

tube and detector crystal translate continuously across the patient, making multiple measurements of the attenuation of the material between the x-ray tube and detector. For the EMI CT 1000 scanner, 160 measurements are made during each translation. Immediately following each translation, the x-ray tube and detector system rotate one degree and the translation process is repeated, thereby generating a second set of 160 measurements. The translate/rotate process is repeated until 180 translations have been completed; that is, until 28,800 (160 × 180) measurements have been made.

Technically, each of the 160 measurements made during translation is called a ray-sum and each of the 180 sets of ray-sums is called a ray-projection. As before, the ray-sums and ray-projections are referred to as the raw-projection data (or raw-data for short).

From a practical point of view, the single-source, single x-ray detector scanner originally designed by EMI has one major disadvantage: it requires 5 minutes to gather the 28,800 ray-sums necessary to form an image. Clinically, this limits its use to body parts that are or can be made immobile, such as the head. On the other hand, the major advantage of the single-source, single-detector system is that x-ray photons as they

pass through the object to be imaged can easily be separated into two forms, those which are scattered in the patient (and thus not seen by the detector), and those that are not scattered (and thus recorded by the detector). Because the detector aperture opening is made very small (2 × 13 mm), the photon acceptance angle into the detector is highly specific and easily eliminates the vast majority of the scattered photons. This ability to avoid including scattered photons in the measurements, as shown in Chapter 14, contributes to high tissue density resolution capabilities. Spatial resolution characteristics, on the other hand, while free of scattered photons, remain poor because the actual number of measurements made of the object allows only an 80 × 80 matrix to be computed. As such, the resulting image has a very coarse and grainy appearance.

To overcome the limitations imposed by a five-minute scan time, manufacturers modified the x-ray collimators so that the x-ray beam was "fan-shaped," having a diverging angle of 3 to 10 degrees. Multiple x-ray detectors were placed juxtaposed to each other in order to intercept the fan-shaped x-ray source. Because more x-ray detectors are utilized, the angular rotation can be made through larger degree increments while gathering the same (or even a greater) number of ray-sums. Through the use of the fan-beam source, multiple detector concept, scanning times have been decreased from 5 min to 2.5 minutes (Ohio Nuclear Delta-50 Scanner), to 18 to 20 seconds (Delta-50 FS, Pfizer ACTA Scanner, EMI CT 5005 Scanner, etc), and finally down to 12 seconds (Picker Synerview Scanner). Thus, the scan time interval is made comparable to a patient's breath-holding ability. Figure 15.8 shows how this reduction in scanning time is accomplished. From the point of view of the reconstruction algorithms, if three x-ray detectors are used per data measurement interval, then three sets of ray-projections are gathered per translation process. This is easily seen by noting that each ray-sum is oriented at an angle slightly oblique to the center ray-sum. Each of the three ray-sums may be grouped independently of the other ray-sums as shown on the right of Figure 15.8. Not only is the single straight-on view (Fig. 15.8.B) produced as it would be by a first generation machine during the one translation of the tube detector assembly, but also views equivalent to those taken at other rotational angles are produced. This allows the scanner to index by larger angles and reduces the number of actual translations required of the mechanism. Though the actual scanning time is reduced, the radiation dose received by the patient may, in fact, be increased. This results from two factors. The first is that even though the number of detectors and therefore the size of the beam is increased the scan time may not be reduced by

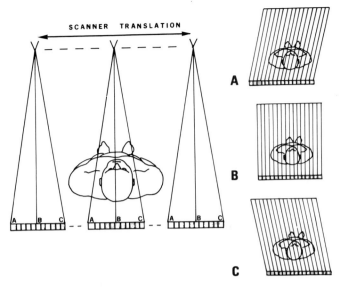

Figure 15.8. Using a translate/rotate scanner and slightly diverging x-ray beam with multiple detectors, the equivalent of multiple angles of view can be obtained during a single translation process by segregation of the detector cell outputs in computer memory. Thus, larger incremental rotational angles may be used, effectively shortening the required scanning time. Because more raw data may also be obtained, better image spatial resolution characteristics may be obtained through larger image matrix size computations.

the same factor, eg, an increase in detectors from 1 to 10 is not matched by a corresponding scan time reduction from 10 minutes to 1 minute. The second problem is that the increased beam size results in the out-of-slice tissue, ie, the tissue on both sides of the area of interest being exposed to a greater amount of scattered radiation during the scan.

ROTATE-ONLY SCANNERS

The next change in CT scanner geometry was to widen the x-ray beam diverging angle to 30 to 90 degrees as shown in Figure 15.9, so it could entirely encompass the object without having to perform any type of translation motion. Thus, a rotate-only scanning motion can be used; however, the larger diverging x-ray beam in turn requires a greater number of x-ray detectors to intercept all of the transmitted x-ray photons. The number of x-ray detectors have been increased from 3 to 10 to 250 to 511 in various scanner models. Each detector in turn required its own amplifier, ADC, etc, increasing the cost of the equipment. The advantage, however, is that a further decrease in the scanning time, down to 3 to 5 seconds is obtained. The rotate-only x-ray tube and detector array is called by some the "Third Generation" scanner because of the chronologically-introduced (compared to the trans-

late/rotate scanners) description of its mechanical motion.

As discussed in Chapter 14, the spatial resolution of the rotate-only scanners is determined primarily by the width of the x-ray detector aperture opening and by the number of angles of view (ie, the number of ray-projections) the scanner makes. The narrow detector aperture opening and large number of x-ray detectors obviates the use of crystal detectors, consequently gas (eg, xenon) detector systems were designed. Because gas is less dense than the scintillation detector crystal, x-ray photon capture efficiency is diminished. This disadvantage is partially compensated for by the fact that the xenon detector produces ion pairs directly in response to the absorption of radiation. These ion pairs are swept out of the detector space by the electric potential applied to the detector and converted immediately to electrical pulses. This is unlike the crystal detectors used in the translate/rotate scanners that require PM tubes to convert the light from the crystal to electrical pulses. The absence of the light-to-electrical conversion process and the PM system itself removes one source of noise and signal distortion in the scanner and compensates somewhat for the lower detection efficiency of the gas detection. The xenon detector photon capture efficiency is dependent upon more than just the presence of xenon gas, but is dependent upon the product of the depth of the xenon detector cell and the pressure of the gas. If short detector cells are used, high-pressure gas requirements are necessitated, with the inherent problem of the gas leaking out of the

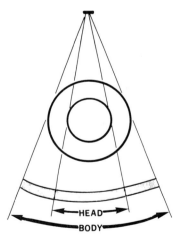

Figure 15.9. Original concept of third generation CT scanners where the diverging angle of the x-ray beam is sufficient to cover the entire object to be imaged without translation. Several hundred closely spaced detectors are required to rotate with the x-ray source around the object in order to record the attenuation profiles of the transmitted x-ray beam. Scan times of 3 to 5 seconds are available with this mechanical geometry.

detector cell length. In general, detectors 5 to 10 cm in depth and gas pressures of 10 to 20 atmospheres are used in order to give a detector depth, gas pressure product of around 100.[13] The overall x-ray photon detector efficiency for this arrangement appears optimal, and thus ranges around 60 to 80 percent, as opposed to crystal capture efficiencies that are on the order of 90 to 100 percent.

An inherent advantage of the longer xenon detector cell is that x-ray scatter rejection capacity becomes "built-in" because an x-ray photon has to travel a finite distance into the detector before it will eventually be "captured." Thus, any x-ray photons entering obliquely are rejected by the detector cell by being absorbed in the metallic spacers dividing the adjacent detectors. This scatter rejection capability results in an increased density resolution for this type scanner. Because spatial resolution is largely a function of the x-ray detector aperture opening, smaller aperture openings are needed in order to attain clinically useful spatial resolution. Consequently, third generation scanner manufacturers have added more detectors with smaller aperture openings to their scanners (eg, GE changed from their original 320 detectors to 511; Searle from 256 to 504 detectors, etc), with the resulting change in just-detectable-diameter values going from 1.75 to 2.0 mm down to 0.75 to 1.0 mm.

In order to diminish the scanning time further, the so-called "Fourth Generation" scanners were introduced by removing detector cells from the rotating gantry and mounting them in stationary positions around the patient volume outside the radius of rotation of the x-ray tube as shown in Figure 15.10. Thus, only the weight of the x-ray tube need be borne by the rotating gantry. This reduction in weight as well as the absence of the necessity of managing the data transfer cables from the rotating gantry reduced scanning times to 1 to 3 seconds. The very short scanning time was felt

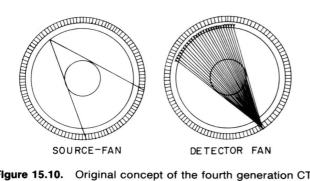

SOURCE-FAN   DETECTOR FAN

Figure 15.10. Original concept of the fourth generation CT scanners, where the diverging angle of the x-ray beam covers the object to be imaged. The detectors, however, are permanently fixed around the periphery of the scanner, so that as the x-ray tube rotates, a different set of detectors records the attenuation profile recordings. Scan times of 1 to 5 seconds are available with the concept.

to be necessary in order to eliminate or minimize involuntary object motion such as intestinal peristalsis. Anywhere from 600 detector units (ie, American Science and Engineering Scanner) through 720 units (Ohio Nuclear Delta 2020 Scanner) to 1088 units (EMI CT 7070 Scanner) were utilized depending upon the scanner manufacturer, and each detector unit employed a crystal detector such as bismuth germanium oxide (BGO) crystal or cesium iodide crystal (EMI CT 7070) in order to obtain a high x-ray photon capture efficiency. Because of the "packing problems" inherent in arranging the 600 to 1088 detector cells and their photo multiplier tubes around the periphery of the scanner, a "dead space," or alternatively a nonsampling region, had to be tolerated between the crystal aperture openings of adjacent detectors. Thus, it is possible for x-ray photons to pass through the object and between the detector cells and not contribute anything toward the image production but still contribute to patient irradiation.

The overall radiation detection efficiency of any detector array is a product of three terms: (1) the ability of the detector to detect a photon if it passes into the detector (photon capture efficiency); (2) the ability of the detector to convert the photon into an electrical signal (conversion efficiency); and (3) the ratio of the area of the detector aperture opening to the total space between any two detector cells (geometrical efficiency). For the fourth generation scanners, the first two conditions are nearly unity while the third is considerably less than unity. For the third generation scanners, as discussed previously, the first term is less than unity while the second and third terms are close to one. Thus, theoretically the detector efficiency for the two scanner generations is approximately the same, ie, in the 60 to 80 percent efficiency region.

While the efficiency of the detectors cannot be changed, the effect of the diminished detector efficiency on the patient can be minimized. The "dead space" effect can be neutralized by prepatient beam collimation, whereby many narrow fan beams are created from the one large fan beam with each narrow fan beam directed toward an individual detector cell (proposed and temporarily implemented by Ohio Nuclear). This prepatient collimation tends to minimize the "extra" patient irradiation but does *not* improve the quality of the final CT image that is generated. The alternate method and the one now used by Ohio Nuclear, plus almost all other scanner manufacturers, is to "harden" the x-ray beam prior to its passing through the patient, thus increasing the ratio of photons absorbed by the detector to those absorbed by the patient.

The third and fourth generation scanners would seem at first glance to be identical in the method that data is collected, with the only difference being that in the former the detectors move while in the latter they are stationary. On closer examination, however, this can be seen as not entirely true. In fact, a very fundamental difference exists in the method whereby the actual data are gathered, and this difference impacts on the type of image produced by each machine. In the rotate-only moving detector systems as seen in Figure 15.9, each detector element has a fixed relationship with the x-ray tube and the fan beam. This relationship remains fixed as the tube-detector assembly rotates and allows the detector to be highly collimated to reduce its detection of scattered radiation. As mentioned earlier, this provides the scanner with the capability of generating images with excellent density discrimination but the fixed geometric relationship makes the system prone to circular rotational artifacts. This type of data collection is referred to as the source-fan concept because it is the fan beam of the x-ray tube, ie, the radiation source, and its motion that determines the data collection resolution.

With the fourth generation machines (Figure 15.10), on the other hand, the detectors cannot be highly collimated as this would force any given detector cell to contribute data only when the x-ray tube was directly opposite it. This would, in turn, severely limit the total number of samples that could be taken about the patient. In the limit of perfect collimation on the detector, in fact, the number of total samples would be limited to the number of detectors. In order to overcome this limitation, the detectors are collimated in such a way as to allow them to gather radiation over a relatively wide range of x-ray tube positions (Fig. 15.10, right). In this configuration, the sampling resolution is determined by the detectors' field of view and is normally termed the detector fan concept. The major advantage of this method of data collection is that a large number of overlapped data measurements can be obtained which, after the overlap effect is mathematically removed, results in a very large number of closely spaced, narrow equivalent ray-sums per ray-projection. This, in turn, leads to very high spatial resolution qualities in the image, but with somewhat diminished density-resolution characteristics, as manifested by an increase in image graininess or noise. Reducing the image noise requires that a moderate increase in patient irradiation, ie, 3 to 10 rads skin dose per cross-sectional image, must occur.

BGO detectors are used on fixed-detector scanners rather than NaI(Tl) detectors, primarily because of "afterglow" phenomena. Afterglow is a phosphorescent effect created by a delayed emission of the crystal's characteristic light when subjected to high radiation flux in the CT scanner. NaI(Tl) has a much longer after-glow effect than the BGO crystals, thus, a longer time interval is required between data measurements in order to allow for the after-glow effect to decay. Since

a one-second total scanning time requires very short intersample time intervals, short after-glow characteristics are necessitated. Otherwise, succeeding data measurements tend to show a gradual background light build-up, which results in a detector output baseline shift during the measurement process. This baseline shift must be corrected before image computation is done and is implemented by measuring a standard material (eg, air) on both the fore and aft side of the object as the x-ray tube rotates past it. In comparison, rotate-only gas detectors do not have this light build-up because ion-pair signal generation does not result in afterglow-like effects. The rotate-only xenon detectors, on the other hand, do require that all of the multiple detector readings are made simultaneously and thus do require that each detector operates at exactly the same zero "voltage base line" and with the same "signal-amplification" characteristics as its neighbor. Rotate-only moving-detector scanners, therefore, require periodic calibration (usually daily or weekly because of the highly stable gas-to-amplifier circuitry used), in order to eliminate any drift in detector characteristics. From an image point of view, if the fixed-detector scanners do not correct for the scan time baseline shifts, streak artifacts will result in the computed cross-sectional image. Similarly, if all the detectors on rotate-only scanners do not have very nearly identical baseline and gain characteristics, ring-artifact will appear in the computed images.

ELECTRONIC MOTION SCANNERS

"Electronic motion" is a misnomer but implies a scanner design where multiple x-ray sources and detectors are all fixed (stationary) around the object and each x-ray source (numbering from 3 to 28) is electronically "fired" in sequence, thus simulating a mechanical motion. Because electronic sequential firing can be accomplished at a much greater rate than by mechanical rotation of an x-ray tube on a fly wheel, an order-of-magnitude reduction in scanning time can be accomplished. One prototype scanner now being built at the Mayo Clinic can gather all the raw data necessary for computation of up to 250 consecutive cross-sectional slices in 16.7 msec.[3] Stop-action cardiac or vascular motion studies are theoretically possible. The trade-off here is that duplication of the x-ray source/multiple detector system of up to 28 or more times is necessary with the corresponding order-of-magnitude increase in scanner costs. Also, just as trade-offs exist between spatial and density image resolution characteristics, temporal resolution trade-offs are present because of severe photon limitation that occurs in the presently available x-ray tubes. Preliminary data on this all-electronic scanner indicates that contrast media needs to be injected into the vascular system in order to separate the blood from the myocardial walls while viewing each of the 250 cross-sectional image sets obtained during the *one* cardiac cycle from diastole through diastole at 60 times per second. For more on all electronic scanners, the reader is referred to Wood et al.[3]

TRADE-OFFS EXPECTED BETWEEN SCANNER DESIGNS

No one scanner may be considered best. Each type of scanner tends to emphasize some features of scanning at the expense of others. These different image features may be summarized as below:

A. SINGLE DETECTOR, PENCIL-BEAM COLLIMATED X-RAY SOURCE

ADVANTAGES
1. Very low to nonexistent susceptibility to scatter radiation image-degrading effects.
2. Slow scanning speeds allow the use of high x-ray photon-detection efficiency NaI crystals.
3. Low data collection rates allow for near simultaneous image reconstruction methods to be used and therefore, minimizes the need for special computer microprocessors to perform the image generation functions of convolution and back projections.

DISADVANTAGES
1. Slow scanning speeds limit images to body parts that can be made "stationary," ie, head-only scanners.
2. Two-motion, ie, translate and rotate, allows for greater mechanical variation in the moving parts and thus, potential inherent reconstruction error.
3. A limited ray-sum and ray-projection data base limits the spatial resolution obtainable.

B. MULTIPLE DETECTORS, LIMITED FAN-BEAM X-RAY SOURCE

ADVANTAGES
1. Faster scanning speeds allow both head and body imaging.
2. A greater number of ray-projections are gathered per translation, therefore, larger matrices and better spatial resolution characteristics may be obtained.
3. Overlapped raw-data measurements may be accomplished leading to even further improved high-spatial resolution images.

DISADVANTAGES
1. Faster scanning speeds require use of less efficient crystals in order to minimize x-ray

detector afterglow effects and results in higher patient irradiation levels.
2. The greater number of accumulated ray-projections requires use of microprocessors in order to minimize reconstruction time, thus increasing scanner costs.
3. Greater susceptibility to scatter radiation is present unless predetector collimators are used.
4. Two-motion scanning allows for larger machine tolerance variations and their potential image artifact generation.

C. MULTIPLE MOVING DETECTORS, SINGLE ROTARY MOTION, FULL-FAN X-RAY SOURCE

ADVANTAGES
1. Short-scanning times (5 seconds or less) minimize motion-induced (both voluntary and involuntary) artifacts.
2. The large number of data measurements allow larger matrix size computations and improved image spatial resolution qualities.
3. Xenon detectors provide inherent collimators, therefore high density resolution images are created.
4. Xenon detectors can be made with narrow detector aperture openings, therefore further improving the spatial resolution image qualities.
5. Single-motion scanning (rotation only) minimizes mechanical tolerance variations.
6. High geometric efficiency of transmitted x-rays occurs because of minimal interdetector dead space, thus minimizing excess patient irradiation.

DISADVANTAGES
1. A large number of ray-projections requires use of microprocessors in order to minimize image reconstruction time.
2. Xenon detectors require very stable interdetector calibration specifications in order to minimize ring-artifacts.
3. Ultimate spatial resolution is determined by xenon detector aperture opening which is fixed in size by engineering design criteria.
4. Xenon gas is the least efficient of available detectors in x-ray absorption efficiency, ie, approximately 60 to 80 percent efficient.

D. MULTIPLE FIXED DETECTORS, SINGLE FULL-FAN X-RAY SOURCE

ADVANTAGES
1. Fast scanning times minimize motion-induced image artifact.

2. Overlapped data collection methods allow for a large number of ray-sum measurements that can be decomposed into a large number of nonoverlapped equivalent ray-sum measurements, thus yielding high spatial resolution image characteristics.
3. The large amount of raw-projection data generated allows very large matrix size reconstructions.
4. Uses moderately high-efficiency crystal x-ray detectors.

DISADVANTAGES

1. Poor geometric efficiency of the transmitted x-ray photons is present because of a large interdetector "dead space." This mandates the use of prepatient collimation in order to avoid high patient irradiation.
2. Intradetector calibration during the course of a scan is mandatory because of afterglow buildup in the detector crystals.
3. Requires extra computer programming steps in order to convert overlapped data measurements into nonoverlapped equivalent measurements prior to convolution and back projection. This increases image noise and, to lesser extent, image reconstruction time.
4. Large matrix computations require microprocessors for back-projection and convolution processes.
5. Inability to collimate scatter radiation from the detector requires either reduced image density resolution or large patient-to-detector spacing (ie, air-gap) in order to minimize the scattered irradiation effects.

FIGURE-OF-MERIT FOR SCANNER COMPARISONS

A convenient figure-of-merit for comparing CT scanners relates to the proportion that exists between the number of data measurements made and the number of matrix elements computed (Fig. 15.11). The number of data measurements made is the product of the number of nonoverlapped (or nonoverlapped equivalent) ray-sums and the number of angles of view (ie, the number of ray-projections). For rotate-only moving-detector scanners, the number of detectors in the scanner is the ray-sum value, while the required number of views is a computer program variable that generally runs from 270 to 1080. For rotate-only fixed-detector scanners, the total number of overlapped measurements made per detector is the required number of nonoverlapped equivalent ray-sums, and the number of fixed-detectors is the required number of views. The number of image pixels making up the matrix that need to be computed during the reconstruc-

tion process is the product of the row-and-column values of the matrix (eg, for 256×256 matrix, $65,536$ pixels need to be computed). The figure-of-merit value that is sought is the ray-sum and ray-projection product divided by the matrix rows and columns product (Fig. 15.11). A value of 1 is required for the image to be computed with any degree of accuracy at all. In general, all scanners on the market have a figure-of-merit greater than unity, and as the figure-of-merit becomes larger, the spatial and density resolution qualities of the image will be higher. (The image will also be more pleasing to the eye, but not necessarily more diagnostic.) However, this figure-of-merit does not take into account any patient irradiation that also goes up with increasing figure-of-merit values or the slice-sensitivity profile characteristics. Also it is only theoretical in that it represents what the scanner is capable of doing, but does not indicate if it achieves the appropriate end.

As an alternative figure-of-merit, General Electric[7] has proposed a graph-type display, which relates image spatial resolution to image density resolution as a function of dose delivered (Fig. 15.12). This also is a good general figure-of-merit device, but it also ignores slice-sensitivity profile changes. This plot of spatial resolution versus density resolution differs from the figure-of-merit above in that it is a plot of measured spatial and density resolution and not theoretical calculations, independent of how the raw data was gathered and/or used in the formation of the image. No slice-sensitivity profile characteristics, to date, have been built into any figure-of-merit criteria for the CT scanners.

ROOM LAYOUT AND EQUIPMENT CONFIGURATION CONSIDERATIONS

Once the manufacturer and type of CT scanner have been decided upon, equipment layout must be accomplished in such a way that it makes the scanner easily accessible to the patients and efficient to operate by the technician. Most companies do offer some architectural and planning assistance, and this help should be sought because these individuals are intimately (or should be) familiar with some of the particulars of their equipment. These include cable length, water and/or air conditioning requirements, etc. Because room renovations will almost always be required, except for possibly a new hospital having a preplanned CT scanner suite, a local architect will also be needed. Another aid one may or may not wish to use is some of the radiology consultant groups that are available around the country with some expertise in CT layout designs.

CT scanners are both expensive to purchase and costly to maintain because of their inherent complexity, mechanical parts, and association with large digital computers. Because of this, considerable attention

Figure 15.11. Figure-of-merit proposal whereby *theoretical* considerations of the "goodness" of CT scanners may be examined. An increase in the number of raw-data measurements is needed to offset an increase in the computational requirements dictated by image matrix size. The "R" values indicate lines where raw-data measurements equal (R=1) or exceed (R=2,4, etc) the matrix size requirements. In general, scanners having R values above 4 give the best, "esthetically gratifying" images; however, very large values do not necessarily result in improved image appearance, but do result in increased patient irradiation.

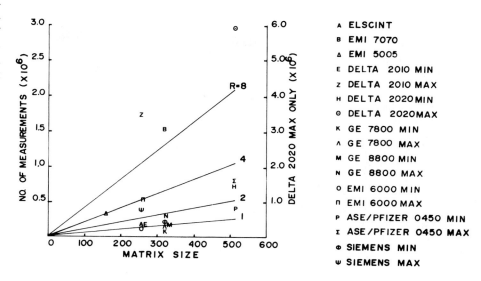

should be given to the efficiency of the overall operation by the radiologists using the facility. This efficiency analysis should begin first with the CT technician, second with the patient, and, finally, with the physician.

The difference between a good and an excellent technician can be based on the number of patient studies done per 8-hour shift. A good technician can do 2 or 3 patient examinations more per 8-hour shift than a poor technician given identical image quality; anything that can be done to make life better for the technician is mandatory. The following ideas represent some that have worked out in the Vanderbilt University Hospital CT environment:

1. All computer equipment (ie, central processing unit,

CPU, disc drives, tape drives, etc) should be housed in a designated room adjacent to, but physically separate from, the scanner room *and* the technician control room in order to maintain this equipment in an air-conditioned environment, and of equal importance, to remove the computer air-conditioning fan noise from the working areas. Other equipment, such as consumable supplies, scanner power supplies, voltage regulators, etc, can also be stored in this highly temperature-regulated, humidity-controlled area (Fig. 15.13).

2. The scanner control room should be separated from the physician interpretation area. This is especially true in any large general or community hospital where friendly consulting staff/house officers are present. The average CT installation will examine

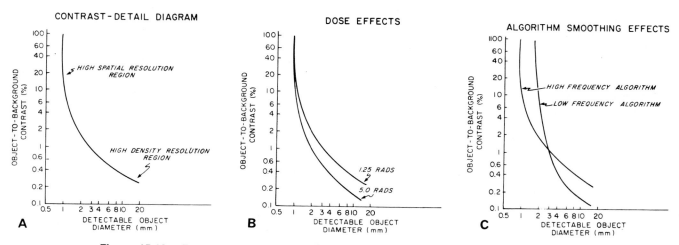

Figure 15.12. Figure-of-merit proposal.[7] **A.** A plot of image-spatial resolution capability against image-density resolution ability as a function of object irradiation dose indicates the *measured* response of the scanner system. **B.** Note that as the irradiation level increases both spatial and density resolution improve (see also Chap. 14) **C.** Changes in convolution filter function also affect spatial and density resolution characteristics.

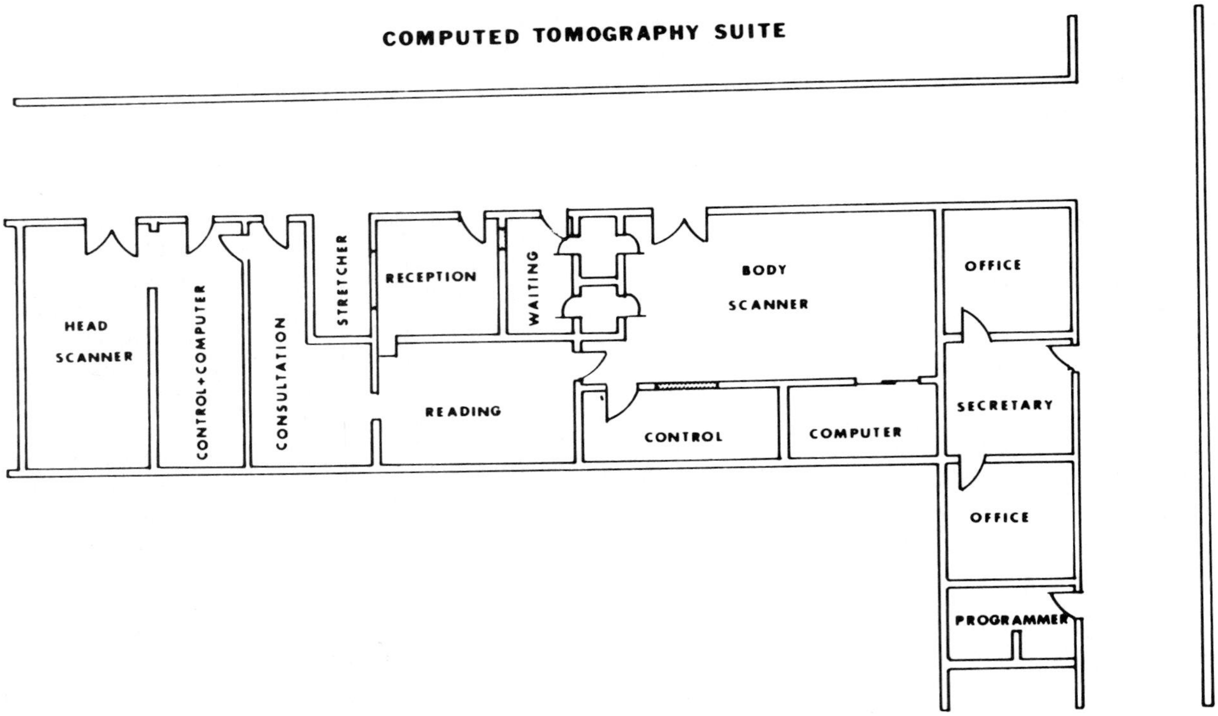

COMPUTED TOMOGRAPHY SUITE

Figure 15.13. CT scanner suite at Vanderbilt University Hospital. The "body scanner" layout represents the recommended multiple room design that maximizes patient output for a two-technician operation and minimizes air-conditioning noise and temperature requirements. The "head scanner" layout represents the standard two-room design that is optimal for a one-technician operation, but maintains a "cold" ambient temperature for both the technician and patient because of the nonisolation of the computer system.

one patient per 45 to 60 minutes of room time at best, so if the physician *and* technician spend 5 to 10 minutes with each curious physician, it means 1 or 2 fewer patient examinations per 8-hour shift.

3. For a one-technician operation, the scanner control console, floppy disc drives, and camera should be in the technician's control room. On the contrary, for a two-technician operation, the camera and floppy disc drives should be more remote so that each technician can work independently, one handling patients and one doing film library work. A two-technician environment will increase the number of patient examinations approximately 50 percent per 8-hour shift.

4. The scanner room should have as much open or free space around the patient couch area as possible because most patients will come to the scanner on beds or on stretchers, especially in the more critical care hospital environments. Alternatively, some scanners have specially designed CT stretchers that do allow for patient transfer outside the scanner suite and for remote IV infusion and/or for water-soluble enema preparations, etc. The end result here is that minimal patient manipulation must occur in

the scanner room itself. This latter option is best but does require "transfer space" and a second technician to supervise the transfer operation, in addition to the other space requirements.

Patient considerations should be directed along three lines: temperature, noise, and privacy.

1. In general, room temperatures around 72 to 75° F are the most comfortable for patients. The scanner gantries generally will operate efficiently at normal room temperatures and if the computer and its specialized air-conditioning requirements have been removed, the air temperature in the scanning room can be made comfortable for the patients. For pediatric patients, especially newborns and premature infants, body-temperature regulation requirements are critical; thus, warming pads and/or heat lamps are mandatory.

2. Because noise distracts the patients and may result in motion-induced image artifact, it must be minimized. Isolation of computer fan noise has been discussed previously and need not be repeated. The remaining sources of noise are the technicians and

doctors during the consulting periods. Whether of a professional or personal nature, such discussions should not occur in either the scanner room or the scanner control rooms.
3. Privacy of the patient's image results and his or her body parts must be maintained under all conditions.

Physician considerations center around the interaction time necessitated by the interpretation console and the time spent consulting with other physicians.

1. The physician interpretation area ideally should be juxtaposed, but separate from, the scanner and technicians' rooms. A quiet area with easy access to the physician display console is required. Display console interaction by the physician is mandatory on most head and body studies, especially where subtle tissue density differences are being evaluated and discussions as to whether to infuse contrast media must be made before the patient leaves the department.
2. The number of consultations per day (and/or per hour) plus the number of visiting physicians will dictate how much space should be available in the interpretation area and how many extra view boxes will be needed for the consultation function. This consultation area should be sealed from the scanner room so the patient does not accidentally hear professional jargon that may be misinterpreted.

INFORMATION STORAGE AND RETRIEVAL

CT images and information can be stored in one or more of the following ways: Polaroid or conventional film, "hard" or "floppy" discs, or magnetic tape. Each of these devices is unique and deserves special considerations, especially relative to the local legal aspects of film storage requirements that are in force. Generally, most statutes require that some record of the patients' examinations will be preserved for 5 to 7 years. For radiologists, the "record" generally means an image, but may also include the interpretation of the image or a method of recreating the image without patient reexposure. At Vanderbilt, the following data storage method is used:

1. Following the examination, the patient's computed images are stored on conventional x-ray film, floppy disc, hard disc, and magnetic tape. Image interpretation occurs predominantly via the film and through the interrogation of the images stored on the hard disc in the computer. The hard disc is erased daily.
2. Floppy discs are stored with the patient's film images for approximately 30 days following the study and are then erased and reused. We have found that we

rarely require access to the discs following 30 days of storage. Floppy discs can be reused for several years if properly stored and cared for, according to the manufacturers' directions. Information stored on floppy discs, while available for manipulation on the physicians' console, many times (depending upon the manufacturer) cannot be reread back into the computer for other types of image-analysis work. Only magnetic tape or "hard disc" have this reread capability.
3. Magnetic tapes are erased and reused after two years of storage. Most tapes are capable of retaining data for five to seven years if they are periodically (eg, monthly) unwound and rewound on their spools. If a tape just sits, the nonuniformity of the magnetic tape winding (ie, the stress and strain on the tape) can alter the physical characteristics of the magnetic oxide allowing information loss and subsequent computer read errors. Because most radiology departments cannot be bothered to wind and unwind tapes, a two-year turn-around time represents a compromise.
4. Conventional x-ray type film is stored for seven years if the patient's examination was abnormal and five years if normal. This time requirement is set by the local statutes. We prefer conventional x-ray film for image storage over the Polaroid film because it has a better gray-scale quality and is less expensive. All discarded film is processed for silver recovery.

EQUIPMENT SERVICE

CT scanners must be considered "brittle" systems in their behavior, which means that the systems are so complex and dependent on each of their components that should any small part fail, the entire system fails and operation comes to a halt. Because the systems are so complex, one does not consider if they are going to fail, but *when* they will fail. This statement is independent also of the manufacturer making the equipment. Furthermore, this equipment is usually housed in a very "hostile" environment (ie, the hospital) where air conditioning and voltage control is at best variable. Next, patients are placed on the equipment who may have blood or other body discharges coming from their wounds and these tissue secretions may drip onto the sensitive electronic parts located under the patient couch. Finally, contrast media and its associated accidents will always be found around the scanner gantries. What this all means is two things: (1) a good, competent serviceman or service agreement with your scanner company is necessary; and (2) routine quality control and calibration performance checks must be done to ensure image quality.[14]

Competent servicing almost always has to be obtained from the company that manufactures the scanner. This is primarily because the instrumentation is so new and is continuously undergoing field changes from the vendor. A nonvendor service organization that does not have privileged access to company information and personnel will be virtually useless. Service contracts generally cost about 6 to 6.5 percent per year of the original cost of the equipment and generally specify that either a serviceman will be stationed in your city and/or a minimum response time per service call will be honored. The contracted service comes in two forms: (1) preventive maintenance and (2) emergency repair. Preventive maintenance is scheduled through the local/regional office while emergency repair is generally initiated by calling the serviceman directly.

Because money is lost in patient revenue by having the preventive maintenance during the normal working hours, we recommend purchasing the service option, if available, for after hours servicing. Emergency call is generally listed in two forms: (1) during working hours (which is usually free) and (2) after working hours (which is not free). After working hours emergency servicing is usually expensive, but necessary if you are to provide emergency CT service to the community and if your scanner must be "ready to go at 8:00 AM tomorrow morning." Thus, your CT budget should contain some "slush" repair money.

Quality control on scanners, using either a company provided or individually purchased phantom, is necessary and should be performed at minimum monthly and at maximum weekly. The frequency of quality control is dependent upon the stability of the scanner. We recommend weekly checks initially, and, if the machine proves stable as indicated by little significant change in the phantom measurements, then lengthening the checks towards the maximum interval length (monthly) can be done. Following any type of major equipment recalibration, overhaul, etc, a quality control is required for new baseline values. Recalibration may be either of two forms, software or hardware. All software recalibration should be done at least daily, unless frequent checks show little change in the calibration values. Hardware checks, such as checks on detector gas pressure, beam hardening correction values, etc, should be done weekly unless extreme stability is noted.

SUMMARY

Commercially available CT scanners are made primarily of three types: (1) tube and detectors that both rotate and translate together, (2) tube and detectors that rotate only, and (3) tube that rotates but detectors that remain stationary. All three different designs have been optimized based upon different image characteristics such as artifact rejection, spatial resolution, and/or density resolution.

Artifact rejection comes in many forms, but primarily relates to minimizing patient motion, equipment miscalibration, x-ray beam hardening effects, and slice-sensitivity profiles. Spatial resolution is dependent upon the aperture opening of the x-ray detector cells, the amount of oversampling employed, the number of angles of view, and the convolution filtering algorithm used. Density resolution is dependent upon patient irradiation, matrix size computed, beam "slice" thickness, and redundancy in the amount of data gathered.

Image reconstruction is done using back-projection techniques in order to form the image, and convolution filtering is required in order to remove or modify the inherent smoothing resulting from the back-projection process. In the order of operation, convolution precedes back-projection. Reconstruction speed is dependent upon the use and/or sophistication of the digital microprocessors employed to perform the back-projection and convolution functions.

CT room layouts or designs should be based more on efficiency of operation and patient comfort than around equipment peculiarities. The computer room, control room, scanner room, and interpretation rooms should be juxtaposed but physically separated.

Equipment preventive maintenance and quality control measures should be instituted and rigidly followed.

REFERENCES

1. Hounsfield GN: Computerized transverse axial scanning (tomography): Part I, Description of system. Br J Radiol 46: 1016–1022, 1973
2. Ambrose J, Hounsfield G: New techniques for diagnostic radiology. Br J Radiol 46: 148–149, 1973
3. Wood EH: New vistas for the study of structural and functional dynamics of the heart, lungs and circulation by non-invasive numerical tomographic vivisection. Circulation 56 (4): 506–520, 1977
4. Gardner NT, Herman GT: Algorithms for reproducing objects from their x-rays. Comput Graph Image Proc 1: 97–106, 1972
5. Gordon R, Herman GT: Three-Dimensional Reconstruction from projections: A review of algorithms. Int Rev Cytol 38: 111–151, 1974
6. Brooks RA, DiChiro G: Theory of image reconstruction in computed tomography. Radiology 117: 561–572, 1975
7. CT/T Technology Continuum: Technical Performance of the CT/T System. General Electric Corporation Medical Systems Division, Milwaukee, Wis., 53201.
8. Phelps ME, Gado MH, Hoffman EJ: Correlation of

effective atomic number and electron density with attenuation coefficients measured with polychromatic x-rays. Radiology 117: 585–588, 1975

9. Zatz LM, Alvarez RE: An inaccuracy in computed tomography: The energy dependence of CT values. Radiology 124: 91–97, 1977

10. Hilal SK, Shepp L, Joseph PM, Stein J: Desirable features for advanced computerized tomography scanners. Ter-Pogossian MM, Phelps MD, Brownell GL, et al (eds) Reconstruction Tomography in Diagnostic Radiology and Nuclear Medicine. Baltimore, University Park Press, 1977, pp 541–549

11. Cormack AM: Sampling the radon transform with beams of finite width. Phys Med Biol 23(6): 1141–1148, 1978

12. McCullough EC, Payne JT: Patient dosage in computed tomography. Radiology 129: 457–463, 1978

13. Yaffe M, Fenster A, Johns HE: Xenon ionization detectors for fan beam computed tomography scanners. J Comput Assist Tomogr 1(4): 419–428, 1977

14. McCullough EC, Payne JT, Baker HL, et al: Performance evaluation and quality assurance of computed tomography scanners, with illustrations from the EMI, ACTA, and DELTA scanners. Radiology 120: 173–188, 1976

CHAPTER 16

Nuclear Medicine Imaging Devices

F. DAVID ROLLO
JAMES A. PATTON

A number of imaging devices have been developed since the first scanning system was built by Benedict Cassen and his colleagues at UCLA in 1950. The rectilinear scanner and scintillation camera are two such devices. Developed over the past three to five years are such devices as the large field scintillation camera, multicrystal whole-body rectilinear scanners, multicrystal cameras, tomographic scanners, positron cameras, and emission computerized axial tomography (CAT) cameras. In this chapter, the theory of operation and characteristics of each of these devices will be briefly presented.

RECTILINEAR SCANNER

The rectilinear scanner is a moving detector imaging system that uses a system of motors and controls to move the detector mechanically in a rectilinear fashion. A shielded NaI(T1) crystal mechanically advances across the field of interest, increments a specific but constant distance (line spacing) down the patient, and then moves back across the patient. During this process, the readout system moves in synchrony with the detector. The pattern is repeated until the small focal region of the focused collimator has swept across the entire field of interest. A single probe rectilinear scanner and its associated electronic components are shown in Figure 16.1.

While the focused collimator is scanned over the distribution of radioactivity, the detector converts the radiation transmitted by the collimator into electrical pulses, which can be further amplified and processed by the electronic components of the scanner. The readout system presents the processed information in a form suitable for visual interpretation. Virtually all scanners in use today have crystal diameters of 12.7 cm, with a thickness of 5.08 cm.

Whole-body rectilinear scanners typically have one probe above the table as well as another below the table. The dual probes are opposed but move in synchrony with one another to provide an anterior as well as a posterior scan of the patient simultaneously.

The collimators used with the rectilinear scanners have multiple holes that are focused at a fixed depth. The field of view of such multihole collimators is simply the superposition of the fields of view of each of the several holes. At the focal plane, the field of view of the holes superimpose quite exactly while everywhere else, the superposition is only partial, depending upon the distance from the focal plane. All collimators have geometric spatial resolutions and efficiencies that are a function of the size of the holes, the hole number, and the thickness and diameter of the collimators.

Those photons that successfully traverse the channels of the collimator, and are subsequently counted, represent the observed concentration of radioactivity at the location of the focused detector. The electrical pulses associated with the activity counted are directed to an output display device such as a photorecorder, paper tapper, or oscilloscope to create an image.

The most common display device for a rectilinear scanner utilizes a light source that is focused as a point or a line on a sheet of photographic film. The light source is mechanically or electronically linked to the scanner's detector. This arrangement causes the detector and light to move in synchrony with one another. Thus, the position of the light at any given time corresponds to the location of the detector. Interactions that occur within the detector are converted to electrical pulses that cause the light to flash. Most scanners create one light flash and, thus, one black dot on the photographic film for some fixed number of input counts. As the detector scans the patient, the light source maps out the activity distribution on photographic film. In most applications, rectilinear scanners provide a one-to-one mapping, ie, the object and image are equal in size. Whole-body imaging devices use a minification feature that permits a whole-body skeletal image to be placed on a single 27.9 cm × 35.6 cm (11 in × 14 in) x-ray film. This typically requires a 5 to 1 minification, ie, each 5 cm on the subject scanned is recorded as 1 cm on the image.

Most scanners use conventional x-ray film as their primary recording medium. This film is characterized by a long contrast scale and is very sensitive to the

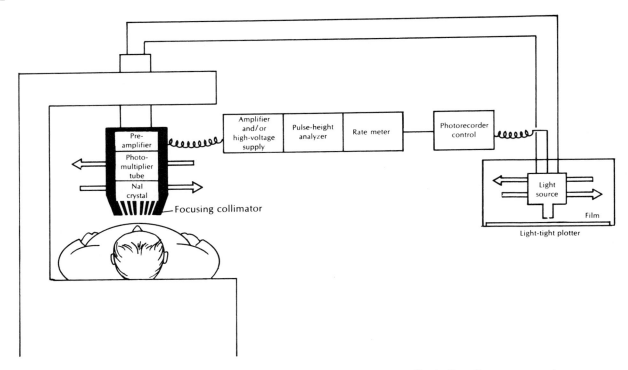

Figure 16.1. Diagram of a single probe rectilinear scanner illustrating the component parts as well as the basic electronics associated with this unit.

photolight used in scanning devices. When properly exposed and developed, this medium provides very satisfactory images.

The chief advantage of rectilinear scanners is their low cost. The thick crystals characteristic of these devices provide very suitable images for high energy radionuclides such as ^{131}I and ^{67}Ga. The principal disadvantages of rectilinear scanners are their relatively low sensitivity and small depth of response in comparison with other devices, such as the scintillation camera. In addition, they are not capable of providing images of rapidly changing distributions.

MULTICRYSTAL WHOLE-BODY SCANNER

The multicrystal whole-body scanner has been available commercially through the name Cleon Whole Body Imager (Union Carbide). The device is similar to the rectilinear scanner in that there is a detector above as well as below the scanning bed and images are obtained by moving the detectors in a rectilinear fashion. The multicrystal whole-body scanner and its console are shown in Figure 16.2. The whole-body imager differs from the conventional rectilinear scanner in that each detector head contains more than one detector. For this imaging system, each detector head consists of 10 NaI(Tl) crystals mounted in a row. Each crystal measures 6.1 cm × 11.4 cm × 2.54 cm and has its own PM tube, amplifier, and pulse height analyzer.

Each detector also has its own multihole collimator that has a focal length of either 9.5 cm or 13.3 cm. In either case, the distance between focal points of adjacent detectors is fixed at 6.1 cm. A scan is made by moving the whole detector array 6.1 cm laterally, while at the same time advancing it slowly along the long axis of the scanner bed. The signals from each detector are accumulated for short intervals and then displayed on a television tube or CRT oscilloscope with a brightness corresponding to the number of photons detected at each point of the scan area. Thus, whole-body images are obtained by means of a modified rectilinear scan pattern.

In normal operation, whole-body images are minified 9 to 1 and recorded on either 20.3 cm × 25.4 cm x-ray film or standard Polaroid film. An optional device allows recording the imaging data on floppy discs. The image may then be replayed for imaging intensity modification and contrast enhancement before being recorded on either x-ray or Polaroid film, using either a 9 to 1 or 4.5 to 1 minification. The 4.5 to 1 minification option is used primarily to obtain double magnification of selected portions of the image.

The standard multicrystal whole-body imager is designed primarily for whole body imaging with ^{99m}Tc. For imaging problems involving the high energy photons of ^{67}Ga, 3.81 cm thick NaI(Tl) crystals and dual energy windows are available as options to increase counting efficiency.

The multicrystal whole-body imager provides ex-

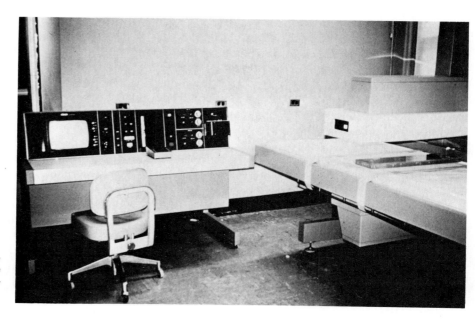

Figure 16.2. The patient table, dual detector heads, and console of the multicrystal whole-body scanner (Cleon) is shown.

cellent bone scans as well as static organ images. The recent increase in crystal thickness, combined with the availability of dual energy window capabilities, have resulted in excellent ^{67}Ga images with this unit. The device is an outstanding unit for whole-body images. It does, however, have the disadvantage of being relatively expensive, does not allow dynamic imaging, is not easily used for small organ imaging such as the thyroid, and is not useful for imaging isotopes with energies above 300 KeV.

MULTICRYSTAL CAMERA

In 1962, Bender and Blau[11] described their autofluoroscope, a multicrystal scintillation camera that has been marketed in a modified version by Baird Atomic Corporation as their System 77 multicrystal scintillation camera.

In the commercial system, a mosaic array of 294 sodium iodide crystals are arranged in 14 columns (Y axis) and 21 rows (X axis). The system utilizes a unique light piping technique that splits the light from each NaI(T1) crystal into two equal parts. A total of 35 PM tubes are arranged in such a way that each detector is covered by two light pipes, providing two output pulses for each event that occurs within a given crystal. With this arrangement, events occurring within a given crystal produce an output pulse that is observed by two PM tubes coupled to that crystal. One PM tube is used to record the X-coordinate while the second records Y-coordinate information. Each PM tube has an associated preamplifier-amplifier circuit. The outputs from all 14 Y-axis and 21 X-axis are added and passed on to a single channel analyzer for pulse height analysis.

A detected event will be recorded at the appropriate XY location of the system's detector if all of the following conditions are met: (1) only one X-and-Y address is registered for the event; (2) the added pulse falls within the selected energy range; and (3) the event is sensed simultaneously by both the column and row phototubes. The positional information is accumulated in a computer memory during the collection mode. The collimator of the system has 294 holes, one corresponding to each crystal of the mosaic pattern.

Thus, the detection of an event and the position of that event are independent of one another. As such, the collimator completely defines the spatial resolution of the system. This design allows the system to operate at extremely high counting rates approaching 400,000 counts per second without saturating the detectors or introducing errors in the position pulses. This feature provides extremely high temporal resolution for cardiac flow studies. The trade-off is a loss of spatial resolution. This occurs because each 8-mm square crystal is individually collimated and, thus, only 294 data points per image are accumulated in dynamic studies. To improve resolution for static images, the multicrystal camera is moved in small increments while obtaining data.

The data stored in the computer during the course of the study can be displayed on a black-and-white or color monitor. A hard copy is provided by either photography or by a printer. The major weakness of the multicrystal scintillation camera, in addition to its poor spatial resolution for dynamic studies, is its poor energy resolution that occurs because of light losses in the long, complicated light guides used for positional information. The advantage of the system resides in its ability to obtain dynamic data of high statistical reliability. This feature allows time separation of heart chamber activity from lung and other background on first-pass cardiac studies. This also allows edge displacements as small as 3 mm to be readily detected under high contrast conditions.

The inherent characteristics of the multicrystal detection system, coupled with its computer capabilities, provide the commercial system with the capability of performing virtually all nuclear cardiology studies. It has not found widespread application in most routine nuclear medicine procedures, however, possibly due to its relatively poor spatial resolution in comparison with conventional scintillation cameras and the poor cosmetic appearance of the mosaiclike images.

STANDARD FIELD SCINTILLATION CAMERA

The scintillation camera is far and away the most innovative and versatile imaging device available. The basic components of the imaging device are shown in Figure 16.3.

The head of the scintillation camera is faced with a collimator. It is the purpose of the collimator to limit the field of view of the detector and provide a 1 to 1 mapping of radiation emanating from the organ or area of interest to displayed events on the readout device. The design of the collimator permits only those gamma rays traveling in the appropriate direction, defined by the holes of the collimator, to interact with the detector. Those gamma rays that successfully traverse the channels of the collimator interact with a NaI(Tl) crystal that serves as the detector of the system. Most standard scintillation cameras have crystal thicknesses of 1.27 cm and diameters of 25.4 cm. When gamma rays interact with the crystal, they lose their energy by photoelectric or Compton interactions, or both. This process produces light photons; the total number produced is directly proportional to the total photon energy absorbed by the crystal by each gamma-photon interaction.

The crystal is optically coupled to a hexagonal array of PM tubes, numbering 37 in most new systems and as high as 91 in at least one commercially available system. A plastic light pipe is optically coupled between the NaI crystal and the PM tubes.

The photons interact with the bi-alkali photocathode surfaces of each PM tube, which then releases electrons. The PM tube multiplies the original number of electrons by a factor of approximately 1 million to produce an output pulse that is directly proportional to the energy incident on the photocathode.

A computing circuit is used in combination with a PM tube array to determine the XY location and energy associated with each scintillation occurring within the crystal. The XY location is determined on the basis of the relative intensity of light seen by each of the phototubes. This information is used by the circuit to determine XY deflection signals for the imaging system's oscilloscope, which will result in a flash of light appearing on the oscilloscope screen at the correct XY location if the energy of the event is appropriate.

The computing circuit also adds the output from all tubes for a single event to determine a Z pulse, ie, an output signal that is proportional to the energy absorbed by the NaI crystal for the event. This signal is applied to the pulse height selection circuit that allows only those pulses that have amplitudes falling within a preselected energy range (ie, within the energy window) to pass on to the data recording portion of the imaging system. If the Z pulse falls outside the window, nothing is displayed on the oscilloscope screen. If it is accepted,

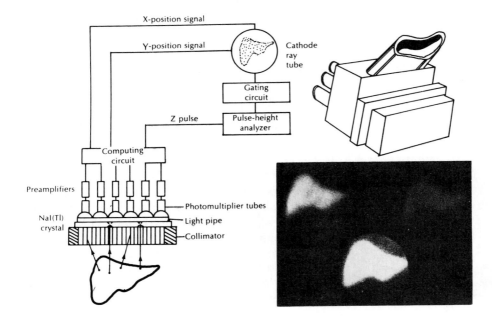

Figure 16.3. Schematic illustration of the component parts of the basic scintillation camera.

a dot is displayed on the oscilloscope screen at the *XY* position determined by the *XY* deflection signal. The phosphor of the display screen has short persistence so that dots produced on the screen are almost instantaneous. This allows permanent images to be recorded using the principle of time-lapse photography; that is, a film is exposed to the flashes of light occurring on the oscilloscope screen for a definite period of time, thereby creating a composite picture corresponding to the organ distribution of activity. One method of recording images uses a Polaroid camera that has three lenses, each with a different f-stop. Thus, each picture has three images of the same event, each having a different exposure. This increases the probability that at least one exposure will have required brightness and contrast to be of diagnostic value. Because of the relatively high cost and limited latitude of Polaroid film, many nuclear medicine laboratories use 35 mm, 70 mm, or various size x-ray film to record the image.

Various manufacturers provide modifications of the basic scintillation camera as described. For example, round PM tubes are generally used for most scintillation cameras. One manufacturer (Picker) uses hexagonally-shaped PM tubes to eliminate the inevitable dead space present between round tubes. Another variation in PM tube technology includes the use of "tea cup" tubes, so named because their inner surface resembles the inside of a tea cup. With this type, the electrons produced from the photocathode surface of the tube are focused toward a collection point by the shaped electric field produced by the parabolic inner surface of the tube. This geometric configuration causes a much higher percentage of the electrons produced in the photocathode surface to be collected than is the case with conventional tubes. The resulting increase in the total number of electrons collected per keV of energy absorbed by the NaI crystal improves the statistical accuracy of localizing an *XY* event within the NaI crystal, thus improving the intrinsic spatial resolution of the imaging device. More and more manufacturers are using this new type of tube.

Another basic difference between different brands of scintillation cameras is the light pipe design. This technology varies from the approach of Ohio Nuclear, which uses essentially no light pipe, to the 3.17 cm thick light pipe used by Searle; Picker uses an intermediate thickness light pipe. The "no light pipe" approach increases sensitivity as well as spatial resolution. This approach is susceptible to nonuniformity when the energy window is not appropriately adjusted, however. Searle has elected to use a thick light pipe to preserve uniformity. They have found that they can also improve sensitivity by placing the PM tube on a "pedestal," formed by cutting V-shaped grooves into the light pipe between adjacent photomultiplier tubes. The grooves reflect light that might otherwise pass between adjacent tubes into the appropriate PM tube.

Picker combines an intermediate thickness light pipe with an optical reflecting technique called variable density filtering to improve both spatial resolution and sensitivity. Basically, they apply opaque paint in a variety of patterns (varying from "snowflake-like" patterns to concentric rings) to the light pipe surface. These patterns serve as "light masks" which absorb undesirable light and transmit favorable light from the crystal onto the photosensitive surface of the hexagonally shaped tube. This technique directs the light produced within the crystal to the appropriate phototube, thereby improving spatial resolution without sacrificing sensitivity.

The most recent variation in scintillation camera design regards the thickness of the crystal used. Various manufacturers have noted that a decrease in crystal thickness to 0.64 cm results in a decrease of approximately 18 percent in counting efficiency for ^{99m}Tc. A subsequent increase of approximately 30 percent occurs in the intrinsic spatial resolution performance of these devices. This is due primarily to the improvement in the spatial localization of events within the crystal associated with these thinner crystals. Imaging devices having thin crystals are designed exclusively for low energy imaging. This requires less shielding, thereby decreasing the overall weight of the imaging system. Therefore, the practice of using thin crystals is applied primarily to portable scintillation camera devices that can take advantage of the inherent decreased weight.

The standard scintillation camera has the advantage of relatively low cost, excellent spatial resolution performance, and reliable and stable electronic circuitry. The system is capable of providing dynamic as well as static imaging, and is easily interfaced to computer systems for purposes of providing important dynamic information such as that available from nuclear cardiology studies.

LARGE FIELD SCINTILLATION CAMERAS

Large field scintillation cameras are characterized by having from 37 to 91 photomultiplier tubes, arranged in a hexagonal array above a 1.27 cm thick NaI crystal having a useful field of view diameter of approximately 38 cm. All manufacturers providing this type camera use the basic Anger camera principle to generate images. As is the case with standard field cameras, variations in PM tubes to include the use of hexagonally shaped tubes or tea cup tubes or variations in light pipe design are also used.

All large field cameras offer a significant advantage in being able to encompass entire organ structures such as the liver or lung in one view. They also offer a significant reduction in the time required to perform whole-body images. Preliminary evaluation by

TABLE 16.1. **Scintillation Camera Performance**

Manufacturer and Model	Field of View (cm)	Intrinsic Resolution (FWHM) (mm)	Spectral Energy Resolution (%)	Paralyzing Deadtime (μsec)	Usable Counting Rate ($\sim$10% loss, cps)
Ohio Nuclear					
100	25 (hex)	5	15 (140 keV)	8.5	68,000
110	37 (hex)	6.5	15 (140 keV)	7.5	68,000
410	37 (hex)	5.0	15 (140 keV)	7.0	68,000
Picker					
4–11	28	3.6	12 (140 keV)	5.0	75,000
4–15	38	4.7	12 (140 keV)	5.0	68,000
Searle Radiographics					
IV	25	6	15 (140 keV)	13.0*	64,000
LFOV	39	6.5	15 (140 keV)	5.5*	70,000
General Electric					
Max I, II	38	5.0	15 (140 keV)	5.0	70,000
Toshiba					
GCA 301	25	3.8	14 (140 keV)	5.0	68,000
GCA 401, 402	35	4.7	14 (140 keV)	7.0	70,000

From Hine, Paras[3]; Hine, Kirch[4]; Lem, Hoffer, Rollo.[5]
*With microdot

many laboratories indicates that these devices can be used with converging collimators to obtain brain as well as cardiac images.[1,2] Most large field cameras now have spatial resolutions comparable to that of standard cameras.[3–5] This fact is demonstrated in Table 16.1. The main disadvantage of these devices is the relatively high cost. The large field camera has now become accepted as a useful imaging device for routine imaging, and is considered by many leading authorities to be the imaging device of choice if only one imaging system is to be purchased by a nuclear medicine laboratory.

SCINTILLATION CAMERAS WITH WHOLE-BODY IMAGING TABLES

Most scintillation camera devices are compatible with one of two types of whole-body imaging tables. In one system, the patient table remains stationary while the camera head moves along a track to scan the full length of the patient from either above or below the table. At the completion of each longitudinal pass, the table is incremented transversely by a fixed distance and a scan performed in the opposite direction. This process is continued until the entire body is imaged. This system has the advantage of requiring a space only slightly larger than the size of the imaging table for performing whole-body imaging.

The second method utilizes a table that moves in a longitudinal direction relative to a stationary camera

head. The camera head can be placed either above or below the table. At the completion of each pass, the table increments transverse a fixed distance and a scan pass is made in the opposite direction. This whole-body imaging technique has the disadvantage of requiring a room that is at least twice the length of the scanning bed in order to perform scans.

With either scanning bed type, standard field cameras require three passes to complete a whole-body image. Large field scintillation cameras require only two passes when parallel hole collimators are used. Recently, diverging collimators have been made available for large field scintillation cameras that allow the whole-body image to be completed in a single pass. Unfortunately, diverging collimators are characterized by a loss in spatial resolution with depth and variation in sensitivity across the collimator face. This results in some distortion of the image as well as poor spatial resolution when compared with parallel hole collimator images. For these reasons, diverging collimators are not generally accepted for use with whole-body imaging devices. The addition of whole-body imaging accessories has allowed the scintillation camera to replace the rectilinear scanner as the basic instrument of choice in whole-body imaging. The introduction of up to three pulse height analyzers on scintillation camera devices allows these systems to image efficiently higher energy radionuclides such as ^{67}Ga. When three energy windows are used in conjunction with high energy parallel hole collimators, excellent ^{67}Ga whole-body images are obtained.

The introduction of whole-body imaging tables allows the scintillation camera to provide total diagnostic imaging capabilities. A principal disadvantage is that the unit is a single detector device. The patient or the detector, therefore, must be moved between anterior and posterior imaging passes. This requires additional time, but even so, the total time required to obtain a whole-body image is generally less than that required on a rectilinear scanner. Another disadvantage is a small loss in spatial resolution when using a scintillation camera in the scanning mode versus the static mode. For this reason, some nuclear medicine laboratories prefer to take multiple spot images of the body, rather than using the scanning bed, to obtain the maximum spatial resolution. When a system is properly calibrated, the spatial resolution in a scanning mode should only be minimally different from that observed when obtaining static images.

TOMOGRAPHIC SCANNER

The tomographic scanner is a device that provides images of several longitudinal tomographic planes simultaneously. The basic system consists of an Anger scintillation camera faced with a focused collimator that scans the patient in the same fashion as a rectilinear scanner. In the original instrument designed by Hal Anger, images were displayed on a oscilloscope in conventional Anger camera fashion. The images were viewed by an array of lenses each having different focal lengths that projected the images onto a film that moved in synchrony with the gamma ray probe.[6]

The new commercial version, referred to as the Pho/Con Model 192 (Searle Radiographics), has dual detectors, each consisting of a 23.6 cm diameter by 1.25 cm thick NaI(Tl) scintillation crystal. Each crystal is viewed by 19 PM tubes. The tubes and their associated circuitry are used to generate signals that localize scintillations within the crystal and measure the total amount of energy deposited there. Each probe is faced with a focused collimator that has a focal length of either 8.89 cm or 11.4 cm. The detectors are directly opposed and move in a rectilinear fashion over the object being scanned.

In the Pho/Con, the oscilloscope, lenses, and moving film of the original device are replaced by a multi-image format device (Microdot) and by the appropriate electronics for displaying information for twelve images (6 for each probe) simultaneously on separate sections of the CRT display.

The tomographic capabilities of the scanner are based on the principles shown in Figure 16.4. The geometry of the focused collimator is such that the field of view seen by the detector decreases as a function of collimator-source distance down to the focal plane of

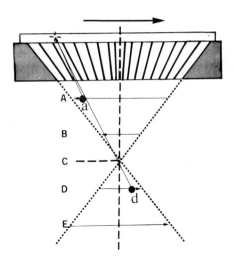

Figure 16.4. Schematic illustration of the operation of the tomographic scanner. The field of view seen by the detector decreases with increasing depth down to the focal plane C. Beyond C, the field of view again increases. The length and direction of the arrow shown in planes A, B, D, and E indicate the relative exposure time and direction a point source within that plane would appear to have to the detector when the detector is moving from left to right. The length of time the source would be seen by the detector decreases as a source plane approaches the focal plane in either direction.

the collimator. Beyond this plane, the field of view increases. A photon originating at point d and interacting in the crystal defines a straight line as shown in the diagram. The instrument cannot determine where along that line the photon originated. However, by knowing the coordinates of the center of the detector in its rectilinear raster, the coordinates of the point of interaction within crystal, the focal length of the collimator, and the distance from the focal plane of each plane being reconstructed, the systems can determine the possible origin of the photon in each plane (A, B, C, D, and E) and display it at each point. The simple back-projection technique results in reinforcement of the information from a particular plane while blurring information from other planes in the image for that plane.

When a three-dimensional activity source is scanned, photons that are traveling in the appropriate direction can traverse the channels of the collimator and interact with the detector where the Anger detection principle is used to localize the event. The geometry of the focused collimator, however, is such that the XY location of the interaction within the crystal may not correspond with the XY location from which the photon originated. For example, as shown in Figure 16.4, photons originating from point a and d have different XY coordinates within the activity source than they have in the detector. Further, even though they produce a scintillation at the same XY position within the detector, they originated not only from different XY positions but also from different depths. Since the purpose of the tomographic scanner is to correctly localize events, both with respect to XY location and depth, a position correction computation must be performed. Basically, this involves a transformation of coordinates calculation that converts the coordinates of the detected event within the crystal into the true coordinates of photon origin within the activity source. The computation takes into account the speed-depth relationship as well as direction of travel associated with the plane. A transformation of coordinates is performed and recorded for each event detected in the crystal for six preselected planes of interest.

The spatial distribution of activity located in any of the preselected planes will be faithfully reproduced in the image of that plane. The spatial distribution of activity outside of that image plane will be distorted or blurred due to the apparent motion of the activity with relation to the spatial coordinates of that plane. This out-of-plane blurring results in a tomographic effect; that is, objects in the image plane are clearly imaged while objects out of the image plane are blurred and thereby obscured.

The tomographic planes are spaced symmetrically about the geometric focal plane of the collimator and can be varied to match the overall thickness of the patient and/or organ being viewed. After determining the thickness of the patient, it is possible to set the plane separation so the twelve planes are equally spaced throughout the patient.

The Pho/Con has an advantage over the Anger camera system equipped with a whole body imaging table in that it can image fields up to 65 cm $\times$ 130 cm on one film. In addition, its rectilinear scanning motion provides an inherently uniform field. Perhaps the greatest value of the tomographic scanner lies in situations where underlying and/or overlying activity is minimal or absent, such as in hot lesion detection problems. For this reason, it is especially effective in bone imaging with ^{99m}Tc as well as tumor scanning with agents such as ^{67}Ga citrate or ^{111}In bleomycin.

The tomographic scanner has the disadvantage of being relatively expensive and is not capable of providing dynamic imaging. In addition, the simultaneous generation of six images from each detector increases the dead time of the instrument and, therefore, limits the maximum count rate capability. It has also been demonstrated that well-circumscribed distributions of activity having very high count rates can develop a doughnut appearance in off focal planes that may result in erroneous characterization of lesions.

Current research activities include interfacing the

Pho/Con to a computer system. It is expected that this practice will eliminate the dead time problem and will allow image planes of interest to be selected after the data collection process is completed. In addition, it will be possible to reconstruct transverse as well as longitudinal images from data collected.

EMISSION COMPUTED AXIAL TOMOGRAPHY

Emission computed axial tomography (CAT) is a relatively old technique that has received renewed emphasis due to the recent development of x-ray transmission CT systems. This technique is used to provide images of transverse or cross-sectional slices of radionuclide distributions within the body. In single-photon counting, this is accomplished by either collecting multiple images about the region of interest with a single detector or by using multiple detectors to obtain the data. Computer algorithms are then used to project as accurately as possible each detected event back to its point of origin in an image space corresponding to the activity distribution being studied. Its requirements are uniform detector resolution and sensitivity with depth, accurate detector positioning and sampling, correction for photon attenuation, high sensitivity, and a computer for data collection and image reconstruction. Much of the original work in this area was performed by Kuhl and Edwards.[7] The latest version of their system, the Mark IV, is optimized for brain scanning and consists of four linear arrays, each containing eight detectors arranged in a square frame. The detectors are fixed in place and different projections are obtained by rotating the entire frame such that the fields of view of the detectors are interlaced.

A system for single-photon counting was commercially available from Cleon (Union Carbide).[8] The brain image consisted of twelve 8 in $\times$ 5 in $\times$ 1 in NaI(Tl) detectors (10 detectors for body imager) with 6 in focal length collimators (17 in focal length for body imager) positioned symmetrically about the scan field. Data were collected by axial movement of the detectors coupled with rotational movement of the gantry. Tomographic images were produced by optimizing the focal point response of each detector, which repeatedly moves from the center to the outer edge of the head during the scanning interval.

The scintillation camera is also under study as a possible device for emission CAT. This can be accomplished by coupling the camera to a computer and using the parallel hole collimator to collect static views at multiple angles about the patient. Advantages of the scintillation camera are high sensitivity, ability to record images simultaneously from multiple planes, and capability for using the system in routine frontal plane

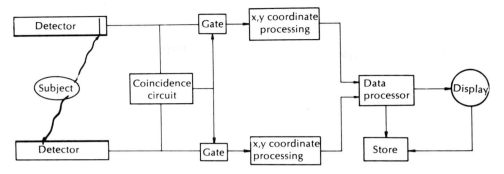

Figure 16.5. Schematic illustration of a basic camera-type detector system used for positron imaging.

imaging. The disadvantage is loss of spatial resolution with depth.

POSITRON IMAGING SYSTEMS

There are three general reasons for an interest in positron imaging. First, because of their unique method of localizing events, positron imaging systems do not require collimators; therefore, these systems characteristically have relatively high detection efficiency as well as good spatial resolution. Second, because better than one-half of all available radionuclides are positron emitters, it should be theoretically possible to find a positron emitter for virtually any imaging problem of interest. The third reason is that positron emissions are inherently tomographic in nature. In the past several years, different types of positron systems have been introduced. These can be classified into two groups: camera-type instruments and multidetector systems. The camera-type instruments currently under study

include positron cameras consisting of: (1) two opposing Anger scintillation cameras; (2) two opposing crystal mosaic plane arrays; and (3) two opposing multidetector proportional chambers with lead converters. A block diagram of these systems is shown in Figure 16.5. The second type consists of annular or hexagonal arrays of detectors which encircle the patient, as shown in Figure 16.6.

Independent of the instrument type, the basic principles of detection are the same. Isotopes such as ^{11}C, ^{13}N, ^{15}O, ^{52}Fe, or ^{82}Ru decay by emission of a positive electron. This positron moves a few millimeters away from the point of isotope decay while undergoing a series of collisions with surrounding matter. Through these collisions, the kinetic energy is reduced to a few electron volts. At low or zero kinetic energy, the positron is captured by an electron (matter and antimatter interaction) and an annihilation process results in the emission of two 511 keV photons at an angle of 180 degrees relative to one another. As shown in Figure 16.5, two camera-type detectors placed on opposite

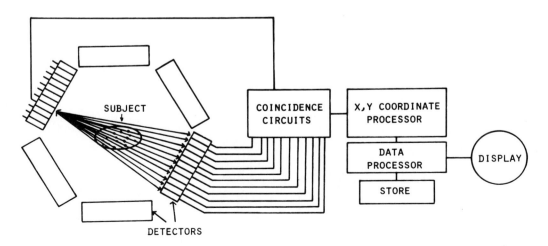

Figure 16.6. Schematic illustration of a multidetector system used for positron imaging.

TABLE 16.2. Comparison of Positron Cameras

Camera	Type	Dimensions	Sensitivity (counts/min/μCi)	Effective Count Rate (counts/sec)	Comments	Spatial Resolution (FWHM) in air (mm)
Searle Radiographics— University of Chicago	Parallel detectors, single crystals	Circular detectors, 1 in thick NaI ~25 cm diameter	12,000	8,000	Measurements with test objects and patients	10.5
Massachusetts General Hospital	Parallel detectors, multicrystal arrays	Square arrays of 127 NaI crystals, ~30×30 cm²	1,000	15,000– 20,000	Measurements with test objects and patients	10
Lawrence Berkeley Laboratory— UCSF	Parallel detectors, MWPC-lead converters	Square detectors, 48×48 cm² sensitive area	1,000 / 3,600*	400 / 1,600*	Measurements with test objects and patients	6 to 7
Lawrence Berkeley Laboratory— Donner Laboratory	Ring, multicrystal array	Ring radius, 40 cm, 288 NaI crystals	1,200	6,000– 12,000	Estimation	7
UCLA	Ring, multicrystal array	Ring radius, 30 cm, 72 NaI crystals	2,300	3,800	Estimation and measurements with test objects	10
Washington University, St. Louis (PETT III)	Ring, multicrystal array	Ring radius, 25 cm, 48 NaI crystals	1,800	1,250	Measurements with test objects and patients	12

*Estimated performance with camera modifications
From Rollo.[10]

sides of the source can be used to detect the two emitted photons simultaneously. When this occurs, the origin of the annihilation can be said to occur along the line between the two detectors. An image of the activity distribution can be obtained by projecting a line of intersection of each set of recorded events to a given plane in the object. As with a single-photon system, this back projection technique results in a reinforcement of the plane of interest while blurring contributions from other planes. Thus, camera-type systems can produce images of longitudinal sections of radioactive distributions within the body. By rotating the camera heads, images of transverse sections or cross-sectional slices may be produced. Multidetector systems are optimized for transverse sectional imaging. A single detector is used in a coincidence circuit with each of a group of detectors on the opposite side of the patient, as shown in Figure 16.6, to produce a fan beam type of geometry for data collection; additional sampling positions may be obtained by translation and rotation of the detector array. A positron imaging system consisting of 66 detectors in a hexagonal array (ECAT) is currently available from Ortec, Inc.[9]

A summary of the characteristics of the various positron systems currently under development is shown in Table 16.2.

The primary limitation to application of positron cameras in the future will be the availability of positron emitters on a routine basis. This will require having inexpensive accelerators, such as "table top" cyclotrons or positron emitter generators, in or close to the nuclear medicine laboratory. Currently, two manufacturers are in the process of marketing self-contained, self-shielded "push button" type cyclotrons that will produce short-lived positron emitters for routine clinical use: the Japanese Steel Works and the Cyclotron Corporation of America. At this point, the technology of developing positron cameras as well as practical cyclotrons is considered in the evaluation stage. Significant improvements in existing technology will be required before positron imaging will become a routine imaging procedure.

SUMMARY

A number of different imaging devices are currently available. Each has advantages as well as disadvantages with regard to clinical application, cost, and dynamic as well as static imaging potential. Currently, the basic Anger scintillation camera combines the best of all possible features. Because ^{99m}Tc imaging appears to be the most practical methodology that will be available over the next five years it suggests that the Anger type scintillation camera will continue to be the main imaging device in nuclear medicine laboratories during this time period.

REFERENCES

1. Burdine J, Murphy P: Clinical efficacy of a large-field-of-view scintillation camera. J Nucl Med 16: 1150–1165, 1975
2. Murphy P, Burdine J, Moyer R: Converging collimator and a large-field-of-view scintillation camera. J Nucl Med 16: 1152–1157, 1975
3. Hine CJ, Paras P: Performance of scintillation cameras. J Nucl Med 16: 1206–1207, 1975
4. Hine GJ, Kirch DL: Recent advances in gamma cameras. Appl Radiol 6: 194–200, 1977
5. Lem C, Hoffer PB, Rollo FD: Performance evaluations of recent wide field scintillation gamma cameras. J Nucl Med 19: 936–941, 1978
6. Beck R: Current status of diagnostic counting of imaging techniques used in nuclear medicine: a sketch. IEEE Trans Nucl Sci 25: 434, 1974
7. Kuhl DW, Edwards R, Ricci AB, et al: The Mark IV system for radionuclide computed tomography of the brain. Radiology 121: 405–413, 1976
8. Product Information Bulletin. Cleon Corporation, Needham, Mass.
9. Product Information Bulletin. Ortec, Inc., Oak Ridge, Tenn.
10. Rollo FD (ed): Nuclear Medicine Physics, Instrumentation and Agents. St. Louis, Mosby, 1977
11. Bender MA, Blau M: The clinical use of the autofluoroscope. J Nucl Med 3: 202, 1962

CHAPTER 17

Nuclear Magnetic Resonance Imaging

C. LEON PARTAIN
RONALD R. PRICE
JON J. ERICKSON
JAMES A. PATTON
CRAIG M. COULAM
A. EVERETTE JAMES, JR.

Nuclear magnetic resonance (NMR) imaging is an extension of traditional NMR spectroscopy in which the quantitative chemical analysis of a homogeneous sample may be determined by the application of magnetic fields. In medical diagnostic imaging, this technology may also be used to produce cross-sectional or transverse images of the spatial distribution of selected nuclei (in particular, hydrogen) at any anatomic level. NMR contrasts with more traditional clinical radiography where images are produced based upon the interaction of x-rays with electrons surrounding atoms and traditional nuclear medicine images where internal concentrations of radiopharmaceuticals are detected.

The concept of using NMR techniques in tumor detection was first introduced by Raymond Damadian[1] in 1971, when quantitative NMR parameters were measured and found to be different in solid malignant tumors than in normal tissue. Damadian patented this approach in 1972.[2] NMR phantom images were published by P. C. Lauterbur[3,4] in 1973, demonstrating two-dimensional transverse images, generated from four, one-dimensional, projections (a very similar approach to the back-projection reconstruction algorithms currently used in conventional x-ray transmission CT).

Damadian presented additional data on in vitro human tumor detection by NMR in 1974.[4] Following these early results, rapid development of NMR imaging then led to the visualization of a tumor in a live animal and finally to the first image of a normal live human torso in 1977.[6,7]

Several different imaging schemes have been recently proposed.[8-14] Each of these methods has interesting and unusual features for data collection and image formation. The clinical potential of NMR imaging is considered in several recent articles.[15-17] Significant current effort is also presently being devoted to improved computer algorithms for image reconstruction[19] as well as to the consideration of possible adverse physiologic effects arising secondary to the use of radiofrequency (RF) and magnetic fields used in NMR imaging.[20]

There is currently great interest in NMR imaging because NMR is non-ionizing, noninvasive, without known risk, and in addition allows tomographic imaging based on the chemistry and metabolism within thin sections. It is apparent that NMR imaging is developing into a technique of major importance in medical diagnosis and biochemical research. Therefore, the purpose of this chapter is to describe the technique and clinical potential of NMR imaging for the practicing radiologist and radiologic physicist.

Because most of the literature to date has assumed a significant prior knowledge of electromagnetic field theory, atomic physics, and computer-based image reconstruction, we will briefly review these concepts and concentrate on a nonrigorous description of the technique with emphasis upon its medical imaging potential. The selected references will allow a deeper study of the physical and mathematical principles of NMR imaging.

PHYSICAL BASIS

NMR has been used since 1946 to obtain nuclear and molecular level information in solids, liquids, and gases (Fig. 17.1).[21] The application of this technology in producing a medical image may be described as the repeated application of four basic steps in different anatomic regions as follows:

Step 1. Place patient in static magnetic field, approximate field strength of 500 Gauss.

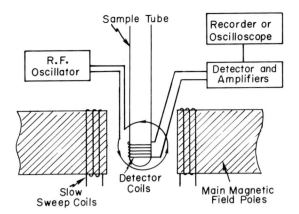

Figure 17.1. Schematic of a NMR spectrometer.

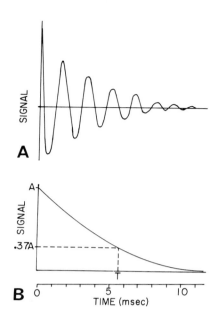

Figure 17.3. Typical NMR signal. **A**. Detector response just off resonance. **B**. Detector response, a decay echo envelope at resonance, ie, at the Larmor frequency. The maximum amplitude, *A*, is proportional to the nuclear concentration at the anatomic point of interest. The decay echo envelope is characterized by *T*. The relaxation time or the time required for the envelope to decay in amplitude by a factor of $1/e$ or approximately 37 percent.

This causes certain nuclei to precess (rotate like "spinning top") about the direction of the magnetic field (Fig. 17.2).

Step 2. Add energy to the selected nuclei by the application of RF energy at just the correct phase and frequency to create a resonance condition. This phenomenon occurs for a given nucleus and magnetic field strength only at one particular frequency; hence the name *nuclear magnetic resonance*.

Step 3. Remove the RF stimulation and observe the response in a receiver coil (Fig. 17.3). This response is measured as an echo envelope and may be characterized by quantitative parameters that can be measured for each anatomic point of interest.

Step 4. Generate transverse total body image based upon nuclear concentration of the selected nucleus or the relaxation time, using an interactive computer-based imaging system (Fig. 17.4).

Certain nuclei with nonzero magnetic moment in a uniform and constant magnetic field will precess simi-

lar to a spinning toy top at a characteristic frequency (Larmor) proportional to the strength of the applied field. If the sample is irradiated with RF electromagnetic radiation at this (resonant) frequency, the nuclei of the selected atomic element (eg, hydrogen) will absorb some of the RF energy. Following RF irradiation, the nuclei will reemit this RF energy and the resulting (NMR) signal can be detected and analyzed. Variations in the molecular environment (eg, methyl, CH_3, or hydroxyl, OH^- ions) cause the resonance condition of the nuclei to occur at slightly different frequencies. This also causes the nuclei to relax, or give up their energy, at different rates, a phenomenon called *chemical shift*. The NMR signal and its descriptive parameters (spin-lattice relaxation [T_1], spin-spin relaxation [T_2], and density of nuclei [ρ]), under appropriate conditions, should be able to provide detailed and possibly specific pathologic information of interest to physicians, physicists, chemists, and biologists.

Magnetic fields can be created such that the resonant condition will exist only at specified spatial locations. Thus, by making NMR measurements at selected regions in heterogeneous samples, it is possible to produce a map of the internal spatial distribution of selected "magnetic" nuclei.

As the name implies, NMR is a nuclear rather than an atomic phenomenon. The nuclei of all elements are composed of charged particles (protons). These par-

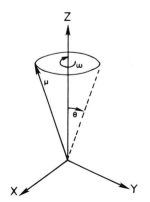

Figure 17.2. Precessing proton with magnetic moment, μ, in a static field, B_0.

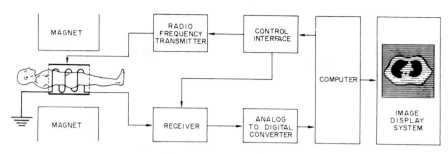

Figure 17.4. Components of a typical NMR Imaging System.

ticles possess angular momentum resulting from their spin, and a spinning charged particle generates a magnetic field. The strength and direction of a magnetic field is defined by a vector quantity called the *magnetic moment*. Most elements exhibit magnetic properties and are therefore capable of being identified by NMR. A certain class of nuclei, however, have an even number of protons, and an even number of neutrons (even-even nuclei) have zero angular momentum and thus do not exhibit magnetic properties. Table 17.1 shows a partial list of the approximately 150 nuclei possessing a magnetic moment. In quantum physics terms, spinning nuclei with spherically shaped charge distributions are assigned a spin quantum number (I) of $1/2$. Nuclei with more complex charge distributions are assigned spin values of I or greater in increments of $1/2$. The number of possible spin states is equal to $2I + 1$.

We will consider first the nuclei with spin $1/2$, such as the hydrogen ion. If an aggregate of spinning nuclei is placed within a strong magnetic field, B_o, the nuclear magnets will tend to orient themselves with the field. These magnets can only assume two possible orientations (spin states): either parallel or antiparallel to the applied static magnetic field. The number of nuclei that will be oriented parallel with (along) the field will be larger than the number oriented against the field. The direction along the field orientation corresponds to the lowest energy state. This can be understood by the analogy of a small bar magnet in a magnetic field. Nuclei with greater spin quantum states (eg, $3/2$, $5/2$, etc) will have more possible orientations within the field. The energy difference between adjacent spin states is directly proportional to the magnetic moment of the nuclei and the applied field and inversely proportional to the spin.

In higher spin nuclei, the differences in population of nuclei in each state will be less. This is an important consideration because the NMR signal that will be measured represents an average effect over the entire sensitive region of the material under study and depends upon the number of nuclei that make transitions between energy states. If the RF energy is supplied to the aligned nuclei at the proper phase and frequency, then the nuclei can absorb energy and thus make a transition between energy states. If the RF source is then turned off the nuclei will reestablish the original population distribution. The time it takes to reestablish this distribution is called the relaxation time and is characteristic of the particular nuclei and its chemical environment.

For example, if a small quantity of water is placed in a constant field B_o in the z direction, we could attempt to bring about NMR with the hydrogen nuclei through the proper application of a second magnetic field, B_1. The hydrogen nucleus consists of a single proton of spin $1/2$. Hydrogen because of its low spin and large magnetic moment can produce a particularly strong NMR signal.

Because the hydrogen nucleus (proton) may be described as a spinning charge distribution, it will behave as a small magnet. The magnetic moment of all the hydrogen nuclei in the water will align themselves

TABLE 17.1. **Resonance Frequencies at 10,000 Gauss, and Related Data for Selected Nuclei**

Nucleus	Spin Quantum Number(I)	Magnetic Moment (μ)	Resonance (Larmor) Frequency (MHz)	Natural Abundance (%)
$_1H^1$	1/2	2.793	42.5759	99.985
$_1H^2$	1	0.85742	6.53566	0.015
$_6C^{13}$	1/2	0.7024	10.705	1.11
$_7N^{14}$	1	0.4036	3.076	99.635
$_7N^{15}$	1/2	−0.2831	4.315	0.365
$_8O^{17}$	5/2	−1.8937	5.772	0.037
$_9F^{19}$	1/2	2.6288	40.055	100
$_{11}Na^{23}$	3/2	2.2175	11.262	100
$_{12}Mg^{25}$	5/2	−0.8553	2.606	10.13
$_{13}Al^{27}$	5/2	3.6414	11.094	100
$_{15}P^{31}$	1/2	1.1317	17.235	100
$_{16}S^{33}$	3/2	0.6433	3.266	0.76
$_{17}Cl^{35}$	3/2	0.82183	4.172	75.4
$_{17}Cl^{37}$	3/2	0.68411	3.472	24.47
$_{19}K^{39}$	3/2	0.3914	1.987	93.1

From Handbook of Chemistry and Physics.[33]

at an angle with respect to the applied magnetic field and will precess or rotate about the z direction with a frequency that is proportional to the magnetic field strength (Table 17.1). The frequency of precession ω_L is given by

$$\omega_L = \gamma B_0 \qquad (1)$$

where γ is a constant called the *gyromagnetic ratio*. The frequency ω_L is referred to as the *Larmor frequency*. If a second magnetic field B_1 is now applied at right angles to B_0 and oscillates at the specific Larmor frequency (determined for a particular nuclei in the static B_0 field) $\omega = \omega_L$, then the B_1 will be in phase with the precession of the hydrogen nucleus (proton) and the effect will be to add energy to the nucleus. This interaction will cause the magnetic moment to flip to the opposite orientation with respect to B_0. When the magnetic moment flips it will induce a current of frequency ω_L into a fixed coil constructed to lie in a plane parallel to B_0 and perpendicular to B_1. The fixed coil is called the *detector* or *pick-up coil*, and it is the interaction phenomenon measured by this coil which generates the NMR "signal."

When a fixed and uniform magnetic field is used, the resonance phenomenon is critically dependent upon the RF being exactly equal to the Larmor frequency. Variations in either the strength of the magnetic field or the applied RF will preclude resonance. Similarly for a fixed frequency, the range of values of the magnetic field strength that permits nuclear magnetic resonance to occur is narrow.

Because different nuclei have different values of magnetic moment and spin, they will undergo resonance at slightly different frequencies when placed in the same magnetic field. As was noted earlier, the signal strength decreases with decreasing magnetic moment and increasing spin. Also because we are observing an average over the sensitive volume of the material, the signal will be proportional to the abundance of the nuclei. The signal strength can be increased by raising the concentration of the nuclei of interest (adding a contrast agent) or by signal averaging. Signal averaging implies scanning the substance many times and adding the results. Because the strength of the signal is being detected where some signal variation or "noise" is present and because this noise is random in nature, the summation process will tend to reduce the noise while increasing the signal.

As was mentioned earlier, the NMR signal can be described by the parameters T_1, T_2, and ρ. These parameters characterize different relaxation processes known as spin-lattice (T_1) and spin-spin (T_2), and describe the magnetic volume density (ρ) of the material. Spin-lattice relaxation implies the transfer of energy to the aggregate of atoms under study in the form of thermal energy. This relaxation time is denoted T_1.

Spin-spin relaxation implies the transfer of energy directly to neighboring nuclei. This measurement is called the T_2 relaxation time.

T_1, SPIN-LATTICE RELAXATION TIME

T_1, spin-lattice relaxation time, is the time required for the bulk magnetization state of the material to return to equilibrium after RF stimulation. Thus, T_1 will be dependent upon the viscosity, temperature, and concentration of the material.

T_2, SPIN-SPIN RELAXATION TIME

At equilibrium all chemically identical nuclei precess about the z direction at exactly the same frequency. Their phase of rotation is random; however, the B_1 field, 90 degrees out of phase from the direction of nuclear precession, creates a coherence in the precessing nuclei and thus generates a small net magnetization in the B_1 direction. When B_1 passes through the resonance point a reorientation of the spins will take place leading to the equilibrium state where there is no net magnetization in the B_1 direction. The rate of relaxation of this magnetic field in the B_1 direction is the phenomenon called *spin-spin relaxation*, characterized by the spin-spin relaxation time, T_2.[21]

Any process that tends to destroy phase coherence will contribute to an increased relaxation speed. A short T_2 implies a reduced time to be detected and will thus introduce an uncertainty in the NMR signal. Highly viscous materials (solids) will have neighborhood variations that will tend to destroy coherence. Classic papers describing the physical and chemical basis, as well as the procedure for calculating T_1 and T_2, were published by Carr and Purcell[23] and by Freeman and Hill.[24]

NUCLEAR MAGNETIC VOLUME DENSITY (ρ)

The size of the NMR signal following RF irradiation is determined by T_1, T_2, and the volume density (number of resonating nuclei per unit volume). In conventional fluoroscopy and CT, the signal output is directly related to fractional transmission of x-rays or inversely related to attenuation or density. In nuclear medicine, the signal is proportional to the quantity of radioactivity in a particular region. Similarly, in NMR, the signal is proportional to the nuclear volume density.

INSTRUMENTATION

A schematic drawing illustrating the various components of the NMR system used for transverse section imaging is shown in Figure 17.4. The single biggest difference between this instrument (in addition to size) and the instruments used in the chemical labortory is the design of the magnet which produces the static B_0 field and the imaging system (Fig. 17.5). The requirement for NMR imaging is the selective resonance of a small volume of tissue or material within the patient. This implies that a selected volume can be chosen through a unique configuration and orientation of B_0 and RF fields, such that all other volume elements are excluded. The spatial extent of this unique volume thus determines the spatial resolution of the system.

A number of approaches are available to select the volume element to be excited. The earliest NMR imaging devices used an inhomogeneous field in which the RF energy was tuned to a very small region at the center (Fig. 17.5). This created a sensitive volume from which resonance was detected. This sensitive volume was then mechanically scanned throughout the body by having the patient on a scanning bed.[1] Other approaches have attempted to scan the sensitive volume throughout the body by reshaping the magnetic field electrically.[2] Still others have approached the problem by creating a field in which there is a linear gradient

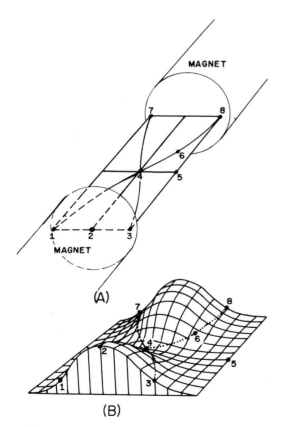

Figure 17.5. NMR static magnetic field. **A.** Coordinate system for central plane between magnetic poles. **B.** Isometric plot of magnetic field strength at multiple points, numbered 1 to 6, corresponding to central plane above. Dashed line represents lines of equal magnetic field.

that results in a resonance condition along a line that extends entirely through the patient at selectable orientations. In this configuration, the signal results from the sum of all resonant nuclei along a line at a particular orientation. Thus, it is necessary to reverse the line integration process mathematically. This requires the techniques of image reconstruction using back-projection and convolution algorithms described in Chapter 14. Techniques to shape the RF field in order to better define the sensitive volume are also being developed.[4]

STATE OF THE ART

Current imaging parameters for one system are summarized in Table 17.2. This system moves the simple sensitive point to multiple positions in two dimensions by utilizing movement of the patient through a scanning matrix.[18]

Alternatively, a reconstruction approach allowing the patient to remain in a fixed position has demonstrated images of the head with improved anatomical resolution and decreased scan time in normal volunteers and patients.[17, 34-36] In addition, whole body, human in vivo T_1 images are beginning to appear in the literature.[14, 37]

TABLE 17.2. NMR Imaging Parameters in 1980

Parameter	Value
Scan time	2–10 min
Anatomic resolution	4–6 mm
Frequency	2–80 MHz
Magnetic field	500–20,000 Gauss

From Damadian.[18]

FUTURE EXPECTATIONS

It is reasonable to expect that in future generations of NMR scanners, scan time may be reduced to seconds, anatomic resolution to 2 mm, and magnetic field to 150 G by optimization of design parameters. NMR, like all imaging techniques, has trade-offs between resolution and imaging time. One basic limitation in NMR imaging is the potential for artifact production as a result of unknown field nonuniformities and attenuation of the RF penetration of thick biologic tissue. This problem is similar to the beam hardening problem in x-ray CT and the attenuation problem in emission CT.

The required control panel and computer-based imaging system appear similar to those required for conventional CT scan systems. The initial capital cost of the total system is comparable to CT systems.

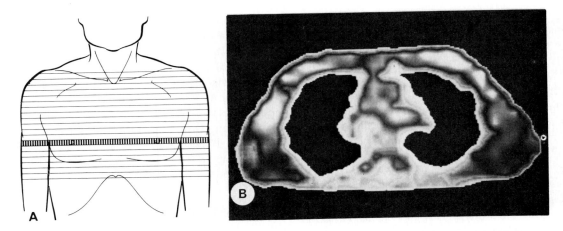

Figure 17.6. **A**. Anatomic level of 8th thoracic vertebrae. **B**. Thorax NMR image at level of T-8. (From Damadian R: Model QED-8; FONAR Corp., 103 Ames Court, Plainview, N. Y., 11803.)

EXAMPLES

Recent NMR images of the thorax and head are shown in Figures 17.6 and 17.7. In the thoracic image, the skeletal and mediastinal soft tissue (water and proton density) are well delineated and clearly differentiated from the lungs. The transverse images of the head demonstrate interfaces between brain, skull, ventricles, and orbits. While the anatomic resolution is limited at this time, the ability to generate a transverse image of in vivo normal human bodies using magnetic field interaction with certain nuclei is in itself remarkable. Future improvements in resolution, sensitivity, and specificity are anticipated and will be a welcomed addition to diagnostic imaging.

CLINICAL POTENTIAL

CHEMICAL VERSUS ANATOMIC BASIS FOR DIAGNOSIS

Since the original paper by Damadian[1] and the first image by Lauterbur,[3] many investigations have shown that neoplastic or otherwise damaged tissue exhibits larger values of T_2 and T_1 compared to "normal" tissue by measurement on excised tissue.[5,26,27] Other investigations have demonstrated conflicting data.[38,39] Diagnosis of the presence and extent of cancer by NMR is currently an active area of research. At this stage in the development of NMR imaging, clinical trials utilizing currently available technology as well as further refinement in the technique are anticipated.

Another area of clinical interest is the use of proton NMR in the diagnosis of diseases related to water content and movement, such as edema, heart disease, and circulation abnormalities. Methods to enhance the NMR signal using intravenous paramagnetic pharmaceuticals are under consideration. This approach is similar to the injection of contrast material in conventional radiography. One ion that has been tried in the visualization of the heart with some success is manganese.

Another potential area of clinical application more closely related to human metabolism than water concentration is the energy cycle of the cell. This kind of study involves changes in the chemical state of the element phosphorus that can also be imaged using NMR. NMR can measure the concentration of phosphorus and in addition provide significant information regarding the chemical environment of the atom.[28] Therefore, if abnormalities in basic cellular energy metabolism can be related to particular diseases (including those that have not yet manifested themselves clinically), NMR images will likely be able to provide much useful information and may eventually be an effective and useful screening technique. One difficulty in using NMR to image phosphorus metabolism is that the signal from phosphorus is much smaller than that from water, and is more difficult to apply to whole-body imaging.

NMR systems are being designed that eliminate all moving parts. Scanning of the sensitive volume and image formation will be completely electrical, avoiding the expense and restrictive rotating gantries of CT scanners. The imaging plane can be in any orientation or position with respect to the sample. Thick-section images can be provided giving the potential to collect a full three-dimensional array of data and to display any thin section or projection as chosen by physician-computer interaction.

The exciting potential of NMR imaging is illustrated by the intriguing opportunity to use high resolution, noninvasive NMR spectra to perform an extensive chemical analysis of one or more specific regions of the body, including for example hydrogen, phosphorus, sodium, carbon, and nitrogen. If this can be done quickly, cheaply, and with minimal or no risk to the patient, and if there is specific clinical correla-

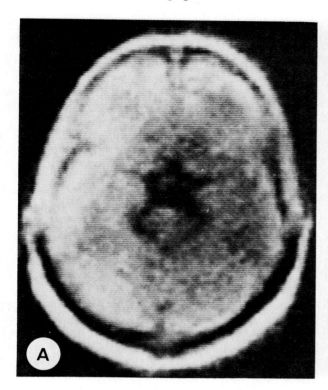
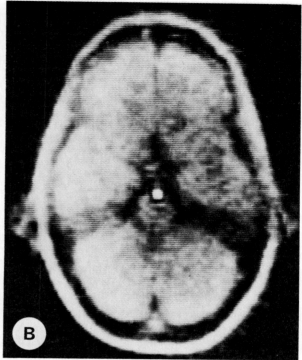

Figure 17.7. **A.** NMR image of head. Brain, skull, and inter-hemispheric fissure can be distinguished. **B.** Image at lower anatomic level showing cerebellum and suprasellar cisterns. (From Holland GN, Moore WS: Department of Physics, University of Nottingham, Nottingham, England.)

tion, then NMR imaging is sure to provide another "quantum leap" in medical imaging and diagnosis much like the added capability provided by x-ray transmission CT.

Because of the difficulty in making accurate forecasts about the realistic and practical use of NMR in diagnosis, however, its proponents emphasize the safety of the method as compared to x-ray and radioisotopic techniques, both of which require ionizing radiation.

EVALUATION OF RISKS

The NMR imaging technique imposes two different conditions on the patient: a high magnetic field and a pulse of RF energy. Budinger[20] lists three aspects of NMR body imaging that could conceivably affect health:

1. Heating due to RF power
2. The static magnetic field
3. The electric current induction due to rapid changes in magnetic field

The first two potential hazards are believed by most investigators to be insignificant. Studies have shown that below certain levels, no adverse biologic effect has

been demonstrated[25]; it should not be difficult to keep within these power levels in NMR imaging. The third potential hazard is receiving further attention. Budinger suggests that magnetic fields should not vary faster than 3×10^{-4} Gauss per second. This limitation may affect some of the techniques used in generating NMR images.

With sensible precautions, current knowledge indicates that NMR is safer than x-ray techniques currently used in diagnosis. With any new modality, however, added caution is necessary because of the possibility of long-term teratogenic or oncogenic potential such as exists with ionizing radiation.

SUMMARY

The next several years should see major advances in both the techniques and applications of NMR imaging. Several research groups have NMR systems large enough to accommodate the whole body, and whole-body images are beginning to appear in the literature.[7, 17, 18, 29] Detailed clinical efficacy and cost-benefit studies are now needed.

An extensive NMR imaging bibliography has been recently published.[30] Research in this imaging modality has to date concentrated upon the following:

1. Design and development of large magnets and RF transmitter-receiver coils
2. Development of techniques for transforming NMR signals into images
3. Definition of NMR parameters for normal and diseased tissue
4. Definition of distinctive image contrast in comparing normal and diseased tissue

As we begin clinical studies and the search for realistic solutions to basic problems, the next sequence of concerns include evaluation of the effects of the following:

1. Flow and motion on images
2. Static and modulated magnetic fields on human beings
3. Continuous and pulsed RF electromagnetic fields on human beings.

The first problem above may be used to advantage in studying blood flow and organ motion. Also, it seems likely at this time that the hazards associated with NMR imaging can be made negligible if even extreme values of the field parameters are avoided.

In spite of several problem areas in the current state of the art in NMR imaging, the data and images that have been already generated are, at least, an adequate stimulus for the serious and aggressive considerations and evaluation of this new imaging modality. Initial studies correlating NMR and CT total body human images have recently been published.[31-32]

ACKNOWLEDGEMENTS

The authors gratefully acknowledge the technical assistance of W. H. Stephens, the clerical contributions of Lori Todd and Betty Burnside, and the photographic assistance of John Bobbitt and Sandy Strohl. The chest NMR image was generated at the FONAR Corporation laboratory, and was provided through the courtesy of Dr. Raymond Damadian. The head NMR image was generated at the University of Nottingham, and was provided through the courtesy of Mr. G.N. Hollard and Dr. W.S. Moore.

REFERENCES

1. Damadian R: Tumor detection by nuclear magnetic resonance. Science 171: 1151–1153, 1971
2. Damadian R: Apparatus and method for detecting cancer in tissue. U.S. Patent No. 3,789,832, March 17, 1972
3. Lauterbur PC: Image formation by induced local interactions: Examples of employing nuclear magnetic resonance. Nature (London) 242: 190–191, 1973
4. Lauterbur PC: Magnetic resonance zeumatography. Pure Appl Chem 40: 149–157, 1974
5. Damadian R, Zaner K, Hor D, DiMaio T: Human tumors detected by nuclear magnetic resonance. Proc Natl Acad Sci 71 (4): 1471–1473, 1974
6. Damadian R: Field focussing nuclear magnetic resonance (FONAR): Visualization of a tumor in a live animal. Science 194: 1430–1432, 1976.
7. Damadian R, Goldsmith M, Minkoff L: NMR in cancer: XV. Fonar image of the live human body. Physiol Chem Phys 9 (1): 97–108, 1977
8. Hinshaw WS, Andrew ER, Bottomley PA, et al: Display of cross-sectional anatomy by nuclear magnetic resonance imaging. Br J Radiol 51: 273–280, 1978
9. Hinshaw WS: Image formation by nuclear magnetic resonance: The sensitive point method. J Appl Phys 47: 3709–3721, 1976
10. Kumar A, Welti D, Ernst RR: NMR Fourier zeumatography. J Mag Res 18: 69, 1975.
11. Hoult DI: Zeumatography: A criticism of the concept of a selective pulse in the presence of a field gradient. J Mag Res 26: 165–167, 1976
12. Crooks LE, Grover TP, Kaufman L, Singer JR: Tomographic imaging with nuclear magnetic resonance. Invest Radiol 13: 63, 1978
13. Damadian R, Minkoff L, Goldsmith M, Koutcher JA: Field-focussing nuclear magnetic resonance (FONAR). Formation of chemical scans in man. Naturwissenschaften 65: 250–252, 1978
14. Hutchinson JMS, Mallard JR, Gold CC: In vivo imaging of body structures using proton resonance. Proc 18th Amp Cong 1: 283, 1975
15. Mansfield P, Maudsley AA: Medical imaging by NMR. Br J Radiol 50: 188–194, 1977
16. Mansfield P, Morris PG, Ordidge R: Carcinoma of the breast imaged by nuclear magnetic resonance (NMR). Br J Radiol 52: 242–243, 1979
17. Holland GN, Moore WS, Hawkes RC: Nuclear magnetic resonance tomography of the brain. J Comput Assist Tomogr 4 (1): 1–3, 1980
18. Damadian R: Field focussing NMR (FONAR) and the formation of chemical images in man. Phil Trans Radiol Svc London B (In press).
19. Shepp LA: Computerized tomography and nuclear magnetic resonance. J Comput Assist Tomogr 4 (1): 94–107, 1980
20. Budinger TF: Thresholds for physiologica effects due to RF and magnetic fields used in NMR imaging. IEEE Trans Nucl Sci NS-26: 2821–2825, 1979
21. Lambert JB, Shurvell HF, Verbit L, et al.: Organic Structural Analysis. New York, Macmillan, 1976
22. Brooks RA, DiChiro G: Theory of image reconstruction in computed tomography. Radiology 117: 561–572, 1975
23. Carr HY, Purcell EM: Effects of diffusion on free precession in nuclear magnetic resonance experiments. Phys Rev 94 (3): 630–638, 1954
24. Freeman R, Hill HDW: Fourier transform study of NMR

spin-lattice relaxation by "progressive saturation." J Chem Phys 54 (8): 3367–3377, 1971

25. Barnothy MF (ed):Biological Effects of Magnetic Fields. New York, Plenning, 1964, p 17

26. Frey HE, Knispel RR, Kruuv J, et al.: Proton spin-lattice relaxation studies at non-malignant tissues of tumorous mice. J Natl Can Inst 49: 903–906, 1972

27. Weissman ID, Bennett LH, Maxwell LR, et al.: Recognition of cancer *in vivo* by nuclear magnetic resonance. Science 173: 1288–1289, 1972

28. Hollis DP, Nunnally RL, Taylor GJ, et al.: Phosphorus nuclear magnetic resonance studies of heart physiology. J Mag Res 29: 319–330, 1978

29. Pickett IL, Mansfield P: A live scan image study of a tumorous rat leg by NMR. Phys Med Biol 23 (5): 961–967, 1978

30. Lauterbur PC: Medical imaging by nuclear magnetic resonance zeumatography. IEEE Trans Nucl Sci NS-26 (2): 2808–2811, 1979

31. James AE, Partain CL, Rollo FD, et al.: Nuclear magnetic resonance (NMR) imaging of the human chest and abdomen. JAMA (in press).

32. Partain CL, James AE, Watson JT, et al.: Nuclear magnetic resonance and computed tomography: Comparison of normal human total body images. Radiology 36: 767–770, September 1980

33. Handbook of Chemistry and Physics. Cleveland, The Chemical Rubber Co., 1973, p B247

34. Moore WS, Holland GN, Kreel L: The NMR CAT scanner—a new look at the brain. CT 4: 1–7, 1980

35. Holland GN, Hawkes RC, Moore WS: Nuclear magnetic resonance (NMR) tomography of the brain: coronal and sagittal sections. J Comput Assist Tomos 4: 429–433, 1980

36. Hawkes RC, Holland GN, Moore WS, Worthington BS: Nuclear magnetic resonance (NMR) tomography of the brain: a preliminary clinical assessment with demonstration of pathology. J Comput Assist Tomos 4:577–586, 1980

37. Mallard JR, Hutchinson JMS, Foster MA, et al.: Medical imaging by nuclear magnetic resonance—a review of the Aberdeen physical and biological programme. IAEA-Sm-247/201. Symposium of Medical Radioisotope Imaging, Transactions. Heidelberg, Germany, 1980

38. McLachlin LA: Cancer-induced decreases in human plasma proton NMR relaxation rates. Phys Med Biol 25: 309–315, 1980

39. Eggleston JC, Saryan LA, Hollis DP: Nuclear magnetic resonance investigations of human neoplastic and abnormal tissues. Cancer Res 35: 1326–1332, 1975

CHAPTER 18

Emission Tomography

JAMES A. PATTON

Radionuclide emission tomography is a technique that grew out of procedures developed for diagnostic x-ray systems to obtain images of selected planes within the body. Recently, it has received renewed emphasis because of another development in diagnostic radiology, the arrival of high resolution x-ray transmission computerized tomography (CT) systems. The purpose of this chapter is to describe briefly emission tomography, to explore the various techniques and emission tomography systems that are currently available, and finally to consider imaging needs relative to the current availability of ultra-high-resolution x-ray transmission tomography systems.

EMISSION TOMOGRAPHY

Emission tomography is a technique that is used to obtain images of planes or sections of radionuclide distributions within the body. Routine radionuclide imaging devices such as scintillation cameras and rectilinear scanners have an inherent limitation in that these systems provide frontal plane images that are projections of three-dimensional distributions into two-dimensional displays. The third dimension, depth, is usually obtained by complementary views at different angles. The difficulty in this circumstance is a result of underlying or overlying activity that prevents an imaging device from obtaining an accurate representation of the plane of interest. Considerable time and effort have been expended in the study and development of emission tomography systems that attempt to provide sectional maps of activity distributions within the body. These systems can be classified into two general types based on the image plane that is visualized (Fig. 18.1).[1] Thus, emission tomography permits the separation of organs into either longitudinal or transverse sectional maps of activity distributions.

As previously stated, routine two-dimensional imaging results in superposition of activity distributions with loss of diagnostic information and reduction in image contrast. A simplified visual example of this concept is shown in Figure 18.2. The tubular arrangement shown in Figure 18.2.C appears as five tubes situated side by side if viewed from position A (Fig. 18.2.A) and three tubes when viewed from position B (Fig. 18.2.B). It is necessary to view the distribution of radioactivity from many angles in order to characterize it accurately. On the other hand, longitudinal section images through planes 1, 2, and 3 (Fig. 18.2.D) more completely reflect the distribution of the tubes. The transverse section image (Fig. 18.2.E) not only characterizes the distribution more completely than the routine frontal plane images (Figs. 18.2.A, B), but also provides additional new information (ie, the tubes are shown to be round). Thus, the major advantages of emission tomography are that depth information is provided and the effects of underlying and overlying activity distributions are eliminated.

REQUIREMENTS

There are many strict requirements imposed on emission tomography systems in order that high-quality images may be obtained.[2] There must be uniform resolution and sensitivity versus depth characteristics for the detector system. Variations in detector response with depth would result in unacceptable image distortions. Accurate corrections for photon attenuation are desirable in order to compare activity concentrations at different depths. Adequate discrimination against scattered radiation is important in all radioisotope image procedures, but is essential in emission tomography to preserve image contrast. Accurate detector positioning and sampling are necessary because most tomography techniques require reconstructions that are geometrical in nature. Also, because of the complexities of most techniques as a result of the large amounts of data that are processed, a computer is generally required for emission tomography. There is also a related need for high-spatial resolution systems in order to reconstruct accurately the distributions under study. Detectors with high sensitivity are required to provide adequate statistics for reconstruction algorithms. Finally, the reconstruction algorithms that are used should

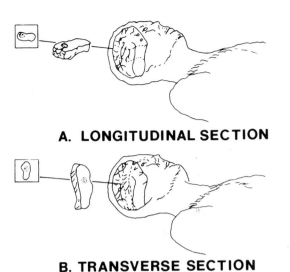

A. LONGITUDINAL SECTION

B. TRANSVERSE SECTION

Figure 18.1. Illustration of the concepts of longitudinal (**A**) and transverse (**B**) section tomography.

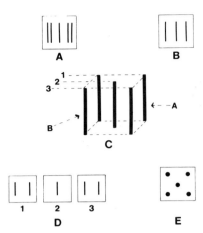

Figure 18.2. A simplified example of the increase in diagnostic information obtained by tomographic techniques. Routine frontal plane images of the tubular arrangement in **C** are shown in **A** and **B**. Longitudinal section images are shown in **D** and a transverse section image in **E**.

provide images that compare quantitatively with the actual distributions.

CATEGORIES OF EMISSION TOMOGRAPHY SYSTEMS

Basically there are two distinct categories of emission tomography systems, each of which has been developed to produce both longitudinal and transverse section images. This division of emission tomography systems is made on the basis of the type of radiations emitted by the radioisotope being imaged. Authorities[2]

have classified these categories as single-photon counting systems (SPC), which make use of routine gamma emitters such as ^{99m}Tc, ^{131}I, ^{123}I, ^{67}Ga, etc, and annihilation coincidence detection systems (ACD) that detect the 511 KeV annihilation radiation from positron emitters such as ^{11}C, ^{13}N, ^{15}O, ^{18}Fl, ^{68}Ga, etc. Single-photon counting systems are generally designed to collect data from as large a solid angle as possible about the patient. This is accomplished either through the use of large, position-sensitive detectors or measurements at multiple angles or both. Images of the radioactivity distribution under study are then reconstructed by at-

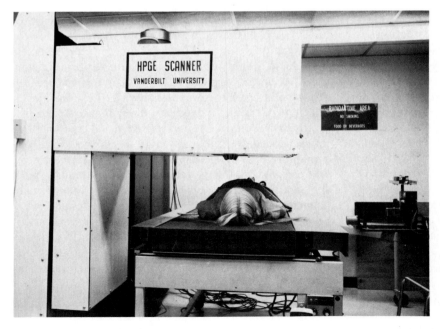

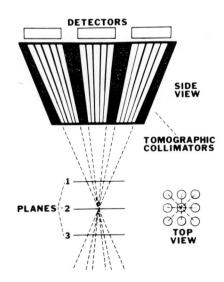

Figure 18.3. An array of 9 high purity germanium detectors with tomography collimators for longitudinal section tomography.

tempting to project as accurately as possible each detected photon back to its point of origin.

SINGLE PHOTON COUNTING

LONGITUDINAL SECTION IMAGING WITH SPS

The 20.3 cm diameter detectors with focused collimators in common use on rectilinear scanners in the late 1960s were actually providing longitudinal section images of planes 1 to 4 cm thick because of the large solid angle and limited depth of response that were characteristic of these detectors. An extension of this concept is the use of multiple detectors with focused collimators utilizing a common focal point. This concept can be illustrated by using the array of nine high-purity germanium detectors[3] constructed at Lawrence Berkeley Laboratory and undergoing evaluation at Vanderbilt University (Fig. 18.3). The system remains stationary while the patient is moved in a rectilinear raster beneath the system with a computer-controlled scanning bed. Data are maintained sep-

arately for each detector; therefore, nine arrays of data are stored in a PDP-11 computer and images are reconstructed after the study has been completed. The nine images shown in Figure 18.4 correspond to the arrays collected by the system when imaging a distribution consisting of a radioactive letter "+" 3.8 cm above the focal plane (F) in plane A and a radioactive letter "O" 3.8 cm below the focal plane in plane B. Image 5 from the central detector corresponds to a routine frontal plane image. The simplest form of image reconstruction of a plane with this technique is back-projection; that is, to project each event back through the image space along the line from which it was detected. Activity in a plane is then reinforced by superposition of data points, and contributions from activity in other planes are blurred. The superposition of back-projections is accomplished by translating the data arrays in the X and Y directions a distance determined by the distance from the plane of interest to the common focal point of the system. The directions of the translations are determined by the relation of the plane of interest to the focal plane (ie, above or below) as shown by the arrows in Figure 18.4. Any type of multidetector arrangement can be used to produce longitudinal section images by this technique.

This multidetector concept is actually a special case of the generalized theory of longitudinal section tomography or focal plane tomography developed by Anger for position-sensitive detectors. This technique has been applied to his multiplane tomographic scanner, which is currently being marketed under the trade name Pho/Con by Siemens Gammasonics, Inc.[4] The newest system (Model 192) consists of two 23.6 cm diameter scintillation cameras (each with 19 PM tubes and an intrinsic resolution of 6.5 mm) that scan in a rectilinear raster for simultaneous anterior and posterior imaging (Fig. 18.5). By electronically determining the coordinates of the detector's geometrical center at the time an acceptable event occurs and the coordinates of the event within the scintillation camera itself,

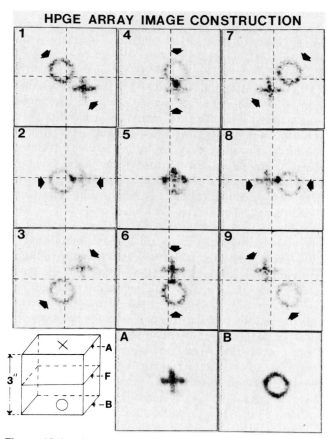

HPGE ARRAY IMAGE CONSTRUCTION

Figure 18.4. An example of image reconstruction by linear superposition of back-projections from a 9 detector array.

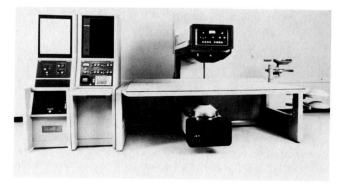

Figure 18.5. The Pho/Con tomographic scanner manufactured by Siemens Gammasonics, Inc.

it is possible by means of analog circuitry to use the back-projection technique to reconstruct multiple planes from a single scan. In practice, 12 longitudinal section planes, 6 from each detector, are produced for each scan with the separation between planes selected by the operator before starting the procedure. A set of images of the liver and spleen obtained from a patient injected with ^{99m}Tc sulfur colloid is shown in Figure 18.6 to demonstrate the separation between planes and the quality of the images obtained with this system.

In years past, several attempts have been made to develop tomographic techniques based on the use of the scintillation camera. The reasoning was that the scintillation camera was the instrument of choice for most nuclear medicine studies and virtually all nuclear medicine laboratories possessed at least one camera. Thus the development of the tomographic capability as an accessory to the camera would be both a logical and an economical advancement. A rotating, slant-hole collimator was used with a moving bed to provide longitudinal section images.[5] This system was marketed for a short time, but was not widely accepted because of circular artifacts inherent in this type of data collection process.

Recently, a new technique has been developed based on the use of a seven pinhole collimator coupled to a large-field scintillation camera and optimized for longitudinal section imaging of the myocardium.[6] A schematic of the collimator is shown in Figure 18.7. Data are acquired in a computer from images projected onto seven independent areas of the camera crystal. Images of a point at a standard distance from the center of the collimator and of a uniform plane source are used to establish the imaging characteristics of the system. Images of multiple planes are then reconstructed by a translation and addition-multiplication algorithm. An example of the type of images obtainable with this system is shown in Figure 18.7. This study was made in the 40 degree LAO projection from an exercised patient with normal coronary arteries. The isotope used was ^{201}Tl to image the perfusion of the myocardium.

TRANSVERSE SECTION IMAGING WITH SPC

Transverse section images with SPC are generally obtained by one of two techniques. Either multiple sets of data are obtained about the region of interest with a single detector or multiple detectors are used to obtain the data. An example of the procedure is shown in Figure 18.8 using a point source and an 8 detector research-prototype system.[7] Each detector rotates about its support axis (Fig. 18.8.A) to collect counts versus angle (Fig. 18.8.B) for each detector. The image is then reconstructed by projecting each event back along its line of origin (back-projection) as shown in (Fig. 18.8.C) for a single detector, (Fig. 18.8.D) for four detectors, and (Fig. 18.8.E) for all eight detectors. Background subtraction yields the final image (Fig. 18.8.F). This is a linear superposition of back-projections and is the simplest of transverse section image reconstructions. This technique is also probably the least favorable because the images obtained are relatively low in contrast, may contain artifacts because of summing effects, and are not quantitatively accurate.

There are other techniques for image reconstruction that can be used to obtain higher quality images.[8] One such technique is the iterative (repetitive) reconstruction procedure in which an initial image is generated (such as a simple back-projection image) and corrections are applied successively in order to force the image into better agreement with the raw data. The process continues until the image converges to a final status in which further corrections cause no change in the image. Analytic reconstruction techniques are also available in which exact equations are solved to provide the final image. Filtered back-projection algorithms (computerized mathematical techniques, similar to but slightly different from those used in transmission CT; see Chap. 14) may be used to alter the individual

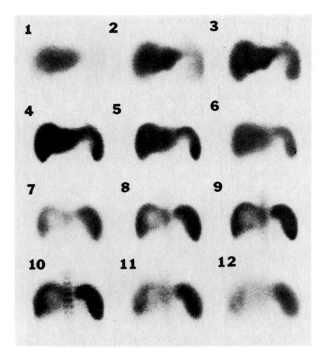

Figure 18.6. A set of images of the liver and spleen obtained from a patient injected with ^{99m}Tc sulfur colloid demonstrating the image quality obtainable with the Siemens Pho/Con tomographic scanner. The first six images were obtained with the anterior probe and the last six images with the posterior probe.

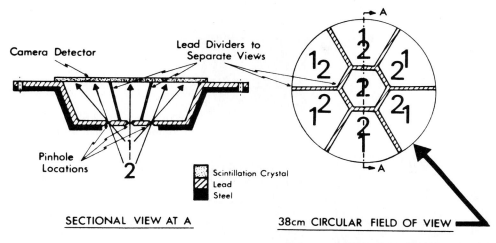

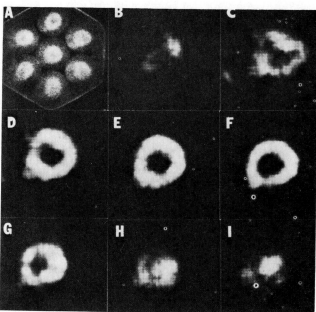

Figure 18.7. Top. Diagram of the 7 pinhole collimator used with the scintillation camera for longitudinal section tomography. Bottom. An example of a normal ²⁰¹Tl study imaging the perfusion of the myocardium of a patient in the 40 degree LAO projection.

projections by applying mathematical correction factors to them before they are projected back into the image array where they are again summed together. Two-dimensional Fourier reconstruction algorithms may also be implemented by taking the one-dimensional transform of each projection and plotting it in the Fourier plane. Interpolation is then used to provide a two-dimensional array of Fourier coefficients. The final image is obtained by taking the inverse two-dimensional transform of this array.

In order to make the reconstructed images quantitatively accurate, it is necessary to correct for the attenuation of photons due to tissue lying between their points of origin and the detector. In SPC, this problem has been approached in several ways. The more successful techniques have involved the use of a phantom corresponding to the area under study which can be scanned to obtain a correction matrix to be applied to

the reconstructed images.[9] Conjugate views (complementary opposed views) and transmission scans can also be used to develop correction factors to apply to the original projection data.

Much of the original work in transverse section radionuclide tomography by SPC was performed by Kuhl and Edwards.[9] The latest version of their system, the Mark IV, is shown in Figure 18.9 and is optimized for brain scanning. The detectors are fixed in place and different projections obtained by rotating the entire frame such that the fields of view of the detectors are interlaced. Images are reconstructed by an iterative technique called *cumulative additive tangent correction* (CATV), an additive correction process in which corrections are based on pairs of orthogonal projections. Nonuniformities in count rates from different detectors are corrected by data obtained from a plane source placed in front of each detector. Attenuation correc-

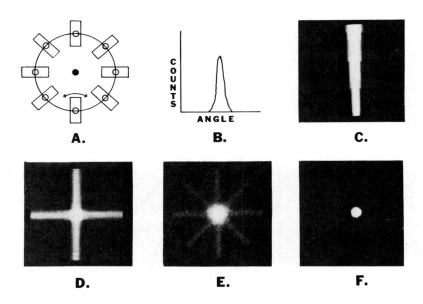

Figure 18.8. Image reconstruction of a point source by linear superposition of back-projections from data obtained with the Vanderbilt University Tomographic Scanner. Each detector rotates about its support axis (**A**) to collect counts versus angle (**B**) data for each detector. The image is then reconstructed by projecting each event back along its line of origin as shown in (**C**) for a single detector, (**D**) for four detectors, and (**E**) for all eight detectors. Background subtraction yields the final image (**F**).

tions are also made using data obtained daily by scanning an 18-cm diameter plastic cylinder of activity. An example of the type of data obtainable with this system is shown in Figure 18.10. The x-ray computed tomography (XCT) image demonstrates the presence of a dense intracerebral hematoma. The XCT scan with contrast and the emission computer tomography (ECT) image obtained with ^{99m}Tc pertechnetate shows a ring of uptake due to alteration of the blood-brain barrier in the surrounding damaged brain tissue. The ECT scan with ^{99m}Tc-labeled red blood cells shows reduced blood volume at the lesion site and in the entire edematous ipsilateral hemisphere.

Kuhl's clinical results indicate that section scanning is most helpful in the basal regions of the brain, by virtue of improved image separation and statistics, as compared to rectilinear scanning. It was also concluded that more precise location and definition of

lesions was particularly useful, often leading to improved ability to make a definitive diagnosis.

One transverse section imaging device for SPC was marketed for a time with two models available.[10] The head imager consisted of twelve 20.3 cm × 12.7 cm × 2.54 cm in NaI(Tl) detectors with focused collimators (15.2-cm focal length), and the body imager consists of ten detectors also with focused collimators positioned symmetrically in a gantry about the scan field. Data were collected by axial movement of the detectors coupled with rotational movement of the gantry. Tomographic images were produced by optimizing the focal point response of each detector, which repeatedly moves from the center to the outer edge of the field during the scanning interval. Another system,[11] the Tomogscanner 2, consists of two opposed detectors mounted in a gantry with rotational movement permitted for data collection. Data may be summed from

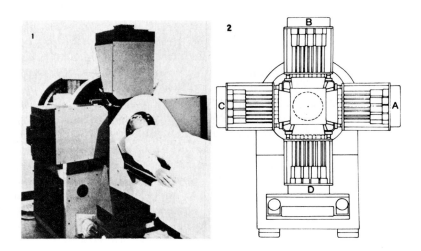

Figure 18.9. The Mark IV transverse section tomographic scanner optimized for imaging of the brain.

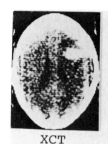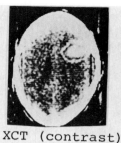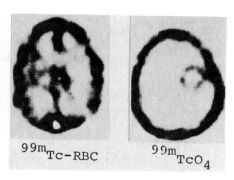

XCT   XCT (contrast) ^{99m}Tc-RBC ^{99m}TcO$_4$

Figure 18.10. Images obtained by XCT and ECT of a patient with a dense intracerebral hematoma.

the two detectors providing a cylindrical response of 15 mm in diameter.

Transverse section imaging has been accomplished by several investigators using the parallel hole collimator with the scintillation camera coupled to a computer.[12-15] Static images are collected at multiple angles about the patient. These data are then used to reconstruct multiple sections through the patient, employing the various reconstruction techniques described earlier. Problems associated with registration of the multiple images have been overcome by mounting the scintillation camera on a rotating frame (Fig. 18.11). Advantages of using the scintillation camera are the ability to record images simultaneously from multiple planes and the capability of using the system in routine frontal plane imaging. The disadvantage is loss of spatial resolution and sensitivity with depth.

A new system that appears to have significantly improved capabilities of camera-type systems has recently been reported.[16] This device consists of two opposed large-field-of-view scintillation cameras that can be used with either conventional parallel-hole collimators or specially designed one-dimensional converging collimators. The system makes use of filtered back-projection reconstruction algorithms and attenuation correction techniques to provide excellent resolution uniformity with variations in sensitivity of only 10 percent throughout a 30×21 cm elliptical scan field.

ANNIHILATION COINCIDENCE DETECTION (ACD)

THEORY

The use of positron emitters lends itself very well to applications in ECT. This is because a positron (positively charged electron) has an extremely short lifetime. When a positron is emitted from a nucleus, it travels only a very short distance before losing its kinetic energy and then uniting with a negatively charged electron. The masses of the two particles are then converted into energy in the form of two 511 KeV gamma rays. These two photons leave the site of their production in opposite directions. If they are detected simultaneously in two opposed detectors, it is known that their point of origin lies somewhere along a straight line drawn between the two detectors (Fig. 18.12). This

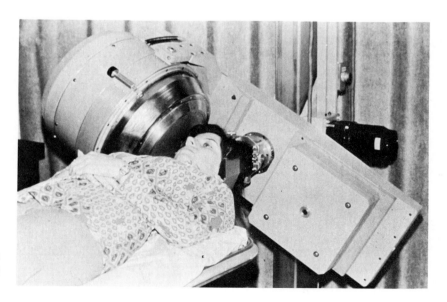

Figure 18.11. A scintillation camera mounted on a rotating frame for transverse section tomography.

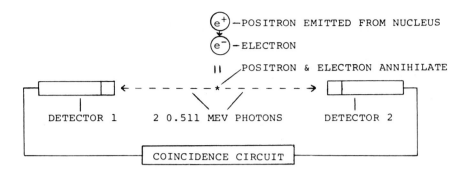

Figure 18.12. A demonstration of the coincidence technique for counting the 511 KeV photons resulting from the annihilation of a positron and electron pair.

phenomenon can be used in longitudinal and transverse section imaging because locating each recorded pair of 511 KeV gamma rays is immediately reduced to a one-dimensional problem in determining the point at which they were produced and therefore the origin of the positron decay. Because the origin of the detected emissions is determined by the physical characteristics of the annihilation process, the need for conventional radionuclide collimators is eliminated (ie, only "electronic collimation" is necessary).

LONGITUDINAL SECTION IMAGING WITH ACD

As in the case with single-photon emission tomography, camera-type devices have also been used for longitudinal and transverse section tomography with positrons. A conceptual diagram of such a system is shown in Figure 18.13. The two detectors record the coordinates of the two 511 KeV photons that arrive in coincidence, and these coordinates are then used to project a line back through the image space. Thus, by the linear superposition of these back-projections, it is possible to create the image of a longitudinal plane while blurring out off-plane information. Using the more complex mathematical techniques described earlier, one can obtain a more complete mapping of the three-dimensional distribution of a radionuclide within the organ. The main features of a positron camera device are (1) no collimators are used in the imaging process, (2) more than one detector are necessary, and

(3) more sophisticated electronics are required in order to perform the coincidence detection.

There are several camera-type imaging devices that are being developed as positron tomography systems. One such system is the MGH positron camera that was developed at the Massachusetts General Hospital as shown in Figure 18.14 and is currently being marketed.[17] The latest version of the system, the PC-II, consists of two opposed detector arrays, each containing 144 small NaI(Tl) detectors arranged in a square array. Each crystal is wired in coincidence with 25 crystals in the opposite array. Thus, as a stationary imaging system, the detector arrays can produce images of longitudinal sections. Sampling problems have been reduced by scanning in the vertical and horizontal direction.

The multiwire proportional-chamber detectors (MWPC) with lead converters are very suitable for a large area positron camera because of relatively low cost for large area detectors, good spatial resolution, and good uniformity of response. Disadvantages presently encountered are low detection efficiency and long resolving times. A MWPC camera has been built consisting of two detectors each with a sensitive area of 48×48 cm and with a single converter for each chamber.[18]

The scintillation camera can also be modified and used as a detector for positron tomography; this task has been accomplished as a joint venture by a group of investigators.[19] The system consists of two large-field-of-view cameras with 2.54-cm thick NaI crystals. The

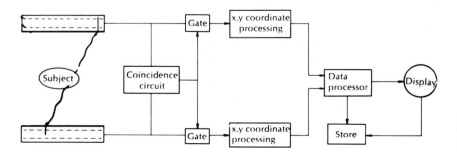

Figure 18.13. A conceptual diagram of camera type systems used for longitudinal and transverse sectional tomography with positron emitters.

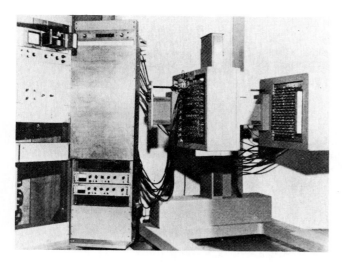

Figure 18.14. The MGH positron camera.

detector electronics have been modified so that each individual camera can record a higher count rate. Coincidence circuitry has been designed such that each positron in one crystal is in coincidence with the entire crystal of the opposed detector.

TRANSVERSE SECTION IMAGING WITH ACD

Transverse section images of positron-emitting distributions can be obtained with the camera-type devices by rotating the systems about the patient. Both the MGH PC-II system and the Siemens Positron Camera can be operated in either the longitudinal or transverse mode. In addition to these systems, specialized devices making use of multiple detectors have been constructed for transverse-section imaging. The first system was constructed from 32 stationary detectors arranged in a circle with corresponding coincidence circuitry.[20] A slightly different system was developed consisting of a ring of 64 detectors with rotational capability.[21] Each detector is coupled in coincidence

with 23 opposed detectors creating a fan beam geometry with a central cross-sectional field of 25 cm.

One system (ECAT) is commercially available and is an undated version of the PETT III system built by Phelps, Hoffman, Ter-Pogossian, and co-workers.[22,23] The system is shown schematically in Figures 18.14 and 18.15 and consists of 66 detectors arranged in a hexagonal array with 11 detectors in each of 6 banks. Each of the 11 detectors in a bank is wired in coincidence with the 11 detectors in the opposite bank. Thus, there are a total of 363 lines of response for the system. The resolution of the system is increased by collecting data as the detector banks are moved in synchrony to perform linear scans over a distance of 3.5 cm. The system is then rotated 5 degrees, and the linear scan is repeated. This process is continued until the entire system has been rotated 60 degrees and an image is then reconstructed using the Fourier techniques of linearly superimposing filtered back projections. The only collimation employed are slit shields whose purpose is to reduce the coincidence count rate from scattered radiation and singles count rate that produces random coincidences. Photon attenuation corrections are performed either by using geometrical factors determined for the head or abdomen or by actually measuring the attenuation with an external ring source of a positron emitter. Scan times are variable from 10 seconds to multiple minutes per view. Resolution is also from 9 mm to 1.8 cm by selection. The system can also perform rectilinear scans which provide three simultaneous views (anterior, 60 degrees LAO, and 60 degrees RAO).

An extension of the PETT III is the PETT IV that was recently completed.[24] This instrument makes use of elongated (Tl) crystals with two PM tubes per crystal and position logic to provide four simultaneous slices each approximately 8 mm thick.

Another system has been developed with the goal of obtaining tomographic images of rapidly changing distributions (dynamic tomography).[25] The system con-

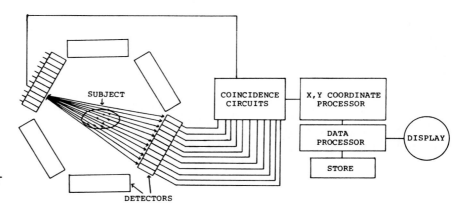

Figure 18.15. A schematic of the ECAT system.

sists of a circular array of 280 detectors with a 31-cm diameter field of view. The system does not move and has 14,000 coincidence lines of response. Because of the geometry of the sampling procedure, the resolution of this system is circular at the center of the image field (8 mm FWHM) and becomes elliptical away from the center (8×13 mm at 10 cm).

An example of the type of information obtainable with the annihilation coincidence detection systems is shown in Figure 18.16. These transverse section studies were performed on a 63-year-old woman with a right occipital cerebral infarct using the Ortec ECAT system.[26] The $^{13}NH_3$ study demonstrates a reduction in perfusion and the ^{18}F-Deoxyglucose (FDG) study shows a glucose metabolism deficit in the right occipital cortex. The ^{68}Ga EDTA study clearly demonstrates an alteration of the blood-brain barrier in this region. XCT (EMI) scans with and without contrast were negative. A distinct advantage of the ACD systems is the availability of the isotopes ^{11}C, ^{13}N, ^{15}O, ^{18}F, and ^{68}Ga, which can be used as radiotracers in labeling a wide variety of metabolically active compounds.[20] Unfortunately, with the exception of ^{18}F, these isotopes have short half-lives and therefore must be obtained from a source close at hand, such as a small on-site cyclotron or an isotope generator (^{68}Ga). On the other hand, SPC systems use radiopharmaceuticals that are readily available and are in common use. The radiopharmaceuticals currently available, however, are not as "physiologically active" as the positron emitters mentioned above.[27] This condition may change in the future with the development of new and improved radiopharmaceuticals.

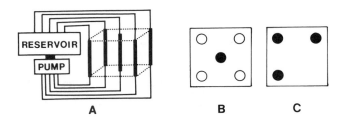

Figure 18.17. A demonstration that transmission and emission tomography are complementary studies (ie, transmission tomography provides anatomic information and emission tomography yields information on the function status of the region under study).

WHY EMISSION TOMOGRAPHY?

Since x-ray transmission tomography images are vastly superior in resolution to radionuclide emission tomography, the question may arise as to why one should be interested in performing emission tomography. The differences in the information content between transverse section images obtained by the two techniques can be demonstrated by again considering the five tube example in Figure 18.2. Suppose that the tubes are connected to a pump and reservoir as shown in Figure 18.17, and it is desirable to know the physical state and functional status of each tube (ie, the anatomy and physiology of the tubes). An x-ray transmission tomograph through the tubes demonstrates that the central tube is solid and the four tubes in the corners are hollow and fluid-filled (Fig. 18.17.B). The functional status of the tubes can be evaluated by placing some radioactive material in the reservoir and allowing the system to reach equilibrium. An emission tomograph through the same region demonstrates that only three of the corner tubes are radioactive and, therefore, flow between the reservoir and the fourth tube must be blocked (Fig. 18.17.C). This simple example demonstrates the important fact that transmission and emission tomography are complementary (ie, transmission tomography provides anatomic information and emission tomography yields information on the functional status of the region under study).

Radionuclide emission tomography, although old in concept, still has not achieved widespread acceptance because of the high cost of equipment necessary to provide most of the capabilities previously described. Even though the market is currently very limited, there are five tomographic systems that are commercially available. These are briefly discussed in Table 18.1. Future developments in radiopharmaceuticals and the outcome of detailed current clinical trials in many laboratories should provide valuable information to determine the cost-benefit relationship for radionuclide tomography as a routine diagnostic procedure.

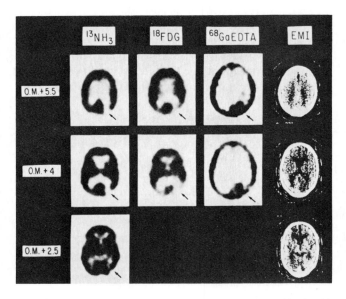

Figure 18.16. Transverse sectional studies obtained with the ECAT system from a patient with a right occipital cerebral infarct.

TABLE 18.1. **Commercially Available Systems**

System	Image Type	Isotope	Detector Description	Spatial Resolution (mm)
Siemens Pho/Con	Longitudinal	Single photon	Two scanning cameras with focused collimators	6.5 (intrinsic)
Union Carbide	Transverse	Single photon	Circular array of 12 detectors with rotational and axial movement	7–8
Tomogscanner	Transverse	Single photon	Two opposed detectors with rotational movement	15
Cyclotron Corp. PC-II (MGH)	Longitudinal and transverse	Positron	Two opposed detector arrays with rotational movement	15
Ortec, Inc., ECAT	Transverse (also recti-linear mode)	Positron	Six banks of 11 detectors each with transitional and rotational movement	9–18

REFERENCES

1. Kuhl DE, Edwards RQ: Image separation radioisotope scanning. Radiology 80 (4): 653–661, 1963
2. Phelps ME, Hoffman EH, Kuhl DE: Physiologic tomography (PT). In Medical Radionuclide Imaging, IAEA-SM-210/303, 1977, pp 233–253
3. Patton JA, Price RR, Brill AB: A mosaic intrinsic germanium radioisotope scanning device with longitudinal section scanning capability. IAEA-SM-210/165, 1977
4. Anger HO: Tomographic gamma-ray scanner with simultaneous readant of several planes. In Fundamental Problems in Scanning. Springfield, Ill., Thomas, 1971, pp 195–211
5. Muehllehner G: A tomographic scintillation camera. Phys Med Biol 16(1): 87–96, 1971
6. Vogel RA, Kirch D, LeFree M, et al.: A new method of multiplanar emission tomography using a seven pinhole collimator and an Anger scintillation camera. J Nucl Med 19: 648–654, 1978
7. Patton JA, Brill AB, King PH: Transverse section brain scanning with a multicrystal cylindrical imaging device. In Tomographic Imaging in Nuclear Medicine. New York, Society of Nuclear Medicine, 1972, pp 28–43
8. Brooks RA, Di Chiro G: Principles of computer assisted tomography (CAT) in radiographic and radioisotopic imaging. Phys Med Biol 21: 689–732, 1976
9. Kuhl DW, Edwards RI, Ricci AB, et al.: The Mark IV system for radionuclide computed tomography of the brain. Radiology 121: 405–413, 1976
10. Advertising brochure. Union Carbide Imaging Systems, Inc. Norwood, Mass., 1978
11. Wooley JL, Williams B, Penkatesh S: Cranial isotopic section scanning. Clin Radiol 28: 519–528, 1977
12. Freedman G: Tomography with gamma camera. J Nucl Med 11: 602–606, 1970
13. Jaszczak R, Huard D, Murphy P, et al.: Radionuclide emission computer tomography with a scintillation camera. J Nucl Med 17: 551, 1976
14. Keyes JW, Orlandea N, Heetderks WJ, et al.: The humogotron—a gamma camera transaxial tomography. J Nucl Med 17: 552, 1976
15. Budinger TF, Gullberg GT, McRae J, et al.: Isotope distribution reconstruction from multiple gamma camera views. J Nucl Med 15: 480, 1974
16. Murphy P, Burdine J, Moore M, et al.: Single photon emission computed tomography (ECT) of the body. J Nucl Med 19: 683, 1978
17. Burnham CA, Brownell GL: A multi-crystal positron camera. IEEE Trans Nucl Sci NS-19: 201–205, 1972
18. Kaplan SN, Kaufman L, Perez-Mendez V, et al.: Multi-line proportional chambers for biomedical applications. Nucl Inst Methods 106: 397–406, 1973
19. Muehllehner G, Buchin MP, Dudek JH: Performance parameters of a positron imaging camera. IEEE Trans Nucl Sci NS-23: 528, 1976
20. Robertson JS, Marr RB, Rosenblum M, et al.: 32 Crystal Positron Transverse Section Detector. In Tomographic Imaging in Nuclear Medicine. New York, Society of Nuclear Medicine, 1973, pp 142–153
21. Cho TH, Chan J, Ericksson L: Circular ring transaxial positron camera for 3-D reconstruction of radionuclide distributors. IEEE Trans Nucl Sci NS-23: 613–622, 1976
22. Hoffman EJ, Phelps ME, Mullani NA, et al.: Design and performance characteristics of a whole body transaxial tomography. J Nucl Med 17: 493–502, 1976
23. Phelps ME, Hoffman EJ, Coble CS, et al.: Some Performance and Design Characteristics for the PETT III. In Reconstruction Tomography in Diagnostic Radiology and Nuclear Medicine. Baltimore, University Park Press, 1977
24. Ter-Pogossian MM: Basic principles of computed axial tomography. Semin Nucl Med 7: 109–128, 1977
25. Derenzo SE, Buddinger TF, Cahoon JL, et al.: High resolution computed tomography of positron emitters. IEEE Nucl Sci 24: 554–558, 1977
26. Advertising brochure. Ortec, Inc. Oak Ridge, Tenn.
27. Phelps ME: Emission computed tomography. Semin Nucl Med 7: 337–365, 1977

CHAPTER 19

Xeroradiography and Electron Radiography

PANOS P. FATOUROS
GOPALA U. V. RAO

In recent years, two electrostatic imaging techniques have been introduced in radiology: xeroradiography (XR) and ionography (also called electron radiography). The use of XR in medicine was pioneered by Wolfe[1] in 1966 at the Hutzel Hospital in Detroit. Electron radiography (ERG) was developed in the early 1970s simultaneously by Johns, Boag, and coworkers and Xonics Incorporated. The image-forming properties of these modalities[2, 3, 4] are fundamentally different from those of the conventional silver halide process and offer new insights and challenges to the radiologist. In xeroradiography, the image receptor consists of a charged selenium plate upon which the input radiological pattern is "imprinted" and subsequently made visible by a powder cloud development process. In ionography, the transmitted x-rays are absorbed by a layer of high-pressure gas or liquid contained between two electrodes. The absorbed x-rays create ions, which are collected on an insulating foil covering one of the electrodes. The charge image may then be visualized by a powder or liquid developer.

In this chapter the xeroradiographic process, which is extensively used in mammography, will be analyzed in detail with particular emphasis on its peculiar image characteristics. The ERG system, which currently has not gained widespread acceptance, will also be discussed briefly and compared to XR.

GENERAL PRINCIPLES

Xeroradiography derives its name from *xeros* (Greek for dry), *radius* (Latin for ray), and *graphein* (Greek for writing). As the name implies, it is a completely dry process in contrast to the "wet chemistry" process of film development. The xeroradiographic system consists of two units: the *conditioner* and the *processor* (Fig. 19.1). Both of these units comprise the Xerox 125 System.* The process is not only dry but requires no

* Xerox Corporation, Pasadena, California.

darkroom as all the processing takes place within the two light-tight units. The basic element of xeroradiography is a thin layer (~ 130 μm) of a photoconducting material (amorphous selenium) placed on a metal substrate. The photoconductor is first covered in the conditioner with a uniform positive charge by corona charging. Selenium (Se) is an excellent insulator in the dark and will hold the "priming" charge for a sufficient time to make an exposure. The sensitized plate is then loaded automatically into a light-tight cassette, and an image is made in the same way as with a conventional screen–film system. The x-rays absorbed in the selenium layer induce a current that alters the uniform surface charge distribution leaving an electrostatic latent image. The sealed cassette with the exposed plate inside is inserted into the processor, where the plate is automatically removed from the cassette and transported to the development chamber. There, the image is made visible by spraying the plate with a cloud of charged, colored particles, which adhere mostly in regions of high electric field strength. The developed powder image is then made permanent by transferring and fixing it to a special white paper. Any residual powder and charge are subsequently cleaned automatically from the plate, which is then ready to be used again.

As outlined above, there are three steps in the xeroradiographic process that are independently controlled: (1) charging, (2) exposure, and (3) development. In the following, we will discuss these stages separately.

CHARGING

The plate is sensitized by corona charging to an initial uniform charge. This is done by passing the plate under an ion-generating device (scorotron), as shown in Figure 19.2. The fine ion-generating wires are held at high potential causing electrical breakdown of the surrounding air. If the wires are biased positively, the repelled

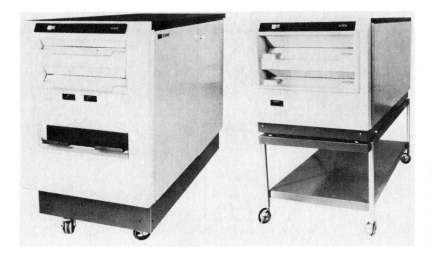

Figure 19.1. The processor (left) and conditioner units of the Xerox 125 System. An empty cassette is inserted in the conditioner and is loaded with a charged Se plate. The exposed cassette is then unloaded in the processor, where development takes place.

positive ions drift towards the grounded Se plate. The screen wires act like a grid, controlling the ion flow and hence the amount of charge deposited and its uniformity. The standard initial charge densities σ_0 on the Se plate for the Xerox 125 System range from about 40 to 70 μ coulombs/cm^2. In Figure 19.3, a uniformly charged unexposed Se layer is shown. During charging, a uniform charge equal in magnitude but opposite in sign is attracted through the metal base to the lower surface of the photoconductor. The resulting "sandwich" resembles a parallel-plate capacitor filled with the selenium dielectric. The electric field lines are essentially limited to the selenium layer, where they are parallel to each other, uniform in density, and directed towards the metal substrate. The field above the uniformly charged Se surface is zero. The fringe fields, which may be quite strong, are confined to a narrow region near the capacitor edges. The internal electric field E_i, the equivalent potential V, and surface charge density are connected by the following familiar equations:

$$E_i = \frac{V}{L} \tag{1}$$

$$\sigma = \frac{K\epsilon_0 V}{L} \tag{2}$$

where K, the dielectric constant of Se, and L, its thickness, equal 6.3 and 130 μm respectively, and ϵ_0, the permittivity of free space, is 8.85×10^{-12} F/m. From the range of σ_0 values given above, equation 2 yields a range for V_0 of 1,000 to 1,600 V. The highest available surface potential of 1,600 V represents an internal field E_i of about 12 V/μm to be compared with a value of 30 V/μm required to cause breakdown in the selenium layer. As will be discussed later, a high initial potential results in more contrasty images, a condition important in mammography, with its inherently low-contrast details. On the other hand, when imaging high-contrast interfaces (eg, bone–soft-tissue) a low initial charge is desirable to reduce the excessive edge delineation.

EXPOSURE: BROAD AREA

Following the corona charging, the photoconducting plate is exposed to the x-rays emerging from the object imaged. The absorbed x-rays in the Se layer produce

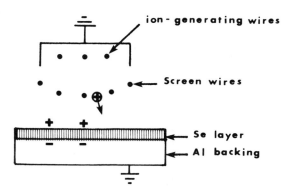

Figure 19.2. The ion-generating wires ionize the surrounding air causing a stream of charges to be deposited on the Se layer. The flow of the positive ions is controlled by the screen wires.

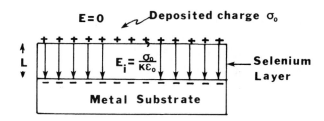

Figure 19.3. The uniformly charged Se plate resembles a parallel plate capacitor. Notice that all the field lines are confined within the Se bulk and that the field above the layer is zero.

charge pairs, which are separated by the strong internal electric field and drift towards the charged surface or the aluminum substrate depending on their sign. The surface charge is thus neutralized by an amount proportional to the amount of radiation incident in different areas of the plate, and the radiological image is converted into an electrostatic image. The mechanism of absorption is mainly the photoelectric effect, although some Compton interactions also take place. The photoelectrons or recoil electrons that result from the interaction of a primary photon with a Se atom have sufficient kinetic energy to create many more charge pairs along their track. On the average, it takes about 7 eV of absorbed energy from ionizing radiation for a pair of charge carriers to be formed. For example, a 35 keV absorbed x-ray can produce as many as 5,000 ion pairs. Of the pairs formed, only the fraction reaching the Se surface contribute to the image-forming process. This charge transport to the surface depends on the applied internal electric field and is more efficient at high field strength. The collection efficiency (η), defined as the fraction of charge that succeeds in reaching the surface, is deduced from experiments[4,5] to be

$$\eta \simeq 10^{-4} V \qquad (3)$$

where V is the surface potential. This equation is valid over the mammographic and radiographic x-ray spectra [30 to 120 kVp] with a Se thickness of 130 μm. An example will illustrate its use. If V is 1,600 volts, the collection efficiency is found from equation 3 to be $10^{-4} \times 1,600 = 0.16$. For the above example of 35 keV photon absorbed in the Se layer, only 16 percent of the 5,000 charge pairs will contribute to the image. For V equal to 1,000 volts the efficiency falls to 10 percent. The electric field (E_i) is reduced from $1,600/130 = 12.3$ V/μm to $1,000/130 = 7.7$ V/μm. Notice that the selenium plate must be given a sufficiently high priming charge in order to maintain good photoconductive efficiency.

PLATE DISCHARGE

A uniformly charged Se plate subject to a continuous irradiation will discharge in an exponential fashion:

$$\sigma = \sigma_0 e^{-R/R_0} \qquad (4)$$

or since σ is proportional to V (see equation 2):

$$V = V_0 e^{-R/R_0} \qquad (5)$$

R is the incident x-ray exposure and R_0 a constant that depends on the beam quality and the Se thickness; σ

(or V) is the surface charge density (or voltage) remaining on the plate following the exposure R. These equations can be shown to follow from the observed field dependence of η (equation 3).[4]

SPEED

The *speed* or *sensitivity* of the Se plates will be defined as the reciprocal of R_0:

$$S = \frac{1}{R_0} \qquad (6)$$

If $R = R_0$ in equation 5

$$V = \frac{V_0}{e} \cong 590 \text{ volts} \qquad (7)$$

assuming an initial voltage V_0 of 1,600 volts. Notice that R_0 is the exposure that reduces the voltage (or charge) to $1/e$ of its initial value. An exposure $R = R_0$ appears to yield an optimal xeromammographic image. In Figure 19.4, calculated values[4] of S (in mR^{-1}) are shown as a function of beam energy. It is seen that Se sensitivity increases with energy and reaches a maximum at about 40 keV, where it equals 0.014 mR^{-1}, or from equation 6, $R_0 = 1/S \cong 70$ mR. This value may be compared with a receptor exposure of about 25 mR required for the Lo-dose I mammographic screen–film system. The currently acceptable kilovoltage (35 to 50 kVp) and filtration levels (1.0 to 2.0 mm Al) lead to lower effective beam energy (20 to 30 keV) and hence a larger exposure level (90 to 180 mR). Harder beams with the resulting reduced image contrasts seem to be clinically acceptable provided that a lower potential is used during development. As the quoted receptor exposure levels indicate, the xeroradiographic method suffers from lack of sensitivity and hence has been largely confined to imaging peripheral parts of the body. On the other hand, ionography has achieved higher sensitivity and promises a wider choice of operating parameters.

In Figure 19.5, the energy absorbed, E_{abs}, per unit area per incident roentgen in the Se layer is plotted against energy. E_{abs} has been calculated by the following formula:

$$E_{abs} = \frac{86.9}{(\mu_{en}/\rho)_{air}} [1 - e^{-(\mu_{en}/\rho)_{Se}\rho L}] \frac{\text{ergs}}{R \text{ cm}^2} \qquad (8)$$

where the first factor represents the incident energy fluence per roentgen and the second is the fraction of the energy absorbed by the selenium. The energy absorption coefficients (μ_{en}/ρ) for air and Se are expressed in cm^2/gm, where ρ is the Se density (4.25 gm/cm^3) and L equals 0.013 cm. Notice that E_{abs} and S are proportional to each other. Multiplying R_0 by

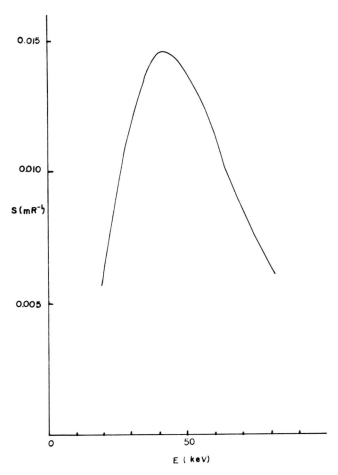

Figure 19.4. The speed of the xeroradiographic plates, $S = R_0^{-1}$, expressed in (milliroentgens)$^{-1}$ as a function of the energy of the incident x-ray beam. The speed continuously increases with energy and reaches a maximum value at about 40 keV.

E_{abs} will yield the energy absorbed by the Se plate following an irradiation $R = R_0$. From Figures 19.4 and 19.5 this product is seen to be about 29 ergs/cm^2.

It would appear that the sensitivity of the Se layers can be increased by increasing the Se thickness; there will be a concomitant increase in absorbed energy (Fig. 19.5). However, a thicker Se layer will lead to an unacceptable loss of resolution. Speed and resolution are always in some inverse relationship regardless of the imaging modality considered.

Thus far we have discussed receptor sensitivity. For a given beam quality (kVp and HVL) the receptor exposure resulting in an optimal image is the one that discharges the Se plate to about 37 percent of its original charge. The next issue of particular importance is the quantification of the carcinogenic risk to the breast following an optimal exposure. The present thinking is that such a risk must expressed in terms of

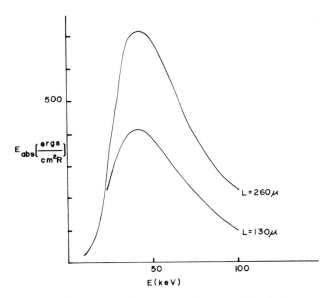

Figure 19.5. The x-ray energy absorbed in the Se layer per incident roentgen as a function of energy for two Se thickness.

absorbed dose of the tissues at risk, ie, the epithelial cells lining the ducts and acini of the breast. In particular, the common practice of quoting the entrance exposure to the breast should be discontinued.

EXPOSURE: DETAIL FORMATION

In the previous section we considered the irradiation of an extended, uniformly charged area and calculated the sensitivity of the Se plates. In this section we will consider the irradiation of some detail represented by an edge in Figure 19.6. Xeroradiography is mainly a contouring process; hence edge response represents its key characteristic. This edge may idealize, for example, the interface between a tumor in the breast and the surrounding soft tissue. During irradiation, the incident x-ray beam is modulated by the edge, producing a voltage discontinuity $\Delta V = V_1 - V$. The exposure R_1 is less than R due to some absorption by the edge. This

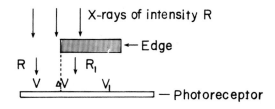

Figure 19.6. The radiological problem: and incident x-ray beam is modulated by an edge producing a step ΔV on the plate.

results in less charge neutralization directly below the edge and hence a larger potential V_1 compared to V. The differential absorption of x-rays by the edge can be described by the edge (or subject) contrast C defined as:

$$C = \frac{R - R_1}{R} \qquad (9)$$

The corresponding voltage step ΔV can be found with the help of equation 5:

$$\Delta V = V_1 - V = V_0(e^{-R_1/R_0} - e^{-R/R_0})$$

$$= V_0 e^{-R/R_0}(e^{(R-R_1)/R_0} - 1)$$

or

$$\Delta V = V_0 e^{-R/R_0}(e^{CR/R_0} - 1) \qquad (10)$$

In the last step equation 9 was used. This last expression for ΔV contains a great deal of information. ΔV is proportional to V_0, the initial surface voltage, and hence the highest setting (1,600 volts) should be used with the imaging of low contrast details. Its dependence on the exposure level R is shown in Figure 19.7. For a given contrast C (eg, given microcalcification in the breast) the potential step ΔV rises initially with exposure until it reaches a maximum value at $R = R_0$. Exposure beyond this point will lead to signal loss. An exposure R equal to R_0 will discharge on the average the Se plate to $1/e$ of its initial charge as was discussed earlier. This will be called the optimal exposure R_{opt}. The two curves in Figure 19.7 indicate the dependence of ΔV on the subject contrast C: the larger the input radiological contrast, the larger the resulting potential step. Notice that both curves essentially peak at $R = R_0$, ie, one exposure will simultaneously optimize all low-contrast details. When $R = R_0$, equation 10 becomes

$$(\Delta V)_{max} = \frac{V_0}{e}(e^C - 1)$$

$$\simeq \frac{CV_0}{e} \qquad (11)$$

where the exponential, $e^C \simeq 1 + C$ has been expanded, since C is small. V is the maximum step, corresponding to an optimal exposure R_0, is directly proportional to the input subject contrast C and the initial voltage (or charge). R_0, which has been discussed previously, depends both on the beam quality (HVL) and the Se thickness. The latter is fixed at 130 μm, and hence one can control only the kVp and the filtration. High beam qualities reduce R (see Fig. 19.4) and thus also reduce patient exposure. Unfortunately, this also leads to reduced subject contrast and therefore reduced detail

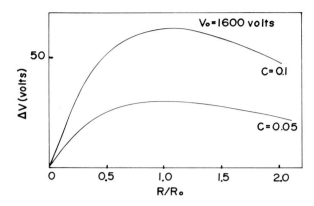

Figure 19.7. The potential step ΔV for two low-contrast edges as a function of exposure. Notice that there exists an optimal exposure, $R/R_0 = 1$, at which ΔV is maximal.

visibility. This is illustrated by a consideration of a bone–soft-tissue interface. The subject contrast, C (equation 9), can be shown to be

$$C = 1 - e^{-d(\Delta\mu)} \qquad (12)$$

where $\Delta\mu = \mu$ (bone) $- \mu$ (tissue) and d is the thickness. In Figure 19.8, C is plotted against energy for $d = 50$ μm. C, and hence $(\Delta V)_{max}$ (equation 11), is seen to fall rapidly with energy. Some of the lost contrast can be retrieved during development by reducing the bias potential. This effect will be discussed later.

FIELD BENDING

The simplified model of image formation discussed above brings out the main features, but it neglects an important consideration: field bending. The signal ΔV initially increases in magnitude with increasing exposure, as shown in Figure 19.7, while the uniform charge background exponentially decays (equation 4). As the exposure continues, the signal alters the uniform surface charge, disturbing the parallelism of the field lines, as shown in Figure 19.9. The charge carriers are then deflected laterally as they travel toward the surface, smearing the input radiological pattern. The field-bending effect becomes more pronounced with increasing Se thickness; this feature limits the use of thick plates for dose reduction. In addition, for a given Se thickness, field bending becomes more important at high exposures, ie, at high plate discharges. The optimal exposure $R_{opt} = R_0$, introduced above, represents a compromise whereby the signal has grown sufficiently and yet has not been distorted greatly by field bending. Thus it is seen that the evolution of the image step inhibits its own further growth.

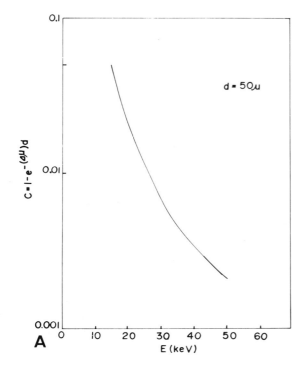
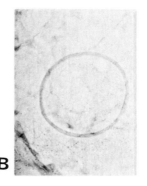
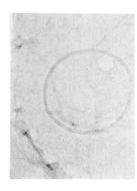

Fig. 19.8. **A.** The subject contrast of a soft-tissue–bone interface as a function of x-ray energy. Contrast falls very rapidly with increasing energy due to the decreasing number of photoelectric interactions. **B.** Xeroradiographs made at 40 (left) and 70 kVp (right) exposures demonstrate contrast changes as a function of energy.

DEVELOPMENT: BROAD AREA

Following the irradiation of the edge, as shown in Figure 19.6, the partially discharged plate is inserted in the processor for development. The plate is automatically removed from its light-tight cassette and is clamped face down over the open development cham-

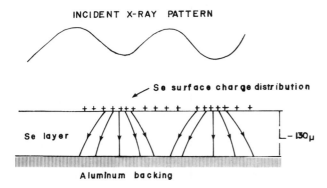

Figure 19.9. An incident sinusoidal x-ray beam alters the uniform charge distribution on the Se surface. As the signal grows, the bulk electric field lines are distorted, displacing the bulk-generated charges as they move towards the surface. The field bending is important for high discharges and for thick plates.

ber (Fig. 19.10). An aspirator-type powder generator introduces a cloud of charged fine particles into the chamber. The toner, as these particles are called, has been charged through particle-to-particle contact electrification as it is injected through a fine nozzle into the chamber. The toner overall is electrically neutral, containing equal numbers of positively and negatively charged particles. Air introduced through the side of the chamber helps to diffuse the powder cloud. Hence toner particle motion is completely controlled and disordered by air motion everywhere in the chamber except in the immediate vicinity of the photoreceptor surface. In this boundary layer the electric fields resulting from the image charge distribution take over and determine toner deposition. In this section we will be concerned with broad-area development, ie, development in regions away from the charge discontinuity. These regions are characterized by surface potentials V and V_1 (Fig. 19.6). As was remarked earlier, the electric fields above these extended, uniformly charged areas are essentially zero: all the field lines are confined within the Se layer. This means that a light toner deposition will occur in these regions regardless of the absolute charge present. These observations explain the so-called wide-recording latitude of xeroradiography, whereby a highly discharged region (soft-tissue irradia-

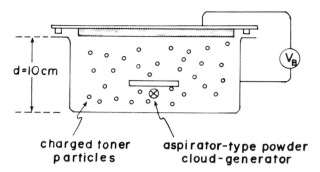

Figure 19.10. The development chamber. The Se plate carrying the latent electrostatic image is sprayed with a cloud of pigmented toner particles in the presence of a bias potential V_B.

tion) will be equally "bluish" as a less discharged area (bone irradiation). Xeroradiography responds to charge gradients and not to absolute charge levels.

In practice, improved toner delivery to an extended, uniformly charged area is achieved by applying a bias potential V_B between the aluminum backing of the selenium layer and the development box, as shown in Figure 19.10. This has the effect of creating above the plate a uniform electric field, whose polarity is determined by a thumbwheel switch on the control panel of the processor.

POSITIVE DEVELOPMENT

The metal plate back is biased positively (Fig. 19.11) with respect to the chamber at a bias voltage V_B of about 2,000 volts. The resulting electric field strength (following an optimal exposure $R = R_0$), E_B, may be found by dividing the total voltage across the chamber by the box depth:

$$E_B = \frac{V_a + V_B}{d} \simeq 0.026 \text{ V}/\mu \tag{13}$$

where V_a, the average plate potential $(V + V_1)/2$, is about 600 volts (equation 7) and d is 10 cm. In this mode of development negatively charged toner particles arrive preferentially at the plate. In the final image, bone appears dark blue and soft tissue slightly lighter.

NEGATIVE DEVELOPMENT

In this mode the biasing is reversed by means of the thumbwheel selector. The bias potential V_B is now about $-3,400$ volts and the average DC field is

$$E_B = \frac{V_a + V_B}{d} \simeq -0.026 \text{ V}/\mu \tag{14}$$

where V_a is about 800 V. As shown in Figure 19.12, positive toner particles are now arriving at the Se surface. In the final image bone appears white and surrounding tissue dark blue.

It should be noted that in some older units a sorting grid was also present in the development chamber about 3 cm away from the plate. Its function was to control toner flow by the application of proper voltages.

BROAD AREA DENSITOMETRY

As was discussed, the electric field above the Se layer controls the toner deposition. However, the electric field above extended, uniformly charged areas is very weak and must be assisted by the application of a bias field. Nevertheless, tone accumulation is expected to be limited regardless of the mode of development. The H

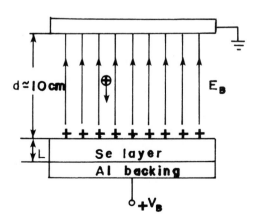

Figure 19.11. Positive development: negative toner particles are arriving preferentially at the Se layer.

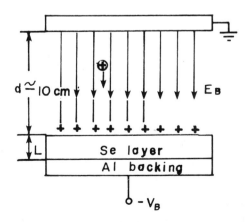

Figure 19.12. Negative development: positive toner particles are accumulating over the plate.

and D curves for the xeroradiographic system are shown in Figure 19.13. These curves were obtained by measuring the reflection density of large uniformly exposed and developed areas of the image. The total output density ranges from 0.2 to 0.4 with a maximum value for gamma of 0.15. The low macro response is evident when compared with the characteristic curve of a typical screen–film system also shown in Figure 19.13. This behavior illustrates again the wide recording latitude of xeroradiography and emphasizes at the same time the need and importance of edge enhancement.

EDGE ENHANCEMENT

The result of irradiating an abrupt edge is a voltage (or charge) discontinuity ΔV on the Se surface. It was shown that ΔV attains its maximal value when the radiation exposure is equal to R_0. The potential step gives rise to strong fringing fields, which dramatically alter the toner distribution during development. In Figures 19.14 and 19.15 the electric field components E_x and E_y are plotted at various heights y above the plate for a potential step of 100 volts. E_y is the electric field component perpendicular to the plate (the normal component) and E_x the horizontal component. Some features of these plots deserve attention since they immediately explain the peculiar characteristics of the xeroradiographic image. E_y is seen to change sign as

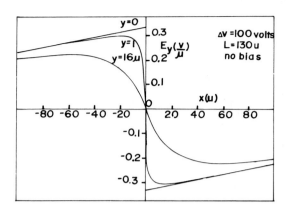

Figure 19.14. The electric field component normal to the Se and due to a potential step of 100 volts as a function of distance across the edge and at various heights above the plate. Notice that the fields are very strong around the edge and of opposite polarity. The higher charge extends to the left of 0.

one moves across the charge discontinuity and to reach its maximum and minimum values on either side of the edge. The horizontal component E_x (Fig. 19.15) is peaked symmetrically at the origin. In all cases, the electric field decreases rapidly with increasing distance from the edge or increasing height; the strong electrostatic fields are confined in the vicinity of the edge. With respect to the image formation, toner particles are deposited in proportion to the vector sum of the E_y and E_x electrostatic fields, as described below.

OPEN CHAMBER DEVELOPMENT

If the plate is exposed to a stream of negative toner particles, there will be accumulation of toner on the positive side of the edge and depletion on the other due to the opposing negative normal field ($E_y[V/\mu]$ effect).

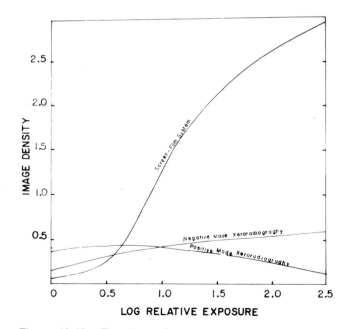

Figure 19.13. The H and D curves for positive and negative xeroradiography. Notice that the two curves are mirror images of each other and that they are essentially flat. For comparison, a curve for a typical screen–film system is shown.

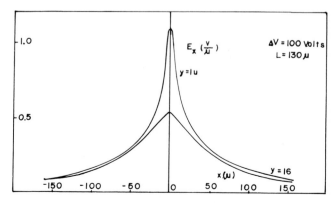

Figure 19.15. The horizontal component of the electric field due to a 100-volt step. The field is again strong at the edge and decreases rapidly away from the edge.

Far away from the edge, on either side, the fields are very weak and the powder will randomly adhere to the plate by friction. This mode of development, where no bias is present, is termed the "open-chamber cloud development" and is capable of delineating small differences in surface charge. Since it responds primarily to density gradients and not to the absolute charges present, it gives rise to a wide exposure latitude.

ELECTRODE DEVELOPMENT

If production of an image whose density is directly related to the amount of charge present is required, a development electrode is used. This electrode placed parallel to the selenium layer and very close to it enhances the electric field above the photoconductor and results in improved solid-area development. The close-electrode development is suitable for continuous-tone reproduction and produces images similar to a silver halide image. As discussed previously, the grounded development chamber (Figure 19.10) resembles a remote electrode, and one obtains intermediate effects, that is, exaggerated density gradients and some limited gray scale.

WHITE GAPS

Remote electrode development in the presence of a bias field alters the normal field component:

$$E_\perp = E_B + E_y \qquad (15)$$

where $E_\perp$ is the total normal component, E_B the bias field (equations 13 and 14) and E_y the normal fringing field (Figure 19.14). In Figure 19.16, the normal field component ($E_\perp$), corresponding to $\Delta V = 100$ volts and $V_a + V_B = 2,600$ volts, is plotted against distance X across the edge. Note that the field is enhanced for $X < 0$ while for $X > 0$ it changes from negative to positive again at $X = X_R$. For points far away from the edge, the total field approaches asymptotically the bias field E_B. If the plate now undergoes positive powder cloud development, the negative toner particles (which are preferentially arriving at the plate due to the applied bias potential) will be deposited in the region $X < 0$ and $X > X_R$, where E is attractive, and repelled in the segment between $X = 0$ and $X = X_R$. The point X_R marks the right-hand edge of the white gap. This forbidden zone, where no toner can land, is better illustrated by plotting the lines of force near the edge (Fig. 19.17). The white gap width δ is defined as the extent $X_R - X_L$ of the "maximal" field line. δ is found to depend not only on the step ΔV but also on the total potential $V_a + V_B$:

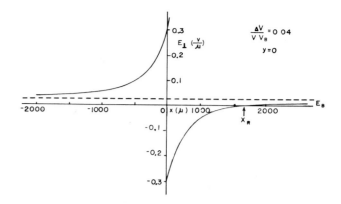

Figure 19.16. The total normal electric field component above the Se plate due to a step discontinuity. $E_\perp$ is positive everywhere except in the region $(0, X_R)$ which defines a depletion zone (white gap).

$$\delta = A \frac{\Delta V}{(V_a + V_B)} \qquad (16)$$

where A is a constant dependent on the chamber geometry. δ is seen to be proportional to the quantity $\Delta V/(V_a + V_B)$, which by analogy with equation 9 may be called the electrostatic contrast C_E.

The difference between positive and negative development of a step discontinuity is shown in Figure 19.18. The step is located at the origin with the higher charge extending to the left of 0. Negative (for positive development) and positive (for negative development) toner particles are driven into the shaded areas in amounts dependent on the local $E_\perp$. The region $0A$ represents the white gap and Δ the maximum edge difference. Notice that the white gap occurs on opposite sides of the edge for the two cases. For example, when a bone-air interface is imaged, the white gap appears on the air side of the edge (low-charge side) for positive and on the bone side for negative development. The toner accumulates on the adjacent side for each case.

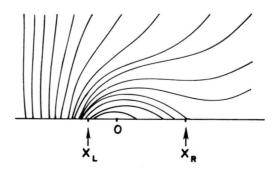

Figure 19.17. The electric field lines indicating the extent of the white gap. No toner can land in the region (X_L, X_R) where the field lines are arching back to the plate.

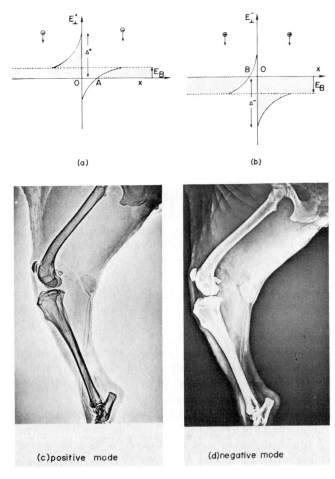

(a)   (b)

Figure 19.18. **A.** During positive development the negative toner particles accumulate in proportion to the local positive electric field. The maximum density Δ^+ occurs on the high-charge side of the edge. **B.** During negative development the reverse is true. **C.** Xeroradiographic exposure of an animal's leg in positive node. **D.** Exposure in negative node.

OPTIMAL EXPOSURES

The white gap for a low-contrast edge and positive development is plotted in Figure 19.19 against the normalized exposure R/R_0. Its maximum value occurs at $R = 1.2\ R_0$, which is 20 percent larger than the value R_0 required for maximizing ΔV. For negative development, optimizing the white gap leads to an exposure equal to $0.8\ R_0$. What constitutes an optimal xeromammographic image from the clinical viewpoint is presently unclear. Some radiologists prefer slightly dark (more blue) images ($R = 0.8\ R_0$ and $R = 1.0\ R_0$) and some insist on brighter images ($R = 1.2\ R_0$). Notice that all three optimal exposures are expressed in terms of R_0, which is the exposure required to discharge the plate to $1/e$ of its initial charge. R_0 depends on the beam quality and the selenium thickness. The use of positive versus negative development depends also on

the information desired. For example, subtle densities are incompletely developed in the positive mode especially if they are in the proximity of a high-contrast object (eg, a densely calcified fibroadenoma). In the negative mode, the low-charge areas develop first and high-charge areas (calcifications, masses) develop last.

DOSE REDUCTION

Dose reduction is a matter of continued concern both to the radiologist and the general public. This is especially true in mammography in connection with screening programs. Some possible ways of reducing doses follow.

SELENIUM THICKNESS

Increasing the photoreceptor thickness will increase x-ray absorption and hence allow one to reduce the incident exposures. This avenue is rather limited because of field bending, which leads to loss of resolution. The present thickness of about 130 microns appears to be optimal.

HARDER BEAMS

For a given Se thickness we have seen that the plate sensitivity increases with increasing energy to a maximum at 40 keV (Fig. 19.4). The drawback with this approach is a greatly reduced image contrast.

LOWER BIAS POTENTIAL

One of the parameters affecting the white gap is the bias potential V_B (see equation 16). As V_B is lowered, the electrostatic contrast and hence the gap width increases. The increased visibility afforded by a greater gap width was substantiated clinically by Van de Riet and Wolfe.[6] These authors achieved significant dose reductions with increased filtration and were able to restore some lost edge contrast by a lower bias potential.

NEGATIVE MODE DEVELOPMENT

The bias potential in this development mode is approximately $-3,400$ volts compared to approximately 2,000 volts in positive mode. The total potential, $V_B + \sigma L/KE_0$, in the region of the optimal exposure ($V = V_0/e \simeq 600\ V$) is about $2,000 + 600 = 2,600\ V$ for positive development and $-3,400 + 800 = -2600\ V$ for negative. The average electric field, extending across the chamber, is then the same for both modes of development in the image of the middle section of the breast and is the normalizing point for a good overall

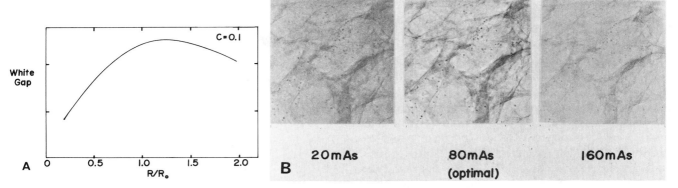

Figure 19.19. **A.** The white gap of a low-contrast edge as a function of exposure level. The white gap reaches its maximum when $R/R_0 = 1.2$. **B.** Xeroradiographs made at exposures of 20 mA, 80 mA, and 160 mA indicating changes in white gap and edge contrast.

contrast level. Its value, as shown earlier, is about 0.026 V/μm. The required higher image potential (800 V) for negative development results in a smaller exposure ($R \simeq 0.7\,R_0$).

RESOLUTION

The response of the xeroradiographic system is fundamentally different from that of conventional screen–film systems. As was stressed earlier, edge gradients are especially accentuated while subtle large area density differences are generally suppressed. Because of the edge enhancement, the traditional tools of resolution characterization (eg, the modulation transfer function, or MTF) are not strictly applicable. It should be recalled that the MTF describes the fidelity of transmission of spatially sinusoidal signals through a linear system. For the special case of mammography, the encountered subject contrasts are generally small leading to small or no white gaps. Under these conditions it is legitimate to develop an MTF-type descriptor. A calculated MTF curve[4] for the xeromammographic system is shown in Figure 19.20. Two features are apparent: a marked decrease of the low-frequency response and a peak at a frequency of about 1 cycle/mm. The first observation is the basic reason for the poor differentiation of subtle broad-area changes, which gives rise to wide recording latitude. The peaked response at one cycle/mm resembles the human eye threshold detectability of sinusoid peaks, a fact that largely explains the diagnostic success of this modality.

A similar behavior can be obtained with ordinary transparent films by diffuse masking: the original transparency is contact printed through some diffusing medium onto new film. This in turn is processed and registered with the original transparency to remove broad area density changes.

IONOGRAPHY

The discussion thus far has revealed the following characteristics for the xeroradiographic process: good edge contrast, limited gray scale, and low sensitivity. The last feature makes this modality inadequate for imaging thick body sections; it would require excessive radiation levels. The low sensitivity follows both from the recording stage and the development process. During the latent image formation a high surface charge must be present to ensure good photoconductive efficiency. As we have already seen the surface charge is exponentially depleted with exposure, resulting in reduced photoconductivity. During development a sufficient number of fine aerosol particles must be brought without much turbulence into the vicinity of the Se plate for the toner deposition to map faithfully the charge distribution. Finally, no toner should be lost during the image transfer from the plate to the special

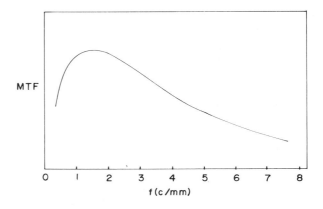

Figure 19.20. The modulation transfer function for the xeroradiographic system. The curve peaks at about one cycle/mm and has a subdued low-frequency response.

Xerox paper. In reality as much as 40 percent of the toner remains on the Se plate.

Ionography [7-9] is an alternate electrostatic method for capturing the x-ray image. A schematic diagram of a high-pressure gas chamber is shown in Figure 19.21. The incident x-ray beam is absorbed in the high-Z gas (usually xenon or Freon) principally through photoelectric interaction. The ions produced are swept across the chamber by an electric field and form a charge pattern on an insulating foil covering the upper electrode. The spherical geometry eliminates any geometrical loss of resolution since the electric field lines coincide with the photon paths. The high pressure gas (about 10 atmospheres) ensures good absorption efficiency as well as good resolution by limiting the photoelectrons to their point of origin. The electrode spacing is usually confined to 1 to 2 cm to reduce recombination between positive and negative ions, which becomes important as the spacing is increased. The applied voltage is about 10,000 volts.

Following irradiation, the chamber is depressurized and the film carrying the charge image is removed from the chamber and developed by a variety of methods. The powder cloud method is similar to the xeroradiographic development and shows good edge contrast. Liquid developers show less contrast and produce continuous tone images. A schematic of liquid development as used by Xonics Inc is shown in Figure 19.22. The electrostatic image is exposed to a colloidal suspension of positively charged black toner particles in an insulating liquid. The collected electrons on the foil attract the toner particles in proportion to the local charge density. The visible image is subsequently fixed or made permanent by a plastic overcoat.

In gaseous ionography high pressures are necessary with the accompanying mechanical problems. Another possibility is the use of liquids containing one or more heavy atoms in their molecule as the x-ray absorbers.

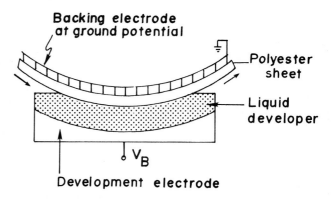

Figure 19.22. The ERG image processor. The electrostatic image is passing through a colloidal suspension of charged toner particles. The negative image charges attract the positive toner particles in proportion to the local charge density on the foil.

With liquid absorbers, high quantum efficiency and good resolution are possible. The main drawback, however, is the low imaging efficiency due to the recombination of positive and negative ions initially formed in close proximity. The use of liquid absorbers in radiography appears limited at present.

From the radiological point of view, gaseous ionography with liquid development offers exciting possibilities. The process is very sensitive (comparable to a high-speed screen–film system), shows high resolution, and allows the possibility of variable edge enhancement. Control of edge contrast is achieved by altering the development conditions. A major disadvantage with ionography, as of now, is the mechanical complexity of the system, which has prevented its taking its rightful place in a modern radiology department.

SUMMARY

Xeroradiography is an electrostatic imaging process that exhibits very limited macro response and relies principally on border exaggeration for detail detection. The subdued response leads to a wide recording latitude, which permits the simultaneous display in the case of mammography of skin, vessels, ducts, tumor masses, and microcalcifications. The edge enhancement, which is primarily responsible for the visualization of soft-tissue details, occurs whenever there is an abrupt difference in the radiation transmitted through adjacent anatomical structures. Such sudden variations in the transmitted x-ray intensity cause "steps" or edges of discontinuity in the originally uniform charge distribution on the selenium layer. This in turn gives rise to strong, rapidly varying fringe electrostatic fields. The amount of toner deposited during development is proportional to the local normal electric field component,

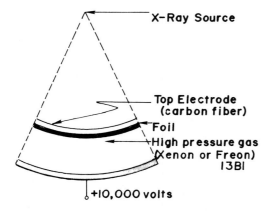

Figure 19.21. Schematic of an ionography chamber. X-rays generate ions in the high-pressure gas, which are swept by the electric field across the chamber and deposited on the foil.

which accumulates toner on one side of the edge and removes it from the other, thus delineating sharply the different borders. Away from boundaries the electric fields are weak and essentially constant regardless of the absolute charge present, leading to uniform light deposition of blue powder. The use of an electrode in the development chamber enhances the overall density, but extended areas are still depicted in a xeroradiogram with almost the same density, resulting in a characteristic curve that is almost flat.

Edge enhancement is manifested as toner accumulation adjacent to a depletion zone (white gap). For a given contrast, edge enhancement of details and hence detail visibility are maximized when the exposure reaches an optimal value R_{opt}. For positive development R_{opt} equals R_0 or $1.2\ R_0$ depending on whether the density profile or the white gap is maximized. R_0 is the exposure that will discharge the Se plate to 37 percent of its original charge. For negative development R_{opt} equals $0.7\ R_0$, which indicates additional dose savings if this mode is used. It should be noted that an exposure R_{opt} will optimize simultaneously *all* low-contrast details in a xeromammogram.

The xeroradiographic process is relatively insensitive compared to film–screen systems; thus its use is largely confined to the imaging of extremities. The sensitivity increases with energy suggesting a possible means for dose reduction. When this is done the bias potential during development must be lowered in order to retrieve some lost contrast. Xeroradiography is a contouring process with resolution characteristics resembling those of the eye: a sharp peak response at information presented at about one cycle/mm. The low-frequency response, which carries little informa-

tion, is effectively suppressed. The detection of microcalcifications and the sunburst pattern of breast carcinomas do not require the presence of low frequencies in the imaging system.

Another method that appears to have the advantages of xeroradiography, but at reduced exposures, is ionography or electron radiography. This is a charge-collection technique in contrast to xeroradiography, in which the latent image is formed by subtraction from a priming charge. With ionography a variety of development methods are possible allowing different ways of presenting the final image. This system is not yet reliable enough for routine use.

REFERENCES

1. Wolfe JN: Xeroradiography of the Breast, Springfield, Ill., Charles C Thomas, 1972
2. Schaffert RM: Electrophotography, 2nd ed. New York, Focal Press, John Wiley, 1975
3. Boag JW: Xeroradiography. Phys Med Biol 18: 3, 1973
4. Fatouros PP: Detail visibility in xeromammography. In Haus AG (ed): The Physics of Medical Imaging: Recording System Measurements and Techniques. New York: American Institute of Physics, 1979, pp 239–287
5. Fender WD: Quantification of xeroradiographic discharge curve. SPIE 70: 364, 1975
6. Van de Riet WG, Wolfe JN: Dose reduction in xeroradiography of the breast. Am J Roentgenol 128: 821, 1977
7. Johns HE, Fenster A, Plewes D: New methods of imaging in diagnostic radiology. Radiology 116: 415, 1975
8. Dance DR, Boag JW: Optimization of design parameters in ionography. J Phot Sci 25: 135, 1977
9. Stanton L, Brady LW, et al: Image characteristics of liquid developed electron radiographs. Radiology 120: 421, 1976

CHAPTER 20

Image Processing Considerations

MALCOLM SLOAN
CHARLES ROBINETTE
MAX I. SHAFF

Film quality is essential to the practice of radiology. Consistently reproducible films of good quality are dependent on quality control and maintenance of the processing equipment. This chapter deals with facets of darkroom practice and emphasizes the importance of quality control and preventive maintenance of the processor and chemicals. Aspects of silver recovery are considered and the newer daylight processing systems are also discussed, as well as inline processing.

DARKROOM CONSIDERATIONS

Adequate processing facilities are essential to the operation of radiographic departments. Processing facilities, both central and dispersed, must provide constant and reproducible results. In addition, high-quality processing must be achieved in a reasonable time and at an acceptable cost. The three basic approaches to the processing of x-ray films are: (1) a centralized darkroom, (2) dispersed darkrooms, and (3) daylight processing. The choice of the appropriate processing facility is influenced by cost and available space. In addition, the facility must be designed to cope with the increased workload of peak processing periods.

A centralized processing area should be located close to all the radiographic rooms, and pass boxes should be placed on at least two sides of the darkroom. Figure 20.1 shows a centralized darkroom. The third darkroom between the two adjacent darkrooms can be used for copying or subtraction. This is an important feature and caters to the increased demand for subtraction in angiographic practice. The principle advantage of centralized processing is the low initial cost. However, this early advantage is offset by the cost of employing an extra darkroom technologist. The light side of this processing area may be used to assemble film series and to assign them to their corresponding film jackets. The disadvantage of the centralized system is the congestion caused by physicians and technologists viewing their films, as well as by films being brought from other areas for processing.

The dispersed or isolated darkroom is usually located between two radiographic rooms (Fig. 20.2). This darkroom is provided with a pass box on either side of the room. These pass boxes provide each radiographic room with easy access to the darkroom. The advantage of the darkroom's being situated between two radiographic rooms is that the technologist does not have to leave the patient unattended in the radiographic room in order to deliver films for developing. As each film is exposed it can be passed directly into the processing darkroom, and at the end of the examination the first films are already available for viewing. Consequently, by the time the patient leaves the room, the examination is complete and the technologist is assured that radiographs will not have to be repeated. The efficiency of both technologist and radiographic room is, therefore, increased. Another advantage of this type of darkroom is that fewer cassettes are used, since the recycling of cassettes is more rapid than with the centralized darkroom facilities. The main disadvantage of dispersed darkrooms is the expense of operating multiple processing rooms.

The accepted size of a darkroom fitted with a through-the-wall processor is 80 to 100 square feet. These dimensions provide adequate storage space for a week's supply of unexposed film. In addition, freedom of movement is provided without compromising the ease of transferring films from the pass box to the processor. It is essential that the darkroom be clean and well ventilated. Humidity must be greater than 40 percent or static electricity will build up in the area. The amount of shelving should be limited to basic essential requirements in order to minimize the accumulation of dust. Dusting, when performed, should be done with antistatic solutions. The feed tray should be dusted daily and the shelves at weekly intervals.

Several types of processors can be used for radiographic film processing. They range in price from $4,000 to $15,000. Price and dependability are the controlling factors in choosing the processor. Because processors

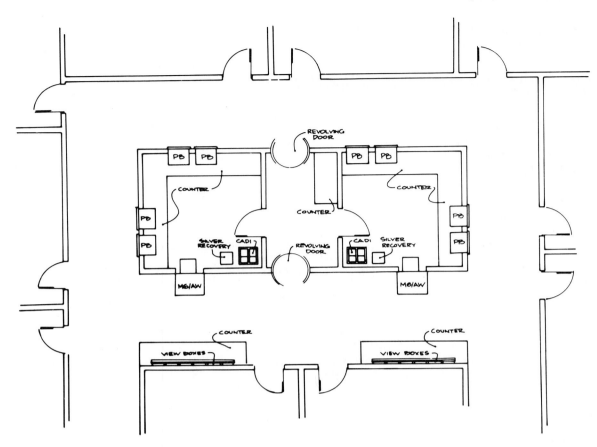

Figure 20.1. Centralized darkroom, utilizing revolving doors. Also note middle room, which can be used for subtraction and duplication.

are used for up to 18 hours per day in a high volume department, only the entrance tray should be placed inside the darkroom. This design allows independent maintenance of the rollers on the outside of the processor while the loading and unloading of cassettes is in progress in the darkroom. It is not recommended that two processors be utilized in one darkroom unless the darkroom is large enough for a partition between the processors.

Since the advent of blue- and green-sensitive films, processor lighting in darkrooms has changed significantly. Departments using blue- and green-sensitive films require a safe light with a GBX filter, which is recommended for both types of film. When only the blue-sensitive film is in use, the sodium vapor lamp is recommended and provides nearly normal brightness. The use of this light produces better working conditions for darkroom technologists and facilitates the placement of patient identification name cards.

Proper patient identification on the x-ray film is an integral part of the patient's examination. In addition to the patient's name and identifying number, the date and time of the exposure should be present on the film. Manual printers are available that transfer the time of

day to the film at the same time as the patient identification. However, with few exceptions these printers are very delicate and unsuitable for prolonged use. Other types of printers will be discussed under the section dealing with daylight systems processing.

Unused films should be stored in the darkroom only if the humidity and temperature are kept at proper levels. They should be stored on end or on side, but not flat, because of the possibility of producing pressure marks and artifacts. Only the minimum amount of film necessary to ensure an uninterrupted supply should be stored in the darkroom. Generally, an amount equal to 7 to 10 days usage is sufficient. Films should be rotated so that the oldest is used first. Films should be stored at 50° to 70°F to prevent fogging and must be stored above floor level to avoid water damage in the event of faulty plumbing.

QUALITY CONTROL

Quality control guidelines must be established to ensure adequate functioning and maintenance of equipment. Table 20.1 outlines the minimum checks and

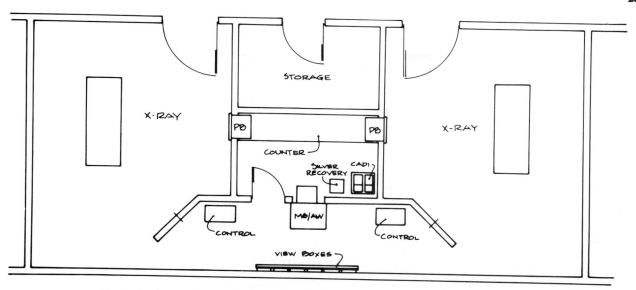

Figure 20.2. Dispersed darkroom accommodating two radiography darkrooms.

preventive maintenance procedures that should be performed. The area that lends itself best to rigorous care and precise control is the processor. Proper film density and contrast are dependent upon optimal processing conditions, and the following details should be attended to if optimal film density and control are to be achieved. Ideally, a single individual should be responsible for the daily monitoring of the inlet water temperature, the developing and drying temperatures, as well as the replenishment and circulation of solution. Developer temperatures are charted daily and the incoming water temperature should be maintained between 80° and 85° F unless cold water processors are used. Temperatures should be checked periodically throughout the day since there is always some variation in the temperature of the water supply. Constant dryer temperature is also essential for the adequate drying of films. Replenishment systems should be checked in the mornings and adjusted when necessary. Solutions in the replenishment tanks, the automatic mixers, and the processor tanks also should be checked daily.

Standardized contrast and density are achieved by

sensitometric methods. This involves the exposure of a film by calibrated sensitometric light for each processor in the department and the comparison of this film with a control film that has previously been established for the department. The data obtained from the sensitometric control film are charted on graph paper, on which lines showing acceptable and unacceptable levels of processing have been previously plotted (Figs. 20.3.A, B, C). In this way, variations in the processing can be detected. These checks should be performed daily at a fixed time of day. However, if at any time the quality control technologist or radiologist observes differences in film quality, sensitometry must be repeated and comparison again made with the departmental control film. These simple checks will allow one to determine immediately if the bad film quality is the fault of the radiographic room or the processor. At quarterly intervals, an exposed strip from each processor is returned to the film manufacturer for complete analysis including a (H and D) film characterization curve and hyporetension, contrast, and speed performance estimations. Chemicals in the processor are not changed unless there is variation from the control film.

When new screens and cassettes are put into service, tests should be done to establish that there is good film-screen contact. Each film should be labeled or numbered on the outside and in one of the corners of the screen to enable immediate identification of a faulty cassette. Monthly cleaning and inspection of cassettes for artifacts produced by dirt or scratches should be performed. This inspection should be recorded to permit continuing evaluation of screen performance and identification of problem areas. As previously mentioned, the numbering of all cassettes and screens is essential. Annual checks for screen–film contact are

TABLE 20.1. Quality Control Checks and Maintenance

Daily	Weekly
Water temperature	Processor cleaning
Developing temperature/ dryer temperature	
Solution levels	
Solution circulation	
Sensitometry	
Processor cleaning	

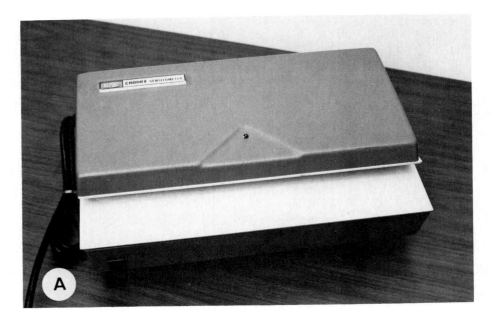

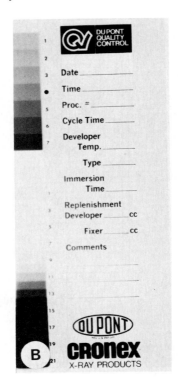

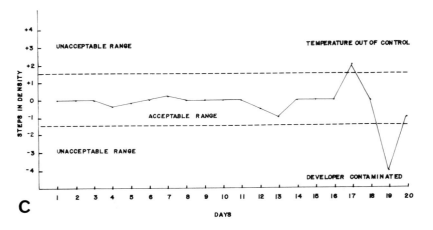

Figure 20.3. **A**. Dupont Cronex sensitometer used for checking density and contrast from film processor. **B**. Test film from the sensitometer after processing showing density and contrast ranges of the chemical. **C**. Graph showing the results of the sensitometer test film. The test is done daily.

also performed but should be done at shorter intervals if poor screen contact is suspected. Commercially available contact screen grids may be used. However, a simple but effective device for testing screen–film contact can be constructed by gluing paper clips on a 14-by 17-inch film. In many cases, poor screen contact is more apparent when using this system (Figs. 20.4.A, B). A simple step wedge exposure done annually on each cassette will identify speed problems (Fig. 20.4.C). The screen should also be examined visually under an ultraviolet light. This is particularly true for screens of calcium tungstate that show a diminished fluorescence in worn areas. Cleaning of screens should be done with the manufacturer's recommended screen cleaners, which have antistatic solutions incorporated within them.

Artifacts are extremely difficult to prevent. Most artifacts occur in the darkroom and result from the handling of films. The most effective means of eliminating darkroom artifacts lie in the instruction of darkroom personnel and in regular monitoring of the darkroom conditions and procedures. The most common artifact is static (Figs. 20.5.A, B, C). Regardless of the excellence of the quality control program, static artifacts will appear from time to time. These artifacts may be minimized by grounding all surfaces that come into contact with the film or cassette, cleaning the screens with antistatic solution, and making sure that the humidity in the darkroom is above 40 percent. The degree of humidity is not easily perceived, and if static continues to be a problem in the darkroom humidity should be accurately measured. Ideal humidity is 70 percent. When no reason for the presence of static can be detected, the darkroom attendant's clothing must be suspected as the source of static. Kink marks and surface markings (Fig. 20.6) are caused by inap-

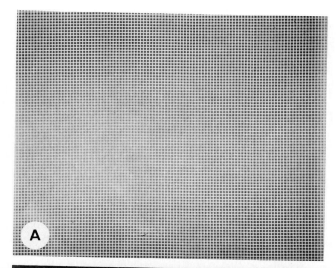

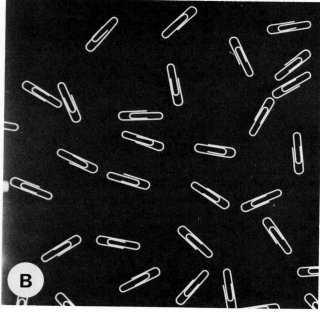

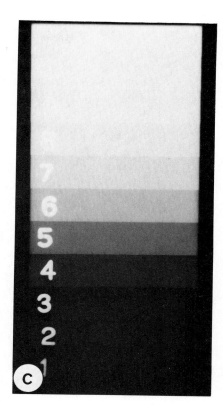

Figure 20.4. **A.** Commercial screen grid used for testing screen–film contact. **B.** Paper clip glued to clear film for checking screen–film contact. This is generally thought to be the easier method for detecting poor contact. **C.** Step wedge used to check the consistency of the x-ray machines from day to day and room to room.

propriate handling of the films. Surface markings are caused by the dirt on hands. Perspiration and hand lotions are often sources of artifacts. Kinks are caused by one's holding the film and causing it to bend at the fingernail. Kink marks may be either black on a clear film background or white on a dark film background. Black marks occur if the defect is caused before exposure of the radiograph while white marks occur after exposure of the radiograph.

A common cause of artifacts occurring in the processor are marks from scratches caused in the turnarounds (Figs. 20.7.A,B). These marks are usually evenly spaced and tend to appear on leading or trailing edges. Occasionally, they extend from one end of the film to the other. A less frequently observed artifact is the plain flame pattern (Fig. 20.8), which is caused by noncirculation of the developer. The microgroove line

also occurs in the processor and is due to the accumulation of material or a groove pattern in the earlier master rollers (Fig. 20.9). Dryer pin scratches (Fig. 20.10) were more common in the older type of processors and are seldom found at the present time. Hesitation marks (Fig. 20.11) occur when the guide shoes are out of alignment, or when there is malfunction of the rack drive components. They may also be caused by an accumulation of chemicals on the roller. Delay streaks (Fig. 20.12.A) appear at random intervals, usually have an increased density, and appear as narrow bands of varying width. They begin at the leading edge of the film and progress in the direction in which the film travels. Delay streaks may be prevented by cleaning the developer rack. Low solution levels in the tank can also cause delay streaks. Another common artifact is surface marks from the finger while passing the film over the entrance tray (Fig. 20.12.B). Also noted are fingerprints caused by moisture on the fingers.

Quality control should include daily and weekly preventive maintenance and cleaning of the processor. The crossovers should be cleaned and dried daily and

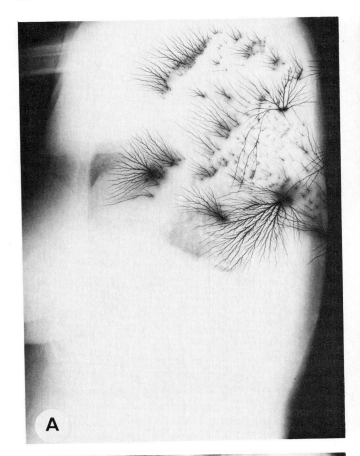

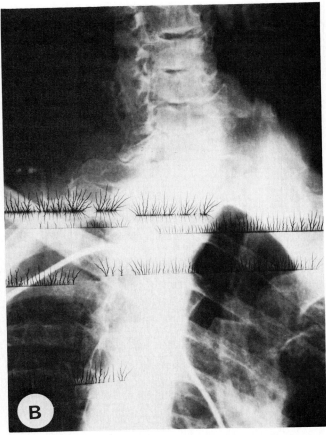

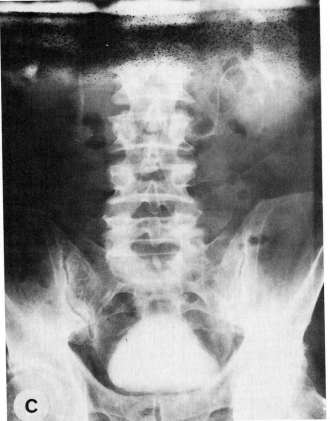

Figure 20.5. **A.** Tree static caused by negatively charged particle on film handling surface. To correct, film handling surface area should be cleaned with antistatic solution. **B.** Tree static caused by negative charge on equipment coming into contact with undeveloped film. To correct, the equipment should be grounded. **C.** Smudge static, caused by low-energy negatively charged particles dissipated over a large surface area.

placed on top of the processor at the end of the day. The processor top should be left open to permit ventilation and to prevent condensation on rollers that are not submerged in chemicals. Wash tanks should always be drained at night. All rollers and racks should be removed from the processor and cleaned at weekly intervals. Developer system cleaner is used to clean the developing racks. All other rollers and racks are cleaned with a mild synthetic abrasive, eg, thin green Scotchbrite pads. Rinsing and thorough washing of racks after use of system cleaner is essential since even a small amount of remaining cleaner will contaminate the developer. At this time, all moving parts should be checked for smooth operation. Blower and dryer belts should be checked and any chemical buildup should be removed. Racks must be scrutinized for roller wear. Rollers should be checked for residue and sediment. Replenishment rates should also be checked. Meticulous attention to these

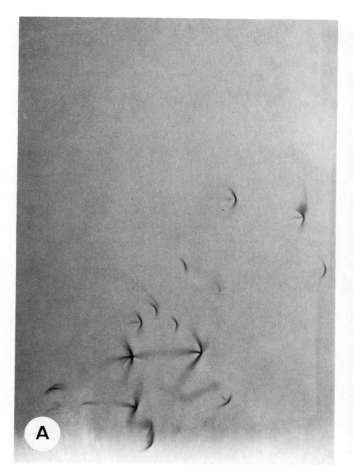
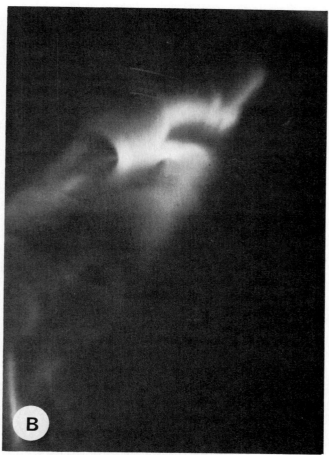

Figure 20.6. **A**. Kink marks of increased density. **B**. Kink marks of reduced density. Occurring at random, these marks are caused by improper handling of the film.

details significantly reduces equipment downtime. The appendix at the end of this chapter gives details of minimum suggested quality control procedures required for optimum film production.

CHEMICALS

Advances in chemical technology have made three choices of chemicals available. These are automatic chemical mixers, inhouse mixing, and solution service. The automatic chemical mixer is clean and alleviates the danger of contamination since the chemicals are untouched by hand. Furthermore, since only small amounts of chemical are mixed at any one time, fresh chemicals are assured. This method also requires less space than the larger tanks.

Inhouse mixing in small quantities is probably the second most popular method available. Volumes of 30 to 40 gallons of chemicals are mixed at a time. The possibility of human error in the mixing process is a disadvantage of this method. Oxidation and con-

tamination occur if the tanks are not properly sealed. This volume of chemical will generally last a week in a small department. Mixing chemicals in large quantities or centralized mixing has the disadvantage of increasing the risk of contamination, which, at present, requires that the entire volume of chemical be discarded. Solution services are costly, generally unnecessary, and not recommended since delegation of this important function of quality control then falls outside the departmental sphere of influence.

SILVER RECOVERY

Silver recovery is undertaken for three principle reasons, the first of which is related to simple economics. In 1969, for example, the average New York commodities price for silver was $1.40 per ounce. In early 1979, the silver prices skyrocketed to $9.00 per ounce, and by late 1979 silver was being sold for over $38.00 per ounce (Fig. 20.13). Silver is recovered both from scrap

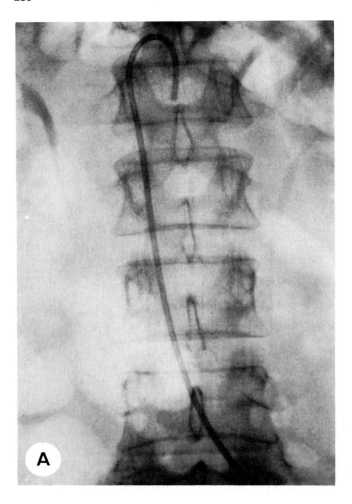

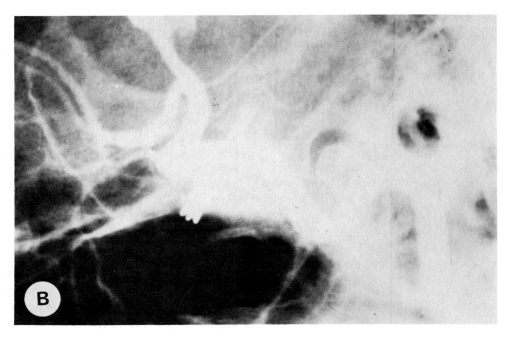

Figure 20.7. Shoe marks are increased or decreased density scratches running in the direction that the film travels. **A.** Increased density. **B** Decreased density. Decreased density scratches are caused when the emulsion is scratched off the face. Shoe marks are caused when the guide shoe is set too close to the adjacent roller.

Figure 20.8. Flame pattern is caused by poor circulation in the developer tank. The recirculation pump should be checked routinely.

Figure 20.9. Microgroove lines are in the direction that the film travels. They are parallel and appear as fine increased-density lines. These lines are caused by the grooved pattern on the early type master roller at the bottom of the rack or by buildup of material on the master roller.

x-ray film and from fixer solution. In 1969, a pound of mixed scrap film contained $0.41 of silver. In late 1979, that same pound would yield $4.05 of silver, even though the actual silver content per film had diminished.

The second reason for recovering silver from the darkroom is the conservation of a valuable resource. The photographic industry in the United States consumes approximately 60 million troy ounces of silver per year. The entire free world's silver use is approximately 400 million ounces annually, and the silver mine production is 250 million ounces annually. The recycling of silver from industrial scrap is, therefore, an important source of this valuable metal. An equally important consideration in recovering silver is the protection of community water supplies. Silver is a heavy metal and discharge of such metals is controlled by federal, state, and local codes and regulations. The silver in x-ray fixer solutions is in the form of silver thiosulfate complexes, which have not been found to have adverse effects on biological systems; however,

local, state, and federal codes govern the discharge of silver without regard to its form. Reduction in the amount of discharge is, therefore, often required in order to meet local codes.

TERMINAL ELECTROLYTIC RECOVERY

The three common methods of recovering silver from fixer solutions are terminal electrolytic recovery, ionic exchange cartridges, and batch recovery. In addition, there are three methods of electrolytic recovery: the terminal electrolytic revolving cathode method, terminal electrolytic revolving anode method, and recirculation devices. All of these methods routinely recover 98 percent or more of the available silver from the fixing solutions. The terminal mode (Fig. 20.14)

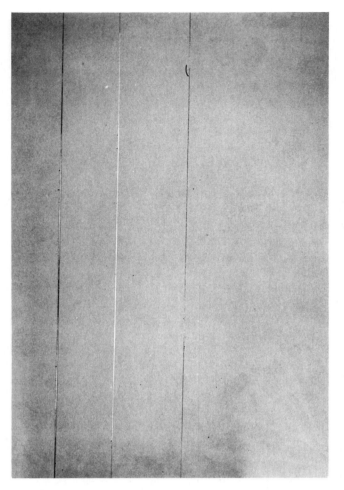

Figure 20.10. Dry pin scratches occur when the dryer air tubes or the dryer rollers are out of position. This is not a problem with later model processors.

Figure 20.11. Film hesitation marks are at right angles to film travel. They are increased density and are regularly spaced at intervals of 0.25 to 0.5 in. They are caused when the guide shoes are out of adjustment or the rack drive components malfunction.

extracts the silver from the tank overflow before it is drained off. The recirculation devices (Fig. 20.15) operate in a closed circuit and maintain the fixer solution with a low silver concentration. It should be noted that recirculation is not a simple process and most major film and chemical manufacturers stress that care must be taken to maintain the chemical standards by careful monitoring and proper chemical additions. Electrolytic plating reduces the sulfate and lowers the pH of the fixer, which, if not properly maintained, markedly shortens the archival life of x-ray images.

There are many regional and specialized manufacturers of electrolytic equipment. Major manufacturers offer national distribution, which assures the availability of spare parts. In general, cost of this equipment is calculated according to the number of ounces per hour of silver recovered. In 1979, a 0.5 ounce per hour capacity system cost between $400 and $700 and a three ounce per hour recovery cost between $900 and $1,400. Generally, silver recovery and service compa-

nies, as well as equipment dealers, offer complete installation packages that include lease-purchase, maintenance, and equipment sales.

A number of considerations should be taken into account before purchasing a terminal silver recovery unit. The better units are equipped with power selection, which would provide a degree of flexibility with respect to the volume of fixer processed. An ammeter provides a quick visual confirmation of the unit's function. As the price of silver is no longer inconsiderable, a locking device to discourage loss by theft is an advantage. Some units are sealed to eliminate fumes. The method used to provide the terminal drive is of great importance. Ideally the cathode should not be directly supported by the gear reduction box since the weight of the cathode may cause abnormal wear. A modularly designed power head allows easy assembly and disassembly. The cathode contact pressure should have a

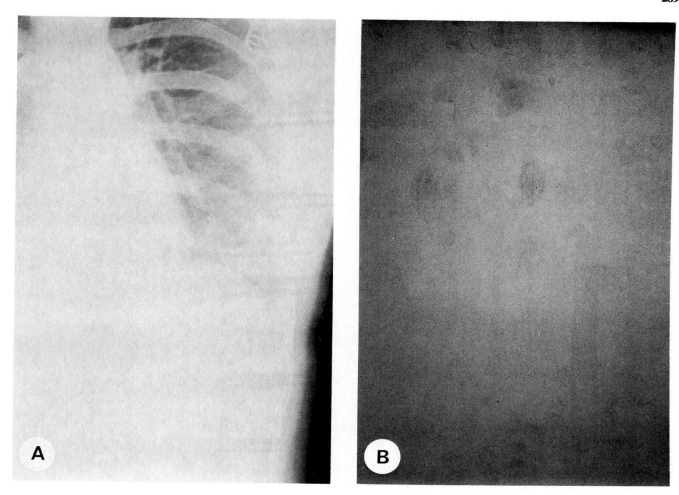

Figure 20.12. **A.** Delay streaks occur at random intervals and are usually of increased density. They begin at the leading edge and run in the direction of the film. The cause is chemical buildup on the developer rewet roller. **B.** Surface marks appear as plus density, and occur at random. They are caused by a dirty or rough entrance tray.

reasonably long life expectancy, and the cathode coupler should allow the shaft to become freely mobile when the lock screw is untightened. Nevertheless, the coupler must keep the cathode in correct alignment to minimize splashing of chemicals. The cathode itself should be of cylindrical design and the tank must be crack resistant and extremely strong. For this purpose, linear polyethylene is preferred. In addition, the tank fitting should be leakproof, and factory-installed fittings are recommended. The tank fitting should be located to prevent fixer from spilling over the top of the tank. Three-quarter-inch tubing is recommended to eliminate air locks and chemical backups caused by kinks in the tubing. Carbon anodes should be bolted to the side of the tank and not to the power supply itself to reduce the weight of the power supply. The anode–cathode support should hold these terminals in place and minimize cathode wobble. It should also be possible to collect any silver that may fall from the cathode.

The anode ground strap should be located on the outside of the tank, where it is not exposed to corrosive fixer fumes. The entire installation should be mounted in a tray to protect carpets and floors in the event of leakage.

IONIC EXCHANGE CARTRIDGES

Ionic exchange cartridges are inserted into the drainline in a similar way to the installation of a terminal device (Fig. 20.16). Ionic exchange takes place when iron in the cartridge comes into contact with the silver thiosulfate fixer. The active metallic ions react with this complex and go into solution. The silver is displaced and settles to the bottom of the cartridge. The disadvantage of these cartridges is that they have a tendency to block when used under conditions of low flow. Silver content is difficult to estimate prior to being sent to the refineries. However, high-efficiency as

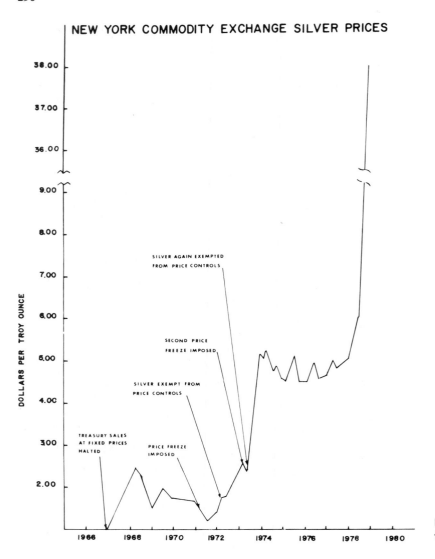

NEW YORK COMMODITY EXCHANGE SILVER PRICES

Figure 20.13. Graph illustrating the fluctuation of silver prices over a four-year period.

well as low-cost silver recovery are distinct advantages. In addition, the new cartridges make excellent tailing units when electrolytic systems are used. Table 20.2 compares the advantages and disadvantages of cartridges and electrolytic units. Cartridges cost between $20 and $60, but the price depends on the volume used and the terms that may be obtained from the equipment suppliers with respect to volume purchases.

BATCH RECOVERY

The third silver recovery method is batch recovery. This method involves the physical removal of silver-bearing fixer from the processor. It is most frequently used in multiprocessor locations, where solutions can be brought to a central point, collected, and sampled for silver content. The silver is then recovered by electroplating or precipitation methods. This method of

silver recovery requires a large working area and is wasteful in terms of time and personnel. Consequently, it is not favored.

X-ray film and silver solutions will be purchased by either silver service companies, solution service/processor maintenance companies or equipment dealers. Written quotations should be provided by the prospective purchasers. References from people in your local area should be collected, and positive identification of all parties must be obtained. When x-ray film is sold, unprocessed virgin film, which has a higher commercial value, should be separated from developed film whenever possible. It should be recalled that films from 1976 and earlier have higher silver values than films manufactured after 1976. The weight of the films should be recorded by hospital staff and the buyer's representative independently. Signed receipts for films should be obtained, and the dates on which the film is priced must be as close to the date of

TABLE 20.2. Advantages and Disadvantages of Metallic Replacement Cartridge and Electrolytic Recovery Cells

Metallic Replacement	Electrolytic Systems
Initial capital expenditure is approximately $25 to $50	Capital expenditure $150 to $15,000
Installation requires a simple plumbing connection	Electrical as well as plumbing connection
Yields a silver sludge that varies in silver content, resulting in higher shipping and refining costs	Yields silver with a high degree of purity
Does not permit reuse of fixer	A reduction in silver concentration to 500 mg/L in a single pass may be the best that can be achieved
Requires little monitoring and uses simple analytical procedures	Requires frequent monitoring for maximum efficiency
Can be used for recovery of silver from wash water	Is not suitable for recovery from wash water
Cannot be used in a continuous circulating system	When incorporated with a continuous circulating system, more silver is available for recovery; less silver is carried into the following wash

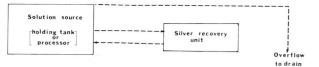

Figure 20.15. Diagram of flow of fixer in the recirculation mode. Dotted lines show the flow of fixer solution.

occurred. The electrolytic machines should be kept locked or sealed at all times. Similarly, harvested chips should be stored in a secure and safe place.

Cartridges are rarely purchased directly. Only a few specialized processors in the country can estimate the silver contained.

In summary, the recovery and ultimate sale of the silver-bearing materials are becoming important revenue-producing areas of an x-ray department. Currently, approximately 0.3 to 0.5 ounces of silver can be recovered from each gallon of fixer solution used, and the silver contained in the scrap film is approximately 23 percent of its bulk weight. Besides the importance of conserving a natural resource and assuring the radiological profession of an adequate supply of silver, silver recovery is a key factor in cost containment. Extreme care should, therefore, be excercised in this often neglected cost effective area.

DAYLIGHT PROCESSING

In the same way that automatic processors represented an advance over wet-tank processing, dispersed processing systems superceded centralized processing. Daylight systems now represent the state of the art.

The daylight system brings a new dimension to the

pickup as possible. If the film is sold at public auction, ensure that the place and date of the auction are adequately publicized. Bids and purchase prices that greatly exceed prices customarily offered in one's area should be viewed with suspicion.

The same type of company that purchases film also purchases electrolytic chips, and the above precautions apply to this type of material as well. However, due to the extremely high value of this form of silver, additional precautions should be taken. The reputation of the company one is selling to must be impeccable since cases of misrepresentation at the time of pickup have

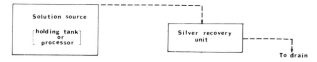

Figure 20.14. Diagram of flow of fixer in a terminal-mode silver recovery system. Dotted lines show flow of fixer solution.

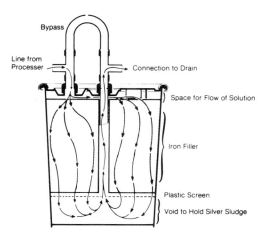

Figure 20.16. Illustration of the flow of fixer through the Kodak® chemical recovery cartridge type P.

operation of x-ray departments since it automates film handling in normal room light. The darkroom is eliminated and the handling of cassettes is accelerated. Patient identification is automatic and is recorded at the time of film processing.

Compared with the conventional darkroom system, the daylight system improves efficiency. Examination time may be reduced by as much as 30 percent without increasing the amount of space or the number of personnel required. The ability to do examinations more quickly results in less patient waiting time. This is particularly important when large numbers of patients are radiographed each day. In this way, faster and better patient care is provided and physician time is more efficiently utilized. Furthermore, the technologist is never required to leave the patient unattended, since the processing area is only a few steps from the x-ray table. Because the films are not handled at any stage of packaging or processing, artifacts are virtually eliminated, resulting in higher quality, clean radiographs. Screen life is extended because the frequency of cleaning is less than that required for darkroom use. Because all film processing is done in or near the diagnostic room, darkroom bottlenecks and the need to wait at pass boxes for cassettes are eliminated. In addition, the daylight system enables the technologist performing the examination to personally identify the films. In centralized darkroom or dispersed film-processing areas, there is always the possibility that error in identification may occur because films from a number of different patients are being processed simultaneously.

Currently, the price of a four-room daylight system would be approximately $50,000. This would include processing and identifying equipment and two film dispensers in each of 8 in×10 in, 10 in×12 in, 11 in×14 in, and 14 in×17 in sizes. Cassettes and screens in corresponding sizes would also be required. An equivalent four-room radiographic department would need four pass boxes, two film bins, two film identifiers, one large processor, and approximately 50 to 60 cassettes. The construction area needed for a darkroom would be 80 to 100 square feet. Additionally, $1\frac{1}{2}$ darkroom technologists would be needed. The initial investment required for a four-room darkroom department would be approximately $30,000, and if the salaries of the darkroom technicians are added, the initial outlay would be at least $45,000 in the first year alone. Because the daylight system requires fewer technologists and eliminates darkroom personnel, the cost of operation is low, with a savings in excess of $80,000 over a five-year period. The darkroom concept is further hampered by the fact that darkroom technicians usually work eight-hour shifts. This means that after hours and over weekends technologists are required to run their own darkrooms.

At the Vanderbilt University Medical Center, three radiographic rooms and three technologists were required to perform hypertensive urograms using conventional centralized darkroom processing. These radiographic rooms were 20 feet to 60 feet from the centralized processing area. In addition to the inconvenience of having to walk this distance, additional personnel were required to remain with the patient in the absence

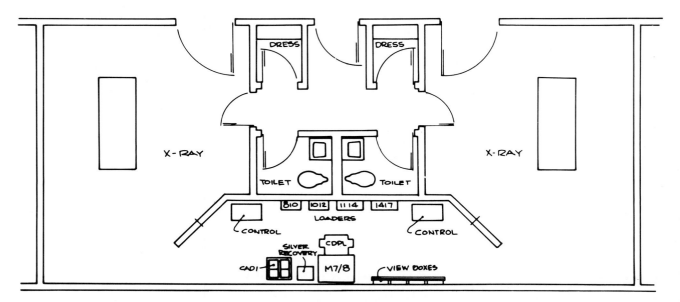

Figure 20.17. Diagram illustrating daylight system accommodating two x-ray rooms. This configuration could be used as the building block for additional radiography rooms.

of the technologist. Approximately 15 to 20 cassettes were required to service these three rooms. After installing a daylight system (Fig. 20.17) only two radiographic rooms, two technologists, and two to four cassettes were used for the identical workload. The expense of these examinations had been reduced, and the time involved in each procedure had been halved.

In-line processing is an extension of the daylight system in which the processor is adapted to the radiographic table (Fig. 20.18). The films are automatically fed into position between the screens and then transferred directly into the processor. Chest rooms are frequently adapted with in-line processing (Fig. 20.19). This is of particular advantage when there is a large patient volume. However, in-line processing is unsuitable for nongrid techniques. A combination of in-line and daylight processing would constitute an ideal system. This facility is especially valuable where the department functions on a 24-hour schedule.

A number of features mutually advantageous to both patient and examining staff are inherent in daylight processing systems. Waiting periods prior to examination are brief, and the duration of procedures is shortened. The technologist remains in close contact with the patient at all times. Each specialized area has total capability. Darkroom delays are eliminated and patient identification is more consistently accurate. Fewer film artifacts occur, and there is increased flexi-

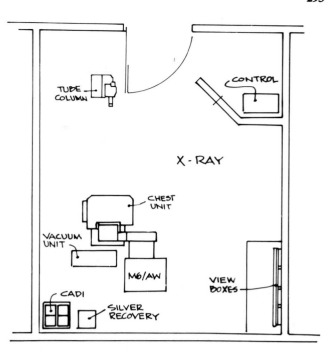

Figure 20.19. In-line processing for the chest radiography in automatic chest changer. This is very efficient for volumes.

bility in the choice of film-screen combinations and chemistry in each processing area.

The design of the entire area is facilitated by the efficient use of floor space and equipment. Items once peculiar to x-ray departments, such as pass boxes, film bins, safe lights, darkroom walls and doors, intercoms, and counters are entirely eliminated. In addition, daylight processors are smaller, fewer cassettes are needed, and darkroom personnel are not required.

ACKNOWLEDGEMENTS

The authors would like to acknowledge the valuable assistance of the following people in the writing of this chapter: Anthony George, President, National Refining Company, Gallatin, Tennessee; James Wall, Technical Representative, E. I. DuPont DeNemours and Company, Alanta, Georgia; Dave Reeves, Technical Representative, E. I. DuPont DeNemours and Company, Atlanta, Georgia; James P. Arendall, Eastman Kodak Company, Atlanta, Georgia.

APPENDIX

I.   **Processor Specialist**
     The selection of this person should take into consideration mechanical aptitude as well as

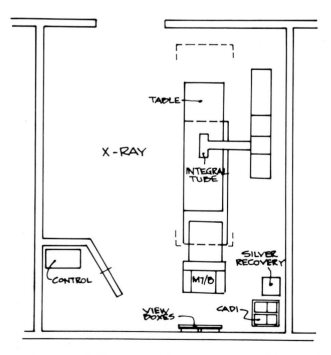

Figure 20.18. In-line processing in processor integrated with radiography table. This method used with the daylight system is very efficient.

self-motivation. Training of selected individuals may take place at processor schools.

II. Solution Checks

Developer—Check temperature three (3) times daily, twice on the day shift, and once on the evening shift. Check solution level in processor at time of temperature check. Check replenishment rates with a beaker for accuracy; DuPont Developer 55 to 60 cc recommended.

Fixer—Check solution level in processor at time of temperature check. Check replenishment rate with a beaker for accuracy; DuPont Fixer 90 to 110 cc recommended.

Water—Check solution level in processor at time of temperature check. Temperature should run 5° to 8°F lower than developer.

III. Recirculation Check

Developer Recirculation—Check micro switches daily to assure replenishment is activated from either side of the feed tray.

Water Flow—Check wash water flow monthly to assure adequate rate. Reduced water flow affects archival quality. Optimum flow—2.5 gallons/minute.

IV. Entrance Feed Tray

The feed tray to the processor is a site for artifacts and static electricity buildup. The feed tray should be cleaned daily with an antistatic solution (DuPont Screen Cleaner).

V. Filter Changes

Developer Filter—The practice has been to replace the developer filter each time the developer chemistry is changed (monthly). It is felt, however, that by changing the developer filter more frequently (bimonthly), that a higher quality of chemistry for a longer period of time can be maintained, thus reducing the frequency of chemistry changes. The chem-

istry in the processor could be replaced quarterly.

Water Filter—Changes in water filters are determined by the quality of incoming water, sediments, and foreign particles. Filters should be changed every four to six weeks for good water flow.

VI. Processor Cleaning

Crossover Racks—Clean crossover rollers daily with a damp cloth to remove solution stains and buildup. Do not submerge.

Deep Racks—The three deep racks should be cleaned bimonthly to remove emulsions and silver buildup. Do not use system cleaner for this cleaning. Use Scotchbright® and mild detergent and rinse well.

Deep Tanks—Internal tanks should be cleaned quarterly at the time of solution changes.

Gear, Chain, and Roller—Bimonthly checks of these parts will give indication for need of replacement or adjustments.

VII. Complete Processor Cleaning

Every six months, the processor should be thoroughly inspected. Processor racks should be completely disassembled and cleaned. Deep tanks should be cleaned with detergent, and a system cleaner should be flushed through the developer system.

VIII. Chemistry Checks

Sensitometric Check—Daily sensitometric exposures should be made and consistency in contrast and density should be checked. Sensitometric exposures should be made available for monthly H and D curve and system evaluation.

Chemical analysis—Analysis should be performed on a quarterly basis for assurance of proper mixing and development.

CHAPTER 21

Image Perception

S. JULIAN GIBBS
RONALD R. PRICE
A. EVERETTE JAMES, JR.

The final steps in a radiologic examination, the importance of which is overlooked in most texts, are perception of diagnostic information from the radiographic images and its integration with other information to arrive at a decision concerning patient management. For the purposes of this discussion, each image is assumed to be technically perfect or as nearly so as possible.

The actions of interpretation of a display of an image are:

1. Detection of those features of interest from the entire image
2. Interaction with the display system to improve the display of those features
3. Description of the significant features of the image
4. Integration with information obtained from other sources
5. Conclusion of the clinical relevance of the integrated information
6. Documentation of the conclusion in such a way as to influence future patient management (or to convince other clinicians)[1]

Actions 1 and 2 involve perception of the image display. Actions 3 through 6 develop a decision, based upon that perception.

PERCEPTION

The image is valuable only if its salient features are perceived by the observer. Observer action required to maximize perception of the image may be determined from the sciences of optic physiology and visual psychophysics. Perception involves four phases of visual acuity, as shown in Figure 21.1.

ATMOSPHERE OF PERCEPTION

An atmosphere free of distraction is required for optimum perception. We cannot deal with multiple signals simultaneously impinging on our sensory system.[2] Some method of selection must be present. Even extraneous visual signals can compete; signals reaching some receptor units in the retina inhibit the response of other receptor units to other signals.[3] Signal perceptibility relates to both familiarity of the signal and motivation of the observer. Familiar visual patterns are more easily recognized. According to filter theory,[2] simultaneous signals are first analyzed by physical characteristics. Each signal is then attenuated differentially, based on its relevance to the principal task of the observer at the moment. Second, all of the signals are fed into a pattern recognition system, which is essentially a dictionary of patterns, each with its own response threshold. Generally, the more familiar the pattern, the lower its threshold. The combination of signal strength and response threshold then selects the stimulus that will be perceived selectively. Only those patterns whose signal strengths exceed their response thresholds will be perceived. Thus more familiar patterns are more easily and more rapidly identified. If we are highly motivated to perceive the information in a radiographic image, we may selectively attenuate other signals, either visual or from other sensory receptors. However, if the number of extraneous signals is reduced, our ability to perceive the desired information may be increased.

Each image must be scanned initially in its entirety in a systematic manner. At any one time, attenuation is focused on only a small portion of the visual field. If the observer's attention is initially drawn to a specific portion of the image display, important information in other parts of the display may be overlooked. Selection of a portion of the image may be the result of extraneous signals, or bias on the part of the observer as to where in the image display the required information might be found.

GRAY-SCALE PERCEPTION

The human visual system can adapt to an enormous range of light intensities; Figure 21.2 indicates a luminance range of approximately 10^{10} from threshold to glare limit. It also shows that for scotopic vision, subjective brightness is a logarithmic function of light intensity.[4] However, at any one time the system cannot operate over such a large range but accommodates to the variation in brightness by adaptation. Pupil diameter ranges from about 2 mm under bright light to 8 mm with dark adaptation[5] and thus accounts for a factor of only 16 in brightness adaptation. Obviously, most adaptation is a central function. As an example, consider an eye adapted to luminance B in Figure 21.3. Discrimination of intensity level is possible only over

the narrow range from B − to B +. Anything below B − is perceived as black. If there are intensities much greater than B +, the adaptation level is shifted upward. Therefore, only a few intensity (gray) levels can be recognized at any one time.

An important visual property for interpretation is the ability to discriminate light intensity, or optical density for a typical radiographic image. E. H. Weber found that the minimum perceptible difference in a stimulus was proportional to the level of the stimulus. Stated in terms of vision, as done by Fechner, it may be written as $\Delta L/L = K$ (Weber ratio) where ΔL is the minimum detectable difference in luminance, L is the luminance, and K is a constant[6]. This relationship has been shown to hold over essentially the entire range of photopic vision. If the eye is adapted to the luminance (L) at which ΔL is determined, that L is a constant, as shown in Figure 21.3.[5] The value of $\Delta L/L$ is shown as approximately 2 percent; however, the precise value may vary with other factors, such as size of the object or the time during which the observer is permitted to view it. If, on the other hand, the subject is adapted to a given level of luminance, then the value of $\Delta L/L$ increases as L deviates from the adaptation level[7] again as shown in Figure 21.4.

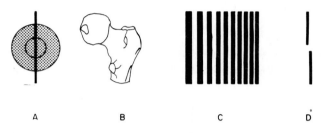

A   B   C   D

Figure 21.1. Perception of a radiographic image display. **A.** Detection of a single thin line. **B.** Recognition of a pattern. **C.** Resolution of detail. **D.** Localization of pattern in the two-dimensional image of the three-dimensional subject. (After Todd-Pokropek and Pizer.[1])

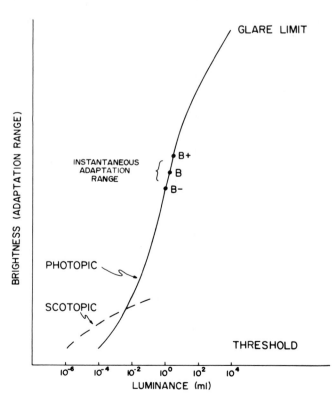

Figure 21.2. Subjective brightness adaptation. Scotopic, retinal rod vision; photopic, cone vision. After Gonzalez and Wintz.[4] (From Gibbs SJ: Principles of radiographic interpretation. In White SC, Goepp RA, Goaz P: Dental Radiology: Principles and Interpretation. CV Mosby, 1980. Used by permission.)

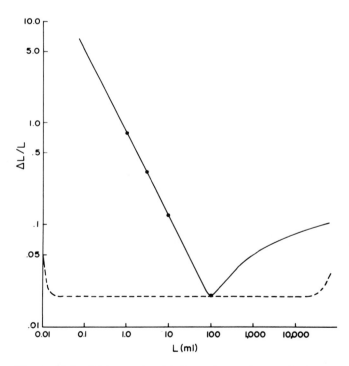

Figure 21.3. Weber ratio, $\Delta L/L$, versus L. ΔL, minimal detectable luminance difference; L, luminance. Broken curve: $\Delta L/L$ constant over a wide range of L, when subject is adapted to L. Solid curve: subject adapted to L of 100 millilamberts; $\Delta L/L$ increases as L deviates from adaptation level. Data of Davson [5] and Heinemann.[7] (From Gibbs SJ: Principles of radiographic interpretation. In: White SC, Goepp RA, Goaz P: Dental Radiology: Principles and Interpretation. CV Mosby, 1980. Used by permission.)

In radiologic interpretation, the observation that the Weber ratio increases as luminance deviates from the adaptation level is of prime importance. For maximum gray-level discrimination, the viewer's eye should be adapted to the luminance level of the image. For example, Figure 21.4 shows how the minimal detectable difference in optical density of a radiograph varies with the luminance adaptation level of the viewer. The standard viewbox provides a luminance of approximately 170 millilamberts at its surface. The usable optical density range of a radiograph is approximately 0.25 to 2.0. If the optical density of a typical area of a radiograph is 1.0, then the luminance of that area is 10 percent of the viewbox illumination, or 17 millilamberts. If the viewer is accommodated to that luminance, then the Weber ratio should be approximately 2 percent, and a difference in density of approximately 0.01 optical density units should be detectable. If, however, the viewer is adapted to the unattenuated luminance of the viewbox (170 mL), then the minimal perceptible difference in optical density is approximately 0.05 optical density units. These data apply quantitatively to sharply defined differences between large areas, each of uniform optical density. In real situations, minimal detectable differences will probably be greater. Differences in optical density may be gradual, and density levels may vary significantly across an image of finite size, confusing the adaption level.

These data provide the scientific basis for the recommendation that all areas of the viewbox not covered by the radiographic image should be masked with opaque material, and for reduction of room illumina-tion such that the viewer will adapt to the luminance level of the radiographic image.

Edge enhancement, or increased perceptibility along an image boundary between two structures, is generally regarded as important only in xeroradiography. However, it also occurs with conventional films and in the visual system (Fig. 21.5). In film, it is called adjacency or edge effect,[8] and can be explained by the development process. Areas of high exposure need more developer to develop their more numerous exposed grains than do areas of low exposure with few exposed grains. Along a line of sharp demarcation between areas of high and low exposure, more fresh chemical is available to the edge of the area of high exposure. The result is a line of incresed density along the edge of the dense area. These effects can be detected by a densitometer. In the absence of edge effects in the image, the visual system may introduce a similar phenomenon of edge enhancement, known as Mach bands.[9] While image edge effects occur only along sharply defined boundaries, Mach bands can occur along either sharp or gradual transitions in density (Fig. 21.5). Mach bands can be a factor in radiography.[10]

COLOR VISION

Previous discussions have ignored the wavelength of the light and how it affects visual perception. Cones

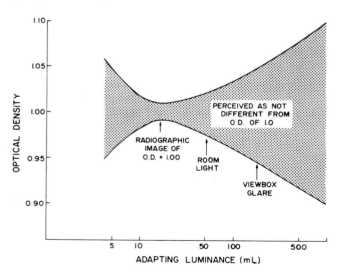

Figure 21.4. Minimum perceptible change in optical density of radiograph versus luminance adaptation level of viewer. Shaded area between the curves cannot be perceived as different from optical density of 1.00. See text for explanation. Calculated from date of Heinemann.[7] (From Gibbs SJ: Principles of radiographic interpretation. In White SC, Goepp RA, Goaz P: Dental Radiology: Principles and Interpretation. CV Mosby, 1980. Used by permission.)

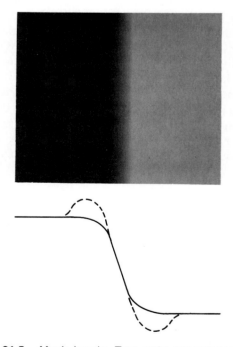

Figure 21.5. Mach bands. Top: note appearance of dark band along edge of denser portion and light band along edge of less dense portion. Bottom: densitometer trace. Solid curve, actual density; broken curve, perceived density. (From Gibbs SJ: Principles of radiographic interpretation. In White SC, Goepp RA, Goaz P: Dental Radiology: Principles and Interpretation. CV Mosby, 1980. Used by permission.)

are the primary color receptors. The cones are not uniformly distributed on the retina; their density is greatest as the center of the retina (fovea) and rapidly declines with distance from the center.

The human eye can perceive a relatively small number of shades of gray. However, the eye may be capable of distinguishing thousands of different colors. Color-coded images thus have the potential of providing the eye with more information than is currently provided by conventional gray-scale images.

With gray-scale vision, we discussed perceptibility in terms of brightness or intensity. For color perception, we introduce in addition to brightness, the terms hue and saturation. Brightness is the aspect of perception that varies with the light intensity (photons per second per unit of retinal area). Hue is the perception aspect that varies as the wavelength of the light changes. Saturation is the aspect that varies as white light is added to pure monochromatic light.

Even human beings whose retinas contain only rods have some capacity for color discrimination. This capacity can be understood from an examination of the absorption spectrum of the rods shown in Figure 21.6. As illustrated, the absorption of light in the rods is wavelength dependent. Thus, a subject presented with two different color patches (different wavelengths) would be able to distinguish between the two as long as their intensities were such as to result in different numbers of absorbed photons. Because of this capability, color discrimination is usually defined as the ability to discriminate on the basis of wavelength alone, independent of other factors such as intensity. With this definition, then, individuals with only rod vision do not possess the capability of color discrimination.

To understand the mechanisms of color vision, let us first consider the absorption spectra of two different hypothetical receptors located in the retina (Fig. 21.7). In this example, the absorption spectra do not overlap. A subject presented with two light patches, one patch

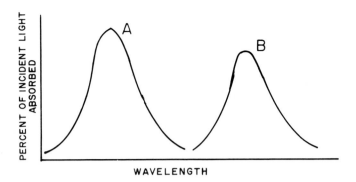

Figure 21.7. Absorption spectra of two hypothetical receptors in the retina.

whose wavelength lay under curve A and the other whose wavelength lay under curve B, would be able to discriminate between the two patches regardless of their relative intensities. Thus according to our definition, this subject would prossess the capability of color discrimination. However, if both light patches had wavelengths under curve A or under curve B, the subject would only be capable of perceiving color in the same manner as with pure rod vision.

There is considerable evidence that the absorption spectra of the various color receptors in the retina all have similar shapes (Fig. 21.8) and differ primarily by being shifted relative to each other along the wavelength axis. There is almost complete overlap of the wavelengths for which the receptors are sensitive, thus eliminating the rod vision condition. All experimental findings seem to establish that there are at least three distinctly different classes of cones in the normal human retina, a condition known as trichomacy. The rods and the three types of cones indicate that the retina contains at least four types of receptors.

A normal human subject with a trichromatic system is capable of distinguishing two patches of light, one of which contains a pure wavelength and the other a mixture of two wavelengths, regardless of their relative intensities. However, the trichromatic system is far

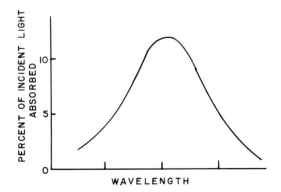

Figure 21.6. Absorption spectrum of the rods. Peak absorption takes place at about 500 mm. However, right quanta at other wavelengths may result in the same response due to different incident intensities.

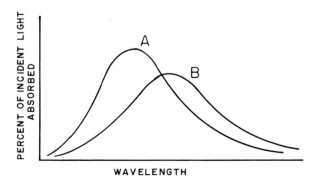

Figure 21.8. Absorption spectra of two different color receptors in the retina. Note that both are sensitive to the same wavelengths but to different degrees.

from perfect and loses an enormous amount of wavelength information. Two light patches that are completely different in wavelength composition can be made to appear indistinguishable from each other to the normal eye. If a subject is presented with two light patches, one of which is a pure wavelength and the other is a mixture of three wavelengths, it will always be possible to make the two patches indistinguishable from each other by varying the intensities of the mixture.

Similar to gray-scale vision, the subject's perception of color can be strongly influenced by background illumination and by adapting the retina to lights of different colors. The perceptions of hue, brightness, and saturation are also affected when the intensity is extremely high or low. The visual threshold for cone vision during dark adaptation is virtually complete by five minutes, whereas rod vision requires from 15 to 30 minutes, a possible advantage of color viewing.

SPATIAL RESOLUTION

The modulation transfer function (MTF) has become the standard expression for resolution of points in space by an optical or imaging system. It is the ratio of contrast in the image to contrast in the subject, plotted against spatial frequency of the subject. For the human visual system, we have no means of measuring contrast in the cortical image. Therefore, standard Fourier analysis is not possible. However, an analogous function to express visual acuity has been developed; since it is not an exact analog, it must be interpreted with some caution.[11] The usual procedure is to allow a subject to view parallel grating patterns of defined spatial frequencies. The contrast of each pattern is varied until the subject perceives it; threshold contrast is thus determined for each spatial frequency, which is usually expressed in cycles per unit of arc as measured at the focal point of the optic lens, since this is independent of viewing distance. A plot of reciprocal threshold, or modulation sensitivity, in arbitrary units, versus spatial frequency, is shown in Figure 21.9. At luminances sufficient for photopic vision, modulation sensitivity is independent of illumination wavelength (color). Note that, at higher luminances, modulation sensitivity peaks at a spatial frequency of 3 to 5 cycles per degree.[12] Other studies, concentrating on higher spatial frequencies, have reported peak modulation sensitivities as high as 10 cycles per degree.[13] The visual system therefore acts as a band-pass filter, tuned to central frequency of 5 to 10 cycles per degree.[15] The decreased sensitivity as high spatial frequencies is in part optical.

The modulation sensitivity at a given spatial frequency is affected by other factors, such as object size,[14] pupil diameter, involuntary eye movement, or eccentric fixation.[5] Modulation sensitivity is greatest at

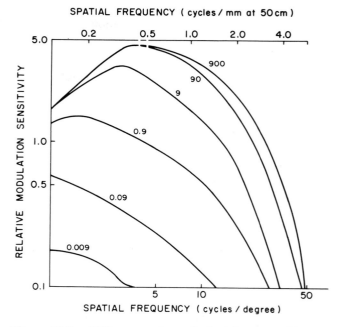

Figure 21.9. MTF curves for a typical human subject at different light intensities. Numbers along curves indicate retinal illuminance in trolands (td, candles/m² times pupil area in mm²). Illuminance for radiographic interpretation lies between curves for 9 and 90 td. Lower abscissa, spatial frequency in cycles/degree of arc at lens; upper abscissa, spatial frequency at normal viewing distance of 50 cm. See text. Data from Van Nes and Bouman.[12] (From Gibbs SJ: Principles of radiographic interpretation. In White SC, Goepp RA, Goaz P: Dental Radiology: Principles and Interpretation. CV Mosby, 1980. Used by permission.)

the center of the visual field. At the normal viewing distance of 50 cm, peak modulation sensitivities occur for subject spatial frequencies of approximately 0.4 to 1.1 cycles per mm. Some images contain information of higher spatial frequency, and magnification is often required for optimum perception. Conversely, the decreased modulation sensitivity at low spatial frequencies suggests need for measures to increase perception of such information. The common method of accomplishing this is to view the image display at an acute angle. This serves the purpose of increasing the spatial frequency in one dimension, in terms of cycles per degree at the eye. The procedure is an example of the deliberate rendering of high spatial frequency information imperceptible, so as to improve the perception of low spatial frequencies.

Factors of both gray-scale discrimination and point resolution indicate the need for the ability to modify display conditions. Perhaps the most useful adjunct is the availability of variable luminance from the viewbox and of a high-intensity illuminating system ("hot light"). Reduced luminance may permit better visualization of areas of low optical density. Intense illumination provides better visualization of areas of high optical density. These two adjuncts may allow perception of required information from marginally overexposed films, and thus eliminate retakes. No known modification of viewing conditions, however, can make possible the use of underexposed films.

STEREOSCOPY

The need for the third dimension in the radiographic image has led to several methods for its display. Stereoradiography involves the obtaining of two images in essentially the same projection, with only a slight movement of the tube between exposures, with the patient remaining absolutely motionless. Viewers can learn to fuse the two images, when viewing them in appropriate configuration, to form a single three-dimensional image. However, a sizeable portion of the population cannot achieve stereopsis under these conditions, even with optical aids. Failure is probably related to loss of several cues, both monocular and binocular, for depth perception: interposition, perspective, monocular movement parallax, shading, accommodation, and convergence.[16] Further, the cue of relative size is aberrant, and relates to distance from the object to the film rather than to the observer. Thus only stereopsis, or the cortical analysis of the difference in the images from the two retinas, is functional. However, it is sufficient for perception of three dimensions, as demonstrated by random-dot stereograms.[2,5] For those viewers who can achieve stereopsis, with or without optical aids, stereoradiography provides reasonably quantitative information in the third dimension.

Clearly the most direct approach to obtaining three-dimensional information is use of two projections at right angles to each other. The location of an object in three-dimensional space is then established by triangulation. Occasionally, three orthogonal projections are useful. Quantitative accuracy of the right-angle method is limited by ability of the observer and by geometric distortion in the radiographic image, the result of the divergent beam.

DECISION MAKING

The ultimate value of diagnostic information obtained from a radiologic or any other source is its contribution to a decision regarding patient management. The process of decision making in health care recently has been the subject of extensive investigation.[17,18] Analysis of decision making includes not only diagnostic probability but also questions of cost–benefit relations, risks, and values.[17] Considerations of quality assurance and cost containment have directed attention to the radiologist and efficacious use of diagnostic information in patient management. The

radiologist must consider not only the results of a decision, but also the process of making a decision.

EXAMINATIONS AND FILMS

The obvious first step of decision making from radiologic information is the description of the significant features of each image in the examination. These features must then be categorized as normal, variant of normal, artifact of the procedure, abnormal, or the result of prior treatment. Each feature on each image must be correlated with other available projections, for confirmation or refutation. This does not imply a requirement of multiple views of all areas. Instead, it means that when a feature is visible on more than one film, information from all views must be utilized in arriving at a decision.

INTEGRATION

Only after presumptive decisions have been reached from the results of the radiologic information alone should this information be related to and integrated with other available information. Prior studies, if available, must be compared with current films to determine rate of progression of signs. Radiologic results should be compared with history, physical examination, laboratory procedures, biopsy, etc. If the results of all diagnostic procedures are mutually confirmatory and provide for exclusion of all but one entity in the differential diagnosis, then the diagnosis may be regarded as established. If not, then additional diagnostic procedures must be prescribed.

In the decision to apply a given diagnostic procedure, the efficacy of that procedure must be considered.[17] Efficacy must not be confused with yield, or the frequency that a given diagnostic procedure provides positive results. For example, a negative result may provide for a better direction of subsequent diagnostic procedures, spare the patient unnecessary treatment, or even rule out the need for further study. Efficacy may be considered at three levels. Diagnostic efficacy refers to the information derived from a procedure, whether or not that information is useful to the management of the patient. That is, it refers to the extent to which the physician is led to change his thinking about the patient's condition as a result of a procedure. Management efficacy refers to the usefulness of diagnostic information in terms of influencing decisions on patient management. It can refer not only to decisions of indicated treatment, but also to the need for further diagnostic information, to deferral of treatment, or even to the recommendation of no treatment. That is, it refers to the clinical relevance of the diagnostic information. Ultimate efficacy, more global in outlook, refers, then, to the prognosis of the patient. It deals with the ultimate outcome of the patient's condition, with or without definitive treatment.

Quantitative analysis of the efficacy, especially the diagnostic efficacy, of a procedure may be obtained from elements of signal detection theory, particularly receiver operating characteristic (ROC) curves.[19] The ROC curve is a plot of true positive versus false positive ratios for a given procedure (Fig. 21.10). For a yes–no process, such as determination of presence or absence of signs of a given abnormality on a image, the points of the ROC curve are established from true and false positive ratios obtained at various magnitudes of the sign of abnormality accepted as cutoff.

ROC analysis provides a method for formalizing and quantitating intuitively obvious concepts—and some that are not so obvious. Since both the abscissa and ordinate of ROC curves are probabilities, both range between 0 and 1. True ROC curves are never upwardly concave.[23] Thus the false positive ratio is directly proportional to the true positive ratio. This means that if we want a maximum true positive ratio, we must accept a maximum false positive ratio. Conversely, if we want to minimize the false positive ratio, we must accept a low true positive ratio. We cannot have simultaneous high sensitivity and high specificity.

ROC analysis assists not only in the designation of grounds for treatment, but also in the design of our diagnostic workups. If we wish to maximize the probability of a correct decision, then we must accept a point midway along the ROC curve, and accept a given level

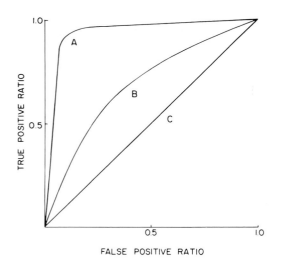

Figure 21.10. ROC curves (hypothetical), of true and false positive results of diagnostic procedures. Curve A represents a procedure in which the signal is almost always distinguishable from noise. Curve B is from a procedure in which the signal is usually detectable. Curve C is random, in which the signal cannot be distinguished from noise. (From Gibbs SJ: Principles of radiographic interpretation. In White SC, Goepp RA, Goaz P: Dental Radiology: Principles and Interpretation. CV Mosby, 1980. Used by permission.)

of false positives (unnecessary treatment). If we are conservative and wish to minimize unnecessary treatment, we must accept a low true positive ratio (frequent misses). Our decision (cutoff level) may be influenced by other values, such as current or ultimate patient discomfort, cost, or patient history.

DOCUMENTATION

Results of the radiologic procedure must be documented such that they influence future patient management and meet medico-legal requirements. The report should include the date, the examination performed, and projections obtained. It should note any compromises with technical perfection of the study as a result of the patient's anatomy or other extenuating circumstances. The radiographic appearance of clinically relevant features should be described in detail, including location, nature (lucency, opacity, discontinuity of structure, etc), shape, size, nature of the margins, and anatomy involved. The report should conclude with an estimate of the clinical or biologic significance of the findings and a differential diagnosis of possible the disease entities that could result in these findings. In cases in which the patient may be referred, or in an institutional setting, a hard copy of the complete radiologic report is essential.

SUMMARY

The scientific basis of several familiar recommendations for the process of radiologic interpretation has been developed as follows:

1. Examine image in a logical, systematic manner to minimize the probability of observer bias in the detection of abnormality.
2. Examine image in a distraction-free environment to minimize competing stimuli.
3. Reduce room illumination to obtain maximum gray-level discrimination in the image by matching brightness adaptation to luminance of the displayed image.
4. Cover all unused portions of the viewbox with opaque material, again to obtain maximum gray-level discrimination.
5. Use a magnifying lens to maximize perception of high spatial frequency information.
6. Employ variable-intensity viewbox illumination and "hot light" to increase both gray-scale discrimination and point resolution, especially at the extremes of image density, and to enable use of radiographs of suboptimal exposure.

Adherence to these recommendations will not guarantee the correctness of decisions based on radiologic evidence. No diagnostic procedure—a technically perfect examination or even a biopsy—exhibits perfect sensitivity and selectivity. Signal detection theory demonstrates that highly sensitive diagnostic procedures have inherently low specificity. Conversely, highly specific procedures have relatively low sensitivity. The conditional probability that a patient has a disease, given a positive radiologic sign (or, more specifically, a sign perceived as positive) relates not only to these factors, but also to the incidence of the disease in the population. Therefore, radiologic findings constitute an aid to diagnosis, not a mechanism for establishing a conclusive diagnosis.

REFERENCES

1. Todd-Pokropek AE, Pizer SM: Displays in scintigraphy. In Medical Radionuclide Imaging. Proceedings of an International Symposium, Los Angeles, Oct 25–29, 1976. Vienna, International Atomic Energy Agency 1:505–537, 1977

2. Davidoff JB: Differences in Visual Perception. New York, Academic Press, 1975

3. Hartline HK, Ratliff F: Inhibitory interaction of receptor units in the eye of limulus. J Gen Physiol 40:357–376, 1957

4. Gonzalez RC, Wintz P: Digital Image Processing. Reading, Mass., Addison-Wesley Publishing Co, 1977. Chapter 2

5. Davson H: The Physiology of the Eye, 3rd ed. New York, Academic Press, 1972

6. Rubin ML, Walls GL: Fundamentals of Visual Science. Springfield, Ill., CC Thomas, 1969

7. Heinemann EG: Simultaneous brightness induction. In Jameson D, Hurvich LM (eds): Visual Psychophysics. Handbook of Sensory Physiology, 7(4). New York, Springer Verlag, 1972

8. Perrin FH: The structure of the developed image. In Mees CEK, James TH (eds): The Theory of the Photographic Process, 3rd ed. New York, Macmillan, 1966

9. Fiorentini A: Mach band phenomena. In Jameson D, Hurvich LM (eds): Visual Psychophysics. Handbook of Sensory Physiology, 7(4), New York, Springer Verlag, 1972, pp 188–201

10. Randall PA: Mach bands in coronary arteriography. Radiology 129:65–66, 1978

11. Cornsweet TN: Visual Perception. New York, Academic Press, 1970

12. Van Nes FL, and Bouman MA: Spatial modulation transfer in the human eye. J Opt Soc Am 57:401–406, 1967

13. Campbell FW, Green DG: Optical and retinal factors affecting visual perception. J Physiol 181:576–593, 1965

14. Blackwell HR: Luminance difference thresholds. In Jameson D, Hurvich LM (eds): Visual Psychophysics. Handbook of Sensory Physiology, 7(4). New York, Springer Verlag, 1972, pp 78–101

15. Westheimer G: Visual acuity and spatial modulation thresholds. In Jameson D, Hurvich LM (eds): Visual Psychophysics. Handbook of Sensory Physiology, 7(4). New York, Springer Verlag, 1972, pp 170–187

16. Graham CH: Vision and Visual Perception. New York, John Wiley & Sons, 1965.

17. Lusted LB, Loop J: An analysis of medical decision making with comments on efficacy studies. In Hill NS (ed): Effective Performance in the Dynamic Health Care Environment. Minneapolis, Society for Computer Medicine, 1977 section 4.2, pp 1–18

18. Lusted LB: Introduction to Medical Decision Making. Springfield, Ill., CC Thomas, 1968

19. Egan JP: Signal Detection Theory and ROC Analysis. New York, Academic Press, 1975

CHAPTER 22

Radiation Protection in Diagnostic Radiology

JOHN W. PAGEL

Medical radiation sources are unquestionably one of medicine's most important diagnostic tools. Because of its diagnostic value, the medical use of x-rays has expanded so that it now accounts for 90 percent of the man-made radiation dose to which the US population is exposed. Since radiation carries with it elements of risk it is important to obtain this diagnostic benefit with minimum exposure to the patient, the radiologic personnel concerned, and the general public. This chapter describes the radiation hazards attendant to the operation of x-ray equipment, and regulations and guidance for the use of this equipment.

RADIATION UNITS

The principal radiation units in current use at this time are defined in Table 22.1. The first of these, the roentgen, is the special unit for exposure. The exposure is a measure of the amount of ionization produced in a unit mass of air and is thus proportional to the quantity of x- or gamma-ray photons incident upon the air mass. The concept of exposure is functionally useful since it is relatively easy to measure. However, it is not defined for particulate radiations such as alpha or beta rays.

TABLE 22.1. **Radiation Units**

Unit	Description
R	The roentgen is the unit of exposure of x- or gamma radiation and is a measure of the amount of ionization produced in air. An exposure of 1 R produces 2.58×10^{-4} coulombs of charge per kg of air (or 1 esu per cm^3 of air at STP).
rad	The rad is the unit of absorbed dose. One rad is the absorption of 0.01 joule per kg (100 ergs per gram) in any irradiated material.
rem	The rem is the unit of dose equivalence and is numerically equivalent to the absorbed dose in rads multiplied by the quality factor and any other necessary modifying factors.

Another limitation of the roentgen that must be borne in mind is that it is not a measure of the total amount of radiation present. For example, an exposure of 1 R to a 100 cm^2 area of the body during an x-ray exam involves only half as much radiation as a 1 R exposure to a 200 cm^2 area. A roentgen-area product unit (such as R-cm^2) is sometimes employed to provide a more complete specification of the total quantity of radiation present.

The rad is a measure of the energy actually absorbed per unit mass of any material, and applies to any type of radiation. For x- and gamma rays, the absorbed dose per roentgen in soft tissues such as muscle or fat is about one rad; in other words, the number of roentgens is approximately equal to the number of rads. On the other hand, for tissues of higher atomic number such as bone, the amount of energy absorbed is dependent on the energy of the radiation. For 50 keV the rad/R ratio is 3.6; at this energy bone absorbs 3.6 times as much energy per gram as does soft tissue. At 100 keV this ratio is 1.5; above 150 keV, the ratio of rad/R is approximately 1.

Consider the practical problem of evaluating the absorbed dose to a patient from a diagnostic x-ray procedure. The absorbed dose is usually determined indirectly from measurements of the entrance exposure, that is, the exposure at the points of entrance of the radiation into the patient's body. If we are interested only in the soft-tissue dose, the rad/R factor can be taken to be 1 and the number of roentgens equals the number of rads. In evaluating the absorbed dose from entrance exposure measurements, however, several other factors must be considered. First, the radiation is attenuated as it passes through the patient. Thus the absorbed dose progressively decreases with depth (dose at exit side of the body may be only a few percent of that at the entrance side). Second, if more than one film is made or if fluoroscopy is performed, and if the same body area is not irradiated for all exposures, the total absorbed dose is not equal to the sum of the individual absorbed doses since the energy will be absorbed in different masses within the body. Absorbed doses are additive only if they refer to the same irradiated mass. This applies particularly when fluoroscopy is performed; for example, fluoroscopy for 5 minutes at an entrance exposure rate of 2 R/min does not result in an absorbed dose of 10 rads unless the beam position is stationary throughout the entire procedure.

Another point to remember is that the total amount of energy absorbed (and thus the potential biological harm) is dependent on the field size as well as the absorbed dose, since the latter is defined as energy absorbed per unit mass. For this reason, it is always desirable during an x-ray exam to maintain the smallest field size consistent with achieving the objectives of the exam.

The rem is the unit of dose equivalence and is used for purposes of radiation protection. The dose equivalence reflects the effectiveness of different radiations in producing the delayed biologic effects of radiation (cancer, genetic effects). For equal absorbed doses in rads, the greatest amount of damage will be produced by those radiations that release the largest amount of energy per unit track length, ie, have the greatest linear energy transfer (LET). The quality factor (Q) is the LET-dependent factor by which absorbed doses are multiplied to obtain the dose equivalent:

$$H(\text{rem}) = D(\text{rads}) \cdot Q \qquad (1)$$

Quality factors are listed in Table 22.2 for different types of radiation. An equal degree of biological risk should result from one rad of alpha particles or 10 rads of x-rays, since both are equal to 10 rem. Maximum allowable radiation doses are given in terms of rems; thus if a mixture of radiations has to be considered, allowance is made for their differing biologic effectiveness.

In experimental radiation biology, the term RBE (relative biologic effectiveness) is used instead of the quality factor. The RBE value depends not only on the type of radiation, but also on the particular biologic endpoint and organism investigated and the experimental conditions employed.

The units described above are those in current use at this time. However, in order to conform to the International System of Units, these units are scheduled to be replaced by new units in the 1980s. The roentgen is to be replaced by the coulomb per kilogram (1 R = 2.58×10^{-4} Ckg^{-1}), the rad replaced by the gray (1Gy = 1 joule kg^{-1} = 100 rads) and the rem is to be replaced by the sievert (1 Sv = 100 rem).

BIOLOGIC EFFECTS OF RADIATION

Roentgen announced his discovery of x-rays on January 4, 1896, and it was soon discovered that ionizing radiation produces harmful biologic effects. For example, consider the following experience related in *Science*:[10]

TO THE EDITOR OF SCIENCE:

As opportunity offered, experiments have been made in our laboratory with the x-rays since a few days after the appearance of Prof. Roentgen's paper.

The most interesting observation is a physiological effect of the x-rays. A month ago we were asked to undertake the location of a bullet in the head of a child that had been accidentally shot. On the 29th of February, Dr. William L. Dudley and I decided to make a preliminary test of photographing through the head with our rather weak apparatus before undertaking the surgical case. Accordingly, Dr. Dudley, with his characteristic devotion to the cause of science, lent himself to the experiment.

The tube was about one-half inch distant from his hair, and the exposure was one hour. The plate developed nothing; but yesterday, 21 days after the experiment, all the hair came out over the space under the x-ray discharge. The spot is now perfectly bald. We, and especially Dr. Dudley, shall watch with interest the ultimate effect.

JOHN DANIEL
PHYSICAL LABORATORY
VANDERBILT UNIVERSITY
MARCH 23, 1896

Epilation is an example of an acute effect of radiation, that is, an effect that occurs within the first month or two after irradiation. Other such early effects are listed in Table 22.3. Note that all of these require large doses of radiation and are unlikely to occur as the result of exposures received by patient or staff from diagnostic medical procedures. A possible exception is exposure to patients from extended fluoroscopies, or exposures from

TABLE 22.2. **Quality Factors For Various Radiations**[4]

Radiation	Q
X-rays, gamma rays, and electrons	1
Thermal neutrons	2.3
Neutrons, protons, and singly charged particles	10
Alpha particles and multiply charged particles	20

TABLE 22.3. **Acute Effects* of Radiation Exposure**

Organ/System	Dose (rads)	Effect
Gonads	50	May result in reduced fertility
	200	May produce temporary sterility (12 to 18 months)
	600–800	Permanent sterility
Skin	200	Erythema (first degree burn). Transient erythema may appear within hours, but major reddening appears in 2 to 3 weeks.
Hair	200	Epilation (loss of hair). Becomes apparent only 2 to 3 weeks after exposure.
	600	Hair may not regrow.
Blood	50	25 percent drop in platelet levels. Other changes in blood cell levels are also observed.
Whole body	300–400	$LD_{50/60}$ (lethal dose within 60 days to 50 percent of the population)—if whole body is exposed, and minimal treatment is given.
	500	$LD_{50/60}$—careful supportive treatment
	1000	LD_{100}—100 percent lethality, minimal treatment

*An acute or short-term effect is one which occurs within a month or two after exposure to radiation.

beryllium window x-ray tubes when the added filtration has been accidentally removed.

CARCINOGENIC EFFECTS OF RADIATION

The long-term or late effects of radiation exposure are generally of more concern since they may be induced by low levels of radiation. Probably the most significant of these effects is the increased likelihood of an irradiated individual developing a fatal malignancy. The appearance of a malignancy follows a latent period that averages about 2 years for leukemias and 15 years for solid tumors.[11] Current best estimates[4] place the risk of developing a fatal cancer at 10^{-4} per rad following whole body irradiation, or one fatal cancer per 10,000 man-rads of absorbed dose. Table 22.4 gives a breakdown of the risk with respect to cancer site. These risk factors are derived primarily from follow-up studies on the effects of rather large doses of radiation (generally more than 100 rads absorbed dose) on human population groups such as the Japanese survivors in Hiroshima and Nagasaki, and patients treated therapeutically for various conditions (thymic enlargement,

tinea capitis, ankylosing spondylitis, hyperthyroidism, cervical cancer, etc). The linearity hypothesis states that the risk per rad is the same at low doses as at high doses. This is probably an oversimplification, which results in an overestimate of the risk since it does not take into account a presumed greater efficiency of cellular repair processes at low doses and/or dose rates. For lack of definite evidence to the contrary, however, the estimates given in Table 22.4 should be assumed to apply regardless of the magnitude of the dose. Another conservative assumption is that there is no threshold for the induction of cancer by radiation; that is, any dose of radiation, no matter how small, carries with it some risk. This is the underlying rationale behind a basic operating principle in radiation protection, the ALARA philosophy, which states that all radiation exposures should be kept As Low As Reasonably Achievable.

GENETIC EFFECTS OF RADIATION

When cells are exposed to ionizing radiation, gene mutations and chromosome aberrations are produced.

TABLE 22.4. **Risk of Cancer for Various Organs**[4]

Cancer Site	Number of Fatal Cancers per Million per Rad
Leukemia	20
Breast	50 (females)
Lung	20
Thyroid	5
Bone	5
Other organs or tissues	50

Note: Average risk rate for both sexes and all ages is about 100×10^{-6} per rad; ie, 1 rad delivered to each of 1,000,000 people will result in 100 cancer deaths, which would be a 0.2 percent increase in the spontaneous death rate from cancer.

When such changes are induced in the germ cells of an individual, harmful effects may become evident in the descendants of the irradiated individual. Mutations, of course, also occur "spontaneously" in organisms, and every individual carries defective genes that tend to reduce his fitness to some degree. The effect of radiation on this natural mutation rate can be expressed by means of the doubling dose, which is the absorbed dose necessary to produce a mutation rate equal to that which occurs naturally. The United Nations Scientific Committee on the Effects of Atomic Radiation in its 1977 report has taken the doubling dose to be 100 rads, and has used this value to derive the risk estimates shown in Table 22.5. Due to a lack of human evidence of genetic effects, the results obtained with experimen-

tal animals, especially mice, form the basis for these risk assessments.

It is known that the female (mouse) is much less sensitive to genetic effects of radiation than is the male.[1] It has also been found that exposure at high dose rates produces more mutations per rad than exposure at a low or chronic dose rate. This is evidence of the repair mechanisms that occur within the cell nucleus. As is the case for the carcinogenic effects of radiation, it is assumed there is no radiation threshold for the induction of genetic effects.

RADIATION EFFECTS ON PRENATAL DEVELOPMENT

An individual in the prenatal stage of life is especially sensitive to the effects of ionizing radiation. A wide range of defects may result, the type of change produced being dependent on the stage of prenatal development at which irradiation occurs.

Prior to implantation of the conceptus in the uterine wall, the main risk from radiation is failure of implantation and death of the embryo. The risk factor for embryo death listed in Table 22.6 corresponds to a lethal dose to 50 percent of the population (LD_{50}) of 60 rem. There is little evidence of an increased frequency of induced abnormalities for this period.

During the period of major organogenesis, death of the embryo may still occur at high dose levels, but impairment of growth and the production of malformations are the major risks. As many as 24 types of abnormalities have been reported among children

TABLE 22.5. **Estimated Effect of 1 Rad per Generation of Low-Dose, Low-Dose-Rate, Low-Let Irradiation on a Population of One Million Live-Born Individuals*[11]**

Disease Classification	Current Incidence	Effect of 1 Rad per Generation	
		First Generation	Equilibrium
Autosomal dominant and X-linked diseases	10,000	20	100
Recessive diseases	1,100	Relatively slight	Very slow increase
Chromosomal diseases	4,000	38	40
Congenital anomalies Anomalies expressed later Constitutional and degenerative diseases	90,000	5	45
Total	105,200	63	185
Percentage of current incidence		0.06	0.17

*Assumed doubling dose, 100 rad

TABLE 22.6. **Risk Factors In Pregnancy**[13]

Period of Pregnancy	Major Risk	Risk Factor*
Preimplantation (0–8 days pc)	Death of embryo	80×10^{-4}
Organogenesis (9–40 days pc)	Malformations	50×10^{-4}
Fetal period (40–270 days pc)	Fatal malignancies in early childhood	2.3×10^{-4}

*Number of effects per rad dose. For example, exposure of 10^4 embryos to 1 rem each results in 80 embryo deaths.

irradiated in utero with relatively large doses; reduced head size (microcephaly) and mental retardation are the most commonly reported defects. The risk factor for the development of abnormalities is given in Table 22.6. This estimate is based on effects observed following doses of the order of 50 rads or more. The risk per rad for low doses is most likely considerably less, since studies of the effects of exposure during radiologic procedures have not shown a significantly increased incidence of malformations, and animal studies indicate there is less effect per rad at low doses than at high doses.

Irradiation with diagnostic x-rays during the fetal period of development has been shown to cause an increased death rate from malignant disease during the first 10 years of life. It may also result in some reduction in subsequent growth, in addition to microcephaly if the doses are high. The cancer risk for a fetus is about 50 percent greater than that for a female adult; a dose of 2 to 4 rads doubles the risk of a fatal cancer in the first ten years of life. Half of the malignancies are leukemias and about one-fourth are tumors of the nervous system.

RADIATION CATARACTS

Exposure of the lens of the eye to ionizing radiation may result in the formation of lens opacities, or cataracts. This is a well-known effect after therapeutic irradiations in the region of the orbit. For x-rays or gamma rays, the minimum cataractogenic dose is 200 to 500 rads when delivered in a single exposure, whereas a dose of more than 1,000 rads is required if the radiation is delivered over a period of time.[1] The latent period ranges from a couple of years to 10 years or more. The lower the dose, the longer the time after irradiation before onset of cataracts. Following small doses much below those necessary to impair vision, lens opacities of a minor degree may be detected by skilled examination. These minor opacities usually do

not progress in severity and may disappear with the passage of time.

MAXIMUM PERMISSIBLE OCCUPATIONAL DOSE

DOSE STANDARDS

Advisory agencies such as the ICRP (International Commission on Radiological Protection) and the NCRP (National Council on Radiation Protection and Measurements) have developed recommendations for maximum permissible dose equivalents (MPDs) for occupationally exposed workers. Review of numerous studies on effects of radiation forms the basis for these limits, which are designed to prevent all acute or threshold radiation injuries and reduce to acceptable levels all nonthreshold effects (cancer and genetic effects). The ICRP has the following to say concerning acceptable levels of risk:

> The Commission believes that for the forseeable future a valid method of judging the acceptability of the level of risk in radiation work is by comparing this risk with that for other occupations recognized as having high standards of safety, which are generally considered to be those in which the average mortality due to occupational hazards does not exceed 10^{-4}.
>
> In most occupations, fatalities, whether due to accidents or disease, are accompanied by a much larger number of less severe consequences. Radiation exposure, on the other hand, at levels imposed by adherence to recommended dose-equivalent limits, is expected to cause very few injuries or illnesses in exposed workers other than any malignant diseases which may be induced. In assessing the implication of dose-equivalent limits therefore the Commission believes that the calculated rate at which fatal malignancies might be induced by occupational exposure to radiation should in any case not exceed the occupational fatality rate of industries recognized as having high standards of safety.[4]

ICRP and NCRP recommendations form the basis for the dose standards established by state and federal regulatory agencies, as listed in Figure 22.1. Also shown in the figure are the dose limits for unrestricted areas and members of the public. The values for occupational exposure and members of the public exclude any dose received by an individual as a patient or from natural background radiation.

The risk to individuals exposed to the maximum permissible dose is very small. However, since it is assumed there is no dose threshold for certain effects,

Occupational Exposure: Whole body, head and trunk, active blood-forming organs, gonads, lens of eyes	Rems per Calendar Qtr. 1.25
Hands and forearms, feet and ankles	18.75
Skin of whole body	7.5
Minors (< 18 yrs of age)	10% of above limits
Fetus (from exposure of mother)*	0.5 in gestation period

Permissible Radiation Levels in Unrestricted Areas:
2 mrem/hr and 100 mrem/week

Population Dose Limits: Individual member of public	Rems per Year: 0.5
Population as a whole*	0.17

Figure 22.1. Dose standards or maximum permissible doses, as given by Nuclear Regulatory Commission regulations and suggested State Regulations for Control of Radiation. Additional NCRP recommendations are indicated by an asterisk.[14]

efforts should be made to reduce all exposures to a level as low as reasonably achievable (ALARA).

MONITORING REQUIREMENTS

All individuals who are likely to receive a dose in any calendar quarter in excess of 25 percent of the dose standards are required by regulation to be furnished with personnel monitoring equipment. In practice, most radiation workers will receive less than this. The mean annual dose for monitored workers in 1970 was only 200 mrem. It is strongly recommended, however, that personnel monitoring badges be furnished to each person who operates x-ray equipment or works in close proximity to such equipment. In addition to a body badge, a ring badge should be used if the fingers are close to the primary beam for any reason.

TYPES OF MONITORING BADGES

The principal types of personnel monitoring badges are the film badge and the TLD badge. For the former, the film density is proportional to the radiation dose; for the TLD (thermoluminescent dosimeter), the amount of light emitted by the heated TLD crystal is proportional to the amount of radiation energy absorbed. Film response is relatively energy dependent compared to TLD. For proper interpretation of the film density, a knowledge of the radiation energy is therefore needed. This is obtained by placing filters in the film holder to provide differential attenuation of the incident radiation. The relative amounts of attenuation are dependent on the radiation energy. Filters serve the additional function, for both the film and TLD badges, of distinguishing penetrating from nonpenetrating radiation, and thus provide values for both skin dose and whole body (penetrating) dose. Since TLDs do not require filters for energy determination purposes, they are preferable to film for ring badges, in which space for filters is limited.

Both film and TLD are capable of measuring absorbed doses from about 10 mrad to thousands of rads, and commercial suppliers of both types can achieve measurement accuracies as good as ±10 percent. However, the TLD badge is consistently more accurate than the film badge. The average reported value is within ±20 percent of the true value for TLD and about ±30 percent for film, as found in a study of commercial and in-house processors conducted by P. Plato in 1976.[15]

If a TLD reader is available on the premises, a TLD has the added advantages of providing fast readout capability for emergency situations and serving as a dosimetry system for monitoring patient exposures and making other exposure measurements. The TLD is also less likely to give false readings due to environmental perturbations such as heat, light, or pressure. On the other hand, film badge systems are less expensive and provide a permanent film record of exposures, which can be stored for possible future reference and reevaluation.

RECORD KEEPING

Records of radiation exposure of all individuals for whom personnel monitoring is required must be maintained indefinitely. At the request of any worker, personnel monitoring results must be made available to the worker at least annually. It is recommended that badge reports be posted on a monthly basis. Former radiation workers requesting a report of their exposure must be supplied this information within 30 days.

FUNCTIONS OF PERSONNEL MONITORING

The main pupose for monitoring is to obtain occupational absorbed dose information and provide assurance that dose limits are not exceeded. In addition, personnel monitoring can be used to observe trends in exposure, to serve as a check on working practice, to assess efforts to reduce exposure, and to assess the effectiveness of programs designed to maintain exposures ALARA.

PROTECTIVE BARRIERS

The walls, floor, and ceiling of an x-ray room must be of sufficient thickness to prevent personnel outside the room from receiving more than their applicable maximum permissible doses: 0.1 rem/wk (5 rem/yr) for occupationally exposed persons (controlled areas); 0.01 rem/wk (0.5 rem/yr) for noncontrolled areas (an area in which the exposure of persons to radiation is not controlled by a radiation protection supervisor).

Areas that are not part of the radiology department should not be declared controlled areas for the purpose of permitting a reduction in the protection requirements. It has been shown, in fact, that the cost of shielding will increase only 25 percent if all areas are shielded to a maximum dose of 0.01 rem per week.

Protective barriers can be classified as primary or secondary. A primary barrier is one that must provide protection against the useful (primary) beam. A secondary barrier must provide protection against only scattered radiation and the leakage radiation that has passed through the tube housing (Fig. 22.2).

The amount of radiation produced is directly proportional to the workload (W) of the room, expressed as mA-min per week of operation, and is also a function of the kilovoltage (kVp). Typical weekly workloads for (very) busy installations are given in Table 22.7. An operating potential of 100 kVp is generally assumed. When potentials greater than 100 kVp are used, the increased barrier transmission is normally offset by a reduction in the workload, since for a higher kVp fewer mA-seconds are required for an exposure.

The fraction of the workload for which the primary beam strikes a given barrier is the use factor (U). If the primary beam does not strike a barrier ($U=0$) or strikes it for only a fraction of the time, the shielding requirements are reduced. In determining the value of U,

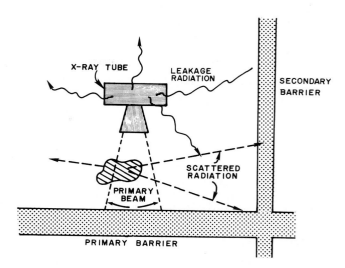

Figure 22.2. Sources of radiation in x-ray room and types of protective barriers. A primary barrier is one that can be struck by the primary beam; a secondary barrier is struck only by scattered and leakage radiation.

consideration needs to be given to the location of vertical cassette holders and the use of horizontal beam techniques. If specific values of U cannot be predicted when designing an x-ray room, the values given in Table 22.8 should be used. Note that use of values in Table 22.8 results in a total use factor of more than 1 ($U=2$ for a room with 4 walls and floor), meaning that some barriers will have more shielding than is really necessary. However, this does allow greater flexibility in future use of the room by allowing procedures not originally anticipated to be safely conducted.

If the primary beam never strikes the barrier, the use factor is 0 for the primary beam and only a secondary barrier is required. This will be the case for fluoroscopic units since the image intensifier system

TABLE 22.7. **Typical Weekly Workloads for Busy Installations[8]**

	Daily Patient Load	Weekly workload (W) mA-min		
		100 kV or less	125 kV	1250 kV
Admission chest (Miniature, with photo-timing grid)	100	100	—	—
Chest (14×17″, 3 films per patient, no grid)	60	150	—	—
Cystoscopy	8	600	—	—
Fluoroscopy including spot filming	24	1,500	600	300
Fluoroscopy without spot filming	24	1,000	400	200
Fluoroscopy with image intensification including spot filming	24	750	300	150
General radiography	24	1,000	400	200
Special procedures	8	700	280	140

TABLE 22.8. **Use Factors for Primary Protective Barriers*†§**

	Radiographic Installations	Therapy Installations
Floor	1	1
Walls	1/4	1/4
Ceiling	—‡	—§

*The use factor for secondary protective barriers is usually 1.

†To be used only if specific values for a given installation are not available.

‡The shielding requirements for the ceiling of a radiographic installation are determined by the secondary barrier requirements rather than by the use factor, which is generally extremely low.

§The use factor for the ceiling of a therapy installation depends on the type of equipment and techniques used, but usually is not more than 1/4.

serves as the primary barrier. The use factor is unity ($U = 1$) for scattered and leakage radiation since barriers in all directions will be irradiated by these sources of radiation, regardless of the direction of the primary beam.

Also to be considered is the fraction of the time that the area being shielded is occupied. Figure 22.3 should be consulted for values of the occupancy factor (T). For occupationally exposed persons in controlled areas the value of T is to taken to be 1. The effective workload for a given barrier is obtained by multiplying W by U and T, ie, WUT.

The distance from the source to the areas to be protected is another important factor since the exposure rate decreases as the square of the distance (inverse square law). If this distance is great enough, no shielding may be required.

After the above factors have been ascertained, the barrier requirements can be determined by using Tables 22.9, 22.10, and 22.11. If more than one source of radiation exists within the room, the barrier thickness must be increased. If the sources are of similar energy this is done by increasing the barrier thickness by one half-value layer (an HVL is the thickness required to reduce the exposure rate of a beam of radiation to one half). Half-value layers are listed in Table 22.13. If the required barrier thicknesses differ by at least one tenth-value layer (a TVL reduces exposure rate by a factor of 10), the thicker of the two will be adequate. Shielding requirements for rooms containing both radiographic and fluoroscopic equipment are usually determined by the radiographic requirements.

For situations not covered by the tables or for more precise determinations, the methods of computation given in Appendix B of NCRP Report No 49 should be used. For example, Tables 22.9 to 22.11 assume an average x-ray field area of 400 cm^2; if the actual field size is only 40 cm^2, the amount of radiation

scattered from the patient will be reduced by a factor of 10. Taking this into account can lead to smaller barrier thickness and cost savings.

In any case, it is best to have a qualified expert review all plans before construction commences to avoid expensive alterations thereafter. Commonly, diagnostic x-ray rooms are overshielded. As a rule of thumb, secondary barriers may require 1/32 in (0.8 mm) lead equivalent, and primary barriers, 1/16 in (1.6 mm). However, there are many cases in which less is required, and there is no requirement that the shielding be made of lead. Frequently the structural walls and floor are adequate (three to four inches of concrete is approximately equivalent to 1/32 in of lead).

The shielding must be installed so that there is no impairment of the protection at joints, openings for conduits and service boxes, etc. Shielding replaced or diminished by such openings must be compensated for. If lead is used, an overlap at joints of at least 1 cm is required. The shielding need not necessarily extend to the ceiling, but a minimum height of 7 feet is required.

The shielded operator's booth should be designed with several radiation safety requirements in mind. There should be adequate space for all control equipment and for several people. The operator should be able to see the patient from within the protected area for all radiographic exams to be performed within the

---

Full Occupancy (T = 1)

Work areas such as offices, laboratories, shops, wards, nurses' stations, living quarters, children's play areas, and occupied space in nearby building.

Partial Occupancy (T = 1/4)

Corridors, rest rooms, elevators using operators, unattended parking lots.

Occasional Occupancy (T = 1/16)

Waiting rooms, toilets, stairways, unattended elevators, janitors' closets, outside areas used only for pedestrians or vehicular traffic.

Figure 22.3. Occupancy factors for non-occupationally exposed persons.[8] The occupancy factor of occupationally exposed persons, in general, may be assumed to be one. It is advantageous in shielding design to take into account that the occupancy factor in areas adjacent to the radiation room usually is zero for any space more than 2.1 m (7 feet) above the floor, as the height of most individuals is less. It is possible, therefore, to reduce the thickness of the wall shielding above this height provided the radiation source is below 2.1 m (7 feet). In determining the shielding requirements for wall areas above 2.1 m (7 feet), consideration must be given to the protection of any persons occupying the floor above the area adjacent to the radiation room. This figure is for use as a guide in planning shielding where other occupancy data are not available.

TABLE 22.9. Minimum Shielding Requirements for Radiographic Installations[8]

WUT* in mA-min			Distance from Source to Occupied Area (m)										
100 kV[†]	125 kV[†]	150 kV[†]											
1,000	400	200	1.5	2.1	3.0	4.2	6.1	8.4	12.2				
500	200	100		1.5	2.1	3.0	4.2	6.1	8.4	12.2			
250	100	50			1.5	2.1	3.0	4.2	6.1	8.4	12.2		
125	50	25				1.5	2.1	3.0	4.2	6.1	8.4	12.2	
62.5	25	12.5					1.5	2.1	3.0	4.2	6.1	8.4	12.2

Type of Area	Material	Primary Protective Barrier Thickness[‖]										
Controlled	Lead, mm[‡]	1.95	1.65	1.4	1.15	0.9	0.65	0.45	0.3	0.2	0.1	0.1
Noncontrolled	Lead, mm[‡]	2.9	2.6	2.3	2.05	1.75	1.5	1.2	0.95	0.75	0.55	0.35
Controlled	Concrete, cm[§]	18.0	15.5	13.5	11.5	9.5	7.0	5.5	4.0	2.5	1.5	0.5
Noncontrolled	Concrete, cm[§]	25.0	23.0	20.5	18.5	16.5	14.0	12.0	10.0	8.0		

Type of Area	Material	Secondary Protective Barrier Thickness[‖]										
Controlled	Lead, mm[‡]	0.55	0.45	0.35	0.3	0	0	0	0	0	0	0
Noncontrolled	Lead, mm[‡]	1.3	1.05	0.75	0.55	0.45	0.35	0.3	0.05	0	0	0
Controlled	Concrete, cm[§]	5.0	3.5	2.5	2.0	0	0	0	0	0	0	0
Noncontrolled	Concrete, cm[§]	11.5	9.5	7.5	5.5	4	3	2	0.5	0	0	0

*W—weekly workload in mA min, U—use factor, T—occupancy factor.
[†]Peak pulsating x-ray tube potential.
[‡]See Table 22.12 for conversion of thickness in millimeters to inches.
[§]Thickness based on concrete density of 2.35 g-cm^{-3} (147 lb-ft^{-3}).
[‖]Barrier thickness based on 150 kV.

x-ray room. He or she should also be able to view any entry into the room. The viewing window should not be too close to the edge of the booth (a minimum of 18 in is recommended), and the exposure switches should be so located that they cannot be conveniently operated outside the booth. A door should be provided if the opening is so located that the radiation is not scattered at least twice before reaching the operator (ie, scattered from the patient and at least one other object such as the wall). In particular, consideration should be given to the proper location of chest stands and Franklin skull units.

TABLE 22.10. Shielding Requirements for Radiographic Film*[8]

Storage Period	Barrier Type	Distance from Source to Stored Film							
		2.1 m (7 ft)		3.0 m (10 ft)		4.2 m (14 ft)		6.1 m (20 ft)	
		Lead (mm)	Concrete[†] (cm)	Lead (mm)	Concrete[†] (cm)	Lead (mm)	Concrete[†] (cm)	Lead (mm)	Concrete[†] (cm)
1 day	Primary with use factor, U, of 1/16	2.3	19.5	2.1	18.0	1.8	15.5	1.5	13.5
1 week		3.0	24.0	2.7	22.0	2.4	20.5	2.2	18.5
1 month		3.7	29.0	3.4	27.0	3.1	24.0	2.8	23.0
1 day	Secondary with use factor, U, of 1	1.7	15.0	1.5	13.0	1.2	11.0	1.0	9.0
1 week		2.4	19.5	2.1	17.5	1.8	16.0	1.5	13.5
1 month		3.0	24.0	2.8	22.0	2.5	20.0	2.2	18.5

Note: In the absence of specific information as to the length of film storage period to be expected, it is suggested that the shielding value for the 1 month's storage period be used.
*Indicated thickness required to reduce radiation to 0.2 mR for a weekly workload of 1,000 mA min at 100 kV, 400 mA min at 125 kV, or 200 mA min at 150 kV (peak pulsating x-ray tube potential).
[†]Thickness based on concrete density of 2.35 g-cm^{-3} (147 lb-ft^{-3}).

TABLE 22.11. **Minimum Shielding Requirements for Fluoroscopic Installations[8]**

| WT* in mA-min | | | Distance from Source to Occupied Area (m) | | | | | | | | | | | |
100 kV†	125 kV†	150 kV†												
2,000	800	400	1.5	2.1	3.0	4.2	6.1	8.4	12.2					
1,000	400	200		1.5	2.1	3.0	4.2	6.1	8.4	12.2				
500	200	100			1.5	2.1	3.0	4.2	6.1	8.4	12.2			
250	100	50				1.5	2.1	3.0	4.2	6.1	8.4	12.2		
125	50	25					1.5	2.1	3.0	4.2	6.1	8.4	12.2	
62.5	25	12.5						1.5	2.1	3.0	4.2	6.1	8.4	12.2

Type of Area	Material	Secondary Protective Barrier Thickness											
Controlled	Lead, mm‡	0.75	0.6	0.45	0.35	0.3	0.05	0	0	0	0	0	0
Noncontrolled	Lead, mm‡	1.6	1.3	1.05	0.75	0.6	0.45	0.4	0.35	0.05	0	0	0
Controlled	Concrete, cm§	7.5	5.5	4	3	2.5	0.5	0	0	0	0	0	0
Noncontrolled	Concrete, cm§	14	12	10	8	6	4.5	3.5	2.5	0.5	0	0	0

*W—weekly workload in mA min, T—occupancy factor.
†Peak pulsating x-ray tube potential.
‡See Table 22.12 for conversion of thickness in millimeters to inches.
§Thickness based on concrete density of 2.35 g-cm^{-3} (147 lb-ft^{-3}).

Viewing windows are generally made of lead glass. Ordinary plate glass should be used only if the protection requirements are minimal, since the thickness required may be considerable. The composition and density of plate glass are similar to those of concrete, and the thicknesses required are therefore about the same as those calculated for concrete. This means that for the rule-of-thumb secondary barrier thickness of 1/32 in Pb, or 3 in concrete, the required glass thickness is 3 in.

Following construction, all new or modified installations require a radiation protection survey to document that the shielding is adequate and is in compliance with applicable regulations. A resurvey must be made after every change that might significantly decrease the radiation protection.

RADIATION PROTECTION RULES AND GUIDELINES

When doses are maintained below the maximum permissible levels, the biologic effects of radiation that are of concern are assumed for radiation protection purposes to have no threshold; that is, there is no absolutely safe level of radiation. Therefore it is prudent to maintain all doses ALARA, even though the absolute risk is considered to be very small.

Sources of Stray Radiation in the X-ray Room. Stray radiation is defined as the sum of scattered radiation plus tube leakage radiation. The principal source of stray radiation is the Compton scattering of the primary beam by the patient. In other words, *the irradiated area of the patient* is an x-ray source, and radiation protection efforts are to a large extent di-

rected at reducing the exposure from this source. Figures 22.4 and 22.5 show some typical stray radiation levels encountered during fluoroscopy procedures. It is obvious that the maximum permissible dose (MPD) of 100 mrem per week can be exceeded easily if proper precautionary efforts are not taken. Three key concepts

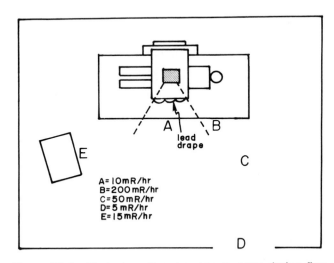

A = 10 mR/hr
B = 200 mR/hr
C = 50 mR/hr
D = 5 mR/hr
E = 15 mR/hr

Figure 22.4. Typical scattered exposure rates during fluoroscopy. Primary beam is incident on shaded area of patient, which acts as source of scattered radiation. The lead drapes provide protection for individuals positioned between the dashed lines. A person positioned at B could reduce their exposure by moving into the shielded area, using a lead drape that extends around the side of the image intensifier stand, using a mobile screen, or simply stepping back to position C. The equipment operator at E may often have their back to the radiation source and should take steps to shield their back (eg, wraparound apron). The door at D should always be closed.

in dose reduction are summarized by the words *time*, *distance*, and *shielding*. These will be explained and developed below.

PROTECTIVE APPAREL AND OTHER SHIELDING DEVICES

Each person in the x-ray room during an x-ray exposure must be shielded by protective aprons or whole body barriers; in addition, lead gloves should always be used during any procedures in which the hands approach the primary beam. Protective aprons and gloves must be of at least 0.25 mm lead equivalency, meaning that the attenuation factor will be 10 to 50 or more, depending on radiation energy. Proper care and handling of aprons will prolong their useful life. Aprons should never be folded, since this can lead to creases and ultimately cracks. The Joint Commission on Accreditation of Hospitals requires that aprons, gonadal shields, and leaded gloves be inspected at least annually for safety defects. Fluoroscopic examination of these items will reveal cracks and pinholes not

TABLE 22.13. Half-Value and Tenth-Value Layers*[8]

| Peak Voltage (kV) | Attenuation Material | | | |
| | Lead (mm) | | Concrete (cm) | |
	HVL	TVL	HVL	TVL
50	0.06	0.17	0.43	1.5
70	0.17	0.52	0.84	2.8
100	0.27	0.88	1.6	5.3
125	0.28	0.93	2.0	6.6
150	0.30	0.99	2.24	7.4
200	0.52	1.7	2.5	8.4

*Approximate values obtained at high attenuation for the indicated peak voltage values under broad-beam conditions; with low attenuation these values will be significantly less.

otherwise visible. The pinholes are relatively insignificant. The most serious deficiency in an apron is an inadequate or missing apron strap, since lack of a secure means of keeping an apron in place can allow a much larger portion of the wearer's body to be exposed to radiation than a hundred cracks or pinholes.

Supplementing the requirements for protective apparel are equipment design requirements. Fluoroscopic tables must have shielding devices such as lead drapes or folding panels (minimum 0.25-mm lead equivalent), which will intercept radiation scattered from above the table. An exception to this requirement is allowed for some special procedures in which a sterile field is necessary, but only if sterilized prefitted covers cannot be used for the barriers. A large amount of scattered

TABLE 22.12. Commercial Lead Sheets[8]

| Thickness | | Weight (lb) for 1 Ft² Section | |
Inches	Millimeters	Nominal Weight	Actual Weight
1/64	0.40	1	0.92
3/128	0.60	1.5	1.38
1/32	0.79	2	1.85
5/128	1.00	2.5	2.31
3/64	1.19	3	2.76
7/128	1.39	3.5	3.22
—	1.50	—	3.48
1/16	1.58	4	3.69
5/64	1.98	5	4.60
3/32	2.38	6	5.53
—	2.50	—	5.80
—	3.00	—	6.98
1/8	3.17	8	7.38
5/32	3.97	10	9.22
3/16	4.76	12	11.06
7/32	5.55	14	12.90
1/4	6.35	16	14.75
1/3	8.47	20	19.66
2/5	10.76	24	23.60
1/2	12.70	30	29.50
2/3	16.93	40	39.33
1	25.40	60	59.00

1. The density of commercially rolled lead is 11.36 g/cm^{-3}.*
2. The commercial tolerances are ±0.005 inches for lead up to 7/128 and ±1/32 for heavier sheets.*
3. It should be noted that lead sheet less than 1/32 inch thick is frequently more expensive than heavier sheet in cost of material and cost of installation.

*Lead Industries Association, Inc, New York, New York.

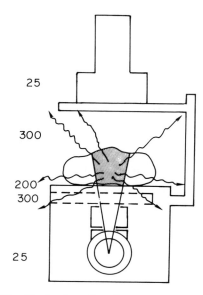

Figure 22.5. Vertical profile of exposure rates next to fluoroscopy table. Numbers give exposure rates in mR/hr. The primary beam rate, at patient skin entrance, is typically 1 to 3 R/min (60,000 to 180,000 mR/hr), but may be as high as 10 R/min (600,000 mR/hr).

radiation also occurs beneath the tabletop level. Since primary beam exposure rate is much greater at the beam entrance or lower part of the patient than the beam exit side of the patient, the amount of scattered radiation produced by the underside of the patient is also much greater. A shield or cone extending from the tube housing to tabletop level can be used to intercept this radiation. If the table has a Bucky tray, the exposure rate through the Bucky slot, which is at approximately gonad level, can be quite high. A Bucky slot cover is required and should always be used during fluoroscopy.

Proper utilization of this existing shielding will aid in keeping exposure of the eyes to a low level. The area directly above the image intensifier assembly, for example, is a shielded area. The important operational rule is to avoid looking directly at the area of the patient that is producing the scattered radiation. Since both light and x-rays travel in a straight line, if an individual is positioned so that the irradiated area of the patient can be seen, then the radiation scattered from the patient is reaching the observer's eyes (Fig. 22.5). Auxiliary eye shielding is often desirable for individuals, whether student or staff, who must be in a position to observe lengthy procedures. Eyeglasses with lead glass lenses are commercially available; these are designed to attenuate more than 90 percent of incident radiation. Ordinary eyeglasses, if they have glass lenses, will attenuate diagnostic quality x-radiation by 30 to 40 percent. Mobile screens with viewing windows are an excellent means of providing shielding for the eyes and the entire body.

TUBE LEAKAGE

Leakage radiation is radiation that penetrates the protective housing surrounding the x-ray tube. For a diagnostic x-ray tube, the tube housing assembly must be so constructed that the leakage radiation at a distance of one meter in any direction from the tube target is less than 100 mR in one hour, when the x-ray tube is operated at its maximum continuous tube current for the maximum rated tube potential. This means that the leakage radiation will be less than 100 mR in an hour for any of the specified ratings of the tube, and for most operating conditions the amount of leakage will be far less. Cones, diaphragms, or adjustable collimators used to restrict the primary beam must provide the same degree of protection.

UTILIZATION OF TIME TO LIMIT EXPOSURE

The exposure received by operators of x-ray equipment is directly proportional to the duration of an exposure or the time spent near the source of radiation.

Patient exposure is also, of course, proportional to the exposure time and in order to make a fluoroscopist aware of the amount of exposure time, fluoroscopic units are required to be equipped with cumulative timers. The timer may be set for any time up to five minutes; upon completion of the preset time, a continuous audible signal must sound until the timer is reset. (Older timers may be designed to interrupt or terminate the exposure.)

DISTANCE PROTECTION

A very important and effective means of reducing radiation exposure is to increase distance from the radiation source. The inverse square law holds approximately, ie, the exposure rate decreases with the square of the distance. For example, if an individual is originally one foot from a source of radiation, simply increasing this distance to 4 feet will result in a $(4 \text{ ft}/1 \text{ ft})^2 = 16$-fold decrease in the exposure rate. This is the same dose reduction that would result from wearing an additional lead apron, but has the added advantage of reducing exposure to all parts of the body. Changes in distance from the source are most important when near to the radiation source: increasing separation by 3 feet over an initial distance of 12 feet from a source will lead to only a 36 percent decrease in exposure.

INFLUENCE OF FIELD SIZE

The amount of scattered radiation will be directly proportional to the area of the x-ray field. For example, increasing fluoroscopic field size from 3 in×3 in, at tabletop level, to 4 in×4 in, will lead to an increase in the amount of scattered radiation by almost 80 percent, since the area increases by $16 \text{ in}^2/9 \text{ in}^2 = 1.78$. The x-ray field size should never be larger than is diagnostically necessary.

AUTHORIZED PERSONNEL IN X-RAY ROOM

Only persons whose presence is needed should be in the room while an x-ray exposure is being made. During fluoroscopy, the operator should require all nonessential personnel to leave the room, or at least the immediate area, before operating the unit. For radiographic exposures no one ordinarily should be in the x-ray room; the operator is required to remain completely behind the protective barrier.

X-RAY CONTROLS

An x-ray control panel must always be located in a shielded area, either outside the x-ray room or in a shielded control booth, and located so that the operator readily can see the patient during the entire exposure. It is also desirable to have a view of all entrances to the room. Radiographic exposure switches must be arranged so that they cannot be conveniently operated by the technologist outside the shielded area. It is sometimes necessary to chain the switch to the control panel if it is installed with a long exposure cord.

Exposure controls must permit an operator to terminate an exposure prematurely whenever necessary (at least for exposure times exceeding 1/2 second). Usually a radiographic switch is of the dead man type, requiring continuous pressure from the operator to complete an exposure. Fluoroscopic switches are always of the dead man type.

FLUOROSCOPIC BEAM PRIMARY BARRIER

The primary barrier for a fluoroscopic tube is the image intensifier assembly. The beam size consequently must be limited so that its entire cross section is intercepted by the primary barrier. Interlocks or permanent mounting of tube and barrier must assure that no x-rays can be produced unless the primary barrier is in position to intercept the beam.

SPECIAL PROCEDURES

Many special procedure examinations involve extensive use of both fluoroscopy and radiography, which can mean potentially large exposures for participating personnel. For these exams it is particularly important to observe all radiation protection precautions. All personnel whose immediate presence is not needed should maintain as much distance as possible from the patient while x-rays are being produced. Full use should be made of all protective devices, and a mobile protective screen is often desirable. The potential exposure from the radiography portion of the procedure must also be appreciated. For example, consider a renal arteriogram that includes 10 minutes of fluoroscopy at 2 mA and 24 films at 50 mA per film, or 1,200 mA from each mode of operation. If other factors such as beam quality are also the same for the two modes, the amount of scattered radiation will then be proportional only to the solid angles subtended by the x-ray beams, which are much greater for radiography than for fluoroscopy because of the large film size which is used for radiography.

PREGNANT EMPLOYEES

Exposure of a fetus needs to be kept to the lowest practicable level. If a pregnant female must be in the x-ray room while exposures are being made, extra shielding should be utilized (eg, wraparound apron, lead-lined girdle, or simply an apron with greater lead equivalency). Since the bulk of exposure received by x-ray personnel comes from fluoroscopy procedures, fluoroscopy duties should be minimized.

PATIENT HOLDING

When a patient must be held in position for radiography, mechanical supporting or restraining devices should be used whenever possible. It is especially important that such devices be available for pediatric radiography. If the patient must be held by an individual, that individual must be protected with appropriate shielding devices such as protective gloves and apron, and should keep his or her body as far as possible from the edge of the useful beam. Pregnant women and minors must not be used for this purpose, and no individual should be employed on a consistent or routine basis.

MOBILE X-RAY EQUIPMENT

Usage. Mobile equipment should not be used for examinations when it is practical to transfer the patient to a shielded x-ray room.

Other Personnel in Room. Non-necessary personnel should leave the room if possible and verbal warning should be given to alert others prior to the production of x-rays. The x-ray beam should be directed away from other personnel in the room. Patients who cannot be removed from the room should be protected from direct scatter radiation by whole body protective barriers or should be so positioned that they are at least 2 meters from both the tube head and the image receptor (the film or image intensifier).

Apron, Distance. The operator and ancillary personnel should stand as far as possible from the patient and the tube, and must wear protective aprons or stand behind a protective shield.

Collimation. Mobile radiographic units must be equipped with a light localizer, which defines the x-ray field. Proper collimation should be used to restrict the x-ray beam as much as possible to the clinical area of interest and within the dimensions of the image receptor. Under no circumstances should the collimator jaws be fully opened as a method of assuring full film coverage.

Patient or Film Holding. When a patient or film must be held for an exposure, lead aprons and lead gloves (if the hands are near the primary beam) must be worn. Mechanical holding devices should be used whenever possible. It is desirable to maintain a patient holding record to make sure no one person is used to hold film or patient too often. This record should include name of person, exam performed, and date.

Gonad Shielding. Gonadal shielding should be carried with the unit and used with patients who have not passed the reproductive age, for those procedures in which gonads are in the direct beam, except where this would interfere with the diagnostic procedure.

RADIATION QUALITY

The term *radiation quality* refers to the penetrating ability and absorption characteristics of an x-ray beam and is most completely described by means of a spectral distribution giving exposure or number of photons as a function of photon energy. Clinically, however, the usual measure of a beam's quality is its half-value layer (HVL), which is that thickness of a given material required to reduce the exposure rate to one-half. The HVL can in turn be related to an effective beam energy (Fig. 22.6), defined as the energy of a monoenergetic beam, which is attenuated at the same rate as the polyenergetic x-ray beam. The incident beam has an effective energy of 25 to 40 keV for most applications in diagnostic radiology.

TUBE POTENTIAL

Since a kVp increase results in an increase in the maximum and average beam energy, the penetrating power and HVL of the beam also increase. Figure 22.7 illustrates the relationship between half-value layer and peak tube potential.

VOLTAGE WAVEFORM

With a single phase generator the voltage decreases to zero during each pulse, whereas the voltage remains relatively constant with a three-phase generator. This

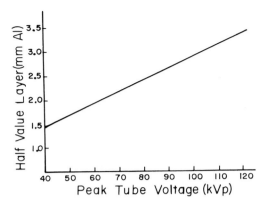

Figure 22.7. HVL is dependent on the peak tube potential. The relationship shown here is for a single-phase generator with 2.5-mm aluminum equivalent filtration in the beam.

results in a greater average energy for the three-phase generator. The HVL is consequently greater (about 15 percent) than for a single-phase generator operated at the same peak potential.

FILTRATION

A filter preferentially attenuates the lower energy components of the x-ray spectrum. This results in an increase in the effective energy and the HVL. Figure 22.8 shows the HVLs obtained with various combinations of filtration and kVp. The total filtration of the beam is defined as the sum of the inherent filtration and any added filtration. Inherent filtration is made up of those materials permanently located in the x-ray

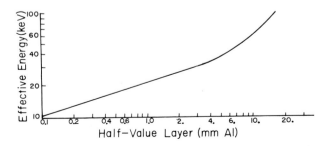

Figure 22.6. Effective energy of x-ray beam as a function of its half-value layer. The effective energy is equal to the energy of a monoenergetic beam of radiation having the same HVL as the x-ray beam.[18]

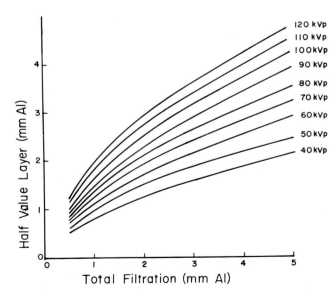

Figure 22.8. Half-value layers as a function of filtration and peak tube potential for single-phase, full-wave rectified units.[19]

beam. For example, the filtration provided by the tube window is generally equivalent to 0.5 to 1 mm Al. Collimators equipped with light localizers, which position mirrors in the path of the beam, may contribute another millimeter or so to the inherent filtration. Added filtration may be necessary to increase the total filtration to at least the minimum level required by the radiation protection regulations shown in Table 22.14.

From a radiation protection standpoint it is desirable to use as much filtration as possible since filtration tends to remove lower energy components of the x-ray beam, which would otherwise be absorbed by the superficial tissues of the patient and contribute little to the diagnostic information reaching the image receptor. Other considerations, however, place practical limits on the amount of filtration that can be added. Since the exposure rate decreases as the amount of filtration in the beam is increased, the mA per exposure would have to be increased somewhat to maintain a constant film exposure. Thus the x-ray generator capacity may be a limiting factor. Another factor is the degree of image contrast required. The radiographic contrast decreases as the HVL increases, and this may reduce the amount of obtainable diagnostic information. Although there are no official upper limits for HVLs, recommendations for reducing beam quality are sometimes in order. For example, the Bureau of Radiological Health's BENT program for assessing mammography techniques and exposures has established a normal range of values according to the following criteria:

IMAGE RECEPTOR	ACCEPTABLE HVL RANGE
Film	0.3-1.0 mm Al
Xeroradiography	0.8-3.0 mm Al

If an x-ray system is to be operated over a range of potentials and filtrations, it is recommended that the system be equipped with filter interlock switches, which will prevent x-ray emission if the minimum required filtration is not in place. Particular care is necessary if the x-ray tube has a beryllium window. Such tubes with no added filtration emit low energy x-rays at very high exposure rates. Patients have received doses of hundreds

TABLE 22.14.[3] Required Filtration for Diagnostic X-ray Units

Operating kVp	Minimum Total Filtration*
<50 kVp	0.5 mm Al
50-70 kVp	1.5 mm Al
>70 kVp	2.5 mm Al

*These requirements may alternatively be expressed in terms of half-value layers. The BRH requires that certified diagnostic equipment have HVLs not less than those shown in Table 22.15.

TABLE 22.15[2]. Half-Value Layer Requirements for Diagnostic X-ray Units

Design Operating Range (kilovolts peak)	Measured Potential (kilovolts peak)	Half-Value Layer (millimeters of aluminum)
<50	30	0.3
	40	0.4
	49	0.5
50 to 70	50	1.2
	60	1.3
	70	1.5
>70	71	2.1
	80	2.3
	90	2.5
	100	2.7
	110	3.0
	120	3.2
	130	3.5
	140	3.8
	150	4.1

of rads, leading to blistering and other skin conditions, when filtration has been inadvertently left off beryllium window tubes.

HALF-VALUE LAYER MEASUREMENT

HVLs are measured by placing varying thicknesses of attenuator between the x-ray tube and an ionization chamber detector positioned to measure the transmitted radiation. An attenuation curve such as that shown in Figure 22.9 can then be drawn, and the HVL can be read from this curve. Here it is seen to be 2.1 mm Al. The second half-value layer, defined as the thickness necessary to reduce the exposure from 50

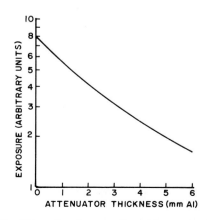

Figure 22.9. Example of x-ray attenuation curve. HVL is 2.1 mm Al. Second HVL is 5.0−2.1 = 2.9 mm Al.

percent to 25 percent of the initial value, is greater than the first HVL because of the beam "hardening" effect of the initial 2.1 mm Al. For a monoenergetic beam no beam hardening occurs, and the first and second HVLs are equal.

When these measurements are performed, narrow beam geometry conditions are necessary so that only radiation in the primary beam is incident on the chamber. If a large field size were to be used, the apparent HVL would be greater due to the increase in the amount of scattered radiation from outlying areas of the attenuator as the attenuator thickness is increased. Narrow-beam geometry is obtained when the field size is only slightly greater than the area of the chamber, and the source–chamber distance is at least 50 cm. The attenuating material should be placed approximately halfway between the source and ion chamber.

PROTECTION OF THE PATIENT

Protection of the patient can be achieved through technical, clinical and administrative means. The general rule is that all radiation exposures should be kept to a minimum and no patient should be exposed unnecessarily.

X-RAY BEAM COLLIMATION AND ALIGNMENT

The x-ray beam should always be limited to the smallest possible size consistent with the clinical objectives of the examination. In no case should it be larger than the film size or the area visible on the television monitor, since any portion of the x-ray field lying outside the image receptor can yield no diagnostic information and represents totally unnecessary patient exposure. Limitation of the x-ray beam is one of the most important and readily effected technical methods for limiting irradiation of a patient. Historically, however, excessive field sizes have been all too common and have been a significant contributor to unnecessary radiation exposure. Data from the 1970 x-ray exposure study of the US Public Health Service[20] showed that the genetically significant dose could be reduced 21 percent if the beam size were reduced to the film size. Reduction of field size also reduces the amount of scatter radiation, thereby improving image detail and contrast.

It is important that the technologist (and radiologist) understand the importance of using proper collimation techniques and that these techniques be routinely practiced. The appearance of an unexposed border on each radiograph has been adopted as a requirement by many institutions as a means of provid-

ing evidence that the x-ray field has been properly limited.

Proper alignment of the x-ray beam is also important, especially if the clinical area of interest lies close to the gonadal area or if infants are being examined (infant gonads are always close to the primary beam). The distance from the nearest edge of the beam to the gonads should be kept as great as possible.

Adjustable Radiographic Collimators. Mobile units and stationary units classified as general purpose (ie, not designed for examination of a specific anatomical region) must be equipped with adjustable collimators that possess beam-defining light fields. The edges of the light field are required to coincide with the edges of the x-ray field to within 2 percent of the source-to-film distance used, as illustrated in Figure 22.10. An additional requirement for stationary units is that they indicate numerically the field size with an accuracy equal to 2 percent of the source-to-film distance. For example, if the field size indicator is set for 8 × 8 in at a 40 in SID, the linear dimensions of the x-ray field can be no less than 7.2 in nor any greater than 8.8 in.

Fixed Collimators or Cones. It is important to label clearly the removable fixed-aperture beam-limiting devices with the combination of the film size and source-to-image-receptor distance (SID) for which they are intended, to help prevent inadvertent use of the wrong cone. A cone designed for an adult chest could provide nearly whole-body exposure if used with a small child. If an assortment of cones is being used with a special-purpose x-ray system, no dimension of the x-ray field can exceed that of the film by more than 2 percent of

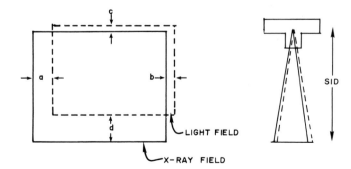

Figure 22.10. Alignment of light field with respect to x-ray field for a radiographic unit equipped with a beam-defining light. Requirement: the total misalignment of the edges of the light field with the respective edges of the x-ray field along either the length or the width shall not exceed 2 percent of the distance from the source to the center of the field, ie, $a + b \leqslant 0.02$ SID and $c + d \leqslant 0.02$ SID, where SID is source-to-image-receptor distance.

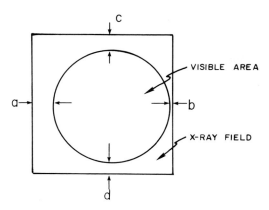

Figure 22.11. Maximum allowable x-ray field size for fluoroscopic x-ray unit. "Visible area" refers to field visible on TV monitor. Requirement: $a + b \leqslant 0.03$ SID, $c + d \leqslant 0.03$ SID, and $a + b + c + d \leqslant 0.04$ SID.

the SID. If the x-ray system is designed for only one image-receptor size at a fixed SID, current regulations permit no overlap of x-ray field with respect to the film.

Positive Beam Limitations. Certified stationary general purpose x-ray equipment must—with certain exceptions—provide positive beam limitations, which will prevent x-ray production when the x-ray field exceeds the dimensions of the image receptor by an excessive amount (the same tolerances as given in Figure 22.11 for fluoroscopic fields).

Collimation and Alignment for Fluoroscopic Systems. For any SID that can be used, neither the length nor the width of the x-ray field shall exceed the visible area by more than 3 percent of the SID, and the sum of the excess length and the excess width shall be no greater than 4 percent of the SID (Fig. 22.11). Provision must also be made to permit further limitation of the field size.

EXPOSURE RATE LIMITS IN FLUOROSCOPY

The exposure as measured at the point where the primary beam enters the patient must not exceed 10 roentgens per minute, except during recording of fluoroscopic images or when there is a provision for optional high-level control. If a high-level control is provided, there is no exposure rate limit; however, in order to exceed 5 R per minute there must be a special means of activation, such as additional pressure applied continuously, in order to avoid accidental use. In addition, there must be a continuous signal audible to the fluoroscopist.

TECHNIQUE FACTORS (kVp, mA, FILTRATION)

Technique factors should have as their objective the minimization of patient dose, consistent with the diagnostic objectives of the study. Tube potential and filtration should be as great as is practical, balanced against the consideration that contrast and resolving power decrease as beam quality increases. Technique protocols, in addition to describing patient preparation requirements and procedures for all standard radiographic projections, also should include technique charts. Knowledge of correct exposure factors will reduce the need for repeat studies.

For radiography, the technique factors to be used during an exposure must be indicated on the control panel prior to the exposure. The technique factors are the conditions of operation and include the peak tube potential in kV, the tube current in mA, and exposure time in seconds, or the quantity of charge in mAs. If the control panel operates more than one radiographic tube, the tube which is energized must be indicated. There must also be a visible indication (light or milliammeter) whenever x-rays are produced and an audible signal to inform the operator that the exposure has been completed.

Although at the present time there are no general regulations governing accuracy of technique factors, it is recommended that they be calibrated to within ± 10 percent of their actual values. For certified equipment the technique factors must not differ from the indicated values by more than whatever limit has been specified by the manufacturer. Certified radiographic equipment must also satisfy requirements for linearity and reproducibility of exposures. The coefficient of variation (standard deviation divided by the mean value) of a series of exposures made with the same technique factors must not exceed 0.05. This means that 95 percent or more of the radiation exposures will be within ± 10 percent of the average. Linearity refers to the x-ray output varying in direct proportion to the tube current setting. The linearity requirement is that the mR/mAs values obtained at any two consecutive tube current settings must not differ by more than 20 percent of the average mR/mAs for the two settings:

$$X_1 - X_2 < 0.2 X_{avg} = 0.2 \frac{(X_1 + X_2)}{2} \qquad (2)$$

where $X_1 = $ mR/mAs at setting 1 and $X_2 = $ mR/mAs at setting 2.

OTHER TECHNICAL FACTORS AFFECTING PATIENT EXPOSURES

Screens and Films. Image recording devices should be as sensitive as possible, consistent with the requirements of the examination. Slow, high-definition screens or nonscreen films should be used only when high resolution is required. Rare-earth screens should definitely be considered; they may reduce patient exposure by 2 to 10 times or more compared to a par speed screen and provide comparable resolution. Their use is especially recommended in situations in which it is particularly important that exposures be kept low, such as pediatric radiography. Inspection and cleaning of screens and cassettes on a regular basis is an important part of an effective quality control program. Damaged screens and faulty cassettes should be repaired or replaced. Tests for screen–film contact should be made for all cassettes of 11 in $\times$ 14 in size or larger.

Grids. The use of grids can improve the diagnostic quality of films by reducing the amount of scattered radiation reaching the film. Since they absorb some of the direct beam radiation, they also increase patient dosage. When grids are used it is recommended that a fast film–screen image recording system be employed. Care is also necessary to properly align focused grids in order to prevent underexposed or shaded films and consequent retakes. If only a small area is being examined, a sufficient amount of scattered radiation reduction can be achieved by simply limiting the field size; in this case a grid is not recommended.

Source-to-Skin Distance (SSD). The smaller the SSD, the greater will be the skin exposure per given exposure to the image receptor (Fig. 22.12). Use of too small an SSD could result potentially in skin exposures of a magnitude that would produce acute skin effects such as erythema and epilation. The SSD employed in a medical exam should be as great as is practical. The minimum SSD must be physically restricted to within the following limits (for certified equipment): mobile radiographic—30 cm; mobile fluoroscopes—30 cm; stationary fluoroscopes—38 cm; fluoroscopes used for specific surgical applications—20 cm.

Automatic Exposure Controls. Any phototiming or other automatic exposure termination control must be able to respond or terminate a radiation exposure within 1/60 second. It must also terminate any radiation exposure when it reaches 600 mAs or 60 kWs (kWs = kVp $\times$ A $\times$ sec).

EXPOSURE OF WOMEN
OF REPRODUCTIVE POTENTIAL

All radiologic examinations should be kept to a minimum during pregnancy. This applies particularly to examinations of the lower abdomen or pelvic area. Examination of the urinary tract, pelvimetry, hysterosalpinography, and radiologic examinations for esti-

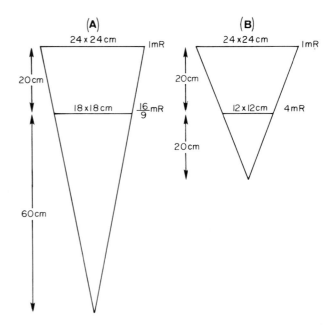

Figure 22.12. Radiation exposure in plane of skin surface for different source–skin distances (SSD). To achieve a value of 1 mR at the image receptor an exposure of 16/9 mR would be necessary at the skin surface for case A: $I_1d_1^2 = I_2d_2^2$ (inverse square law), thus, 1 mR $\times$ (80 cm)^2 = I_2 (60 cm)^2, or $I_2 = \dfrac{I \times 80^2}{60^2} = \dfrac{16 \text{ mR}}{9}$. For case B, a value of 4 mR would be necessary. Thus a relatively short SSD implies a relatively high value for the exposure at the skin surface. The integral dose (Roentgen-area product) is the same in each case, however: (A) (18 $\times$ 18) cm^2 $\times$ 16/9 mR = 576 mR-cm^2 and (B) (12 $\times$ 12) cm^2 $\times$ 4 mR = 576 mR-cm^2. This assumes no attenuation by the patient. If the patient attenuation factor is 100, the values for exposure and integral dose at skin surface should each by multiplied by 100.

mation of fetal maturity should be performed only when there is a clear need. On the other hand, x-ray examinations for breech presentation, multiple pregnancy, and other suspected fetal abnormalities are often fully justified. If an exam is performed on a pregnant patient, special efforts should be made to reduce the fetal dose as much as possible, such as by minimizing the number of views and carefully collimating the x-ray field to the region of interest. Since a patient with a recognized pregnancy is generally at least a month or two pregnant, the major risk to the fetus is that of radiation carcinogenesis. An absorbed dose of 4 rads to the fetus will double the natural probability (1 in 1,000) of a fatal childhood malignancy.

Safeguards must also be observed to prevent accidental irradiation of an early undiagnosed pregnancy. All women of reproductive potential need to be regarded as potentially pregnant. The ICRP has pointed out that the 10-day interval following onset of menstruation is the time when it is least probable that a woman could be pregnant, and has recommended that all examinations of the pelvis and lower abdomen not in connection with the immediate illness of the patient be postponed to this period. This is known as the 10-day rule. It requires that inquiry be made concerning the recent menstrual history of the patient. If one is willing to accept the additional hazard of a possibly increased incidence of early (undetectable) embryonic death from irradiation during the first 11 days postconception, then such exams could be performed at any time during the first 21 days of the menstrual cycle (21-day rule).

It has also been recommended by the NCRP that even for those cases in which pregnancy is not suspected, the patient should be advised that she should not run the risk of pregnancy until two months after an examination of the abdomen or pelvis has been performed.[12]

Every effort should be made to determine if a patient is pregnant before a radiologic exam is performed. However, if a patient who has been irradiated later finds out that she is pregnant, and becomes concerned about the possible hazard, a decision about termination of the pregnancy may have to be made. This decision of course needs to be based on psychological, legal, and emotional considerations as well as on an estimate of the fetal dose and consequent risk. This risk is generally considered to be negligible at doses of 5 rads or less, compared to the normal incidence of congenital defects. Doses of 10 to 15 rads or more provide some justification for therapeutic abortion. It should be noted that the vast majority of radiographic examinations of the pelvis or lower abdomen will result in fetal doses in the range of 0.2 to 4 rads; thus there is generally little reason from a radiation effects standpoint to terminate a pregnancy. However, doses exceeding 10 to 15 rads may result from procedures that include many films combined with extensive fluoroscopy.

GONAD SHIELDING

Gonadal shielding should be provided for patients who have not passed the reproductive age whenever the gonads are within or near the primary beam, unless this would interfere with the clinical objectives of the examination. The male gonads can be shielded for many abdominal x-ray examinations without obscuring features of diagnostic interest, and shields should always be used for examinations of the hip, pelvis, and upper femur. On the other hand, gonad shielding is generally not considered to be practical for female patients, for it will usually interfere with visualization of structures in the gonad area.

A gonad shield may take one of several forms. For example it may be simply a piece of lead rubber cut from an old apron. Another and better type is a shaped contact shield, which will provide lateral coverage against scattered radiation as well as protection against the direct primary beam. A third type is the shadow shield, which is attached to the tube head or the side of the table. This has the advantages of being always readily available and usable in a sterile field. Great thickness or weight is not necessary in a gonad shield: 0.25 mm lead equivalent is sufficient to attenuate the primary beam by 90 percent at 100 kVp.

ADMINISTRATIVE MEASURES TO CONTROL PATIENT EXPOSURE

Prescription of X-ray Studies. The single most important factor in reducing radiation exposure is to avoid the performance of clinically unproductive x-ray examinations. Prescription should be based on clinical indications or past history. All requests for radiologic services should state precisely the reason for the examination. Before the examination proceeds, it should be determined if there were any previous radiologic examinations that would make additional x-rays unnecessary. It is important that radiographic records be available when a patient transfers from one department or hospital to another.

The need for routine or screening examinations should be periodically reviewed. Guidelines for federal agencies from the Environmental Protection Agency and the Department of Health and Human Services state that the following examinations should not be routinely performed, unless justified for specific high risk groups of people:

1. Chest and lower back x-ray examinations in routine physical examinations or as a routine requirement for employment
2. Tuberculosis screening by chest radiography
3. Chest x-rays for routine hospital admission of patients under age 20 or lateral chest x-rays for patients under age 40 unless a clinical indication of chest disease exists
4. Chest radiography in routine prenatal care
5. Mammography examinations of women under age 50 who neither exhibit symptoms nor have a personal or strong family history of breast cancer[7]

Minimum Number of Examinations and Views. Every effort should be made to minimize the number of standard views for any examination. Beyond specified minimum views, an examination should be tailored to a patient's specific needs. Clinically unnecessary and unproductive views should not be performed. The necessity for a repeat examination should also be carefully considered. The diagnostician should always be aware of the quantity and potential risk of the radiation being administered.

TABLE 22.16. Summary of Estimates of Annual Whole-Body Dose Rates in the United States

Source	Average Dose Rate* (mrem/yr)
Environmental	
Natural	102
Global Fallout	4
Subtotal	106
Medical	
Diagnostic	72[†]
Radiopharmaceuticals	1
Subtotal	73
Occupational	0.8
Miscellaneous	2
Total	182

*The numbers shown are average values only. For given segments of the population, dose rates considerably greater than these may be experienced.
[†] Based on the abdominal dose.
From The Effects of Populations of Exposure to Low Levels of Ionizing Radiation. Washington, DC, NAS-NCR BEIR Committee, Nov 1972.

Qualifications of Operators. The fundamental objective of a diagnostic x-ray exam is the obtaining of optimum diagnostic information with minimum patient exposure. This requires, in addition to properly functioning and calibrated equipment, a properly trained operator. Physicians who are not radiologists should be granted radiology privileges only after receiving adequate training in equipment use and radiation protection. Technologists should be licensed or registered, or have received equivalent instruction and training. Evidence obtained from the Nationwide Evaluation of X-ray Trends indicates that credentialed operators, on the average, do in fact conduct their examinations using less radiation exposure than noncredentialed operators. Only properly qualified and supervised individuals should be given permission to operate x-ray equipment.

RADIATION DOSES

POPULATION RADIATION DOSE

Man has always been exposed to radiation from various natural sources, and this natural background remains the largest contributor to the average population dose. Man-made sources of radiation include medical radiation, occupational exposure, consumer products, and fallout from nuclear tests. Average annual dose rates from these sources are summarized in Table 22.16.

Natural Radiation. Naturally occurring radionuclides are present throughout our environment in rocks, soil, water, and air. Table 22.17 provides some idea of just how omnipresent radioactivity is in our world. The average dose from these terrestrial radiation sources is 40 mrem/year. Cosmic radiation contributes an additional 44 mrem/year, and radionuclides within the body, principally potassium 40, contribute an average of 18 mrem/year.

Medical Radiation. Diagnostic radiology accounts for 90 percent of the man-made radiation dose to which the US population is exposed, as derived from Public Health Service data for 1970. The annual per capita dose from this source is 72 mrem. This figure is based on an estimate of the "abdominal dose," which is an index of somatic dose. By comparison, the "genetically significant dose," which is an index of radiation received by the genetic pool, was 20 mrem.

Clinical use of radiopharmaceuticals contributes a lesser but growing amount of radiation exposure—1mrem/year.

TABLE 22.17. Concentration and Amount of ^{40}K, ^{232}Th, and ^{238}U in Typical Soils[9]

Radionuclide	Concentration		Total Amount	
	(ppm)	Ci/g($\times 10^{-12}$)	(1 km^2 ×1 m depth)	1 mi^2 ×1 ft Depth
Potassium 40	1.5	12	24 Ci* or 3,500 kg	19 Ci or 3 tons
Thorium 232	9	1	2 Ci or 18,000 kg	1.6 Ci or 16 tons
Uranium 238	1.8	0.6	1.2 Ci or 3,600 kg	1.0 Ci or 3 tons

*Ci is the abbreviation for curie, the unit of activity. Other major radionuclides present in soil include rubidium 87 and the radioactive daughters of thorium and uranium present in their decay series.

TABLE 22.18. **Radiation Exposure or Absorbed Dose for a "Standard" Patient from Representative X-Ray Exams as Determined by Nationwide Evaluation of X-Ray Trends Program for 1977**

Exam	Ovarian Dose Index (mrad)	Testicular Dose Index (mrad)	Exposure at Skin Entrance (mR)	Surface Exposure Integral (R-cm)	Red Bone Marrow Dose Index (mrad)	Thyroid Dose Index (mrad)	ESEG* (mR)
Chest (A/P)	< .5	< .5	19.2	28.3	1.9	0.6	30
Skull (lat)	< .5	< .5	228	119	7.4	46.8	300
Abd (KUB) (A/P)	134	9.3	592	448	20.9	< .5	750
Retr pyelo (A/P)	188	30.2	725	812	34.7	< .5	900
Thor spine (A/P)	< .5	< .5	814	318	14.6	22.7	900
Cerv spine (A/P)	< .5	< .5	165	90	3.1	121	250
Lum-sac spine (A/P)	164	19.7	736	548	25.5	< .5	1,000
Full spine (A/P)	52.2	18.5	202	730	19.5	170	300
Feet (D/P)	—	—	254	178	—	—	270
Dental BW post			430	14.7	—	—	700
Dental periapical	—	—	429	14.7	—	—	700
Dental ceph (lat)	< .5	< .5	61.5	68.9	2.4	25.2	—

*ESEG is the EPA's recommended maximum exposure value. The standard patient is one with the following body-part thickness: head—15 cm, neck—13 cm, thorax—23 cm, abdomen—23 cm, foot—8 cm.

Occupational Exposure. A 1972 EPA report calculated a mean annual dose of 210 mrem per radiation worker in the United States, or an average per capita dose of 0.8 mrem/year.

Radioactive Fallout. This is mainly a result of the high-megaton yield atmospheric tests conducted by the US and USSR prior to 1963, which introduced large amounts of radioactive material into the stratosphere. The average 1970 per capita dose was 4.0 mrem per year.

Miscellaneous Sources. Included in this category are sources such as nuclear power production, television, wristwatches, and the increased cosmic radiation levels incident to high altitude aircraft travel. These sources contribute about 2.0 mrem per year.

PATIENT RADIATION DOSES FOR INDIVIDUAL EXAMS

The Bureau of Radiological Health in conjunction with various state radiation control agencies conducts an ongoing program, known as the Nationwide Evaluation of X-ray Trends (NEXT), to determine the radiation dose a "standard" patient receives from selected x-ray projections. Data for 1977 are presented in Table 22.18.

The relative genetic risk of an x-ray procedure is proportional to the magnitude of the gonadal dose. The relative somatic risk is more difficult to assess since it depends on the particular organ or organs irradiated and their sensitivity to radiation-induced damage. The red bone marrow dose index and the thyroid dose

index as given in Table 22.18 are indicators of the relative risk for leukemia and thyroid cancer induction. Laws and Rosenstein have developed the somatic risk concept still further.[6] Using the risk coefficients for induction of cancer and the relative severities of these cancers given in Table 22.19, together with information on the dose received by the various body organs from various radiologic examinations, they have computed an equivalent whole body dose and relative somatic detriment for these examinations. These are shown graphically in Figure 22.13. The examinations with the highest somatic dose detriment — mammography, thoracic spine (females), and ribs (females) — all place the female breast in the primary beam.

TABLE 22.19. **Risk Coefficients and Relative Severities for Selected Organs[6]**

Organ or Tissue	Male Risk Coefficient (Cases of cancer or leukemia/10^6 males-yr-rad)	Female Risk Coefficient (Cases of cancer or leukemia/10^6 females-yr-rad)	Relative Severity*
Active bone marrow	1.5	1.0	1.0
Thyroid	1.5	3.0	0.3
Breast	0	6.0	0.65
Lung	1.0	1.0	1.0
Other malignancies	2.0	2.0	1.0

*Relative severities are based on the mortality and morbidity associated with eacy type of malignancy.

The figures in Table 22.19 are representative values only. The NEXT data show that exposures for the same exam vary greatly from facility to facility, depending on the x-ray generator, the processing equipment, films and screens, grids, technique factors, and the skill of the radiographer. Maximum and minimum values found in the NEXT program differ by factors of 50 or more. The number of films per examination also varies (the figures above are for a single film only).

There are currently no dose limits for patients, but the Environmental Protection Agency, which provides guidance for all federal agencies (such as VA hospitals) in the formulation of radiation standards, has stated that steps should be undertaken to evaluate and reduce, where practicable, exposures that exceed the Entrance Skin Exposure Guides (ESEG) listed in Table 22.18. The ESEG represents the third quartile level from the NEXT data; that is, 75 percent of all measured exposures were below this level. Exposures above this level can be considered excessive.

Fluoroscopic Exams. Doses from fluoroscopic exams depend on total fluoro time, the technique factors and equipment, the range of movement of the beam, and the number of spot films made. Thus it is difficult to give numerical values for these exams. It is advisable to record exposure times for high-dose procedures so that exposure estimates can be made at a later time should they be needed. Tabletop exposure rates are limited to 10 R/min for most units and typical values are in the range of 2 to 4 R/min.

Computerized Tomography. Published articles have presented a range of exposure values. Typical are the values given by Parker and Hobday[16] for the EMI CT 5005 whole-body scanner. Using a bolus at 20-second scan speed, the maximum exposure from a single slice is 3.5 R. For eight contiguous slices at 1.5-cm intervals, this increases to 4.8 R due to the scattered radiation from adjacent scans. If this is repeated with contrast media, the exposure doubles to 9.6 R. And if the slow scanning speed is used (70 seconds) the maximum exposure can be as high as 36 R. For body scans at the 20-second scan speed, the estimated maximum skin exposure is 3.2 R (12 to 15 slices, 1.5-cm intervals).

STANDARD-SETTING AND REGULATORY ORGANIZATIONS

REGULATORY AGENCIES

State Radiation Protection Programs. Each of the fifty states has regulations governing the use of x-radiation, patterned in general after the Suggested State Regulations published by the Council of State Govern-

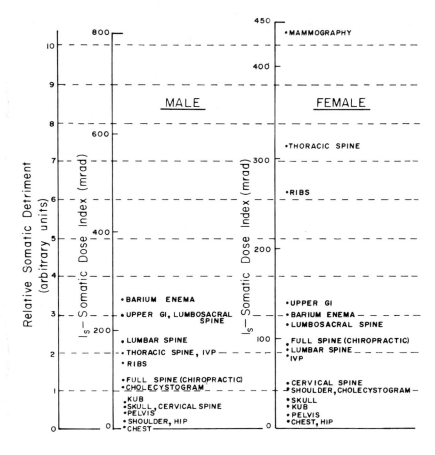

Figure 22.13. The somatic detriment or carcinogenic potential from common radiographic exams is represented by the common scale on the left side of the graph. The internal scales give values of the somatic dose index for the radiographic exams shown; this is essentially the equivalent whole body exposure. For example, a lumbar spine exam (male) is equivalent to a whole body dose of 180 mrad. Since a female is more radiosensitive, a whole body exposure of 100 mrad to a female produces the same somatic detriment as a 180 mrad whole body dose in a male.[6]

ments.[3] These model regulations in turn incorporate recommendations developed by various nongovernment standard-setting bodies and federal agencies. Although there are differences in the various state programs, these model regulations tend to make the regulations of the different states compatible with each other and with those of the federal government.

State regulations cover registration, equipment performance and safety, shielding, operational procedures, and dose standards.

Bureau of Radiological Health. A subagency of the Food and Drug Administration, the BRH develops and enforces performance standards (as contrasted with design requirements) to control the emission of electronic product radiation. These regulations are issued under the authority of the Radiation Control for Health and Safety Act of 1968 and are published in Title 21 of the Code of Federal Regulations, Subchapter J. Manufacturers and assemblers of x-ray equipment must certify that equipment manufactured after August 1, 1974, meets the performance standards. The standards do not regulate the users of x-ray equipment. However, failure to follow the manufacturer's maintenance schedule could relieve the manufacturer of the responsibility for continued compliance. Manufacturers must repair, replace, or refund the cost of certified components that fail to comply with the standard. The BRH contracts with state radiation control agencies to assist in their field inspection programs.

Other functions of the BRH include development of recommendations for users, workshops, and educational programs, quality assurance and imaging activities, and research into the health effects of radiation. The BRH also sponsors the BENT (Breast Exposure: Nationwide Trends) and NEXT (Nationwide Evaluation of X-ray Trends) programs.

Environmental Protection Agency. The EPA advises the President in radiation protection matters and recommends guidance for federal agencies (eg, the military services, Public Health Service, Veterans Administration) in the formulation of radiation standards, including medical uses of diagnostic x-rays.

Other federal agencies with activities and regulations in the field of x-ray protection include the Occupational Safety and Health Administration, the National Bureau of Standards, and the Veterans Administration.

NONGOVERNMENTAL STANDARDS-SETTING OR ADVISORY ORGANIZATIONS

International Commission on Radiological Protection (ICRP). Formed in 1928 by the International Congress of Radiology, the ICRP is recognized as an international authority in preparing recommendations for the safe use of ionizing radiation. Its recommendations on the various aspects of the subject are published in appropriate reports and are used by most of the countries of the world as the basis for their radiation protection standards.

National Council on Radiation Protection and Measurements (NCRP). The NCRP is a nonprofit corporation chartered by Congress in 1964 to collect and analyze information and recommendations about radiation measurements and protection against radiation. The NCRP is organized into a main council and 58 scientific committees. Each of the scientific committees is composed of experts having special competence in the particular area of the committee's interest, and is responsible for the drafting of proposed recommendations for the main council's consideration. Approved recommendations are published as reports of the NCRP. These reports serve as guides to good practice and as guidelines for the establishment of regulatory protection codes.

International Commission on Radiological Units and Measurements (ICRU). The ICRU has as its objective the development of internationally recommended radiation units, measurement procedures, and compilations of physical data required in the application of these procedures.

National Academy of Sciences (NAS). The NAS's advisory committee on the Biological Effects of Ionizing Radiation (BEIR committee) has conducted major reviews of the effects of low levels of ionizing radiation and the scientific basis for the establishment of radiation protection standards.

United Nations Scientific Committee on the Effects of Atomic Radiation (UNSCEAR). UNSCEAR performs a role similar to that of the BEIR committee of the NAS. It has collected, reviewed, and published a wealth of information and data on sources of radiation exposure and the biologic effects of radiation. UNSCEAR reviews new information on radiation effects as it becomes available and publishes this new information along with its conclusions on a periodic basis.

Joint Commission on Accreditation of Hospitals (JCAH). The JCAH has a number of requirements for radiation safety programs in hospitals. It states that the recommendations of the NCRP should be known and applied, and specifies frequencies and requirements for radiation protection surveys. It also recommends that the services of a health or radiation physicist be available for the conducting of periodic radiologic safety testing and participation in educational programs. The

JCAH regularly inspects hospitals for accreditation purposes.

Other Organizations. Private organizations and societies that set standards or develop guidelines for radiation protection include, among others, American Association of Physicists in Medicine (AAPM), American College of Radiology (ACR), American National Standards Institute (ANSI), Health Physics Society (HPS), and National Electrical Manufacturers Association (NEMA).

RADIATION PROTECTION SURVEY PROGRAMS

SURVEY REQUIREMENTS

The Joint Commission on Accreditation of Hospitals requires all diagnostic radiologic equipment to be checked at least annually for compliance with federal and state requirements, unless prevented by the unavailability of qualified personnel (in which case the interval should not exceed two years). In addition, radiation protection surveys and calibrations should be performed when radiologic equipment is initially installed or is altered significantly. Documentation of the surveys and of actions taken to correct deficiencies must be maintained for inspection by the Joint Commission.

The more important tests that should be conducted during a radiation protection survey of radiographic/fluoroscopic equipment are summarized below. Applicable state and federal requirements should be consulted.

Fluoroscopic collimation—beam size and alignment (both fluoro and spot modes)

Radiographic collimation—beam size and alignment, congruence with light field, automatic collimator operation (for certified equipment)

Half-value layer

Protective apparel—availability and integrity of shielding material

Control panel indicators—proper functioning

Minimum source-skin distance

Fluoro output—maximum at tabletop level

Interlocks between fluoro tube and primary barrier

Inspection of shielding devices (drapes, Bucky slot cover)

Linearity and reproducibility of exposures

Illumination of light localizer (certified equipment)

Automatic exposure termination—response time and backup timer

Radiographic timer—accuracy and reproducibility; exposure switch location

Leakage radiation from x-ray tube (if new tube or tube insert)

Adequacy of protective barriers (new rooms or new equipment in old rooms)

The above tests are necessary to verify compliance with government regulations. In addition, certain radiation dose measurements should be made to familiarize the radiographer or fluoroscopist with the radiation characteristics of the equipment.

Fluoroscopic exposure rates should be determined with an attenuator that represents a typical patient (eg, 1.5-in thick aluminum). Increases in exposure rate over a period of time may indicate loss of image intensifier gain or aging of the input phosphor.

Tableside scatter rate measurements are useful in educating the technical staff and alerting them to conditions of high exposure.

Radiographic output measurements made under standard conditions are necessary if outputs in different rooms are to be standardized.

Radiographic exposure measurements for common exams performed in a department should also be made. Comparison can be made with results from the Nationwide Evaluation of X-ray Trends (see Table 22.18).

QUALITY-ASSURANCE PROGRAMS

A quality-assurance program can contribute greatly to the production of images of consistently high quality with minimum patient exposure by aiding in the detection of changes in the image-producing variables before they become clinically observable and adversely affect the quality of the images. A poor image reduces the amount of diagnostic information available to the physician and increases the probability of an incorrect diagnosis. If a diagnosis cannot be made because of a poor image, the radiation exposure the patient received will have been entirely unproductive. If a radiograph is repeated, a patient's exposure is of course doubled. Data from the NEXT surveys indicate that some patients are receiving unnecessary radiation exposure on a routine basis: radiation exposure for a given exam varies widely from facility to facility, by factors of 50 or more.

The Food and Drug Administration therefore has recommended that all diagnostic x-ray facilities establish a quality-assurance program, the type and extent of the program to be commensurate with a facility's needs and resources. One recommended protocol is the AAPM's Basic Quality Control in Diagnostic Radiology.[5] Monitoring should be established for parameters in all four components of the x-ray system:

1. *X-ray generators*
   kVp accuracy
   mA accuracy

Focal-spot size
Automatic brightness controls
2. *Image receptors*
    Screen condition, artifacts
    Film–screen contact
    Resolution, distortion, asymmetry in image-intensified systems
3. *Film processors*
    Solution temperatures and composition
    Sensitometric monitoring (speed, contrast)
    Standardization of all processors in a department
4. *Ancillary equipment*
    Proper grid alignment and focal distance
    Safelight illumination in darkroom
    Uniformity of viewbox illumination

Other items perhaps more traditionally a part of a radiation protection survey program also must be looked upon as necessary to a quality assurance program, eg, half-value layer measurements, reproducibility of output, mA linearity, and collimation checks.

Each of the elements in an x-ray system has a variability associated with it that contributes to the degradation of image quality and the overall retake rate. Improvement of any component therefore will lead to a reduction in the retake rate. A QA program actually can be cost effective by reducing the number of repeat examinations, thus saving on personnel time and film costs.

REFERENCES

1. The effects on Populations of Exposure to Low Levels of Ionizing Radiation. Biological Effects of Ionizing Radiation (BEIR) Report, Washington, DC, National Academy of Sciences, National Research Council, Nov 1972
2. Regulations for the Administration and Enforcement of the Radiation Control for Health and Safety Act of 1968. HEW Publ (FDA)76-8035, Rockville, Md, Bureau of Radiological Health, Jan 1976
3. Suggested State Regulations for Control of Radiation. Rockville, Md, prepared by US Atomic Energy Commission, US Public Health Service, and Conference of Radiation Control Program Directors, Oct 1974
4. Radiation protection. International Commission on Radiological Protection Publication 26, Oxford, England, Jan 1977
5. Basic Quality Control in Diagnostic Radiology. American Association of Physicists. In Medicine Report 4, Chicago, American Association of Physicists in Medicine
6. Laws PW, Rosenstein M: A somatic dose index for diagnostic radiology. Health Physics 35: 629–642, 1978
7. Radiation protection guidance to federal agencies for diagnostic x-rays. Federal Register 43, No 22: 4377-4380. US Environmental Protection Agency and US Department of Health, Education, and Welfare, Feb 1, 1978
8. Structural Shielding Design and Evaluation for Medical Use of X-rays and Gamma Rays of Energies up to 10 MeV. National Council on Radiation Protection and Measurements, Report No 49, 1976
9. Natural background radiation in the United States. NCRP Report No 45, 1975
10. Daniels J: The x-rays. Letter to the Editor. Science N S 3(67): 562-563, 1896.
11. Sources and Effects of Ionizing Radiation. Report to the General Assembly. New York, United Nations Scientific Committee on the Effects of Atomic Radiation, 1977
12. Medical Radiation Exposure of Pregnant and Potentially Pregnant Women. NCRP Report No 54, 1977
13. Problems Involved in Developing an Index of Harm. ICRP Publication 27, Oxford, England, 1977
14. Basic Radiation Protection Criteria. NCRP Report No 39, 1971
15. Plato P: Testing and evaluating personal dosimetry services in 1976. Health Physics 34: 219–223, March 1978
16. Parker RP, Hobday P: Radiation exposure to the patient in computerized tomography. Brit J Radiol 52: 349, 1979
17. Accreditation Manual for Hospitals. Chicago, Joint Commission on Accreditation of Hospitals
18. Radiological Health Handbook. Rockville, Md, US Dept of Health, Education, and Welfare, Jan 1970
19. Gonad Doses and Genetically Significant Dose from Diagnostic Radiology, US, 1964 and 1970. US Dept of Health, Education, and Welfare Publ (FDA) 76-8034, Rockville, Md., Bureau of Radiological Health, 1976.
20. Population Exposure to X-rays, US 1970. Health, Education and Welfare Publ (FDA) 73-8047, Rockville, Md, Bureau of Radiological Health, 1973.
21. Wald N: Radiation injury and its management. In Handbook of Radioactive Nuclides, Part IX. Cleveland Chemical Rubber Co, 1969.

CHAPTER 23

Approaches to Radiation Risk Estimation

S. JULIAN GIBBS

For many years the biologic hazards of ionizing radiations have been known. The first report of biologic injury from exposure to diagnostic x-ray was published within a few months of Roentgen's discovery; the victim was the Dean of the Vanderbilt University School of Medicine.[1] However, there are still essentially no data dealing with the effects of small radiation doses, such as those employed in diagnostic radiology and nuclear medicine. A great deal of effort is now being expended by many institutions and agencies in an attempt to assess low-dose risks to human populations. Results of this effort have been summarized in the reports of the Advisory Committee on the Biological Effects of Ionizing Radiations (BEIR) of the National Academy of Sciences,[2,3] and the United Nations Scientific Committee on the Effects of Atomic Radiation (UNSCEAR).[4] However, in addition to population risks, radiologists are interested in determining the probability of injury to an individual from exposure to a given diagnostic procedure.

RADIATION UNITS

Newly defined SI units are used throughout this chapter. Definitions of these units, and their relationships to conventional units, are given in Table 23.1.

DELAYED EFFECTS OF RADIATION

Radiation delivered in sufficient acute doses to mammals leads to acute lethality via the well-known syndromes. These effects are nonstochastic; ie, a given dose is associated with severity of effect in a given organism, implying the existence of a threshold. Current data suggest a threshold of about 1 Sv for these effects in man.[5] Smaller doses have been associated with delayed effects in mammals: mutation, cancer, effects on the embryo and fetus, nonspecific life-span shortening, and cataracts. Life-span shortening, or so-called radiologic aging, has been demonstrated in animals.[6] However, in Japanese atomic bomb survivors, no premature deaths have been observed except those associated with cancer.[7] Current data suggest that development of progressive, clinically significant cataracts in man requires relatively large x-ray doses, certainly greater than those likely to be encountered in diagnostic procedures.[5] This chapter thus considers radiation-induced mutation and cancer as potential risks of small postnatal doses in man. The mammalian embryo is quite sensitive to relatively small doses of radiation.[8] Observed effects have included prenatal death, congenital abnormalities, growth and mental retardation, and childhood cancer.

These effects of small doses are stochastic in na-

TABLE 23.1. **Radiation Units**

Quantity	Conventional Unit	SI Unit*	Conversion
Exposure	roentgen (R) 2.58×10^{-4} c/kg	coulomb/kilogram (c/kg)	$1 \text{ c/kg} = 3.88 \times 10^3 \text{R}$
Dose	rad 100 ergs/gm	gray (Gy) 1 joule/kg	$1 \text{ Gy} = 100 \text{ rad}$
Dose Equivalent	rem rad × (RBE or QF)	sievert (Sv) Gy × (RBE or QF)	$1 \text{ Sv} = 100 \text{ rem}$
Radioactivity	curie (Ci) 3.7×10^{10} disintegration/s	becquerel (Bq) s^{-1}	$1 \text{ Bq} = 2.7 \times 10^{-11} \text{Ci}$

*Système International d'Unités, or "metric system"

ture. That is, a given dose may be associated only with a probability of effect, implying the absence of a threshold. Further, these radiation-induced diseases in no way differ from those arising from other causes. For example, it is not possible to determine whether the leukemia in a Japanese atomic-bomb survivor was caused by radiation exposure or arose spontaneously. We can only associate radiation exposure with increased incidence of the effect.

DOSE-RESPONSE CURVES

Shapes of dose-response curves for late stochastic effects of radiation are not completely known—especially at low doses. Most available animal data have been obtained at relatively large doses (generally at least 1 Gy) for statistical accuracy with study populations of reasonable size. For a linear dose response, size of the required population varies approximately inversely with the square of the dose.[9] For example, for the same level of statistical accuracy, studies carried out at doses of 1 cGy (1 rad) require populations 10,000 times larger than those needed if the dose is 1 Gy (100 rads). Thus, although reasonably accurate data are available for large doses, animal experiments using doses in the diagnostic range have not been carried out—and probably never will be—because of huge animal costs involved.

Human epidemiologic studies have been performed using study populations whose sizes have been determined on other grounds (Japanese atomic-bomb survivors, patients treated by radiotherapy for benign disease, and so on). Many of these populations have been inadequate for statistical accuracy even at large doses.

Since no data are available, shapes of dose-response curves in the low-dose region must be inferred from available high-dose data and from theoretical considerations. Studies of microdosimetry indicate that the probability of molecular damage leading to a delayed effect (eg, malignant transformation in a somatic cell, mutation in a germ cell) is probably a linear function of dose, especially from small doses of low-LET radiation.[10] The distribution of dose deposition from doses of a few μGy is highly inhomogeneous. For example, from a dose of 1 μGy (0.1 mrad) of 80 kVp x-rays, the probability of an average cell receiving any dose is of the order of 10^{-4}, while 99.9 percent of cells receive no energy. Further, from that 1 μGy, in the microenvironment along the track of the electron ejected by that rare interaction, the local dose may be the equivalent of several grays. Thus the probability of a molecular lesion is actually the probability of an electron track passing within close proximity of a sensitive, important molecule (DNA). Thus, with small doses, our expression of dose in grays, requiring averag-

ing on a macro scale, is inappropriate and may be misleading.

The problem lies in the expression of these molecular lesions. For example, in cultured mammalian cells, transformation rates on the order of 10^{-3}/Gy (10^{-5}/rad) have been demonstrated.[11] If these rates apply to humans in vivo, several malignant transformations per person should occur each minute from background radiation. Obviously expression of these transformations by development of tumor involves other factors, such as repair and immunological capabilities of the host.[12] Thus, microdosimetry accounts for physical, but not biologic, processes.

THE LINEAR HYPOTHESIS

In general, the dose-response function for a delayed stochastic effect of low-LET radiation should be of the form[9]

$$I = (a_0 + a_1 D + a_2 D^2) e^{-(b_1 D + b_2 D^2)} \qquad (1)$$

where I is incidence of the effect, D is dose, and a and b are constants.

The term a_0 represents the intercept, or incidence at zero dose. Induction of the effect is related in terms $a_1 D + a_2 D^2$. At low doses, the dose-square term is probably negligible—a_2 is near zero. The exponential term accounts for killing of affected cells at higher doses. A plot of this function consists of an ascending, upwardly concave portion, reaching a maximum and then declining as affected cells are killed at higher doses, before the late effect can be expressed.

Land and McGregor[9] have applied this function to breast cancer incidence in Japanese atomic-bomb survivors (Table 23.2, Fig. 23.1). Noise in the data is shown in Figure 23.1.A. Fitting the complete function required estimation of five constants (a_0, a_1, a_2, b_1, and b_2), statistically a weak procedure from so few data points confounded by noise. The authors found b_1 to be near zero, and eliminated it. However, the procedure was still statistically weak, so they eliminated other

TABLE 23.2. **Models of Breast Cancer Dose Response***

Model	Function	Constants
Complete	$(a_0 + a_1 D + a_2 D^2) e^{-b_2 D^2}$	4
Linear with killing	$(a_0 + a_1 D) e^{-b_2 D^2}$	3
Quadratic with killing	$(a_0 + a_2 D^2) e^{-b_2 D^2}$	3
Linear and quadratic	$a_0 + a_1 D + a_2 D^2$	3
Linear	$a_0 + a_1 D$	2

*From Land and McGregor.[9]

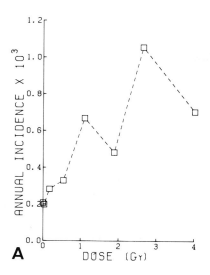

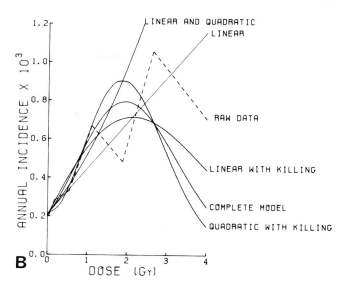

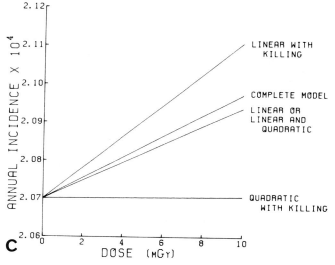

Figure 23.1. Breast cancer in Japanese atomic-bomb survivors. For dose units, 1 Gy = 100 rads, and 10 mGy = 1 rad. **A**. Raw data. There is considerable statistical uncertainty (noise) in annual cancer incidence at each dose level, basically because of the small population. **B**. Fit of several theoretical models (Table 23.2) to raw data (dashed line, reproduced from A). It is not possible to reject any model conclusively. By eye, the linear and linear-with-killing models appear to fit best. **C**. Expanded scale in low-dose region of interest. The low-dose risk estimate will depend strongly on the model chosen. The complete, linear, and linear-with-quadratic models suggest essentially equal low-dose risks. The linear model with killing predicts a substantially greater risk, and the quadratic with killing suggests a near zero low-dose risk. Thus, the linear model may be either an overestimate or an underestimate of the actual risk. Data from Land and McGregor.[9]

terms to increase statistical power (Table 23.2, Fig. 23.1.B). They showed that the noisy data could be fitted reasonably well by simplified versions of the model. Visually, the simple linear model appeared to provide the best fit; next best was linear with killing.

An expanded-scale plot of the low-dose region indicates that the choice of model may have a significant effect on the estimation of low-dose risk (Fig. 23.1.C). The two models that exclude cell killing agree well with the complete model. The quadratic model with killing suggests that the low-dose risk may be near zero. The linear model with killing suggests that the risk may be substantially greater than that predicted by this simple linear model. The real risk probably lies between these extremes. Since several of these models fit the high-dose data reasonably well, there is no clear basis for selection of a model for determination of low-dose risk.

Similar problems have been encountered in analyzing data for many other risks. Both the BEIR and

UNSCEAR committees have utilized the linear model for first approximation of low-dose risks because its simplicity provides the only reasonable means for handling some of the data.[2,4] Both committees provided convincing arguments that the linear model is conservative, that it overestimates the real risk. However, they provided equally convincing arguments that it may be an underestimate. It is simply the best available at present. Pochin has emphasized that fear of being proven wrong at some future date should not deter the providing of risk estimates from the best current data.[13] Estimates of risk in succeeding portions of this chapter are based on the linear model.

RISK COEFFICIENTS

Estimates provided in this section are approximations of average risk, for application to populations. Their use for estimation of risk to an individual is tenuous at best because of other interacting factors, eg, age, sex, genetics, and environment. Calculations required to generate these estimates compound numerous assumptions. Animal data are frequently applied to man—clearly a risky procedure. It may be equally risky to extrapolate data from one human population to another because of differences in genetics, culture, environment, and other factors.

MUTATION

Current knowledge of mammalian radiation genetics has been obtained almost exclusively from studies of mice. No excess genetic disease has been detected in first-generation offspring of Japanese atomic-bomb survivors[14], or in any other human population. Animal data, however, are so convincing that we must assume a genetic effect in man until proven otherwise.

Summarizing available data, the UNSCEAR committee estimated the probability of recessive mutation from irradiation of mature mouse testes is 5×10^{-6} mutants/locus/Sv (5×10^{-8} mutants/locus/rem).[4] In females, the rate is much lower; it has not been accurately determined. No studies with populations of sufficient size for statistical accuracy have been carried out. Using available data, the BEIR committee has estimated the human doubling dose (the dose required to double the spontaneous mutation rate) as 0.2 to 2 Sv (20 to 200 rems).[2] The UNSCEAR committee suggested 1 Sv (100 rems).[4] These estimates may be of correct magnitude for males, but are probably conservative for females. The absence of genetic effects in the Japanese suggests that the doubling dose for human males is at least 1.4 Sv (140 rems), and for females at least 10 Sv (1,000 rems).[4]

Table 23.3 presents the estimates of probability of radiation-induced genetic disease of the UNSCEAR committee, using a doubling dose of 1 Sv (100 rems).[4] These data apply only to liveborn. They do not include lethals, which generally cause embryonic death so early as to be unrecognizable as abortion. These lethals, however, do not contribute—in the strict sense—to propagation of genetic disease.

The data in Table 23.3 are intended for application to populations. For example, the current recommendation for maximum population exposure of 5cSv (5 rems) per generation might be expected to increase the incidence of genetic disease in the first succeeding generation by approximately 0.03 percent, or from the current spontaneous rate of 10.5 percent to 10.53 percent.[2] At genetic equilibrium, after several generations, the increase should be about 0.09 percent, for a total incidence of 10.59 percent. These small increases would be detectable epidemiologically only by studies of extremely large populations. However, these radiation-induced mutations might be expressed as increased incidence of genetic disease over many (perhaps all) succeeding generations. Thus their occurrence, although rare, must not be regarded as trivial.

The data in Table 23.3 cannot be applied necessarily to an individual, to estimate the genetic risk of a diagnostic procedure. The data were derived almost exclusively from studies of male mice. The male data indicate that radiation exposure may lead to mutations carried by any subsequent conception, regardless of the interval between exposure and conception.[4] Thus the probabilities given in Table 23.3 may be reasonable estimates of genetic risks of exposure of young males.

Current data indicate that the genetic risk of exposure of females is significantly less. Irradiation of female mice has led to expressed mutations only if the interval between exposure and conception was less than seven weeks.[15] Thus the data of Table 23.3 probably represents an overestimate (or upper limit) of the genetic risk of exposure of females.

Obviously, the genetic risk is zero in individuals who will not conceive additional offspring. As shown in Table 23.4, birth rates—and genetic risk—decrease sharply for females over 35 years of age and males over 40.

TABLE 23.3. **Genetic Effects of Radiation* Liveborn**

Disease (type)	Current Incidence (%)	Probability of Radiation First Generation	Effect (%/Sv)[†] Equilibrium
Autosomal dominant and X-linked	1.0	0.20	1.0
Recessive	0.11	Slight	Very slow increase
Chromosomal	0.40	0.38	0.40
Complex etiology	9.0	0.05	0.45
Total	10.5	0.63	1.85

*Data from UNSCEAR.[4]
[†]1%/Sv = 0.01%/rem

TABLE 23.4. Birth Rate by Age of Parents, U.S., 1975*

| Age (years) | Live births per 1,000 in age group | |
	Mothers	Fathers
10–14	1.3	—
15–19	56.3	21.1
20–24	114.7	97.8
25–29	110.3	126.6
30–34	53.1	82.7
35–39	19.4	40.1
40–44	4.6	16.6
45–49	0.3	6.1
50–54	—	2.1
55–	—	0.4

*Data from US National Center for Health Statistics.[16]

CANCER

Recent retrospective studies have shown statistically significant associations between diagnostic radiation exposure and leukemia in adult human males and in children.[17,18] These studies, however, do not necessarily demonstrate cause and effect. There is reason to believe that the pathogenesis of leukemia is a prolonged process, involving at times suppression of the immune system.[19] It may therefore be proposed that individuals undergoing leukemogenesis may be more likely to succumb to infectious diseases, seek medical attention, and be exposed to diagnostic procedures.

A large body of evidence has accumulated dealing with increased cancer incidence in human populations exposed to large doses: Japanese atomic-bomb survivors, patients treated with radiation for benign disease (eg, ankylosing spondylitis, postpartum mastitis, tinea capitis, thymic hypertrophy), and patients subjected to repeated high-dose diagnostic procedures with large accumulated doses (eg, multiple pneumothorax, under fluoroscopy, for tuberculosis). The follow-up periods for these studies have been about 20 to 30 years. Estimates of mean radiation risks derived from these studies and summarized by the UNSCEAR committee[4] are presented in Table 23.5, for those organs and tissues for which a radiation risk has been demonstrated. Also given in Table 23.5 are current estimates of the incidence of these tumors, from the American Cancer Society.[20]

The risk estimates in Table 23.5 are based on currently available data, some of which may be incomplete. For example, the most recent report of excess cancer in the Japanese indicates that new cases may still be occurring.[7] Current data may therefore underestimate the real risk in that population. Once again it must be emphasized that these risk estimates cannot be applied to individuals because of the known interactions of radiation with other factors.

TABLE 23.5. Carcinogenic Effects of Radiation

Site	Estimated Incidence US, 1979* (new cases)	Probability of Radiation-Induced Cancer[†] ($\times 10^4$/Sv)[‡]
Esophagus	8,400	2–5
Stomach	23,000	10–20
Colon, rectum	112,000	10–15
Liver	11,600	10–15
Pancreas	23,000	2–5
Lung	112,000	50
Bone	1,900	2–5
Breast	106,900	50–200
Uterus	53,000	7–10
Ovary	17,000	8
Bladder	35,000	4–7
Brain	11,600	5–20
Thyroid	9,000	50–150
Leukemia	21,500	15–25
Lymphoma	38,500	4–12
Salivary glands	—	5–10
Paranasal sinuses	—	2–5

*Data from American Cancer Society.[20]
[†]Data from UNSCEAR.[4]
[‡]($\times 10^{-6}$/rem)

The latent period for radiation-induced leukemia appears to be about 5 to 20 years. It does not vary in a consistent manner with dose.[4] For solid tumors, the latent period may be much longer—perhaps as long as 50 years. It might be reasonable, therefore, to assume that the risk of radiation-induced cancer in the elderly would be negligible, because they are likely to die from other causes before the tumor could develop. That assumption, however, is not always supported by the facts. The high risk of thyroid cancer occurs in young individuals; older thyroid glands appear to be relatively insensitive.[2] The risk in females appears to be approximately twice that in males, and is greatest in young Jewish females.[4]

In the Japanese, leukemia risk appears greater in males than in females. It is greatest in children and the elderly.[4]

Spontaneous lung cancer is known to be highly dependent on age; its occurrence is greatest in the elderly. In the Japanese, excess lung cancer was observed within about 10 years postexposure in individuals aged 50 or over at the time of exposure, within 15 years in those aged 35 to 49, but only after more than 20 years in those less than 35. Thus, the latent period for these tumors appears to vary inversely with age.

These examples point out that we do not yet fully understand how radiation interacts with these other factors in the etiology of cancer. Thus the risk estimates of Table 23.4, tenuous as they are for application to populations, may lead to either gross overestimation or severe underestimation of the risk to an individual—depending on unknown cofactors.

EFFECTS ON EMBRYO AND FETUS

The prenatal mammal is significantly more sensitive to radiation than the adult, or even the growing juvenile.[21] Such might be expected on theoretical grounds. Life *in utero* is characterized by rapid growth. It is well known that rapidly dividing cells are more sensitive to lethal effects of radiation. Experiments dealing with malignant transformation in cultured mammalian cells have suggested that cell division may be required to stabilize the transformed state.[11] Immunological competence develops after birth; immunological factors in carcinogenesis are well known but poorly understood.[19] Diagnostic procedures that expose the pelvic region of the pregnant female usually provide whole-body exposure to the fetus.

Lethal and teratogenic effects of radiation may not be stochastic.[2] Dose-response curves from animal studies are frequently sigmoid, implying the existence of thresholds. Brent and Gorson have suggested minimal effective doses of 25 cSv (25 rems) for death and 10 cSv (10 rems) for malformations.[8] However, malformations have been demonstrated in mice from doses as low as 5 cSv (5 rems).[21] A few cases of microcephaly and mental

retardation have been observed in Japanese atomic-bomb survivors exposed in utero to doses in the 0 to 9 cSv (0 to 9 rems) range.[14] The UNSCEAR committee suggested a risk of 100 percent from a dose of 1 Sv (100 rems) for lethal effects of preimplantation exposure.[4] However, rodent data suggest that the LD$_{50}$ is about 1 Sv (100 rems), for a risk of coefficient of 50 percent/Sv (0.5 percent/rem). It must be emphasized that these data were derived almost totally from studies of rodents. Negative data from the Japanese suggest that the human risk is probably no greater.[4] Therefore, the risk coefficients for these effects (Table 23.6) may overestimate risks of low doses.

Genetic effects of prenatal exposure have not been investigated adequately. Data are insufficient to allow assignment of risk coefficients. Spermatogonia of newborn mice are similar in sensitivity to those of adults; immature oocytes in newborn mice are more sensitive than those in adults, but less sensitive than mature oocytes.[2]

Carcinogenic effects of low-level embryonic irradiation have been extensively investigated in man. Several large-scale epidemiologic studies have shown a highly significant association between diagnostic exposure in utero and childhood cancer, especially leukemia.[4] The large English study conducted by Stewart and associates suggested a risk of $(572 \pm 133) \times 10^{-4}$/Sv ($572 \times 10^{-6}$/rem).[22] A prospective study found a similar risk in whites, but no risk in blacks.[23] Correlation with an immunologic cofactor has been demonstrated.[24] However, no excess cancers have been identified in Japanese atomic-bomb survivors exposed in utero.[25] A major study of children exposed to routine pelvimetry at term also found no excess cancer.[26] Thus the picture is still not totally clear; the risk coefficient in Table 23.6 is a weighted average proposed by the UNSCEAR committee.[4]

The timing (Table 23.6) of radiation exposure during pregnancy is critical to both the nature and extent

TABLE 23.6. Radiation Effects on Embryo and Fetus*

Effect	Period of Maximum Sensitivity	Probability of Effect (%/Sv)†
Prenatal death	Preimplantation	50
Malformation	Organogenesis	50
Growth retardation	First trimester	10
Mental retardation	First trimester	Unknown
Genetic effect	Unknown	Unknown
Childhood cancer	First trimester	2

*Data from Brent and Gorson,[8] Sikov and Mahlum,[21] and UNSCEAR.[4]
†1%/Sv = 0.01%/rem.

of injury.[8] Prenatal death is the dominant effect, and is most likely to occur following preimplantation exposure. The LD_{50} increases as pregnancy progresses, reaching essentially postnatal values during the fetal period. Congenital malformations are most likely to occur following exposure during organogenesis. The period for induction of a specific abnormality is short —exposure must occur during a critical period of development for the particular organ or system; exceptions are growth and mental retardation, abnormalities of which may occur from exposure during any part of organogenesis and, with lesser frequency, during the fetal period. Thus a gross congenital malformation in the absence of growth or mental retardation is unlikely to be radiation-induced. Childhood cancer is more likely to occur from exposure during the first trimester.[22] The risk at term may be little or no greater than that from postnatal exposure.

DOSIMETRY

A major problem in the assessment of risk from diagnostic procedures is nonuniformity of dose distribution within the exposed organism. Most risk coefficients have been developed from data from uniform whole-body exposure. They are designed for application to such exposure.

The most frequently mentioned dosimetric data for diagnostic radiologic procedures have been incident skin exposures in the central axis of the beam. These are not reliable indicators of risk. During many multiprojection examinations, no single area of skin receives the entire exposure. Thus these data frequently are actually total tube output, measured at the plane of skin entry. The skin traditionally has been regarded as a relatively insensitive organ, with skin cancer appearing only in areas of radiodermatitis, which occurs only after rather large doses.[27] Recent animal data, however, indicate that small doses of radiation may interact with other carcinogens to increase the frequency of skin cancer.[28] In any event, we now believe that the risk is related more to exposure of critical target organs (Tables 23.3, 23.5, and 23.6), than of skin.

For nuclear medicine procedures, doses have traditionally been provided for the investigated organs and sometimes the organs receiving the greatest doses.[2,4] These data are not necessarily reliable risk estimates, for reasons analogous to those given for skin exposures in diagnostic radiology.

For nonuniform partial-body exposure, the risk is given by

$$R = \sum D_i C_i \qquad (2)$$

where R is total risk, D_i is dose to ith organ, and C_i is risk coefficient for ith organ. Thus the product $D_i C_i$ is

the probability of adverse effect in the ith organ, and the sum of these products for all organs is the total risk.

DOSES FROM DIAGNOSTIC RADIOLOGY

Rosenstein has recently developed a method for determining doses to certain critical organs (thyroid, active bone marrow, gonads, and embryo) from some common diagnostic radiographic projections.[29] The method allows calculation of doses to these organs if projection geometry, skin entry exposure, and half-value layer are known.

Recently, Laws and Rosenstein have extended the Rosenstein system to include doses to lung and breast.[30] They provided organ doses for common diagnostic procedures rather than for single projections (Table 23.7). These data are certainly a step in the right direction. However, they are inadequate in several respects.

Each examination in Table 23.7 consists of specific projections determined as average in the US national study.[31] For example, the chest examination consists of 0.1 AP, 0.92 PA, 0.5 lateral, and 0.02 oblique films, for a total of 1.5. Organ doses are given for the sums of these fractional projections.

The data assume inadequate collimation. For example, all projections of the lumbar spine are presumed to fill entire 14×17 inch films. Clearly, many organ doses from examinations using well-collimated beams will be significantly less.

Fluoroscopy is not mentioned by Laws and Rosenstein. Presumably, their data exclude organ dose contributions from fluoroscopy.

Finally, the data are incomplete. Doses for many known sensitive organs (Table 23.5) are not given. High-dose special procedures are excluded. Table 23.7 includes data from other sources for several procedures not mentioned by Laws and Rosenstein.

DOSES FROM NUCLEAR MEDICINE

The MIRD committee of the Society of Nuclear Medicine has developed a system for computing absorbed doses to various organs and tissues from numerous commonly administered radionuclides.[35] Specific organ doses for common nuclear medicine procedures can be calculated from the MIRD data. Results of such calculations have been summarized by Roedler, Kaul, and Hine.[35] These data (Table 23.8) are currently even less complete than those for diagnostic radiology.

DIAGNOSTIC RISKS

From the data presented in previous sections, crude estimates of risk may be determined for some situations. Data are not yet sufficiently complete for all

TABLE 23.7. **Specific Organ Doses from Diagnostic Radiology***

Exam*	Films (Number)	Organ Dose (μGy)[‖]						
		Thyroid	Active Marrow	Lung	Breast	Testes	Ovaries	Embryo
Chest	1.5	60	40	200	140	†	0.6	0.6
Skull	4.1	2,200	300	20	†	†	†	†
Cervical spine	3.7	4,000	100	150	†	†	†	†
Ribs	3.0	1,500	450	3,000	4,100	†	4	5
Shoulder	1.8	600	60	350	750	†	†	†
Thoracic spine	2.1	800	450	4,000	5,400	†	10	1
Cholecystogram	3.2	10	650	1,800	†	†	60	50
Lumbar spine	2.9	3	1,200	1,400	†	70	4,000	4,100
Upper GI	4.3	70	1,200	5,000	550	4	450	500
KUB	1.7	0.1	500	100	†	150	2,100	2,600
Barium enema	4.0	2	3,000	500	†	600	7,900	8,200
Lumbosacral spine	3.4	0.5	2,200	350	†	450	6,400	6,400
IVP	5.5	†	1,200	350	†	500	6,400	8,200
Pelvis	1.3	†	250	10	†	550	1,500	2,000
Hip	2.0	†	150	†	†	3,700	800	1,300
Mammography	2.0	‡	‡	‡	1000	‡	‡	‡
Exam§								
Urethrocystography		50	3,000	200	200	20,000	15,000	
Hysterosalpingography		10	1,700	100	50		5,900	
Paranasal sinuses		7,900	1,200	100	100	10	10	
Cerebral angiography		3,000	15,000	100	100	100	100	
Dental	1.0	30	10	1	5	0.1	0.1	
CT brain	5.0		1,400			70	70	
CT abdomen	5.0		4,900			400	400	

*Average exams, US, 1970, excluding contribution of fluoroscopy. Data from Laws and Rosenstein.[30]
†Less than 0.1
‡Considered negligible, compared to dose to breast
§Data from UNSCEAR (4), Gregg[32], and Shrivastava et al.[33]
‖1 mrad = 10 μGy

cases. Alternatively, diagnostic exposures may be related to average exposures from environmental sources (Table 23.9), as estimated by the BEIR[2] and UNSCEAR[4] committees. Risk relative to unavoidable radiation may thus be estimated.

GENETIC RISKS

Since gonadal dose estimates are available for essentially all procedures (Tables 23.7 and 23.8), rough approximations of genetic risks can be determined by multiplying gonad dose by genetic risk coefficients (Table 23.3). Genetic risk per examination computed in this manner ranges from 10^{-10} (for chest, skull, and several other diagnostic procedures) to 10^{-4} (for adrenal scans), with most 10^{-6} or less. These risks can then be weighted by ages for probability of conceiving additional offspring (Table 23.4). For females over 44 years of age and males over 54, genetic risks may be assumed to be zero.

The concept of genetically significant dose (GSD) has been used to assess the genetic risk to populations from diagnostic procedures.[36] The GSD is that dose which, if administered uniformly to the entire population, would carry the same total genetic burden as the doses actually given nonuniformly to parts of the population. It is valid only if the dose-response curve is linear, and all individuals carry uniform sensitivity. Thus it is a first-order approximation. The US GSD for diagnostic radiology was estimated as 200±40 μGy (20±4 mrads) in 1964. The BEIR committee estimated that the genetically significant component of environmental exposure in 1970 was 900 μSv (90 mrem). Thus, it appears that in 1970 diagnostic radiology contributed about 18 percent of the total genetic radiation burden to the American population. The absence of significant increase in the GSD from 1964 to 1970 may be attributed to technologic improvements, since the use of diagnostic x-ray increased about 30 percent in that interval.[31] However, there was still room for improvement. For example, if in 1970 all x-ray beams had been collimated to no larger than the image receptor, the GSD would have been about 25 percent less.[36] It is hoped that continued advances will hold the GSD to no greater than it was in 1970.

No analogous GSD data are available for nuclear

TABLE 23.8. **Specific Organ Doses from Nuclear Medicine**[*]

Exam	Radiopharmaceutical	Activity Administered (MBq)	Organ Dose (μGy)[†]					
			Thyroid	Active Marrow	Lung	Testes	Ovaries	Fetus
Thyroid	[99m]Tc pertechnetate	37	3,400	220		120	170	
	Na[131]I	1.9	1,100,000	210		88	93	
	Na[123]I	7.4	40,000	66		30	42	
Parathyroid	[75]Se methionine	9.3		24,000		21,000	25,000	
Adrenal	[131]I cholesterol	74	500,000	20,000		40,000	60,000	
Placenta	[99m]Tc HSA	37		200			410	200
	[113m]In transferrin	37		100			100	81
Brain	[99m]Tc pertechnetate	440	40,000	2,600		1,400	2,000	
	[99m]Tc DTPA	440		1,100		620	840	
CSF	[131]I HSA	3.7	(2,000, total body)					
	[99m]Tc HSA	37	(3, total body)					
	[169]Yb DTPA	37	(2,000, total body)					
	[111]In DTPA	37	(22, total body)					
Bone	[99m]Tc methylene diphosphonate, polyphosphate, pyrophosphate	370		3,500		1,500	1,500	
Liver	[99m]Tc colloid or phytate	56		410		17	84	
	[198]Au colloid	5.6		4,100		54	210	
	[99m]Tc HIDA	74		400		50	1,000	
	[131]I rose bengal	11		950		420	4,700	
Salivary gland	[99m]Tc pertechnetate	56	5,200	340		180	260	
Tumor, abscess	[67]Ga citrate	74		12,000		4,800	5,600	
Pancreas	[75]Se methionine	10		26,000		23,000	27,000	
GI blood loss	[51]Cr red cells	7.4		4,000		600	600	
GI protein loss	[51]Cr HSA	3.7		520				
Kidney (static)	[99m]Tc DMSA	74		700		280	460	
	[99m]Tc glucoheptonate	74		240		74	140	
	[197]Hg chlormerodrin	7.4		220		56	81	
Kidney (dynamic)	[99m]Tc DTPA	190		490		270	360	
	[99m]Tc glucoheptonate	190		610		190	360	
	[113m]In EDTA	190	(270, total body)					
	[113m]In DTPA	190	(510, total body)				1,400	
	[123]I hippurate	19	250,000			210	320	
Lung perfusion	[99m]Tc microspheres or MAA	74		300	4,200	74	120	
	[131]I microspheres or MAA	11		1,500		1,200	1,300	
Lung ventilation single breath	[133]Xe	37MBq/1		2.6[‡]	59[‡]	2.6[‡]	2.6[‡]	

[*]Computed from data of Roedler, Kaul, and Hine (36)
[†]1 mrad = 10 μGy
[‡]Per liter administered

(cont'd.)

TABLE 23.8. Cont'd.

| Exam | Radiopharmaceutical | Activity Administered (MBq) | Organ Dose (μGy)[†] | | | | | |
			Thyroid	Active Marrow	Lung	Testes	Ovaries	Fetus
Lung ventilation (cont'd.)								
rebreathe, 3 min	[133]Xe	37MBq/1		37[‡]	410[‡]	37[‡]	37[‡]	
Spleen	[99m]Tc colloid	56.0		410			17	84
	[99m]Tc denatured red cells	37.0		(200, total body)				
	[197]Hg BMHP, red cells	11.0		(600, total body)				1,200
	[198]Au colloid	5.6		4,100			53	210
Iron kinetics	[59]Fe citrate or chloride	0.37		1,700			1,600	1,800
Red cell survival time or volume	[51]Cr chromate	3.7		2,000			300	300
Plasma volume	[131]I HSA	0.19		97			87	97
B-12 absorption	[57]Co B-12	0.019		18			22	18
Cardio-vascular (dynamic)	[99m]Tc HSA	560.0		3,000			3,000	3,000
Cardio-vascular (static)	[99m]Tc HSA	190.0		1,000			1,000	1,000
	[113m]In transferrin	190.0		930			660	660
	[131]I HSA	5.6		2,600			3,000	3,000
Myocardium	[201]T1-chloride	74.0		5,000			6,000	6,000
	[99m]Tc pyrophosphate	560.0		5,300			1,500	2,000
Thrombosis test	[125]I fibrinogen	3.7		(20,000, total body)				

[‡]Per liter administered

medicine. Because of the low frequency of procedures, the contribution to the population genetic radiation burden is substantially lower than that of diagnostic radiology.

CANCER RISKS

Available data are not yet sufficiently complete to allow application of equation 2 for all procedures. However, approximations may be generated in some cases. For example, the major risk from mammography is breast cancer, which may be as great as 10^{-3} per examination in young adult females; Gregg estimated 10^{-4}.[32] For chest examinations, the major risks are lung and thyroid cancer, leukemia, and (in females) breast cancer. The sum of risks to these organs is 10^{-6} per chest examination. The risk of lethal cancer is substantially lower. For example, most radiation-induced thyroid cancers are of the follicular epithelial type; about 3 percent are fatal.[13] The risk of fatal cancer from a chest exam is on the order of 10^{-7}. For virtually all procedures, the risk of fatal cancer appears to be 10^{-4} or less. Fortunately, for most common procedures, it is on the order of 10^{-6}.

For leukemia, the caput marrow dose (CMD),

TABLE 23.9. Annual Population Dose from Background Sources

Organ	Annual Dose (μSv)[†][‡]
Whole body*	1,090
Gonads[†]	780
Lung[†]	1,100
Active marrow[†]	920

*United States, 1970; data from BEIR.[2]
[†]World average; data from UNSCEAR.[4]
[‡]1 m + cm = 10μSv

analogous to the GSD, has been developed.[37] The CMD is that dose which, if administered uniformly to the entire population, might be expected to carry the same total risk of leukemia as the actual dose administered nonuniformly to part of the population. The 1970 CMD for diagnostic radiology was estimated as 1030 μGy (103 mrads), up from 830 μGy (83 mrads) in 1964. It appears that diagnostic radiology contributes about half the leukemogenic radiation burden to the American public. No analogous concepts have been developed for nuclear medicine, or for other cancers.

EMBRYONIC RISK

Doses to the embryo have been estimated for many diagnostic radiologic procedures, but few for nuclear medicine. For higher-dose procedures (Table 23.7), it appears that the presumed childhood cancer risk may be as great as 10^{-5} per examination for exposure during the first trimester, and significantly less for the second and third trimesters. Extrapolation of the risk coefficients from Table 23.6 indicates a risk as great as 10^{-3} per study for prenatal death from preimplantation exposure and for congenital anomalies from exposure during organogenesis, and 10^{-4} per exam for growth retardation from exposure during the first trimester. However, since no epidemiologic studies have shown increased incidence of anomalies or growth retardation from low doses, these data may grossly overestimate the risk.

RECOMMENDATIONS

In 1914, Pfahler published the following recommendations for the safe conduct of radiographic examinations[38]:

1. Use as small a quantity of rays as is consistent with the examination.
2. Use a quality of rays that will penetrate the tissues.
3. Make every examination as short as possible.
4. Use intensifying screens when practicable.
5. Use filters for the elimination of the softer rays.
6. Confine the rays to the part actually under examination.

Today we might add:

7. Perform only those examinations for which there is reasonable expectation of health benefit to the patient.

Recent data (unpublished) from the Tennessee Department of Industrial and Radiologic Health indicates that the most frequent grounds for radiologic equipment citation by state regulatory agencies are inade-

quate collimation for radiographic tubes and excessive skin entry dose rates for fluoroscopic apparatus. It appears, therefore, that some of Pfahler's recommendations are still not followed routinely. We must increase our efforts to (1) collimate beams to the area of clinical interest or the size of the image receptor, whichever is smaller; (2) use imaging systems of the highest sensitivity consistent with clinical requirements, such as high-speed rare-earth screens; (3) upgrade quality control to assure consistent images as nearly technically perfect as can be reasonably obtained; and (4) perform only clinically justified examinations.

In nuclear medicine, technology has been advancing so rapidly as to make it difficult to maintain current estimates of patient doses and risks.[34] Comparison of specific organ doses (Table 23.8) from newer and older radiopharmaceuticals indicates that significant dose reductions have been achieved. However, recent developments (eg, dynamic studies, emission tomography) and the current increased use of nuclear medicine procedures must warn us to expand our efforts at continued risk reduction.

PREGNANT AND POTENTIALLY PREGNANT PATIENTS

Because of the well-known higher sensitivity of the embryo, pregnant patients must be regarded as special cases. Every effort must be made to minimize exposure to the uterus. Only those examinations required for current patient management should be performed. For a radiographic examination involving primary-beam exposure of the lower abdomen or pelvis, only those projections required for the specific clinical problem should be obtained. Close cooperation between the radiologist and attending physician is required for sound patient care with minimum risk to the fetus.

In some parts of the world, female patients of child-bearing age are regarded as potentially pregnant unless proven otherwise. The 10-day rule, currently in use in many countries, states that examinations of the lower abdomen and pelvis of such patients will be conducted only during the first 10 days of the menstrual cycle unless there is compelling medical justification to proceed or convincing evidence that the woman is not pregnant.[39] This rule has not been implemented in the United States. The National Council on Radiation Protection and Measurements has recommended that those examinations that contribute to management of current illness should not be postponed.[40] Deferral of examinations for a patient in the last half of the cycle should be considered only if the patient is subsequently determined to be pregnant.

Occasionally a woman is subjected to extensive diagnostic procedures and is subsequently determined to have been pregnant. In such cases the radiologist may be asked whether to recommend therapeutic abortion on grounds of radiation risk. The following general principles may be used as a guide in making that decision.

If the exposure occurred before implantation, the major documented risk is prenatal death, generally leading to early, probably unrecognized, spontaneous abortion. The risk of congenital malformations from preimplantation exposure is now believed to be small. If the exposure occurred during organogenesis, the major concerns are malformations and childhood cancer. The radiologist should first determine dose to the embryo. Data from Tables 23.7 and 23.8 may be used for a first approximation, though the previously expressed deficiencies must be kept in mind.

The following guidelines, modified from Brent and Gorson[8] may be applied:

1. If the dose to the embryo was less than 1 cGy (1 rad), the probability of adverse effect is very small; therapeutic abortion should not be recommended.
2. If the dose was between 2 and 5 cGy (2 to 5 rads), risk of abnormality is now believed to be relatively minor. Therapeutic abortion should not be recommended on grounds of radiation risk alone. If the couple strongly want a baby, they should be advised that there is circumstantial evidence only for increased risk of malformation, and disputed data suggesting increased childhood cancer risk. Risk coefficients (Table 23.6) might be used to generate upper limits of risk.
3. If the dose was between 5 and 10 cGy (5 to 10 rads), risk is greater, but not generally regarded as sufficient to recommend therapeutic abortion unless there are other unrelated reasons to do so. Relatively minor malformations have been demonstrated in animals following doses in this range.
4. If the dose was greater than 10 cGy (10 rads), radiation risk is believed to be sufficient to recommend therapeutic abortion. Data from Table 23.6 suggest that 10 cGy may result in increased risk of malformation as great as 5 percent. However, that implies that the probability of no radiation effect is at least 95 percent. Many normal individuals received at least 10 cGy in utero.

If the dose to the embryo, as estimated from Tables 23.7 and 23.8 falls near a critical level—and particularly if the parents have strong desires for continuing the pregnancy—then more accurate dose determinations for radiographic procedures should be obtained. Examinations should be reconstructed as accurately as possible, with accurate calibration of equipment and measurements on an appropriate phantom.

These guidelines for abortion might be regarded as conservative, when contrasted with recommendations in the section for minimizing exposure to the embryo.

TABLE 23.10.   One-in-a-Million Risks*

Condition or Action	Nature of Risk
Existence	
20 minutes as a 60-year-old man	Heart disease, cancer
2 days in New York	Air pollution
2 months in Denver	Cosmic radiation
2 months in a stone or brick building	Natural radioactivity
1 year drinking Miami water	Chemical carcinogens
10 years near PVC plant	Chemical carcinogens
Travel	
6 minutes by canoe	Accident
10 miles by bicycle	Accident
300 miles by car	Accident
1,000 miles by jet airliner	Accident
6,000 miles by jet airliner	Cosmic radiation
Work	
1 hour in coal mine	Black lung disease
3 hours in coal mine	Accident
10 days of typical factory work	Accident
Miscellaneous	
1.4 cigarettes	Cancer, heart disease
500 cc wine	Cirrhosis of the liver
30 cans diet soda	Chemical carcinogen

*After Pochin[13] and Wilson.[41]

However, the underlying concepts are totally different. Every possible effort must be made to prevent a radiation effect. Abortion, however, is a highly emotional issue. It is frequently difficult for parents to accept. The radiologist should rarely—if ever—be dogmatic in recommending it because of other overriding concerns on the part of the parents.

CONCLUSIONS

For all practical purposes, there are no conclusive data documenting radiation risks from diagnostic doses. However, circumstantial evidence is so compelling that the burden of proof must be placed on those who argue for the safety of such procedures. There is every reason to believe that a small, as yet inadequately quantified, radiation risk from diagnostic procedures exists. Current data associating diagnostic exposures with increased cancer risk deal with procedures carried out many years ago, when doses may have been substantially greater than they are now.

It now appears that the radiation risk for most procedures is of the order of one in a million. We readily accept that level of risk in other areas (Table 23.10), especially if we perceive an attending benefit. Many other accepted medical procedures carry risks of complications at least as high. However, the potential severity of radiation injury is so great as to warrant special consideration. Few other procedures carry the risk of a genetic defect that may be propagated over many generations.

REFERENCES

1. Daniel, J: The x-rays. Science 3: 562–563, 1896
2. The Effects on Populations of Exposure to Low Levels of Ionizing Radiation. Advisory Committee on the Biological Effects of Ionizing Radiations Report. Washington, DC, National Academy of Sciences, National Research Council, 1972
3. Considerations of Health Benefit–Cost Analysis for Activities Involving Ionizing Radiation Exposure and Alternatives. Advisory Committee on the Biological Effects of Ionizing Radiations Report. US Environmental Protection Agency Publication EPA-502/4-77-003, 1977
4. Sources and Effects of Ionizing Radiation. United Nations Scientific Committee on the Effects of Atomic Radiation Report. New York, United Nations, 1977
5. Langham WH (ed): Radiobiological Factors in Manned Space Flight. Washington, DC, National Academy of Sciences, National Research Council, 1967
6. Casarett GW: Similarities and contrasts between radiation and time pathology. In Strehler B (ed): Advances in Gerontological Research. New York, Academic Press, 1964, vol 1, pp 109–163
7. Beebe, GW, Kato H, Land CE: Studies on the mortality of A-bomb survivors. 6. Mortality and radiation dose, 1950–1974. Radiat Res 75: 138–201, 1978
8. Brent RL, Gorson RO: Radiation exposure in pregnancy. Curr Prob Radiol 2: 1–48, 1972
9. Land CE, McGregor DH: Breast cancer incidence among atomic-bomb survivors: Implications for radiobiologic risk at low doses. J US National Cancer Institute 62: 17–21, 1979
10. Kellerer AM: Radiation carcinogenesis at low doses. In Booz J, Ebert HG (eds): *Sixth Symposium on Microdosimetry*, vol 1. London, Harwood Academic Publishers, 1978, pp 405–422
11. Borek C, Hall, EJ: Effect of split doses of x-rays on neoplastic transformation in single cells. Nature 252: 499–501, 1974
12. Yuhas JM, Tennant RW, Regan JD (eds): Biology of Radiation Carcinogenesis. New York, Raven Press, 1976
13. Pochin EE: Why be Quantitative about Radiation Risk Estimates? Washington, DC, National Council on Radiation Protection and Measurements, 1978
14. Okada S, Hamilton HB, Egami N, Okajima S, Russell WJ, Takeshita K: A review of thirty years study of Hiroshima and Nagasaki atomic-bomb survivors. J Radiat Res 16 (supplement), September 1975
15. Prasad KN: Human Radiation Biology. Hagerstown, Md., Harper & Row, 1974
16. Vital Statistics of the United States 1975, vol 1, Natality.

US Department of Health, Education and Welfare Publication (PHS) 78-1113. US National Center for Health Statistics 1978
17. Gibson R, Graham S, Lilienfeld AM, Schuman LM, Dowd JE, Levin ML: Irradiation in the epidemiology of leukemia among adults. J US National Cancer Institute 48: 301–311, 1972
18. Graham S, Levin ML, Lilienfeld AM, Schuman LM, Gibson R, Dowd JE, Hempelmann L: Preconception, intrauterine, and postnatal irradiation as related to leukemia. In Haenszel W (ed): Epidemiological Approaches to the Study of Cancer and Other Chronic Diseases. US National Cancer Institute Monograph 19: 347–371, 1966
19. Duplan JF (ed): Radiation-Induced Leukomogenesis and Related Viruses. Amsterdam, North Holland, 1977
20. American Cancer Society: 1979 Cancer Facts and Figures. New York, American Cancer Society, 1978
21. Sikov MR, Mahlum DD: Radiation Biology of the Fetal and Juvenile Mammal. Springfield, Va., National Technical Information Service, 1969
22. Stewart A: Low-dose radiation cancers in man. Adv Cancer Res 14: 359–390, 1971
23. Diamond EL, Schmerler H, Lilienfeld AM: The relationship of intrauterine radiation to subsequent mortality and development of leukemia in children. Am J Epidemiol 97: 283–313, 1973
24. Bross IDJ, Natarajan N: Genetic damage from diagnostic radiation. J Am Med Assoc 237: 2399–2401, 1977.
25. Jablon S, Kato H: Childhood cancer in relation to prenatal exposure to atomic bomb radiation. Lancet 2: 1000–1003, 1970
26. Oppenheim BE, Griem ML, Meier P: Effects of low-dose prenatal irradiation in humans: analysis of Chicago lying-in data and comparison with other studies. Radiat Res 57: 508–544, 1974
27. Rubin P, Casarett GW: Clinical Radiation Pathology. Philadelphia, WB Saunders, 1968
28. Lurie AG: Enhancement of DMBA tumorigenesis in hamster cheak pouch epithelium by repeated exposures to low-level x-radiation. Radiat Res 72: 499–511, 1977
29. Rosenstein M: Organ Doses in Diagnostic Radiology. US Department of Health, Education and Welfare Publication (FDA) 76-8030, 1976
30. Laws PW, and Rosenstein M: A somatic dose index for diagnostic radiology. Health Physics 35: 629–642, 1978
31. Population Exposure to X-Rays, US 1970. US Department of Health, Education and Welfare Publication (FDA) 73-8047. US Bureau of Radiological Health, 1973
32. Gregg EC: Radiation risks with diagnostic x-rays. Radiology 123: 447–453, 1977
33. Shrivastava PN, Lynn SL, Ting JY: Exposures to patient and personnel in computed axial tomography. Radiology 125: 411–415, 1977
34. Smith EM: Dose estimate techniques. In Rollo FD (ed): Nuclear Medicine Physics, Instrumentation, and Agents. St Louis, CV Mosby, 1977, pp 513–543
35. Roedler HD, Kaul A, Hine GJ: Internal Radiation Dose in Diagnostic Nuclear Medicine. Berlin, Verlag H Hoffmann, 1978
36. Gonad Doses and Genetically Significant Dose from

Diagnostic Radiology US, 1964 and 1970. US Department of Health, Education and Welfare Publication (FDA) 76–8034. US Bureau of Radiologic Health, 1976

37. Shleien B, Tucker TT, Johnson DW: The mean active bone marrow dose to the adult population of the United States from diagnostic radiology. Health Phys 34: 587–601, 1978

38. Pfahler GE: Present-day danger of Roentgen-ray burns and how to avoid them. *JAMA* 62: 189–191, 1914

39. Warrik CK: Radiology now—the 10-day rule. Brit J Radiol 46: 933–934, 1973

40. Medical Exposure of Pregnant and Potentially Pregnant Women. National Council on Radiation Protection and Measurements Report No 54, 1977

41. Wilson R: Risks caused by low levels of pollution. Yale J Biol Med 51: 37–51, 1978

Index